PEDIATRIC CARDIOLOGY BOARD REVIEW

THIRD EDITION

PEDIATRIC CARDIOLOGY BOARD REVIEW

THIRD EDITION

Benjamin W. Eidem, MD, FACC, FASE

Professor of Pediatrics and Medicine
Departments of Cardiovascular Diseases and Pediatrics
Division of Pediatric Cardiology
Mayo Clinic
Rochester, Minnesota

Bryan C. Cannon, MD, FHRS

Associate Professor of Pediatrics
Department of Cardiovascular Diseases
Division of Pediatric Cardiology
Mayo Clinic
Rochester, Minnesota

Anthony C. Chang, MD, MBA, MPH, MS

Chief Intelligence and Innovation Officer
Medical Director
Heart Failure Program
Children's Hospital Orange County
Orange, California

Jonathan N. Johnson, MD

Professor of Pediatrics
Department of Pediatrics
Division of Pediatric Cardiology
Mayo Clinic College of Medicine
Rochester, Minnesota

Paul F. Kantor, MBBCh, MSc

Professor, Pediatric Cardiology
Keck School of Medicine of the
  University of Southern California
Division Chief
Children's Hospital Los Angeles, Heart Institute
Los Angeles, California

Robert E. Shaddy, MD

Professor of Clinical Pediatrics
Department of Cardiology
Keck School of Medicine of the University of
  Southern California
Los Angeles, California

Frank Cetta, MD, FACC, FASE

Professor of Pediatrics and Medicine
Department of Cardiovascular Diseases
Division of Pediatric Cardiology
Mayo Clinic
Rochester, Minnesota

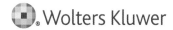

. Wolters Kluwer

Philadelphia • Baltimore • New York • London
Buenos Aires • Hong Kong • Sydney • Tokyo

Acquisitions Editor: James Sherman
Senior Development Editor: Ashley Fischer
Editorial Coordinator: Christopher Rodgers
Marketing Manager: Kirsten Watrud
Senior Production Project Manager: Sadie Buckallew
Manager, Graphic Arts & Design: Stephen Druding
Manufacturing Coordinator: Beth Welsh
Prepress Vendor: Aptara, Inc.

9 8 7 6 5 4 3 2 1

Printed in Mexico

Library of Congress Cataloging-in-Publication Data

Names: Eidem, Benjamin W., editor. | Cannon, Bryan C., editor. | Johnson, Jonathan N., editor. |
    Chang, Anthony C., editor. | Cetta, Frank, editor. | Shaddy, Robert E., editor. |
    Kantor, Paul (Paul F.), editor.
Title: Pediatric cardiology board review / [edited by] Benjamin W. Eidem,
    Bryan C. Cannon, Jonathan N. Johnson, Anthony C. Chang, Frank Cetta,
    Robert E. Shaddy, Paul F. Kantor.
Description: Third edition. | Philadelphia, PA : Wolters Kluwer, [2023] |
    Includes bibliographical references and index.
Identifiers: LCCN 2022005042 | ISBN 9781975180478 (paperback) |
ISBN 9781975196141 (ebook)
Subjects: MESH: Heart Defects, Congenital | Child | Heart Diseases | Infant |
    Adolescent | Examination Questions
Classification: LCC RJ421 | NLM WS 18.2 | DDC 618.92/12043—dc23/eng/20220204
LC record available at https://lccn.loc.gov/2022005042

shop.lww.com

QUADM0722

Dedication

To my wife Jori for all of her love and support and to my fellows and colleagues for all the lessons they have taught me in my career.

—Benjamin W. Eidem

I would like to thank all of my mentors and colleagues who have taught me so much. Thanks to the pioneers in pediatric electrophysiology who inspired my interest and the interest of many generations to come.

—Bryan C. Cannon

I would like to express my gratitude to all the children and families whom I serve as well as all the mentors and clinicians who have taught me through the decades. Teaching is a labor of love and I feel fortunate that I have had the opportunity to continue to do so, especially for my 6-year-old daughter Olivia who insists that she would like to become a pediatric cardiologist someday.

—Anthony C. Chang

Thank you to my wife Alissa and my children Elliana and Nicholas, for their love, patience, and support. I also want to express my deep gratitude for my mentors (including all of my co-editors) for their support of my career, and for their dedication to the education of decades of pediatric cardiology fellows.

—Jonathan N. Johnson

To all fellows and scholars of pediatric cardiology from whom I have learned over the years, for it is by your questions that we all gain wisdom. To all patients, who through their courage have made the pathway easier for those whose journey lies ahead.

—Paul F. Kantor

I dedicate this to all of my mentors, to whom I am forever grateful, and to all of the trainees I had the privilege of learning so much from.

—Robert E. Shaddy

Cate, Michael, Matt: I am so proud of you guys.

—Frank Cetta

Contributors

Katherine Agre, MS, LCGC
Department of Clinical Genomics
Mayo Clinic
Rochester, Minnesota

Thomas G. Allison, PhD, MPH
Professor of Medicine
Consultant, Department of Cardiovascular Medicine
Department of Pediatric and Adolescent Medicine, and
    Division of Preventive Cardiology
Mayo Clinic
Rochester, Minnesota

Jason H. Anderson, MD
Assistant Professor
Division of Pediatric Cardiology
Mayo Clinic
Rochester, Minnesota

Yaniv Bar-Cohen, MD, FHRS, CEPS-P, FACC, FAAP
Professor of Clinical Pediatrics and Medicine
Keck School of Medicine of the
    University of Southern California
Director, Electrophysiology
Co-Director of Southern California Consortium for
    Technology and Innovation in Pediatrics (CTIP)
Children's Hospital Los Angeles
Los Angeles, California

Bryan C. Cannon, MD, FHRS
Associate Professor of Pediatrics
Department of Cardiovascular Diseases
Division of Pediatric Cardiology
Mayo Clinic
Rochester, Minnesota

Adam Cassidy, PhD
Assistant Professor of Psychiatry
Mayo Clinic
Rochester, Minnesota

Frank Cetta, MD, FACC, FASE
Professor of Pediatrics and Medicine
Department of Cardiovascular Diseases
Division of Pediatric Cardiology
Mayo Clinic
Rochester, Minnesota

Anthony C. Chang, MD, MBA, MPH, MS
Chief Intelligence and Innovation Officer
Medical Director
Heart Failure Program
Children's Hospital Orange County
Orange, California

Sheri S. Crow, MD, MS
Consultant Pediatric Critical Care Medicine
Department of Pediatrics and Health Services Research
Mayo Clinic College of Medicine
Department of Pediatric and Adolescent Medicine
Mayo Clinic
Rochester, Minnesota

Sylvia Del Castillo, MD
Clinical Associate Professor of Pediatrics
Keck School of Medicine of the
    University of Southern California
Medical Director
Cardiothoracic Intensive Care Unit
Children's Hospital of Los Angeles
Los Angeles, California

John Detterich, MD
Associate Professor of Clinical Pediatrics, Physiology,
    and Biophysics
Keck School of Medicine
Los Angeles, California

Benjamin W. Eidem, MD, FACC, FASE
Professor of Pediatrics and Medicine
Departments of Cardiovascular Diseases and Pediatrics
Division of Pediatric Cardiology
Mayo Clinic
Rochester, Minnesota

M. Eric Ferguson, MD
Assistant Professor of Pediatrics
Division of Pediatric Cardiology
Emory University School of Medicine
Children's Healthcare of Atlanta
Atlanta, Georgia

Brittany M. Graham, MD
Pediatric Cardiology Fellow
Department of Pediatric and Adolescent Medicine
Division of Pediatric Cardiology
Mayo Clinic
Rochester, Minnesota

Justin M. Horner, MD, MPH
Assistant Professor of Pediatrics
Division of Pediatric Cardiology
Mayo Clinic
Rochester, Minnesota

C. Charles Jain, MD
Assistant Professor of Medicine
Mayo Clinic
Rochester, Minnesota

Jonathan N. Johnson, MD
Professor of Pediatrics
Department of Pediatrics
Division of Pediatric Cardiology
Mayo Clinic College of Medicine
Rochester, Minnesota

Paul F. Kantor, MBBCh, MSc
Professor, Pediatric Cardiology
Keck School of Medicine of the
    University of Southern California
Division Chief
Children's Hospital Los Angeles, Heart Institute
Los Angeles, California

Grace Kung, MD
Clinical Professor of Pediatrics
Keck School of Medicine of the
    University of Southern California
Children's Hospital Los Angeles
Los Angeles, California

Carolina P. Larmeu, MD
Pediatric Cardiology Fellow
Mayo Clinic
Rochester, Minnesota

Emily R. Levy, MD
Senior Associate Consultant, Pediatric Infectious Diseases
Senior Associate Consultant, Pediatric Critical
    Care Medicine
Assistant Professor of Pediatrics
Mayo Clinic College of Medicine
Rochester, Minnesota

Joseph J. Maleszewski, MD
Professor of Laboratory Medicine and Pathology
Professor of Medicine
Consultant, Departments of Laboratory Medicine and
    Pathology and Cardiovascular Medicine
Rochester, Minnesota

Emily Morell, MD
Assistant Professor of Pediatrics
University of California, San Francisco School of Medicine
UCSF Benioff Children's Hospital
San Francisco, California

Talha Niaz, MBBS
Assistant Professor of Pediatrics
Mayo Clinic College of Medicine
Senior Associate Consultant
Department of Pediatrics
Division of Pediatric Cardiology
Mayo Clinic
Rochester, Minnesota

Sabrina D. Phillips, MD
Associate Professor of Medicine
Mayo Clinic
Jacksonville, Florida

Sophia Pillai, MD
Assistant Professor of Pediatrics
Department of Pediatrics
Division of Pediatric Pulmonology
Mayo Clinic
Rochester, Minnesota

Jay D. Pruetz, MD
Associate Professor of Pediatrics and
    Obstetrics and Gynecology
Keck School of Medicine of the
    University of Southern California
Attending Cardiologist and Director of
    Fetal Cardiology
Department of Pediatrics
Children's Hospital of Los Angeles
Los Angeles, California

M. Yasir Qureshi, MBBS, FACC, FASE
Director of Fetal Cardiology
Consultant, Pediatric Cardiology
Associate Professor of Pediatrics
Mayo Clinic College of Medicine
Rochester, Minnesota

Ezequiel Sagray, MD
Pediatric Cardiology Fellow
Mayo Clinic
Rochester, Minnesota

Robert E. Shaddy, MD
Professor of Clinical Pediatrics
Department of Cardiology
Keck School of Medicine of the
    University of Southern California
Los Angeles, California

Nibras E. El Sherif, MBBS
Pediatric Cardiology Fellow
Mayo Clinic
Rochester, Minnesota

Mark Shwayder, MD
Clinical Assistant Professor of Pediatrics
Keck School of Medicine of the
    University of Southern California
Children's Hospital Los Angeles
Los Angeles, California

Elizabeth H. Stephens, MD, PhD
Associate Professor of Surgery
Department of Cardiovascular Surgery
Mayo Clinic
Rochester, Minnesota

Nathaniel W. Taggart, MD
Associate Professor
Division of Pediatric Cardiology
Mayo Clinic
Rochester, Minnesota

Charlotte Van Dorn, MD
Assistant Professor of Pediatrics
Department of Adolescent Medicine
Divisions of Pediatric Cardiology and Pediatric
    Critical Care
Mayo Clinic
Rochester, Minnesota

Philip L. Wackel, MD, FHRS, CEPS-P
Assistant Professor of Pediatrics
Mayo Clinic
Rochester, Minnesota

Preface

The editors are pleased to introduce the 3rd edition of the *Pediatric Cardiology Board Review*. This textbook serves as an adjunct to our Pediatric Cardiology Review courses that we have organized since 2006. Trainees preparing for their board certification examination as well as practicing physicians wishing to refresh their knowledge base of adult and pediatric congenital cardiology have found the previous editions vital to their education.

All of the chapters in our 3rd edition have been expanded and new authors have contributed to many of these chapters. Three new chapters highlighting the role of genetics in congenital heart disease (CHD), fetal and perinatal cardiology, and classic imaging in CHD have been added to the 3rd edition.

This edition has more than 1200 questions and, similar to the previous editions, the answers have full in-depth explanations.

The 3rd edition highlights the collaboration between faculty from Mayo Clinic and Children's Hospital of Los Angeles (CHLA). CHLA now partners with Mayo for the Pediatric Cardiology Review course which is scheduled for in-person and virtual learning in August 2022 in Huntington Beach, California. This textbook provides a nice adjunct to that course. Drs Robert E. Shaddy and Paul F. Kantor have joined the editorial staff and their colleagues from CHLA have made important contributions to the textbook and review course.

We hope that you find the 3rd edition of the *Pediatric Cardiology Board Review academically enriching*.

Abbreviations

AAP	American Academy of Pediatrics
ABG	arterial blood gas
ABP	American Board of Pediatrics
ACCF	American College of Cardiology Foundation
ACE	angiotensin-converting enzyme
ACM	arrhythmogenic cardiomyopathy
ADA	adenine deaminase
ADHD	attention-deficit/hyperactivity disorder
AH	atrium-His
AHA	American Heart Association
AICD	automatic implantable cardioverter-defibrillator
AKI	acute kidney injury
ALC	absolute lymphocyte count
ALCAPA	anomalous left coronary artery from the pulmonary artery
ANCOVA	analysis of covariance
ANOVA	analysis of variance
ANP	atrial natriuretic peptide
AOLCA	anomalous origin of the LCA
AORCA	anomalous origin of RCA
AP	aortopulmonary
APV	absent pulmonary valve
ARB	angiotensin-receptor blocker
ARCAPA	anomalous origin of right coronary artery from pulmonary artery
ARR	absolute risk reduction
ARVC	arrhythmogenic right ventricular cardiomyopathy
AS	aortic stenosis
ASD	atrial septal defect
ASE	American Society of Echocardiography
ATG	antithymocyte globulin
AV	atrioventricular
AVM	arteriovenous malformation
AVSD	atrioventricular septal defect
AVT	acute vasoreactivity testing
AZT	zidovudine
BAS	balloon atrial septostomy
BMI	body mass index
BNP	B-type natriuretic peptide
BP	blood pressure
bpm	beats per minute
BRS	baroreflex sensitivity
BT	Blalock–Taussig
BTT	Blalock–Taussig–Thomas
CABG	coronary artery bypass graft
CARPREG	cardiac disease in pregnancy
CAVC	complete atrioventricular canal

CBA	cost-benefit analysis
CBC	complete blood count
CCA	cost-consequence analysis
CCB	calcium channel blocker
CCTGA	congenitally corrected transposition of the great arteries
CEA	cost-effectiveness analysis
CHB	complete heart block
CHD	congenital heart disease
CHF	congestive heart failure
CHRS	Canadian Heart Rhythm Society
CI	cumulative incidence
CI	confidence interval
CMA	cost-minimization analysis
CMR	cardiac magnetic resonance imaging
CNI	calcineurin inhibitor
CNS	central nervous system
COPE	Colchicine for Acute Pericarditis
CP	constrictive pericarditis
CPAP	continuous positive airway pressure
CPB	cardiopulmonary bypass
CPR	cardiopulmonary resuscitation
CPVT	catecholaminergic polymorphic ventricular tachycardia
CRF	cardiorespiratory fitness
CRP	C-reactive protein
CRT	chronic resynchronization therapy
CS	coronary sinus
CT	computed tomography
CTA	CT angiogram
CTA	computed tomography angiography
CUA	cost-utility analysis
CVA	cost-value analysis
CVP	central venous pressure
CW	continuous wave
CXR	chest x-ray
DALY	disability-adjusted life year
DBP	diastolic blood pressure
DCM	dilated cardiomyopathy
DCMA	dilated cardiomyopathy with ataxia
DCRV	double-chambered right ventricle
df	degrees of freedom
DHCA	deep hypothermic circulatory arrest
DILV	double-inlet left ventricle
DKS	Damus–Kaye–Stansel
DORV	double-outlet right ventricle
DSMB	Data Safety Monitoring Board
d-TGA	d-Transposition of the great arteries

EA	Ebstein anomaly
EBV	Epstein–Barr virus
ECG	electrocardiogram
ECMO	extracorporeal membrane oxygenation
ED	emergency department
EDNO	endothelial-derived nitric oxide
EF	ejection fraction
EFE	endomyocardial fibroelastosis
EHRA	European Heart Rhythm Association
EIAH	exercise-induced arterial hypoxemia
EIB	exercise-induced bronchoconstriction
ERAS	endothelin receptor antagonists
ERI	elective replacement indicator
ERP	effective refractory period
ESC	European Society of Cardiology
ESR	erythrocyte sedimentation rate
FFP	fresh frozen plasma
FiO_2	fraction of inspired oxygen
FISH	fluorescent in situ hybridization
FTAAD	familial thoracic aortic aneurysm and dissection
FXN	frataxin
HCM	hypertrophic cardiomyopathy
HFA	Heart Failure Association
HHT	hereditary hemorrhagic telangiectasia
HITT	heparin-induced thrombocytopenia with thrombosis
HIV	Human immunodeficiency virus
HLHS	hypoplastic left heart syndrome
HOCM	hypertrophic obstructive cardiomyopathy
HPAH	hereditary PAH
HR	heart rate
HRA	high right atrium
HRS	Heart Rhythm Society
HV	His-ventricle
IAA	interrupted aortic arch
IART	intra-atrial reentrant tachycardia
ICD	implantable cardioverter-defibrillator
ICU	intensive care unit
IE	infective endocarditis
IM	intramuscularly
INR	international normalized ratio
IPAH	idiopathic pulmonary arterial hypertension
IQ	intelligence quotient
IRB	Institutional Review Board
ISHLT	International Society for Heart and Lung Transplantation
IV	intravenous
IVC	inferior vena cava
IVIG	intravenous immunoglobulin
IVS	intact ventricular septum
IVUS	intravascular ultrasound
JET	junctional ectopic tachycardia
KD	Kawasaki disease
LA	left atrium
LABA	long-acting beta agonists
LAD	left anterior descending

LAD	left-axis deviation
LAMP2	lysosome-associated membrane protein 2
LBBB	Left bundle branch block
LCA	left coronary artery
LDL	low-density lipoprotein
LFTs	Liver function tests
LIV	left innominate vein
LMWH	low–molecular-weight heparin
LPA	left pulmonary artery
LQTS	long QT syndrome
LSVC	left superior vena cava
LUSB	left upper sternal border
LV	left ventricle
LVEDD	left ventricular end diastolic dimension
LVEDP	left ventricular end diastolic pressure
LVEDV	left ventricular end diastolic volume
LVEF	left ventricular ejection fraction
LVH	left ventricular hypertrophy
LVNC	LV noncompaction
LVOT	left ventricular outflow tract
LVOTO	left ventricular outflow tract obstruction
MAP	mean arterial pressure
MAPCA	major aortopulmonary collateral arteries
MDE	myocardial delayed enhancement
MELAS	mitochondrial encephalopathy, lactic acidosis, and stroke-like episodes syndrome
MFS	Marfan syndrome
MI	myocardial infarction
MIG	maximum instantaneous gradient
MIS-C	multisystem inflammatory syndrome in children
MPA	main pulmonary artery
MPI	myocardial performance index
MR	magnetic resonance
MRI	magnetic resonance imaging
MV	mixed venous
MVC	maximal voluntary contraction
MVP	mitral valve prolapse
MVV	maximal voluntary ventilation
NEC	necrotizing enterocolitis
NICU	neonatal intensive care unit
NIRS	near-infrared spectroscopy
NNT	number needed to treat
NPV	negative predictive value
NSAIDs	nonsteroidal anti-inflammatory drugs
PA	pulmonary valve atresia or pulmonary artery
PACES	Pediatric and Congenital Electrophysiology Society
PACS	premature atrial contractions
PAH	pulmonary arterial hypertension
PA-IVS	pulmonary atresia and intact ventricular septum
PAPVC	partial anomalous pulmonary venous connection
PB	plastic bronchitis
PBF	pulmonary blood flow
PCA	patient-controlled analgesia
pCO_2	partial pressure of CO_2
PCWP	pulmonary capillary wedge pressure

PDA	patent ductus arteriosus	**RUPV**	right upper pulmonary vein
PEA	pulseless electrical activity	**RV**	right ventricle
PEP	positive expiratory pressure	**RVA**	right ventricular apex
PF-4	platelet factor 4	**RVEDP**	right ventricular end-diastolic pressure
PFO	patent foramen ovale	**RVH**	right ventricular hypertrophy
PGE1	prostaglandin E1	**RVOT**	right ventricular outflow tract
PHTN	pulmonary hypertension	**RV-PA**	right ventricle-to-pulmonary artery
PICC	peripherally inserted central catheter	**RVSP**	right ventricular systolic pressure
PICU	pediatric intensive care unit	**SA**	systemic artery
PIG	peak instantaneous gradient	**SABA**	short-acting beta-2 agonists
PJRT	permanent junctional reciprocating tachycardia	**SBP**	systolic blood pressure
PKA	protein kinase A	**SCD**	sudden cardiac death
PKU	phenylketonuria	**SD**	standard deviation
PO	per os (by mouth)	**SEM**	standard error of the mean
POTS	postural orthostatic tachycardia syndrome	**SIDS**	sudden infant death syndrome
PPV	positive pressure ventilation	**SLE**	systemic lupus erythematosus
PPV	positive predictive value	**SPAMM**	spatial modulation of magnetization
PR	pulmonary regurgitation	**SSFP**	steady-state free precession
PRES	posterior reversible encephalopathy syndrome	**SVASD**	sinus venosus atrial septal defect
PRF	pulse repetition frequency	**SVC**	superior vena cava
PS	pulmonary valve stenosis	**SVR**	systemic vascular resistance
PS	pulmonary stenosis	**SVT**	supraventricular tachycardia
PTLD	posttransplant lymphoproliferative disorder	**TAPVC**	total anomalous pulmonary venous connection
PV	pulmonary vein	**TAPVR**	total anomalous pulmonary venous return
PVCs	premature ventricular contractions	**TAR**	thrombocytopenia-absent radii
PVOD	pulmonary vascular occlusive disease	**TDI**	tissue Doppler imaging
PVR	pulmonary vascular resistance	**TEE**	transesophageal echocardiography
PW	pulsed-wave	**TFTs**	thyroid function tests
PWP	pulmonary wedge pressure	**TGF-β**	transforming growth factor beta
RA	right atrium	**TOF**	tetralogy of Fallot
RAP	right atrial pressure	**TRICKS**	time-resolved imaging of contrast kinetics
RCA	right coronary artery	**TSH**	thyroid-stimulating hormone
RCM	restrictive cardiomyopathy	**TTE**	transthoracic echocardiography
RER	respiratory exchange ratio	**TVI**	time velocity integral
RF	radiofrequency	**UVC**	umbilical venous catheter
RF	rheumatic fever	**VAT**	ventilatory anaerobic threshold
RHD	rheumatic heart disease	**VEC**	velocity-encoded cine
RLSB	right lower sternal border	**VF**	ventricular fibrillation
ROC	receiver operating characteristic	**VGAM**	vein of Galen malformation
RPA	right pulmonary artery	**VQ**	ventilatory:perfusion
RPCW	right pulmonary capillary wedge	**VSD**	ventricular septal defect
RRR	relative risk reduction	**VT**	ventricular tachycardia
RSV	respiratory syncytial virus	**WPW**	Wolff–Parkinson–White

Contents

Cardiac Anatomy and Physiology

Brittany M. Graham, Joseph J. Maleszewski, and Jonathan N. Johnson

Questions

1. Left ventricular (LV) isovolumic contraction continues until what cardiac event occurs?

    A. Mitral valve opens
    B. Passive atrial filling
    C. Increased ventricular volume
    D. Aortic valve opens
    E. Aortic pressure greater than left ventricular

2. Many metabolic factors are responsible for regulating coronary arterial blood flow. Which of the following metabolic factors is derived from the breakdown of high-energy phosphates?

    A. Prostaglandin
    B. Nitric oxide
    C. Endothelin-1
    D. Adenosine
    E. Vascular endothelial growth factor

3. **Figure 1.1** was taken from which cardiac chamber?

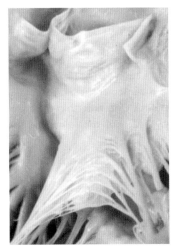

FIGURE 1.1

A. Right atrium
B. Right ventricle
C. Left atrium
D. Left ventricle
E. Coronary Sinus

4. You are evaluating a toddler admitted to the pediatric service due to failure to thrive. There is concern that a vascular ring may be present. Upon completing an echocardiogram, you note that there is a right-sided arch. In combination with a right-sided aortic arch, which of the following would be concerning for a symptomatic vascular ring?

    A. Mirror image branching
    B. An aberrant right subclavian and diverticulum of Kommerell
    C. An aberrant left subclavian and left-sided patent ductus arteriosus
    D. Aberrant right subclavian with a left-sided diverticulum of Kommerell
    E. An aberrant left subclavian with a right-sided patent ductus arteriosus

5. You diagnose a neonate with polysplenia. Which of the following is most likely to be true regarding this patient?

    A. Limb-length abnormalities are present
    B. There are multiple spleens on both the left and right sides
    C. Multiple gallbladders are common
    D. The SVC is interrupted
    E. The IVC is interrupted, with azygos continuation to SVC

6. In the mature cardiac myocytes, the majority of calcium involved in the binding of troponin C and thus the initiation of myocyte contraction is stored in which cellular space?

    A. Extracellular space
    B. T-tubule
    C. Mitochondria
    D. Lysosomes
    E. Sarcoplasmic reticulum

7. The term *straddling* may be applied to which of the following?

    A. Semilunar valves
    B. Atrioventricular valves
    C. Both semilunar and atrioventricular valves
    D. Neither semilunar nor atrioventricular valves
    E. Valve of the fossa ovalis

8. A 15-year-old patient with hypoplastic left heart syndrome had a total cavopulmonary anastomosis (Fontan). In clinic, O_2 saturations are much lower than anticipated. On imaging, there is no obstruction to flow at the level of the Glenn, Fontan, or Branch PAs. Which of the following is the most likely cause of the desaturations?

    A. Venovenous collateral circulation
    B. Aortopulmonary collateral circulation
    C. Venoarterial collateral circulation
    D. Aneurysmal arteriovenous malformation
    E. Coronary fistula

9. A 12-year-old boy is diagnosed with mild aortic stenosis. You suspect that he has an abnormal aortic valve. Echocardiographic imaging demonstrates that his valve is similar to the following pathology image (**Figure 1.2**). Which of the following is the aortic cusp pattern in this patient?

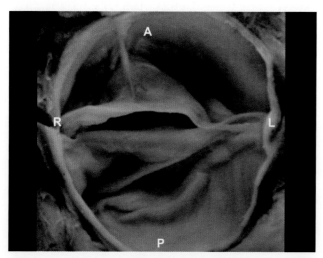

FIGURE 1.2 A, anterior; L, left; P, posterior; R, right. (Image courtesy of Dr. William Edwards, Mayo Clinic.)

A. Bicuspid valve with fusion of the right and noncoronary cusps
B. Quadricuspid valve with a cleft of the left coronary cusp
C. Unicuspid valve with fusion of more than one cusp
D. Bicuspid valve with fusion of the right and left cusps
E. Bicuspid valve with fusion of the left and noncoronary cusps

10. Which *one* of the following pairs is *mismatched*?

    A. Right coronary artery — near tricuspid annulus
    B. Tricuspid valve — direct septal cordal insertions
    C. Right ventricle — crista terminalis
    D. Left ventricle — fine apical trabeculations
    E. Right atrium — limbus of fossa ovalis

11. You are assessing a patient with coarctation of the aorta. The coarctation is discrete with no aortic arch hypoplasia. Surgical repair is planned via a lateral thoracotomy instead of median sternotomy. Which of the following would most accurately determine arch sidedness prior to surgical intervention?

    A. Suprasternal notch echo view of the third branch of the aorta
    B. Subcostal echo view demonstrating the relationship of the spine to the aorta
    C. CT angiogram (CTA) demonstrating the branching pattern of the arch when compared to the branch pulmonary artery
    D. Suprasternal notch echo view demonstrating the relationship between the aortic arch and left pulmonary artery
    E. CT angiogram (CTA) demonstrating the relationship between the aortic arch and the bronchus

12. Which of the following factors has the greatest impact on the pressure change across two points in a vessel?

    A. Vessel radius
    B. Blood viscosity
    C. Vessel length
    D. Maximum velocity of blood flow
    E. Hemoglobin concentration

13. On gross inspection of a heart specimen, there is a defect adjacent to the interventricular component of the membranous septum. You note that there is aortic–tricuspid continuity. Which of the following is the most likely diagnosis?

    A. Perimembranous VSD with inlet extension
    B. Outlet muscular VSD
    C. Anterior muscular VSD
    D. Apical muscular VSD
    E. Doubly committed VSD

14. The normal left aortic arch is primarily derived from which embryologic aortic arch?

    A. Fourth (IV) aortic arch
    B. First (I) aortic arch
    C. Second (II) aortic arch
    D. Third (III) aortic arch
    E. Sixth (VI) aortic arch

15. Embryologically, the ductus arteriosus and the left pulmonary artery arise from the:

    A. Left fourth (IV) aortic arch
    B. Left sixth (VI) and fourth (IV) aortic arches, respectively
    C. Left fourth (IV) and sixth (VI) aortic arches, respectively
    D. Left sixth (VI) aortic arch
    E. Right fifth (V) arch

16. You diagnose a 5-day-old female infant with tetralogy of Fallot. Of the following defects, which is most likely to be seen concurrently on echocardiogram?

    A. Right aortic arch
    B. Aortic stenosis
    C. Atrial septal defect or patent foramen ovale
    D. Coarctation of the aorta
    E. Mitral valve prolapse

17. In contrast to a left-sided aortic arch, a right-sided aortic arch travels over the:

    A. Left atrium
    B. Right pulmonary artery
    C. Right bronchus
    D. Left pulmonary artery
    E. Left bronchus

18. A 4-year-old patient is postoperative day 2 from surgical repair of a moderate to large-sized secundum atrial septal defect. There is a distinct high-frequency "scratching" sound heard throughout the cardiac cycle and diffuse ST elevation on EKG. Which of the following structures is responsible for these findings?

    A. Parietal pleura
    B. Pericardial reflection
    C. Epicardium
    D. Myocardium
    E. Visceral pericardium

19. In the patient mentioned in question 18, the fibrinous pericarditis goes untreated. Several months later the patient returns with difficulty breathing, lower extremity edema, and hepatomegaly. What is the underlying physiology leading to this clinical presentation?

    A. Decreased systolic function due to fibrous deposition within the myocardium
    B. Decreased diastolic function due to excessive strain
    C. Increased afterload secondary to reduced stroke volume
    D. Decreased diastolic function due to constriction
    E. Increased afterload secondary to restriction

20. A newborn female infant presents with cyanosis. The following echocardiogram is obtained (**Figure 1.3**). In patients with this anatomy, which of the following is the most common coronary arterial abnormality?

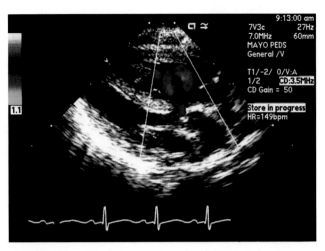

FIGURE 1.3

    A. Intramural left coronary
    B. Left anterior descending from the RCA
    C. Single right coronary artery
    D. Single left coronary artery
    E. Left circumflex from the RCA

21. How does atrial natriuretic peptide (ANP) work on the kidney?

    A. Decreases tubular resorption of sodium
    B. Activates vasopressin receptors
    C. Inhibits ion exchange in the ascending loop of Henle
    D. Inhibition of sodium resorption in the proximal tubule
    E. Dilation of the efferent arteriole

22. In a normal adolescent heart, the average ratio of ventricular septal thickness to left ventricular free wall thickness is:

    A. 1.1
    B. 2.9
    C. 1.9
    D. 0.6
    E. 2.4

23. Cardiac situs is determined by position of which structure?

    A. Cardiac apex
    B. Left atrium
    C. Left ventricle
    D. Right atrium
    E. Right ventricle

24. A 3-year-old boy with a history of a ventricular septal defect (VSD) presents to your office for follow-up. On examination, you hear a diastolic murmur at the apex. Echocardiography is performed (**Figure 1.4**). Prolapse of which aortic cusp is most likely causing the diastolic murmur?

A. Left
B. Anterior
C. Septal
D. Right
E. Noncoronary

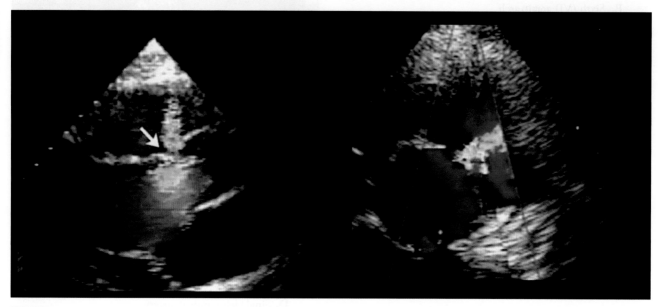

FIGURE 1.4

25. You diagnose a neonate with asplenia. Which of the following is most likely to be present in this patient?

A. The liver is midline with two mirror-image left lobes
B. Descending aorta and IVC on the same side of vertebral column
C. The biliary tree is patent with multiple gallbladders
D. Stomach position is fixed to the right side
E. Normal rotation of the bowels

26. A 16-year-old boy is a long-distance runner for his high school. He has been training all year preparing for the state track meet. How did his resting hemodynamics change from pre- to posttrained state?

A. Increased stroke volume
B. Increased heart rate
C. Decreased blood volume
D. Increased myocardial oxygen demand
E. Increased resting arterial blood pressure

27. Which of these sites contains contractile cardiac myocytes?

A. Proximal aorta
B. Epicardium
C. Proximal main pulmonary artery
D. Proximal pulmonary veins
E. Distal inferior vena cava

28. Identify the arrowed structure in **Figure 1.5**.

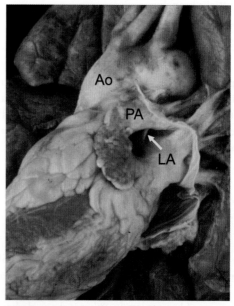

FIGURE 1.5

A. Levoatrial cardinal vein
B. Ligament of Marshall
C. Thebesian vein
D. Eustachian valve
E. Ligamentum arteriosum

29. The valve of the fossa ovalis represents the remnant of which embryologic structure?

    A. Septum primum
    B. Septum secundum
    C. Ostium primum
    D. Ostium secundum
    E. Septum spurium

30. A trauma patient is rushed to the OR due to concern for cardiac tamponade. He was in a rapid deceleration accident. Initially at the scene he was lucid, but coded upon arrival to the ED.

    Which of the following is the most likely area of injury?

    A. Main pulmonary artery
    B. Terminal SVC
    C. Ascending aorta
    D. Descending aorta
    E. Distal IVC

31. Which of the following factors would shift the O_2 dissociation curve to the left?

    A. Increased temperature
    B. Increased pCO_2
    C. Increased 2,3-DPG
    D. Increased pH
    E. Increased fetal hemoglobin concentration

32. A single sinoatrial node in a normal position is typically found in which of the following?

    A. Left juxtaposition of the atrial appendages
    B. Right atrial isomerism
    C. Right juxtaposition of the atrial appendages
    D. Left atrial isomerism
    E. Situs inversus of the atria

33. Systemic arteriolar vasodilation occurs in response to:

    A. Decreased pCO_2
    B. Decreased H^+
    C. Decreased pO_2
    D. Decreased K^+
    E. Decreased Mg^+

34. Which term best describes the type of defect that is characterized by large atrial septal and ventricular septal defects as well as a common atrioventricular valve, but with separate left and right orifices?

    A. Partial AVSD
    B. Intermediate AVSD
    C. Complete AVSD
    D. Transitional AVSD
    E. Membranous VSD

35. Which chamber is shown in **Figure 1.6**?

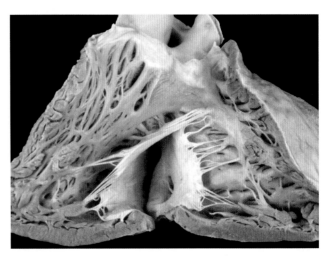

FIGURE 1.6

    A. Right atrium
    B. Right ventricle
    C. Left atrium
    D. Left ventricle

36. Which fetal venous structure has the lowest oxygen saturation?

    A. Ductus venosus
    B. IVC
    C. Left hepatic vein
    D. Coronary sinus
    E. Right pulmonary vein

37. The direction in which blood flows through an ASD primarily is related to the:

    A. Pulmonary vascular resistance
    B. Systemic vascular resistance
    C. Relative compliances of the left and right ventricles
    D. Morphology of the eustachian valve
    E. Redundancy of the atrial septum

38. A newborn male infant is diagnosed with hypoplastic left heart syndrome (HLHS). Of the following, which anatomic form of HLHS will most likely be seen in this patient?

    A. Aortic valve atresia with patent mitral valve
    B. Aortic valve stenosis with patent mitral valve
    C. Aortic valve stenosis with mitral valve stenosis
    D. Aortic valve atresia with mitral valve atresia
    E. Aortic valve atresia with mitral valve regurgitation

39. In the cardiac sarcomere, which of the following named features includes the entirety of the myosin contractile elements?

   A. E-line
   B. A-band
   C. I-band
   D. H-zone
   E. Z-disk

40. A patient with pulmonary atresia is undergoing an operation. While operating, the surgeon wants to find out if there is a remnant of the hypoplastic or atretic main pulmonary artery. Which of the following would be the most helpful landmark?

   A. Coronary sinus
   B. Transverse sinus
   C. Fossa ovalis
   D. SVC
   E. Pericardial reflection

41. Truncus arteriosus is diagnosed in a newborn male infant. Of the following, which truncal valve morphology are you most likely to find?

   A. Unicuspid
   B. Bicuspid
   C. Quadricuspid
   D. Pentacuspid
   E. Sextacuspid

42. The resting potential of which ion is primarily responsible for the baseline (phase 4) resting conductance of cardiac myocytes?

   A. Calcium
   B. Sodium
   C. Potassium
   D. Chloride
   E. Magnesium

43. What is the most common location of the pulmonary artery in patients with truncus arteriosus?

   A. Branch pulmonary arteries arise from posterior sides of the truncus
   B. Branch pulmonary arteries arise from the lateral sides of the truncus
   C. Main pulmonary artery arises from the truncus
   D. Branch pulmonary arteries arise from the descending aorta
   E. Main pulmonary artery arises from the innominate artery

44. Which type of atrial septal defect is shown in **Figure 1.7**?

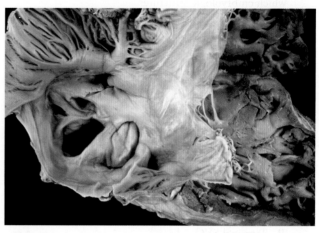

FIGURE 1.7

   A. Primum
   B. Secundum
   C. Coronary sinus
   D. Sinus venosus
   E. Membranous

45. In cardiovascular surgery, if the pericardium is transected, it is usually left open. In addition, chest tubes are placed prior to chest closure. These interventions are primarily to prevent fluid buildup in which of the following?

   A. Anterior mediastinum
   B. Pleural space
   C. Posterior mediastinum
   D. Pericardial space
   E. Lung interstitium

46. The rapid depolarization of cardiac myocytes (phase 0) is driven by the rapid influx of which ion into the myocytes?

   A. Sodium
   B. Potassium
   C. Chloride
   D. Magnesium
   E. Calcium

47. You are called to see a cyanotic neonate in the neonatal intensive care unit. You note that the patient has an oxygen saturation of 69%. His chest x-ray shows decreased vascular markings in the lung fields. Which of the following is the most likely anatomy you will find on examination and echocardiography?

   A. Truncus arteriosus
   B. TAPVC
   C. Critical pulmonary stenosis
   D. HLHS
   E. Tricuspid atresia with transposed great arteries

48. Which is the most abundant nonmyocyte cardiac cell in the mature heart?

A. Fibroblast
B. Pericyte
C. Vascular smooth muscle
D. Macrophage
E. Endothelial

49. A 4-year-old boy is referred for cardiomegaly on a chest x-ray. His four-chamber view is seen in **Figure 1.8**. Of the following, which additional cardiac diagnosis is most likely to be found in this patient?

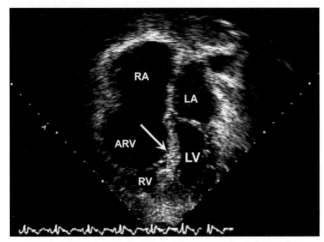

FIGURE 1.8 ARV, atrialized right ventricle; LA, left atrium; LV, left ventricle; RA, right atrium; RV, right ventricle.

A. Ventricular septal defect
B. Pulmonary valve stenosis
C. Patent ductus arteriosus
D. Mitral valve prolapse
E. Atrial septal defect

50. Of the following, which structure in the fetus has the least saturated blood?

A. Superior vena cava
B. Inferior vena cava
C. Patent ductus arteriosus
D. Ductus venosus
E. Ascending aortic arch

51. A 2-year-old boy undergoes repair of coarctation of the aorta. Postoperatively, he is able to be extubated, but develops intermittent stridor. Chest radiography is unremarkable. Which of the following is the most likely structure that was injured during the operation?

A. Left vagus nerve
B. Right recurrent laryngeal nerve
C. Thoracic duct
D. Right vagus nerve
E. Left recurrent laryngeal nerve

52. A fetal echocardiogram is performed and demonstrates double outlet right ventricle. Which of the following positions of the aorta, relative to the pulmonary artery, are you most likely to find on further imaging?

A. Right anterior
B. Left anterior
C. Side by side
D. Left posterior
E. Right posterior

53. The normal right superior vena cava is derived from which of the following embryologic structures?

A. Left anterior cardinal vein
B. Right vitelline vein
C. Right anterior cardinal vein
D. Ductus venosus
E. Left umbilical vein

54. Which structures connect cardiac myocytes end to end, and are responsible for structural integrity and synchronized contraction of cardiac tissue?

A. Dystrophin
B. T-tubules
C. Costameres
D. Intercalated discs
E. Myosin

55. A term neonate presents with tachycardia, poor perfusion, and respiratory failure. The liver is enlarged on examination. Echocardiography reveals dilation of all four heart chambers. You note that the echo-calculated cardiac output is markedly elevated. Which of the following is the most likely source of the high-output cardiac failure?

A. Lower extremity AVM
B. Upper extremity AVM
C. Hepatic AVM
D. Vein of Galen malformation
E. Pulmonary AVM

56. A 5-day-old female infant has an echocardiogram performed (**Figure 1.9**). Of the following abnormal coronary patterns, which are you most likely to find on this echocardiogram?

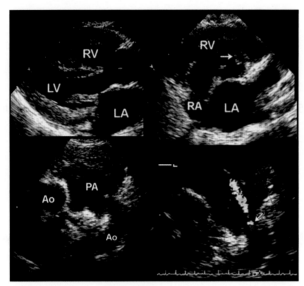

FIGURE 1.9 Ao, aorta; LA, left atrium; LV, left ventricle; PA, pulmonary artery; RA, right atrium; RV, right ventricle.

   A. Intramural left coronary artery
   B. Left anterior descending from the RCA
   C. Left circumflex from the RCA
   D. Single left coronary
   E. Single right coronary

57. Which of the following is an anatomic hallmark of the morphologic right atrium?

   A. Ostium of the IVC
   B. Finger-like atrial appendage
   C. Smooth-surfaced free wall
   D. Ostium of the pulmonary veins
   E. More posterior location than the left atrium

58. A 4-day-old male infant has the following echo performed (**Figure 1.10**). Which of the following great artery relationships are you most likely to find on echocardiography?

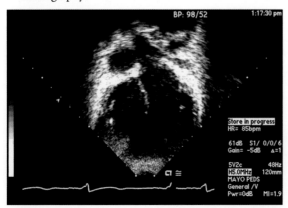

FIGURE 1.10

   A. D-transposition of the great arteries
   B. L-transposition of the great arteries
   C. Left anterior aorta
   D. Right anterior aorta
   E. Normally related great arteries

59. During the relaxation phase of the cardiac muscle contraction, the majority of Ca^{2+} is removed from the sarcoplasm by:

   A. Passive exchange through L-type Ca^{2+} channels
   B. Efflux via Na^+-Ca^{2+} passive exchange
   C. Ca^{2+}-ATPase pumps located on the sarcolemma
   D. Reuptake in the sarcoplasmic reticulum via SERCA pumps
   E. Efflux via K^+-Ca^{2+} passive exchange

60. An infant presents to the emergency department with signs and symptoms of shock. There is no infectious etiology identified. He remains hypoxic. An echocardiogram is obtained. On echocardiogram, the heart is anatomically normal other than a prominence visualized in the right atrium. This prominence is most likely which of the following?

   A. Prominent thebesian valve
   B. Enlarged Chiari network
   C. Prominent eustachian valve
   D. Enlarged tendon of Todaro
   E. Supravalvar mitral rims

61. You are evaluating a 3-week-old male infant with tricuspid atresia, transposition of the great arteries, moderate pulmonary stenosis, and a mildly restrictive ventricular septal defect. In this patient, where is the AV node most likely to be positioned?

   A. Posteriorly behind the ostium of the coronary sinus
   B. Anteriorly along the atrial septum in the right atrium
   C. Floor behind the right atrium
   D. In the left atrium just medial to the left atrioventricular valve annulus
   E. Lateral to the ostium of the IVC in the right atrium

62. Which of the following is true regarding the right ventricle in the normal heart?

   A. Is typically a bipartite chamber
   B. Has small apical trabeculations
   C. Has prominent crista terminalis
   D. Has a coarse septal surface
   E. There is tricuspid-pulmonary continuity

63. A neonate is diagnosed with d-transposition of the great arteries. In addition to the transposed great vessels, the most common concurrent finding on echocardiography in this patient is:
    A. Ventricular septal defect
    B. Mitral valve abnormalities
    C. Coarctation of the aorta
    D. Leftward juxtaposition of the atrial appendages
    E. Left ventricular outflow obstruction

64. You diagnose a neonate with truncus arteriosus. It appears that this patient has a single pulmonary artery. Which artery is most likely to be absent in this patient?
    A. Left pulmonary artery
    B. Right pulmonary artery
    C. The pulmonary artery on the opposite side of the aortic arch
    D. Both right and left pulmonary arteries
    E. The pulmonary artery on the side of the aortic arch

65. A 12-year-old girl presents with cyanosis. An echocardiogram reveals severe Ebstein anomaly with severe tricuspid valve regurgitation. Which of the following is the most likely cause of her cyanosis?
    A. Left-to-right shunt at the atrial level
    B. Right-to-left shunt at the atrial level
    C. Right-to-left shunt at the ventricular level
    D. Coronary fistula
    E. Stenotic outflow to the pulmonary arteries

66. Which of the following is an anatomic hallmark of the morphologic left atrium?
    A. Valve of the fossa ovalis (septum primum)
    B. Limbus of the fossa ovalis
    C. More anterior location compared to the right atrium
    D. Entrance of the inferior vena cava
    E. Connection to the tricuspid valve

67. Which of the following is true regarding fetal hemoglobin?
    A. Is composed of alpha and gamma subunits
    B. Is present in normal children until age 6 years
    C. Is replaced by adult hemoglobin by the 38th week of gestation
    D. Has a lower affinity for oxygen than adult hemoglobin
    E. Interacts more efficiently with 2,3-DPG than adult hemoglobin

68. Through which pathway does norepinephrine activate β1 adrenergic receptors?
    A. Direct activation of Ca^{2+}-ATPase
    B. Gq-dependent activation of phospholipase C
    C. Gs-dependent activation of adenylate cyclase, increasing cAMP
    D. Gi-dependent inhibition of adenylate cyclase, decreasing cAMP
    E. Activation of guanylate cyclase, increasing cGMP

69. Which of the following changes occurs with inspiration in the normal heart and lungs?
    A. Increase in pleural pressure by 3 to 5 cm H_2O
    B. Decrease in intra-abdominal pressure
    C. Increased E' velocity of the tricuspid valve
    D. Increased E' velocity of the mitral valve
    E. Decrease in right ventricular stroke volume

70. A 3-month-old infant presents with a systolic murmur heard best at the apex. An echocardiogram is diagnostic of a mitral arcade. Which of the following would best describe a mitral arcade?
    A. Thickened mitral valve leaflets
    B. Fused papillary muscles
    C. Absent papillary muscle
    D. Absent/abnormal chordal insertions
    E. Decreased interpapillary muscle distance

71. The formation of an ostium primum ASD results from:
    A. Excessive resorption of the septum primum
    B. Insufficient growth of the septum secundum
    C. Abnormal endocardium cushion development
    D. Failure of the common pulmonary vein to connect to the left atrium
    E. Abnormal rotation of the dextrodorsal conal swelling

72. A vessel is noted running lateral and leftward to the pulmonary artery on high parasternal short-axis views, with flow heading inferiorly. The structure is seen again on a transesophageal echocardiogram running between the left pulmonary veins and the left atrial appendage, just posterior and superior to the mitral valve. What does this structure most likely represent?
    A. Membrane of the cor triatriatum
    B. Innominate vein
    C. Total anomalous pulmonary venous return
    D. Descending aorta
    E. Persistence of the left horn of the sinus venosus

73. A 2-month-old female infant presents with cyanosis. Which of the following is true regarding the diagnosis of cyanosis in this patient?

    A. To visualize cyanosis, the patient must have at least 5 g/dL of deoxygenated hemoglobin
    B. This patient most likely has an atrial septal defect
    C. The best indicator of cyanosis in this patient is examination of the nail beds
    D. The patient most likely has rib notching on chest radiography
    E. This patient most likely has a patent ductus arteriosus

74. The sarcomere is the fundamental contractile unit of striated muscle. Which contractile protein binds to calcium, allowing cross-bridges to form and permitting contraction?

    A. Actin
    B. Troponin C
    C. Myosin
    D. Tropomyosin
    E. Troponin I

75. A 3-year-old girl is referred to you for a murmur. You uncover that the patient is a recent immigrant from Bolivia, having arrived here in the last week. She had lived at an altitude of 10,000 ft since her birth. Which of the following are you most likely to find on a hemodynamic evaluation of this patient, compared to a patient living at sea level?

    A. Left atrial enlargement
    B. Decreased LV systolic function (EF~40%)
    C. Elevated pulmonary artery pressure
    D. Decreased tricuspid regurgitant velocity
    E. Elevated systemic blood pressure

76. Baroreceptors are stretch receptors located in the carotid sinus and aortic arch. What is the outcome of increased arterial pressure on these receptors?

    A. Decrease in afferent impulses to the CNS
    B. Decrease in parasympathetic efferent output
    C. Increased sinus atrial stimulus
    D. Increased cardiac output
    E. Decreased heart rate

77. What is the primary mechanism by which the myocardium compensates for increased oxygen demand?

    A. Increased oxygen extraction
    B. Increased parasympathetic stimulus
    C. Decreased adenosine release
    D. Increased coronary blood flow
    E. Decreased cardiac output

78. A neonate is diagnosed with d-transposition of the great arteries. You hear a loud, single second heart sound. What is the explanation behind this examination finding?

    A. Ventricular septal defect
    B. Anterior position of the aorta
    C. Pulmonary atresia
    D. Severe aortic stenosis
    E. Pulmonary vascular obstructive disease

79. A newborn baby is diagnosed with double outlet right ventricle. Which of the following is most likely to also be found?

    A. Secundum atrial septal defect
    B. Right aortic arch
    C. Primum atrial septal defect
    D. Pulmonary stenosis
    E. Subaortic stenosis

80. Which of the following embryologic aortic arches regresses and typically does not contribute to any structure in the normal neonate?

    A. Left fourth arch
    B. Left fifth arch
    C. Right fourth arch
    D. Left third arch
    E. Left sixth arch

81. Left ventricular isovolumic *relaxation* continues until what cardiac event occurs?

    A. Aortic valve opens
    B. Passive atrial filling
    C. Mitral valve opens
    D. Increased ventricular volume
    E. Aortic pressure greater than left ventricular volume

82. The atrioventricular node and proximal portion of the His bundle are located within the triangle of Koch. Which of the following is a border of the triangle of Koch?

    A. Eustachian valve
    B. Anterior leaflet of the tricuspid valve
    C. Ostium of the coronary sinus
    D. Limbus of the fossa ovalis
    E. Crista terminalis

83. You are called by the neonatal intensive care unit regarding a new admission. The neonate's mother had a prior fetal echo which showed concern for total anomalous pulmonary venous return. Which of the following is the most likely type of total anomalous pulmonary venous connection to be found?

    A. Infracardiac
    B. Supracardiac
    C. Infradiaphragmatic
    D. Mixed
    E. Cardiac

84. A 16-month-old toddler whose status post repair of a partial AV canal defect has the following results of a blood gas:

pCO$_2$: 37 mm Hg

HCO$_3$: 33 mm/L

pH: 7.54

Which of the following is the acid–base abnormality present in this patient?

A. Acute respiratory alkalosis
B. Acute respiratory acidosis
C. Acute metabolic acidosis
D. Acute metabolic alkalosis
E. Chronic respiratory acidosis

85. A 15-year-old girl is admitted with chest pain. There is a concern for left ventricular inferior wall motion abnormalities on echocardiography. She admits to using cocaine in the past 24 hours. Which coronary artery typically supplies the inferior left ventricular wall and the posteromedial papillary muscle of the mitral valve?

A. Right coronary
B. Left circumflex
C. Left anterior descending
D. Obtuse marginal
E. Conal branch

86. The AV nodal artery arises from which coronary artery?

A. Right coronary
B. Left anterior descending
C. Left circumflex
D. Posterior descending
E. Marginal

87. The most common coronary artery abnormality seen in patients with otherwise normal hearts is:

A. Anomalous origin of the right coronary artery from the left sinus of Valsalva
B. Anomalous origin of the right coronary artery from the posterior sinus of Valsalva
C. Single coronary artery
D. Anomalous origin of the left circumflex coronary artery from the right main coronary artery
E. Anomalous origin of the left coronary artery from the posterior sinus of Valsalva

88. A 15-year-old boy undergoes a chest CT after direct chest trauma in a car accident. He has no significant past medical history or prior symptoms. The radiologist identifies a congenital abnormality of the aortic arch. Which of the following is the most likely aortic arch malformation in this patient?

A. Right aortic arch with left ductus arteriosus
B. Double aortic arch
C. Left aortic arch with anomalous right subclavian artery
D. Cervical arch
E. Anomalous RPA from ascending aorta

89. A 5-day-old infant presents with cyanosis and lower extremity edema. Hepatomegaly is apparent on physical examination. Echocardiography reveals a normal tricuspid valve, but the right ventricle is thinned and akinetic. Which of the following defects is most likely present?

A. Tricuspid atresia
B. Ebstein anomaly
C. Uhl anomaly
D. Arrhythmogenic right ventricular dysplasia
E. Pulmonary stenosis

90. Which of the following is thought to be most responsible for high pulmonary vascular resistance in the fetus?

A. Low blood and alveolar oxygen tension
B. Fetal secretion of vasoconstrictors (e.g., thromboxane, leukotrienes)
C. Systemic vascular resistance
D. Right-to-left shunting of blood
E. Maternal and placental hormones

91. Around 1 month of gestation in the human embryo, the pulmonary venous plexus establishes a single connection to the sinoatrial portion of the developing heart, called the common pulmonary vein. What is the fate of this structure in the normal heart?

A. Disappears, with eventual independent appearance of the four pulmonary veins
B. Is incorporated into the coronary sinus
C. Is incorporated into the wall of the right atrium
D. Is incorporated into the back wall of the left atrium
E. Becomes the superoposterior portion of the atrial septum

92. Which phase of the cardiac action potential is characterized by entrance of Ca^{2+} into the cell through L-type voltage-gated channels?

A. Phase 0
B. Phase 1
C. Phase 2
D. Phase 3
E. Phase 4

93. A 6-month-old female infant is brought to the emergency room with cyanosis, tachypnea, and irritability. Her father reports that a murmur was heard at her first checkup, but that he missed her appointment that had been scheduled with cardiology. What is most likely causing this patient's cyanosis?

    A. Increased pulmonary blood flow
    B. Increased systemic vascular resistance
    C. Decreased pulmonary vasculature pressure
    D. Increased right-to-left shunting
    E. Increased left-to-right shunting

94. Which of the following will decrease myocardial oxygen consumption?

    A. Decreasing end diastolic volume
    B. Increasing wall tension
    C. Increasing heart rate
    D. Increasing cardiac contractility
    E. Sympathetic activation

95. A 2-month-old infant whose status post repair of a complete AV canal has the following results of a blood gas:

    pCO_2: 36 mm Hg

    HCO_3: 14 mm/L

    pH: 7.21

Which of the following is the acid–base abnormality present in this patient?

    A. Acute respiratory alkalosis
    B. Acute respiratory acidosis
    C. Acute metabolic acidosis
    D. Acute metabolic alkalosis
    E. Chronic respiratory acidosis

96. A 5-month-old infant whose status post repair of an atrioventricular septal defect has the following results on a blood gas:

    pCO_2: 73 mm Hg

    HCO_3: 25 mm/L

    pH: 7.15

Which of the following is the acid–base abnormality present in this patient?

    A. Acute respiratory alkalosis
    B. Acute metabolic acidosis
    C. Acute metabolic alkalosis
    D. Acute respiratory acidosis
    E. Chronic respiratory acidosis

97. Which of the following is true regarding the branching patterns of the right (RPA) and left (LPA) branch pulmonary arteries in a normal patient?

    A. The RPA travels anterior to the right upper lobe bronchus, while the LPA travels posterior to the left upper lobe bronchus
    B. The RPA travels posterior to the right upper lobe bronchus, while the LPA travels anterior to the right upper lobe bronchus
    C. Both LPA and RPA travel inferior to the left and right mainstem bronchi
    D. Both LPA and RPA travel posterior to their respective upper lobe bronchi
    E. Both LPA and RPA travel anterior to their respective upper lobe bronchi

Answers

1. (D) Flow–volume loops are highly likely to be tested on the board examination (see the ICU section of this book for further questions on flow–volume loops). At end diastole, LV filling is complete, and the mitral valve closes. There is a period of isovolumic contraction, after which the aortic valve opens secondary to a lower pressure in the aorta compared to the LV.

2. (D) Adenosine is produced from the breakdown of ATP, which cannot be regenerated at times of low oxygen tension. Therefore, at times of low oxygen tension, AMP is made and then further broken down into adenosine, which causes coronary artery vasodilation. Nitric oxide induces the cyclic guanosine monophosphate which causes muscle relaxation. Endothelin-1 causes tonic vasoconstriction. Prostaglandin induces smooth muscle relaxation.

3. (D) Fibrous continuity of the semilunar and atrioventricular valves is a feature of a morphologic left ventricle. The

aortic valve cusps can be seen in the top of **Figure 1.1** with mitral valve and associated chordae seen at the bottom of the image. Conversely, the morphologic right ventricle exhibits muscular separation of the semilunar and atrioventricular valves.

4. (C) A vascular ring occurs when there is abnormal regression of the embryologic aortic arches. In the setting of a right-sided aortic arch, the combination of an aberrant left subclavian artery and left-sided patent ductus arteriosus will lead to a vascular ring. A diverticulum of Kommerell is specific to a bulbous outpouching of the aorta that appears at the origin of an aberrant subclavian artery. To determine whether there is a vascular ring present, you must know arch sidedness, aortic arch branching, and side/presence of PDA.

5. (E) In polysplenia, the multiple spleens are typically located all on the same side of the vertebral column as the stomach. The gallbladder is typically single, but patients may have concurrent biliary atresia. The abdominal situs is variable and can be normal, mirror image, or indeterminate. The IVC commonly is interrupted with azygos continuation to the SVC.

6. (E) In mature myocytes, the sarcoplasmic reticulum stores the most important source of calcium involved in the initiation of myocyte contraction. Calcium enters the myocyte during the action potential through L-type voltage-gated calcium channels. This calcium then activates the calcium release channel (also called the ryanodine receptor), causing release of calcium from the sarcoplasmic reticulum. In immature cardiac myocytes, the function and organization of the sarcoplasmic reticulum is not yet mature, and activation is more dependent on flow through the L-type calcium channels.

7. (B) Straddling is a feature of a valve's insertion into the ventricles, which is only a feature of atrioventricular valves because of the tensor apparatus (tendinous cords and papillary muscles) necessary for their function. Overriding, a feature of the valve annulus, can be seen in both atrioventricular and semilunar valves.

8. (A) Fontan or stage III palliation includes connection of IVC flow to the pulmonary artery, allowing all pulmonary arterial flow to be passive. Venovenous collaterals lead to direct flow of deoxygenated systemic blood into the pulmonary venous circulation.

Aortopulmonary collaterals develop when there is no sufficient pulmonary blood flow present, and do not result in hypoxemia.

9. (D) Of patients with a bicuspid aortic valve, by far the most common form is fusion of the right and left cusps (75%). The next most common are patients with fusion of the right and noncoronary cusps, followed by those with left and noncoronary cusp fusion. Fusion of more than one cusp can result in a unicuspid valve.

10. (C) The crista terminalis is a right atrial structure, which represents the interface between the sinus portion of the atrium and the embryologic (trabeculated) atrium.

11. (E) While arch sidedness can be determined by echocardiography, CTA allows for a more detailed assessment of the anatomy. Arch sidedness is critical to determine prior to surgical repair via lateral thoracotomy. This is because depending on the side of the arch, surgical planning will change. Whether or not an aortic arch is right or left sided is determined by which bronchus the aortic arch travels over. When assessing by echo, the suprasternal notch will demonstrate the direction the first aortic branch travels. The subcostal views do not allow you to determine arch sidedness.

12. (A) This question refers to the Poiseuille–Hagen relationship, where the resistance R between two points is a function of pressure and flow. This is ultimately described by the equation $R = (8 \times L \times \eta)/(\pi \times r^4)$, where the radius is raised to the fourth power (L = length of the vessel, η = viscosity).

13. (A) There are different names for ventricular septal defects based on their anatomic location. Central perimembranous VSDs can have inlet or outlet components. If there is tricuspid-aortic continuity, then the VSD is a perimembranous inlet VSD. If the lesion extends toward the aortic valve, then it is a perimembranous outlet VSD.

Overall, think of VSDs as perimembranous, inlet, outlet, and muscular. "Central" is another name given in some textbooks to describe perimembranous defects. (See **Figure 1.11**.)

14. (A) The majority of the aortic arch arises from the left fourth aortic arch, while the right fourth aortic arch gives rise to the proximal portion of the right subclavian artery. The pulmonary arteries and ductus arteriosus arise from the left sixth aortic arch.

15. (D) The pulmonary arteries and ductus arteriosus arise from the left sixth aortic arch. The majority of the aortic arch arises from the left fourth aortic arch, while the right fourth aortic arch gives rise to the proximal portion of the right subclavian artery. The fifth aortic arch most typically involutes.

16. (C) An atrial septal defect or a patent foramen ovale is present in over 80% of patients with tetralogy of Fallot (occasionally termed the "pentalogy of Fallot"). Abnormalities of the left side of the heart are rare in patients with tetralogy. A right aortic arch occurs in around 25% of patients.

17. (C) The laterality of the aortic arch is determined by the bronchus it travels over. Both left and right aortic arches travel over the right pulmonary artery. A left aortic arch will travel over the left bronchus and a right aortic arch over a right bronchus.

18. (E) Postoperative atrial septal defect patients are at high risk of developing a friction rub (heard throughout the cardiac cycle). This is secondary to fibrinous pericarditis where fibrin is replaced by fibrovascular granulation tissue. This leads to adherence of the parietal and visceral layers of the heart. The visceral pericardium (epicardium) covers the heart and intrapericardial portions of the great vessels. The parietal pericardium is a strong sac that surrounds the heart.

19. (D) The parietal pericardium is a strong, flask-shaped sac that surrounds the heart. This sac limits diastolic dimensions.

In the setting of chronic pericarditis, there can be further stiffening of the pericardium leading to constriction and elevated ventricular end diastolic pressures.

20. (E) The echocardiographic image (see **Figure 1.3**) represents a patient with d-transposition of the great arteries. Note the immediate posterior course of the great vessel arising from the left ventricle, indicative of the vessel being a pulmonary artery. There is a ventricular septal defect also present in the image. Patients with transposition of the great arteries most commonly have normal coronary anatomy (67%), but approximately 16% of patients will have an anomalous circumflex coronary artery arising from the right

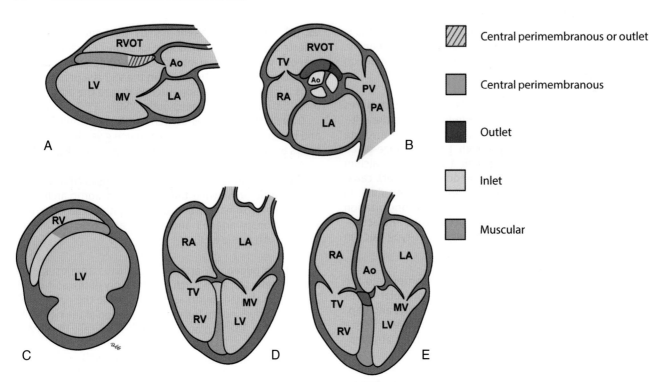

FIGURE 1.11 Diagrammatic representation of ventricular septal defect (VSD) locations as seen in standard echocardiographic views. **A:** Parasternal long-axis view showing trabecular muscular, central perimembranous, and outlet VSDs. **B:** Parasternal short-axis view at the base showing central perimembranous and outlet VSDs. **C:** Parasternal short-axis view at the level of the left ventricular (LV) papillary muscles showing trabecular muscular VSDs. **D:** Apical four-chamber view showing inlet and trabecular muscular VSDs. **E:** Apical five-chamber view showing trabecular muscular and central perimembranous VSDs. Ao, aorta; LA, left atrium; MV, mitral valve; PA, pulmonary artery; PV, pulmonary valve; RA, right atrium; RV, right ventricle; RVOT, right ventricular outflow tract; TV, tricuspid valve. (From Eidem BW, Cetta F, Johnson J, et al. *Echocardiography in Pediatric and Adult Congenital Heart Disease*. 3rd ed. Wolters Kluwer; 2021. Fig 12.3.)

coronary. The next most common abnormalities are a single right coronary artery and an inverted right coronary and left circumflex (inverted origins of the RCA and LCx but normal origin of the LAD from the anterior facing sinus).

21. (A) ANP is released in response to stretch from either atrium. ANP works on the kidney by dilating the afferent arteriole and constricting the efferent arteriole, effectively increasing GFR. It also works on the distal tubules to decrease sodium resorption. ANP also has vasodilator and cardioinhibitory effects.

22. (A) In normal hearts in the first two decades of life, the thickness of the ventricular septum and left free wall are similar (mean = 1.1, range: 0.8 to 1.4). This ratio increases slowly in adulthood and averages greater than 1.2 by age 70. It can also be affected in diseases of asymmetric hypertrophy such as hypertrophic cardiomyopathy. The average ratio between left and right ventricular thickness is 3 (range: 2 to 5). Due to high right-sided pressure in utero, this ratio is lower in fetuses and neonates.

23. (D) The pathologic definition of cardiac sidedness (situs) is the position of the right atrium.

24. (D) The subarterial type of VSD (also called supracristal or infundibular) comprises 5% of VSDs at autopsy, but is

significantly more common in Asian populations. Due to the location of the VSD, there is deficiency of the support structure below the aortic valve, with subsequent herniation of the right coronary leaflet through the defect. This may also occur in some patients with perimembranous defects.

25. (B) In most asplenia patients, the descending aorta and IVC will travel on the same side of the vertebral column. There is a high incidence of bowel malrotation, and the stomach can be located on the left, right, or midline. There is typically only one gallbladder, but it can be variable in position, depending on the site of the liver. Biliary atresia may occur. The liver is most commonly midline with two mirror-image right lobes.

26. (A) Repetitive exercise for prolonged periods of time results in benefits on one's cardiovascular health and increases an individual's work capacity. Changes include increased blood volume and stroke volume and decreased heart rate, resting arterial blood pressure, and myocardial oxygen demand.

27. (D) The pulmonary veins contain cardiac myocytes instead of smooth muscle cells in the last 1 to 3 cm before insertion to the left atrium. This allows them to minimize retrograde flow during atrial systole. This can also be a source of atrial fibrillation, which is why pulmonary vein isolation procedures are often used in adults.

28. (B) The structure shown, a small fibrous ridge traveling anterior to the pulmonary veins and the left pulmonary artery, represents the vestige of the left-sided superior vena cava—otherwise known as the ligament of Marshall.

29. (A) The valve of the fossa ovalis is derived from septum primum, while the limbus of the fossa ovalis is derived from septum secundum.

30. (C) The ascending aorta, main pulmonary artery, and terminal SVC are considered "intrapericardial" structures. Injury to the proximal aorta would lead to a pericardial effusion due to the location of the vessel within the pericardium and not within the mediastinum. In deceleration injuries, the aorta is the most likely structure to be injured. IVC and descending Ao injuries would not lead to cardiac tamponade as these structures do not lie within the pericardium.

31. (D) The hemoglobin–oxygen dissociation curve helps to understand the relationship between pO_2 and oxygen saturations. Increasing the pH (alkalosis), decreasing temperature, and decreasing 2,3-DPG will shift the curve to the left; likewise, acidosis, increased temperature, and increasing 2,3-DPG shift the curve to the right.

32. (C) In patients with right atrial isomerism, bilateral sinus nodes can be encountered. In left atrial isomerism, the sinus node can be absent or malpositioned. In left-sided juxtaposition of the atrial appendages, the sinus node is often displaced anteriorly or inferiorly. Left juxtaposition is associated more with abnormal ventriculoarterial connections, while right-sided juxtaposition is more commonly associated with simpler lesions, like atrial septal defects.

33. (C) Specific tissues are able to regulate local blood flow in response to changing metabolic demands. A decrease in the pO_2 causes a systemic arteriolar vasodilation, as the local tissues attempt to get more oxygen delivery through increased volume of flow. Similarly, *increasing* pCO_2, *increasing* H^+ (acidosis), or *increasing* K^+ will cause local vasodilation. Some tissues will also release adenosine as a vasodilator in response to increased oxygen demand.

34. (B) An intermediate AVSD is a rare subtype of a complete defect where the common AV valve has separate left and right orifices. This is accompanied by a large primum ASD and inlet VSD, and the clinical picture is similar to complete AVSD. Partial AVSD consists of a septum primum ASD and cleft left AV valve anterior leaflet, but the left and right AV valves are separate. Transitional defects are a subtype of partial defects and include a small inlet VSD. See **Figure 1.12**.

AVSD Summary

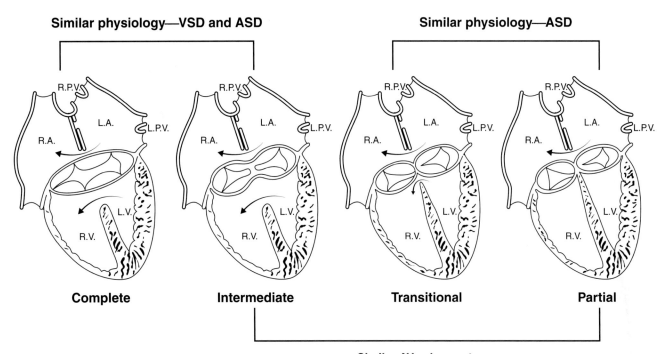

FIGURE 1.12 ASD, atrial septal defect; AVSD, atrioventricular septal defect; LA, left atrium; LPV, left pulmonary vein; LV, left ventricle; RA, right atrium; RPV, right pulmonary vein; RV, right ventricle; VSD, ventricular septal defect. (Image courtesy of Dr. Frank Cetta, MD.)

35. (B) Three characteristic features of a morphologic right ventricle are shown in this example: (1) direct septal cordal insertions onto the ventricular septum; (2) course apical trabeculations; and (3) muscular separation of the atrioventricular and semilunar valves (tricuspid and pulmonary, respectively, in this case).

36. (D) The least saturated blood in the fetus is in the coronary sinus and the superior vena cava, the oxygen having been used by the head/brain or the myocardium. The inferior vena cava, left hepatic vein, and ductus venosus receive some or all of their flow from the umbilical vein, and thus will have higher oxygen saturations.

37. (C) The primary determinant of the direction of blood flow through an atrial septal defect is the relative compliances of the left and right ventricles. In the otherwise normal patient, the right ventricle will be more compliant than the left ventricle, with less resistance to filling from the right atrium, and thus left-to-right shunting across the ASD. The vast majority of patients with ASDs have a relatively normal pulmonary resistance.

38. (D) Aortic atresia with mitral valve atresia occurs in 36% to 46% of patients with HLHS, compared to 13% to 26% of patients with aortic stenosis with mitral stenosis. About 20% to 29% of patients have aortic atresia with a patent mitral valve.

39. (B) The A-band, bisected by the M-line, contains all the myosin contractile elements of the sarcomere. The I-band, bisected by the Z-disk, contains purely actin elements of the sarcomere. The H-zone is a central subsection of the A-band that does not include the areas of myosin–actin overlap.

40. (B) During surgery, the transverse sinus can be used to identify the ascending aorta which can then be used to help identify the remnant of the pulmonary artery.

The transverse sinus is a tunnel-shaped structure that runs between the anterior/superior walls of the atria and posterior/inferior to the great vessels.

41. (C) The truncal valve in truncus arteriosus is most commonly *tricuspid* (~70%). The next most common form of truncal valve is quadricuspid (~20%), followed by bicuspid (~10%), pentacuspid (<1%), and unicommissural (<1%). The valve is in fibrous continuity with the mitral valve in all patients, but can also rarely be in fibrous continuity with the tricuspid valve.

42. (C) The I_{K1} potassium current is the dominant resting conductance of the myocyte. It keeps the myocyte negatively polarized around −85 mV, until an action potential arrives to activate the cell into phase 0. See **Figure 1.13**.

43. (C) 48% to 68% of patients with truncus have type I, with the main pulmonary artery arising from the left posterolateral aspect of the truncus just above the valve. 29% to 48% of patients have type II, with branch pulmonary arteries arising from the posterior surface of the truncus. 6% to 10%

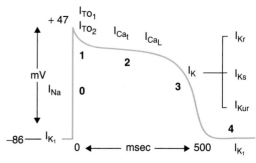

FIGURE 1.13

of patients have type III truncus, with branch pulmonary arteries arising from the lateral sides of the truncus. In type IV truncus, the branch pulmonary arteries arise from descending aorta.

44. (D) The defect is located posterior to the fossa ovalis, in the sinus region of the atrium. This is consistent with a sinus venosus defect.

45. (D) Postoperatively, the pericardium is generally left open so that any blood or serous fluid can drain into a pleural space and then out into a chest tube instead of causing fibrinous buildup within the pericardial space leading to postoperative cardiac tamponade.

46. (A) When an action potential arrives to the cardiac myocyte, the cardiac sodium channels open, resulting in a rapid depolarization of the myocyte (phase 0). Once this primary depolarization has occurred, the sodium channels are inactivated in a time-dependent manner. Potassium and calcium conductance takes over at that point, providing the prolonged phase 1 and 2 depolarization required to achieve muscle contraction. Mutations in the sodium channel gene, *SCN5A*, may cause either type 3 long QT syndrome or Brugada syndrome.

47. (C) This patient is presenting with cyanosis and decreased pulmonary blood flow as evidenced by the lack of vascular markings in the lung fields. Critical pulmonary stenosis can present in this manner. All other options more commonly present with cyanosis and increased pulmonary vascularity.

48. (A) Cardiac fibroblasts are vital for the structural integrity of the heart. They play a large role in remodeling and development. They are responsible for the deposition of the extracellular matrix and also contribute to remodeling through secretion of metalloproteinases. They are also involved in the secretion of cytokines and growth factors which influence neighboring cells. Pericytes are contractile cells that help regulate blood flow in capillaries. Vascular smooth muscle cells are mostly found in medium caliber blood vessels in the heart. Macrophages are scattered throughout the heart. Endothelial cells line the inner wall of the ventricles.

49. (E) The four-chamber view demonstrates Ebstein anomaly, with marked apical displacement of the septal leaflet of the tricuspid valve. The most common additional abnormality seen in patients with Ebstein anomaly is an atrial septal defect, seen in >80% of patients. The next most common associated abnormality is pulmonary stenosis, followed by a ventricular septal defect. The degree of RV outflow obstruction is critical to determine prior to designing treatment plans in the neonate with severe Ebstein anomaly. Functional or true pulmonary atresia may be present in the neonate. Left ventricular noncompaction has been reported in some genetic association studies, but other left-sided lesions are uncommon.

50. (A) The superior vena cava drains deoxygenated blood from the upper body to the right atrium. The inferior vena cava carries blood from the lower body and the placenta. The patent ductus arteriosus carries mixed blood from the pulmonary artery to the descending aorta. The ductus venous carries mixed blood from the hepatic veins to the inferior vena cava. The ascending aortic arch supplies the most oxygen-rich blood to heart and brain. The superior vena cava and coronary sinus have the lowest oxygen saturations of all vascular pathways in the fetus.

51. (E) The left recurrent laryngeal nerve is a branch of the vagus nerve that travels inferiorly around the aortic arch before traveling superiorly to innervate muscles in the larynx. The right recurrent laryngeal nerve takes a similar course but loops around the right subclavian artery. Injury to the left recurrent laryngeal nerve is possible during surgical manipulation of the aortic arch and often results in postoperative hoarseness and stridor.

52. (C) The most common aortic–pulmonary position in patients with double outlet right ventricle (DORV) is the side-by-side configuration (aorta to the right of the pulmonary artery), accounting for around two-thirds of DORV patients. The aorta may arise more anteriorly (right anterior aorta) or posteriorly (right posterior aorta) in some patients or may be leftward and anterior to the pulmonary artery.

53. (C) The right anterior cardinal vein and right common cardinal vein give rise to the right superior vena cava. The left anterior cardinal vein typically regresses but may be persistent as a left superior vena cava. The ductus venosus remnant is termed the ligamentum venosum, and the umbilical vein remnants include the round ligament of the liver.

54. (D) Intercalated discs connect cardiac myocytes and are responsible for maintaining structural integrity and transmission of electric impulses. They are made up of adherens junctions, desmosomes, and gap junctions. Dystrophin and costameres are proteins which connect the myocytes to the extracellular matrix. T-tubules are invaginations of the sarcolemma which allows transmission of the action potential to the inner part of the cell. Myosin is involved in muscle contraction.

55. (D) The vein of Galen malformation is the most common hemodynamically significant extracardiac

arteriovenous malformation in neonates. It affects male infants three times more than female infants. The infants commonly present with high-output cardiac failure soon after birth. A bruit can often be heard through the fontanelles. Other types of cerebral AVMs may also present similarly, but the vein of Galen malformation is the most common.

56. (B) This patient has tetralogy of Fallot; the echo images demonstrate aortic override, the presence of an RV outflow tract with a prominent conus, and a small left-to-right shunting ductus arteriosus. About 5% of patients with tetralogy have an origin of the left anterior descending artery arising from the right coronary artery. This coronary then takes a course anterior to the right ventricular outflow tract. This is an important anomaly to rule out, as the coronary course can prevent the surgeon from using a transannular patch to open the right ventricular outflow tract. 10% to 15% of patients will have an accessory LAD (large conal branch). Other coronary patterns are rare, occurring in less than 5% of patients.

57. (A) Since some patients with congenital heart disease may have absence of the typical left atrial (valve of the fossa ovalis) and right atrial (limbus of the fossa ovalis) characteristics, the next best marker for the right atrium is the ostium of the IVC. The suprahepatic IVC nearly always connects directly to the right atrium. This rule is particularly useful in the evaluation of complex heterotaxy patients. The finger-like atrial appendage and the smooth-surfaced free wall are more common characteristics of the left atrium. Pulmonary vein ostia are a poor predictor of atrial morphology due to the high frequency of anomalous pulmonary venous return in patients with heterotaxy.

58. (E) The infant has tricuspid atresia noted in this four-chamber image. The most common form of tricuspid atresia is type 1, or tricuspid atresia with normally related great arteries. The pulmonary outflow can vary from pulmonary atresia to being widely patent without stenosis. The associated ventricular septal defect is expectedly larger in the presence of a widely patent pulmonary outflow and smaller in patients with pulmonary stenosis. Approximately 70% to 80% of patients with tricuspid atresia have normally related great arteries.

59. (D) About 80% of the calcium that is sequestered during the relaxation phase of the cardiac muscle contraction is done so via Ca^{2+}-ATPase SERCA pumps located on the sarcoplasmic reticulum. The remaining 20% is removed from the cell through Na^+-Ca^{2+} and Ca^{2+}-ATPase pumps located on the sarcolemma.

60. (C) The thebesian valve is a crescent shaped valve that guards the coronary sinus. The tendon of Todaro is a small cord between the IVC and coronary sinus that makes up part of the triangle of Koch. When either the thebesian or eustachian valve is fenestrated, we call this a Chiari network

The eustachian valve is a crescent-shaped small flap of tissue that guards the ostium of the IVC. Rarely, a eustachian valve can be so prominent that it leads to a double chambered right atrium (cor triatriatum dexter).

61. (C) The AV node in tricuspid atresia is on the floor of the blind right atrium. The bundle of His then courses onto the crest of the intraventricular septum (muscular) and runs posterior to the VSD rim. This is important in the eventual repair or palliation of tricuspid atresia, in which care needs to be taken with any surgical procedure involving the VSD for fear of inducing heart block.

62. (D) The right ventricle is typically composed of the inlet, trabecular, and outlet regions (tripartite). There is typically a coarse septal surface, unlike the smooth-walled left ventricular septal wall. There are prominent apical trabeculations. The tricuspid and pulmonary valves are not in continuity in the normal patient, but can be in continuity in patients with tetralogy of Fallot with membranous VSD extension. The crista terminalis is a smooth muscular ridge in the right atrium.

63. (A) A ventricular septal defect occurs in 40% to 45% of patients with d-TGA. The majority of VSDs are of the perimembranous, muscular, or malalignment type. Isolated LV outflow obstruction occurs in ~5% of patients. Coarctation, arch hypoplasia, or interrupted arch occurs in ~5% of patients. Leftward juxtaposition of the atrial appendages occurs in 2% to 5% of d-TGA patients. Around 20% of patients have been shown to have mitral valve abnormalities at autopsy; however, they are rarely functionally significant. Of these, a cleft mitral valve is the most common.

64. (E) In tetralogy of Fallot, when a pulmonary artery is absent, the one affected is most commonly on the *opposite* side of the aortic arch. In contrast, in patients with truncus arteriosus, the absent pulmonary artery is typically on the *same* side of the aortic arch. This is a key distinction between absent pulmonary arteries in these two entities.

65. (B) Most patients (80%) with Ebstein anomaly will also present with an atrial septal defect or patent foramen ovale. Patients with Ebstein and cyanosis often have right-to-left shunting at the atrial level. This cyanosis often will worsen with exercise in older patients.

66. (A) The best and most specific hallmark of the morphologic left atrium is the valve of the fossa ovalis. In contrast, hallmarks of the right atrium include the limbus of the fossa ovalis and the entrance of the inferior vena cava. The left atrium is typically more posterior compared to the right atrium. The left atrial appendage is finger-like and trabeculated, compared to the broad-based appendage of the right atrium.

67. (A) Fetal hemoglobin has a higher affinity for oxygen as compared to adult hemoglobin and is composed of alpha and gamma subunits. Adult hemoglobin meanwhile is composed of alpha and beta subunits. The fetal hemoglobin has to have a higher affinity for oxygen in order for transport of oxygen across the placenta to be achieved. In the normal newborn, fetal hemoglobin is replaced by adult hemoglobin by the age of 3 months.

68. (C) Norepinephrine activates β1 adrenergic receptors by activating the Gs subunit of the G-protein complex which activates adenylate cyclase. This enzyme converts ATP into cAMP, which activates protein kinase A (PKA). PKA phosphorylates are multiple proteins involved in muscle contraction and action potentials of the heart, resulting in increased chronotropy and inotropy.

69. (C) With inspiration, there is a fall in pleural pressure and a rise in intra-abdominal pressure. These changes lead to increased right-sided venous return and increased RV stroke volume. E′ velocity across the tricuspid valve is increased (~5% to 10%), while E′ velocity across the mitral valve is slightly decreased (~5% to 10%).

70. (D) The mitral arcade, or hammock mitral valve, is characterized by absent or abnormal chordal insertions, and the leaflet edges may connect directly to the papillary muscles. The papillary muscles themselves are often small and abnormal. The leaflet edges are often thickened and rolled. Due to this direct insertion of the leaflets, the leaflets are relatively tethered and display poor coaptation. Mitral regurgitation is most common, although functional mitral stenosis can also occur.

71. (C) A primum ASD is located anteriorly to the fossa ovalis in the inlet portion of the septum. Failure of the endocardial cushions to develop is the embryologic basis behind atrioventricular canal defects, including primum ASDs. Anomalous pulmonary venous return occurs when there is failure of the common pulmonary vein to connect to the left atrium. Excessive cell death and resorption of the septum primum, or insufficient growth of the septum secundum, are common etiologies for secundum atrial septal defects.

72. (E) The circular structure seen in this location most commonly represents a dilated coronary sinus (due to a persistent left superior vena cava) which is the remnant of the left horn of the sinus venosus. This can be mistaken for the descending aorta, which should be seen more posteriorly outside the pericardium. The left SVC runs posteriorly along the left atrium before joining the coronary sinus in the left AV groove.

73. (A) In order for the examiner to be able to visualize true cyanosis, there must be at least 5 g/dL of deoxygenated hemoglobin. Thus, in a patient with anemia, a relatively low oxygen saturation may not result in the expected clinical cyanosis. The best indicator of cyanosis is the tongue due to the rich vascular supply and lack of pigmented cells. Rib notching is rare in a 2 year old even in the presence of a significant coarctation of the aorta. Atrial septal defect will rarely cause significant enough right-to-left shunt to produce cyanosis in a 2-year-old patient.

74. (B) Calcium binds to troponin C, changing the tertiary structure of troponin C and other troponin subunits. This allows tropomyosin to shift positions and allows myosin and actin binding, leading to muscle cell contraction.

75. (C) Children living at elevation have been shown to have higher mean pulmonary artery pressures as compared to those living at sea level. This increase in pulmonary pressure is even more exacerbated with exercise. This may have a role in explaining the relatively increased risk of persistence of the patent ductus arteriosus in children living at altitude.

76. (E) Baroreceptors are found in each carotid sinus and aortic arch. These receptors respond to stretch of the arterial walls and send impulses to the brain. This stimulation results in a decreased blood pressure by a decrease in heart rate and vasodilation.

77. (D) Due to high baseline oxygen extraction levels by the myocardium, the coronary oxygen tension is low (about 20 to 25 mm Hg). Increase in oxygen demand is fulfilled by increasing coronary blood flow, and not necessarily by changes in oxygen extraction.

78. (B) The aorta and pulmonary artery are often located in an anterior–posterior position to each other, causing the narrow mediastinum and "egg-on-a-string" image seen on some chest x-rays. Due to the anterior aorta, the second heart sound is often single and loud.

79. (D) Pulmonic stenosis is the most commonly associated cardiac lesion and is seen in roughly 50% of patients with double outlet right ventricle. Atrial septal defects are the next most common; 25% of patients have a secundum defect, while up to 8% may have a primum defect. Subaortic stenosis and right aortic arch may also be seen in these patients, but they are much less common.

80. (B) The fifth aortic arch is typically rudimentary and does not usually develop into any known vessels in the normal neonate. It is not even present in many embryo specimens. Rare cases have been reported of persistence of the fifth arch, which can either be asymptomatic or be associated with other cardiac findings. If the fifth arch persists but there is interruption of the normal fourth arch, the patient may present with a clinical picture of coarctation.

81. (C) At end systole, LV ejection is complete, and the aortic valve closes. This begins the period of isovolumic relaxation, with a subsequent drop in LV pressure. At the end of this period, the mitral valve opens, allowing filling of the ventricle due to lower pressures in the ventricle.

82. (C) The tricuspid valve annulus attaches to the septum slightly lower than the mitral annulus, resulting in a portion of the septum known as the atrioventricular septum. This septum is the location of the triangle of Koch, where the AV node is located. This area is bordered by the tendon of Todaro, the attachment of the septal leaflet of the tricuspid valve, and the ostium of the coronary sinus.

83. (B) Supracardiac total anomalous pulmonary venous connection is the most common type (46%) of TAPVC. The pulmonary veins form a confluence posterior to the left atrium and blood is directed through a venous channel to the left cardinal system. The most common anatomical site is the left innominate vein. Other forms of TAPVC include infracardiac (23%), cardiac (20%), and mixed (11%).

84. (D) The patient has an acute metabolic alkalosis, as evidenced by the elevated pH, relatively normal pCO_2, and high bicarbonate. Causes of metabolic alkalosis can include vomiting, hypokalemia, the use of alkalotic medicines such as bicarbonate, hyperaldosteronism, and rare causes such as Bartter syndrome.

85. (A) While the anterolateral papillary muscle typically has a dual blood supply from the left anterior descending and circumflex coronary arteries, the posteromedial papillary muscle is typically solely supplied by the right coronary artery. The inferior wall of the left ventricle is also typically supplied by the right coronary artery.

86. (A) In 90% of the general population, the AV nodal artery arises from the right coronary artery and supplies the AV node. In the 10% of the general population, the left circumflex artery is dominant, and it supplies the AV nodal artery.

87. (D) Anomalous origin of left circumflex coronary artery from the right main coronary artery is the most common anomaly in patients with no evidence of other congenital heart disease and makes up approximately one-third of major coronary artery anomalies. Anomalous origin of right coronary artery from the left sinus of Valsalva is a close second at just under 30%. Single coronary arteries make up somewhere between 5% and 20% of coronary anomalies. Anomalous origin of the left or right coronary artery from the posterior sinus of Valsalva is a rare finding.

88. (C) The most common abnormality of the aortic arch is an anomalous right subclavian artery from a left aortic arch. This occurs in approximately 0.5% of the general population and is usually asymptomatic. The diagnosis is often made at autopsy or during imaging for another condition. It is seen commonly in patients with Down syndrome who have congenital heart disease (>30%).

89. (C) Uhl anomaly is a rare disorder characterized by partial or complete absence of the right ventricular myocardium with epicardium and pericardium opposed to each other. Valvular morphology is often normal as opposed to Ebstein anomaly. The normal tricuspid valve on echocardiography rules out tricuspid atresia. Arrhythmogenic right ventricular dysplasia is characterized by fatty infiltration and replacement of the right ventricular myocardium and arrhythmias or even sudden cardiac death. Pulmonary stenosis would result in hypertrophy of the right ventricle.

90. (A) The normally low blood and alveolar oxygen tension is most associated with the high pulmonary vascular resistance in the fetus. The fetus also produces vasoconstrictive substances such as thromboxane and leukotrienes, but these do not appear to have as significant of an effect.

91. (D) The common pulmonary vein is the initial connection between the pulmonary venous plexus and the heart.

The vein typically has four (or more) primary feeding veins, which eventually become the left and right upper and lower pulmonary veins. The common pulmonary vein is eventually incorporated into the back wall of the left atrium, with the atrium eventually appearing such that the individual pulmonary veins connect independently to the atrium.

92. (C) Phase 2 (the plateau phase) is characterized by influx of Ca^{2+} into the cell through L-type Ca^{2+} channels. Phase 0 is the rapid depolarization phase due to Na^+ entry. Phase 1 involves early repolarization with K^+ efflux from the cell. Phase 3 is the repolarization phase and is dominated by K^+ efflux from the cell. Phase 4 is the return of the resting membrane potential and is maintained by Na^+/K^+-ATPase channels. See **Figure 1.14**.

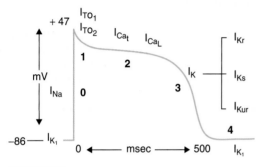

FIGURE 1.14

93. (D) Hypercyanotic ("tet") spells consist of abrupt onset of cyanosis, hypoxemia, dyspnea, and agitation. Events usually occur after the age of 2 months. Crying and agitation lead to increased pulmonary vascular resistance, with increased right-to-left shunting and decreased pulmonary blood flow. Infundibular spasm may also be involved in the limitation of RV outflow to the pulmonary arteries. In the modern era, the presence of hypercyanotic spells is widely considered an indication to proceed to surgical repair of the underlying tetralogy of Fallot.

94. (A) Myocardial oxygen consumption is determined by wall tension which is related to intraventricular pressure and radius. Therefore, decreasing end diastolic volume decreases both the pressure and radius of the ventricle. Increased cardiac contractility increases the work that the ventricle is doing, thereby increasing the wall tension. Increased heart rate results in increased oxygen consumption over time due to an increase in the frequency of generating the pressure needed to overcome aortic pressure in left ventricular contraction. Sympathetic activation results in increased heart rate and contraction.

95. (C) The patient has an acute metabolic acidosis, as evidenced by the low pH, relatively normal pCO_2, and low bicarbonate.

96. (D) The patient has an acute respiratory acidosis, as evidenced by the low pH, elevated pCO_2, and normal bicarbonate. After the acute period of a respiratory acidosis, the bicarbonate will typically begin to increase to compensate and bring the pH closer to normal values.

97. (A) The right pulmonary artery travels anterior to the right upper lobe bronchus, while the left pulmonary artery travels posterior to the left upper lobe bronchus. Answer (**B**) may occur in patients with sinus inversus and mirror-image morphology. The branches may both travel anterior to their respective upper lobe bronchi in patients with bilateral morphologic right lungs, while they may both travel posterior to their respective upper lobe bronchi in patients with bilateral morphologic left lungs.

Congenital Cardiac Malformations

M. Eric Ferguson and Benjamin W. Eidem

Questions

1. A 4-month-old girl is referred to you because of a cardiac murmur. She appears jaundiced. She has a grade 2 to 3/6 systolic ejection murmur along the left upper sternal border that radiates to the back bilaterally. She has prominent facial features including a broad forehead and pointed chin. Her mother has similar features. A defect in which of the following genes would most likely explain her clinical findings?

   A. *NOTCH1*
   B. *PTPN11*
   C. *TBX1*
   D. *JAG1*
   E. *GATA*

2. A 28-year-old woman develops severe rubella infection late in the second month of pregnancy. The fetus is at increased risk for which congenital heart defect?

   A. Complex heterotaxy
   B. Ebstein anomaly
   C. Coarctation of the aorta
   D. d-Transposition of the great arteries (d-TGA)
   E. Valvar and supravalvar pulmonary stenosis

3. A 31-year-old primigravid woman drinks three cups of coffee daily. She is otherwise healthy. The fetus is at increased risk for which congenital heart defect?

   A. Tetralogy of Fallot (TOF)
   B. Tricuspid atresia
   C. Patent foramen ovale
   D. Secundum atrial septal defect
   E. No increased risk of cardiac defects

4. Which of the following defects is most likely to occur in a newborn whose mother had phenylketonuria?

   A. Ebstein anomaly
   B. Tricuspid atresia
   C. Coarctation of the aorta
   D. Anomalous pulmonary venous return
   E. Right aortic arch

5. You are asked to evaluate a 2-year-old boy for a cardiac murmur. You note that the child, for a 2 year old, is quite friendly and has stellate irises, a long philtrum, depressed nasal bridge, prominent lower lip, and enamel hypoplasia. There is a grade 3/6 systolic ejection murmur and no click. Which of the following chromosomal deletions is most likely in this patient?

   A. 18q
   B. 22p
   C. 8p23
   D. 7q11.23
   E. 22q11

6. A 4-month-old boy develops tachypnea and poor feeding. On examination, the blood pressure in the right arm is 110/60 mm Hg, in the left arm 105/60 mm Hg, and in the right leg 108/60 mm Hg. An echocardiogram demonstrates increased left ventricular (LV) wall thickness, moderate supravalvar aortic stenosis with estimated mean outflow gradient of 44 mm Hg, and mild supravalvar pulmonary stenosis. The aortic and pulmonary valves appear normal. The estimated LV ejection fraction (EF) is 20% with evidence of inferior wall hypokinesis. Which of the following is the most likely diagnosis in this patient?

   A. Velocardiofacial syndrome
   B. Down syndrome
   C. Williams syndrome
   D. Rheumatic heart disease
   E. Coarctation of the aorta

7. You are consulted to assess a small-for-gestational-age newborn with a heart murmur. Dysmorphic features include microcephaly, microphthalmia, short palpebral fissures, micrognathia, a prominent occiput, short sternum, and small nipples. The hands are clenched with overlapping fingers, and the feet have a convex shape. Which of the following statements is correct regarding this clinical scenario?

A. Trisomy 13 is the most likely clinical diagnosis
B. Associated congenital heart disease (CHD) occurs in ~50% of patients
C. Ventricular septal defect (VSD) and polyvalvular dysplasia are the most common CHD in this disorder
D. Most patients survive well into the second decade of life without surgery
E. If corrective cardiac surgery is performed successfully, the risk of death is decreased 10-fold

8. An infant presents in the newborn nursery with feeding difficulty and is noted to have cleft palate, hypocalcemia, and lymphopenia. FISH testing is positive for a 22q11 deletion. Among the following, what is his echocardiogram most likely to demonstrate?

A. Ebstein anomaly of the tricuspid valve
B. Pulmonary atresia + intact ventricular septum (IVS)
C. Interruption of aortic arch between the left common carotid and left subclavian arteries
D. Left ventricular diverticulum
E. Double-outlet right atrium

9. You are seeing a female patient for a chief complaint of dyspnea with exertion. You note in her medical chart that she has a history of a large secundum atrial septal defect (ASD) that apparently went unrepaired. She last saw a physician at age 10 years, where the defect was noted to be 18 mm by echocardiography. The patient is now 31 years old. She has not had any cardiovascular interventions in the interim. You listen and fail to appreciate a widely split S_2. In fact, you think the split is narrow and P2 is loud. There is a very short systolic murmur over the left upper sternal border (LUSB). There is no diastolic murmur. What is the most likely cause of the physical findings?

A. Spontaneous closure of the defect
B. Severe mitral valve regurgitation
C. Nonsustained ventricular tachycardia
D. Left ventricular diastolic dysfunction
E. Significant pulmonary hypertension

10. A 19-year-old male patient is found by echocardiogram to have a large sinus venosus defect with partial anomalous pulmonary venous connection with drainage of the right upper and middle pulmonary veins to the superior vena cava. The right ventricle appears severely dilated with moderately decreased function. The ventricular septum appears flattened throughout the cardiac cycle. The tricuspid valve does not leak. There is trace pulmonary insufficiency. What is your recommendation to the patient?

A. Dismiss from follow-up as there is nothing to be done
B. Begin propranolol immediately
C. Start IV epoprostenol
D. Cardiac catheterization with pulmonary vascular reactivity testing
E. Counsel that there is little to do at this point, as he is past the point of medical benefit

11. In a patient with typical auscultatory findings of an atrial septal defect (ASD) and a P-wave axis of <30 degrees on the electrocardiogram, one should think immediately of which of the following types of atrial septal defect?

A. Unroofed coronary sinus
B. Sinus venosus
C. Secundum
D. Primum
E. Patent foramen ovale

12. Which of the following papillary muscle arrangements are seen most commonly with complete atrioventricular canal (septal) defect (AVCD, or AVSD)?

A. The papillary muscles are closer together, the anterior muscle is closer to the septum than normal, and the posterior muscle is farther from the septum than normal
B. The papillary muscles are closer together, the anterior muscle is farther from the septum than normal, and the posterior muscle is closer to the septum than normal
C. The papillary muscles are closer together and positioned clockwise from their normal location
D. The papillary muscles are farther apart, the anterior muscle is closer to the septum than normal, and the posterior muscle is farther from the septum than normal
E. The papillary muscles are farther apart, the anterior muscle is farther from the septum than normal, and the posterior muscle is closer to the septum than normal

13. A 17-year-old male who underwent complete repair of a partial atrioventricular septal defect (AVSD) at 15 months of age presents with progressive shortness of breath. He has a grade 3/6 holosystolic murmur that is loudest over the apex and is less prominent with Valsalva maneuver. Chest x-ray reveals mild cardiomegaly and mildly increased pulmonary vascularity. Which of the following is the most likely cause of these symptoms?

    A. Mitral regurgitation
    B. Primary pulmonary hypertension
    C. Left ventricular outflow tract obstruction
    D. Mitral stenosis
    E. Pulmonary valve stenosis

14. Which of the following is true regarding left ventricular outflow tract (LVOT) obstruction in patients with AVSD?

    A. Obstruction may be due to displacement of the left atrioventricular (AV) valve annulus, resulting in shortening and narrowing of the LVOT
    B. Nearly 30% of patients with AVSD will require reoperation for LVOT obstruction
    C. Progressive LVOT obstruction is more common in patients with two atrioventricular (AV) valve orifices
    D. Preoperative LVOT obstruction is often progressive, while postoperative obstruction is frequently static
    E. LVOT obstruction is the most common indication for reoperation after partial AVSD repair

15. An 18-month-old boy undergoes operative repair of a moderate-sized ASD and moderate-sized mid-muscular ventricular septal defect (VSD). His preoperative chest x-ray revealed borderline cardiomegaly and an ECG at the same time was normal. He remains intubated on post-op day 2, at which time you note a new finding of a widely split S_2 with no murmur. Which of the following is the most likely reason for your findings?

    A. Residual ASD
    B. Residual VSD
    C. Postoperative decrease in pulmonary artery pressure
    D. Right bundle branch block
    E. Mechanical ventilation

16. Which of the following statements is true regarding VSD?

    A. Flow across a large (unrestrictive) VSD is limited primarily by the size of the defect
    B. Frequently, supracristal defects are partially or completely occluded by redundant tricuspid valve tissue
    C. Prominent S_2 splitting is occasionally heard with a small VSD
    D. After VSD repair, the LV mass decreases more prominently than left ventricular end-diastolic volume (LVEDV)
    E. Patients who develop Eisenmenger physiology typically first manifest cyanosis between ages 4 and 6 years

17. You are seeing a 19-year-old female who was diagnosed at age 6 months with a moderate-sized, isolated perimembranous VSD with outlet extension. The patient was then lost to cardiology follow-up. The patient presents for evaluation of a murmur that was noted during her required physical for her new job. She is asymptomatic and plays golf 2 to 3 times per week. On examination, she is acyanotic. There is a grade 2/6 systolic murmur over right upper sternal border and a grade 3/4 high-pitched decrescendo diastolic murmur at the left sternal border. What is the most likely explanation for the murmur?

    A. Prolapse of the left aortic cusp has closed the VSD, and the aortic valve is insufficient
    B. Prolapse of the right aortic cusp has closed the VSD, and the aortic valve is insufficient
    C. Prolapse of the septal leaflet of the tricuspid valve has closed the VSD, and the tricuspid valve is insufficient
    D. Right and left ventricular pressures have equalized, and new pulmonary insufficiency has developed
    E. Left atrial (LA) and LV volumes have increased secondary to unrestricted left-to-right shunting with secondary mitral valve insufficiency

18. What is the relationship of the bundle of His to an inlet VSD?

    A. The bundle passes posterior-inferiorly to the defect
    B. The bundle passes anterior-superiorly to the defect
    C. The bundle courses caudally around the defect
    D. The bundle courses through the right AV groove
    E. The bundle passes laterally to the defect through the left ventricle

19. A 28-week preemie develops persistent abdominal distention, increasing residuals before feedings, blood in the stools, and decreasing bowel sounds. Abdominal x-ray reveals evidence of intramural air in the right lower quadrant. The patient has bounding pulses, and an echocardiogram confirms the presence of a hemodynamically significant patent ductus arteriosus (PDA). What is the best next step in management?

    A. Referral to surgery for immediate surgical closure
    B. Percutaneous closure of PDA with occluding coil
    C. Trial of indomethacin
    D. Trial of ibuprofen
    E. Do nothing

20. You see an 8-year-old child who presents for evaluation of a cardiac murmur. As an infant, he had poor feeding, irritability, and tachypnea. Weight gain was slow. The symptoms gradually resolved after age 3 to 4 months, and he has grown steadily along the third percentile since then. He tires more easily than his peers. He has progressive myalgias, arthralgias, headache, and general malaise. Fever is relapsing and low grade, and his parents report marked diminution in appetite.

On examination, peripheral pulses are full and bounding. The precordium is hyperdynamic, and there is a thrusting apical impulse. A systolic thrill is palpable at the upper left sternal border. S_1 and S_2 are difficult to hear because they are masked by a loud continuous murmur. The murmur is intense and is heard throughout the precordium as well as posteriorly. It has a harsh quality with low-frequency components, and eddy sounds that vary from beat to beat give it a machinery quality. A third heart sound is heard at the apex. Blood cultures are positive for *Streptococcus viridans*. His CXR is shown in **Figure 2.1**.

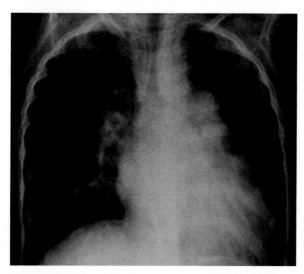

FIGURE 2.1

Which of the following statements is most likely to be true in this clinical setting?

A. Vegetation is likely, and it will be seen on the pulmonary arterial (PA) end of the ductus arteriosus
B. Vegetation is likely, and it will be seen on the aortic end of the ductus
C. *Streptococcus viridans* is very unlikely to cause endocarditis in this setting
D. Abscess is much more common than vegetation in this setting
E. Vegetation is unlikely but, if present, would be seen on the aortic end of the ductus

21. Which of the following events is most responsible for early, functional closure of the ductus arteriosus?

A. Hemorrhage and necrosis in the subintimal region
B. Medial smooth muscle cell migration in the wall of the ductus
C. Equalization of pulmonary and systemic vascular resistance
D. Infolding of the endothelium
E. Thinning of the intimal layer

22. What is the theoretical benefit of ibuprofen over indomethacin for closure of PDA in premature infants?

A. Decreased risk of intraventricular hemorrhage
B. Decreased risk of pulmonary hypertension
C. Decreased risk of gastrointestinal bleeding
D. Greater rate of ductal closure
E. Less effect on cerebral blood flow

23. A 2-week-old infant is found to have anomalous left coronary artery from the pulmonary artery (ALCAPA). Surgical correction is planned. What preoperative comorbidity has been found to be a risk factor for mortality and for late reoperation?

A. Mitral insufficiency
B. Tricuspid insufficiency
C. Aortic valve insufficiency
D. Pulmonary valve insufficiency
E. Patent foramen ovale

24. You examine a 17-year-old male with a 2-year history of progressive dyspnea on exertion and 2 months of orthopnea. Vital signs: pulse 80 beats per minute, BP 118/44 mm Hg, respiratory rate 24 breaths per minute. Physical examination reveals a lift along the left sternal border and a continuous murmur with maximal intensity in the third to fourth intercostal space near the right sternal edge. On the basis of the available information, of the following diagnoses, which is most likely?

A. Sinus of Valsalva fistula from the aorta to the right atrium
B. Sinus of Valsalva fistula from the aorta to the left atrium
C. Anomalous left coronary artery from the pulmonary artery
D. Patent ductus arteriosus
E. Severe isolated aortic regurgitation

25. A 3-week-old infant has had several episodes of acute onset of agitation and crying. During these episodes, the baby is inconsolable. On examination, there is a high-frequency systolic murmur audible at the apex with radiation to the left axilla. Which of the following coronary artery anomalies most likely would be responsible for these symptoms?

A. Anomalous origin of right coronary artery from left sinus of Valsalva
B. Anomalous origin of left main coronary artery from right sinus of Valsalva
C. Anomalous origin of left coronary artery from the pulmonary artery
D. Anomalous origin of left anterior descending artery from the right main coronary artery
E. Origin of left circumflex coronary artery from the right main coronary artery

26. Which of the following is true regarding aneurysms of the sinus of Valsalva?

A. The most common location is the noncoronary sinus
B. There is no gender predilection for aneurysm formation
C. Concomitant VSD is seen up to 50% of the time
D. The most common site of rupture is into the left atrium
E. Most VSDs seen with coronary sinus aneurysms are paramembranous

27. A neonate presents at birth with high-output cardiac failure secondary to a cerebral arteriovenous malformation (AVM). If left untreated, what is the approximate risk of mortality during the first week of life?

A. 3%
B. 15%
C. 30%
D. 50%
E. 90%

28. Which of the following is true regarding pulmonary AVM?

A. Pulmonary AVM in the setting of hereditary hemorrhagic telangiectasia (HHT) tends to shrink as the patient grows older
B. In patients with pulmonary AVM, cardiac output typically is twice that of normal
C. If there are multiple pulmonary AVMs, there is a >80% chance of the patient having HHT
D. Patients with pulmonary AVMs typically are hemodynamically unstable and require significant respiratory support in infancy
E. Most pulmonary AVMs in children are acquired

29. Which of the following statements is correct regarding transcatheter embolization of pulmonary AVM?

A. To avoid device embolization, liquid adhesive is more effective than coil device closure
B. Embolization effectively prevents strokes and transient ischemic attacks, but not brain abscesses
C. Embolization effectively prevents brain abscess but does not prevent strokes
D. Greatest success is achieved by decreasing systemic arterial oxygen tension to <50 mm Hg
E. Embolization provides persistent relief of desaturation but not of orthodeoxia

30. Which of the following measurements has the best potential to distinguish a large AVM from a large PDA in a young infant?

A. Pulse pressure as determined by sphygmomanometry
B. Cardiothoracic ratio on plain chest x-ray
C. Systemic vein oxygen saturation measurements obtained during cardiac catheterization
D. QRS axis on electrocardiogram
E. Liver span by physical examination

31. An 11-year-old boy is evaluated for swallowing difficulty and moderate exercise intolerance. A barium esophagram shows evidence of anterior indentation, and pulmonary function testing shows evidence of obstruction. What is the most likely diagnosis?

A. Retroesophageal left subclavian artery
B. Pulmonary artery sling
C. Tracheoesophageal fistula
D. Innominate artery compression of the trachea
E. Retroesophageal fistula of Phillips

32. A CT scan is done to assess a neck mass in a 3-year-old patient with a history of murmur but no prior cardiac history. This patient has no trouble swallowing and has no history of respiratory problems. The scan incidentally showed a right aortic arch with mirror-image branching. What additional action is warranted?

A. Barium swallow
B. Echocardiography
C. Bronchoscopy
D. Surgical referral
E. No further action needed

33. Which of the following typically results in a vascular ring?

A. Right aortic arch with retroesophageal innominate artery, left patent ductus arteriosus

B. Right aortic arch, retroesophageal left subclavian artery, no patent ductus arteriosus

C. Right aortic arch with mirror-image branching, right ligamentum arteriosus

D. Left aortic arch with cervical origin of right subclavian artery

E. Left aortic arch with retroesophageal right subclavian artery

34. An infant presents with acute cardiovascular collapse on day 3 of life. Physical examination reveals absence of all limb pulses with strong carotid pulses bilaterally. Echocardiography is most likely to reveal which of the following?

A. Critical aortic stenosis

B. Interruption of the aortic arch, type A, with anomalous subclavian artery

C. Interruption of the aortic arch, type B

D. Interruption of the aortic arch type B with anomalous subclavian artery

E. Right aortic arch with retroesophageal diverticulum of Kommerell

35. A 5-month-old girl presents with stridor and wheezing since birth. She has been treated with albuterol and inhaled steroids without any improvement. Her parents have noticed that she has been coughing and gagging since starting baby foods 2 weeks prior. Which of the following diagnoses is most likely?

A. Right aortic arch with retroesophageal diverticulum of Kommerell

B. Left aortic arch with retroesophageal diverticulum of Kommerell

C. Right aortic arch with mirror-image branching

D. Left aortic arch with retroesophageal right subclavian artery

E. Right aortic arch with retroesophageal innominate artery

36. Which of the following statements is true regarding anomalies of pulmonary venous return?

A. An untreated infant born with total anomalous pulmonary venous connection (TAPVC) has a 50% chance of surviving until the age of 1 year

B. The cardiothymic silhouette tends to be shifted leftward in Scimitar syndrome

C. Patients with cor triatriatum have enlargement of the right atrium and right ventricle

D. Normal P-wave size (<2.5 mm) on ECG effectively rules out cor triatriatum

E. Ventricular arrhythmias are common following TAPVC repair

37. A 3-year-old asymptomatic boy has a 2/6 systolic ejection murmur at the left upper sternal border and fixed splitting of S_2. An echocardiogram reveals a sinus venosus ASD. This defect results from which of the following?

A. Deficiency of septum primum

B. Deficiency of septum secundum

C. Excessive resorption of septum primum

D. Anomalous insertion of the superior pulmonary vein

E. Deficiency of the common wall of the superior vena cava and the pulmonary vein

38. What is the catheter course in **Figure 2.2**?

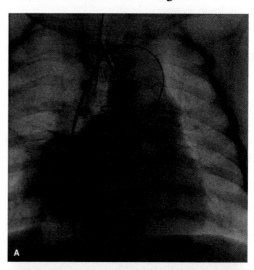

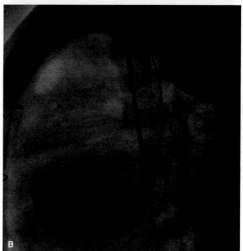

FIGURE 2.2

A. Aorta → right aortic arch → innominate artery → BT shunt → RPA

B. Aorta → right aortic arch → right sinus of Valsalva

C. Scimitar vein → right SVC → innominate vein → left SVC → coronary sinus

D. IVC → right atrium → SVC → innominate vein → left SVC → coronary sinus

E. IVC → right atrium → SVC → innominate vein → vertical vein → anomalous pulmonary venous confluence

39. A newborn is diagnosed with infradiaphragmatic TAPVC to the portal vein. Echocardiography demonstrates high-velocity, continuous, nonphasic venous flow in the anomalous vein. PGE1 has been started. The cardiorespiratory and metabolic states have been optimized. What is the best immediate plan of action?

    A. Supportive therapy for 24 to 48 hours to allow PA pressures to fall before operation
    B. Bedside balloon atrial septostomy
    C. Cardiac catheterization to determine pulmonary vascular resistance (PVR) and to perform blade atrial septostomy if needed
    D. Balloon dilation +/− stent placement in anomalous pulmonary vein
    E. Immediate corrective surgery

40. A 19-year-old female presents with a several-month history of worsening breathlessness. Past medical history is significant for five episodes of pneumonia over her lifetime. Chronic medications include inhaled fluticasone, budesonide, and montelukast. She carries a rescue inhaler of albuterol. Physical examination reveals an RV heave, loud P2, and pulmonary systolic ejection click. There is a soft, blowing systolic murmur along the left sternal border. Echocardiography reveals the following (**Figure 2.3**):

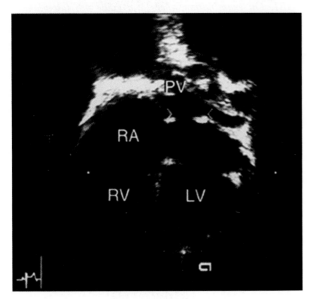

FIGURE 2.3

    What is the most correct statement about this condition?
    A. Surgical correction is universally futile
    B. Medical management offers a better chance of 20-year survival than operative correction
    C. Perioperative risk is low
    D. In patients who survive operative correction, prognosis is excellent
    E. Atrial fibrillation is common

41. Which of the following statements is correct regarding anomalous drainage of the left pulmonary veins to the left innominate vein (LIV)?

    A. The left lung drains typically by a left SVC
    B. A primum ASD is common
    C. The vertical vein represents a persistent embryologic connection between the splanchnic plexus of the lung buds and the cardinal veins
    D. This is a normal variant and found in 0.5% of the general population
    E. This condition has never been described

42. A 3-year-old child has complex single ventricle, bilateral superior vena cavae, and interrupted IVC with azygous continuation to the right SVC. At operation, he has construction of bilateral bidirectional superior vena caval–pulmonary anastomoses. Two months postoperatively his systemic arterial blood oxygen saturation is 87%, and he is doing well. Six months postoperatively his saturation is 82%, and he is doing well. Two years postoperatively his saturation is 75%, and he is a bit more fatigued. Which of the following factors, unique to the operation he had, contributes the most to his progressive desaturation?

    A. Increased coronary sinus drainage
    B. Increased pulmonary arteriolar resistance
    C. Erythrocytosis
    D. Pulmonary arteriovenous fistulae
    E. Decreased chest wall compliance

43. An 8-year-old girl with palpitations has an echocardiogram that demonstrates an outpouching originating in the coronary sinus that has a distinct neck and extends behind the LV. What is the most likely source of her palpitations?

    A. RVOT-origin ventricular tachycardia
    B. Accessory pathway-mediated SVT
    C. AV nodal reentry tachycardia
    D. Torsades de pointes
    E. Brugada syndrome

44. A 14-day-old infant presents with irritability. He has been eating poorly due to tachypnea (RR = 80s) and he is 15% below his birthweight of 3,216 g. Physical examination reveals tachypnea and a loud systolic murmur over his entire precordium. There is a soft low-pitched diastolic murmur at the apex. Distal pulses are slightly diminished. An ABG demonstrates pH = 7.27, pCO_2 = 31, HCO_3 = 16 on room air. Echocardiogram reveals tricuspid atresia, d-TGA, and a moderately restrictive VSD. His aortic arch is moderately hypoplastic, although there is no evidence of a definite posterior shelf at the isthmus. Of the following procedures, what is the best initial surgical palliation option?

A. Modified Blalock–Taussig (BT) shunt only

B. PA banding only

C. Bidirectional cavopulmonary anastomosis

D. Anastomosis between main pulmonary artery (MPA) and ascending aorta (Damus–Kaye–Stansel [DKS]) with aortic arch augmentation and BT shunt

E. VSD closure + patch enlargement of LVOT (modified Konno)

45. Which of the following features are more specific for Uhl anomaly than Ebstein anomaly?

A. The presence of significant cyanosis on physical examination

B. Large P waves and diminished right ventricular voltages on ECG

C. Thin appearing, dysfunctional RV myocardium on echocardiography

D. Similar pressure wave contours in the RA and RV during cardiac catheterization

E. Ventricular endocardial potentials recorded past the expected anatomic tricuspid valve annulus during electrophysiologic assessment

46. An 11-year-old boy with a history of pulmonary stenosis presents for evaluation. His blood pressure at rest is 100/70 mm Hg. Echocardiography reveals normal inspiratory collapse of his IVC. The following Doppler-derived velocities are obtained (at rest):

Tricuspid regurgitation (CW) = 3.5 m/s

Infundibulum (PW) = 2 m/s

RVOT (CW) = 4 m/s

Assume RA pressure is 6 mm Hg. Using traditionally accepted Doppler-derived criteria to determine severity, what degree of pulmonary stenosis is present in this patient?

A. Trivial

B. Mild

C. Moderate

D. Severe

E. Not enough information provided

The following clinical scenario pertains to Questions 47 and 48:

A 1-day-old term newborn is admitted to the NICU with cyanosis and a murmur. He is diagnosed with critical pulmonary stenosis and a moderate-sized PDA. Percutaneous pulmonary valvotomy is performed. Cardiac hemodynamics obtained during the catheterization are shown in **Table 2.1.**

TABLE 2.1 Cardiac Hemodynamics Obtained During Catheterization

	Pre-Valvotomy	Post-Valvotomy
RA (mean)	10	9
RV (systolic/EDP)	100/11	72/10
MPA	35/18	37/20
RPCW (mean)	Not done	7
Systemic BP	51/21	53/25

RA, right atrial; RV, right ventricular; EDP, end-diastolic pressure; MPA, main pulmonary artery; RPCW, right pulmonary capillary wedge pressure.

That night, the baby continues to have low oxygen saturations in the mid-80s despite being mechanically ventilated and on PGE1. On examination, there is a grade 4/6 late-peaking harsh systolic murmur at the left upper sternal border, which is increased in intensity from his admission exam, and a new, soft diastolic murmur. Blood pressure is 52/24 mm Hg. Blood gas reveals a base deficit of −2.

47. Which of the following would be the next best step?

A. Urgent repeat percutaneous valvotomy

B. Urgent open pulmonary valvotomy

C. STAT echocardiogram

D. Increase the PGE dosage

E. Continued close observation

48. Which of the following is the most likely underlying cause of his desaturation?

A. Pulmonary vein stenosis

B. Infundibular RVOT obstruction

C. Right-to-left shunting across the PDA

D. Undiagnosed VSD

E. Severe pulmonary regurgitation

49. You are performing an echocardiogram on an asymptomatic 4-month-old girl referred for a cardiac murmur. You note discrete stenosis of the proximal LPA, measuring 2 mm. The distal LPA is 6 mm. The RPA is 8 mm. The pulmonary valve and MPA are normal. There is no ASD or VSD. Peak Doppler velocity across the LPA stenosis is 2.0 m/s. Right ventricular systolic pressure (RVSP) is estimated to be 25 mm Hg. There is mild RV hypertrophy. Which of the following statements is true?

    A. The degree of LPA stenosis is mild
    B. RVSP is likely underestimated considering the degree of LPA narrowing
    C. Invasive pressure measurements would be likely to show an MPA-to-LPA gradient that is much higher than that estimated by Doppler flow velocity.
    D. If angioplasty is performed, a 6- to 8-mm balloon should be used
    E. The risk of restenosis after angioplasty is approximately 3% to 5%

50. A newborn infant is cyanotic, and echocardiography reveals pulmonary atresia with intact ventricular septum. The right ventricle is bipartite and quite small. The baby is receiving PGE1. Which of the following is the next step in the management of this patient?

    A. Balloon atrial septostomy
    B. Surgical outflow tract reconstruction
    C. Cardiac catheterization and angiography
    D. Cardiac CT scan
    E. Cardiac MRI

51. Which of the following anatomical substrates most likely predicts a successful decompression of the RV using radiofrequency ablation and balloon pulmonary valvotomy in patients with pulmonary atresia with intact ventricular septum?

    A. Unipartite RV
    B. Muscular pulmonary atresia
    C. RV-dependent coronary circulation
    D. Severe tricuspid stenosis
    E. Tricuspid valve Z-score = −2

52. The angiogram demonstrated in **Figure 2.4** is performed in a 9-month-old boy with pulmonary atresia and intact ventricular septum.

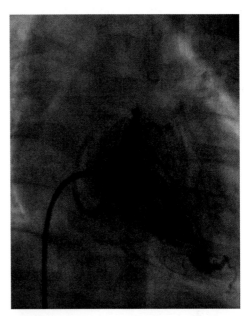

FIGURE 2.4

Which of the following operations is best for this patient?

    A. Bidirectional Glenn alone
    B. RV–PA conduit with a bidirectional Glenn
    C. RV–PA conduit alone
    D. Pulmonary valvotomy alone
    E. Pulmonary valvotomy with a bidirectional Glenn

53. For the above patient, a takedown of his BT shunt is performed along with the placement of an RV–PA conduit. That evening he develops congestive heart failure (CHF). Which of the following ECG findings would you most likely see in this patient at this time?

    A. Complete heart block
    B. Left bundle branch block
    C. ST-segment elevation in I, aVL
    D. ST-segment elevation in II, III, aVF
    E. Increased voltages in V1, V2, V3

54. You are seeing a 4-day-old infant with cyanosis. Echocardiography reveals pulmonary atresia with intact ventricular septum. There is significant subpulmonary (infundibular) obstruction. The RV appears tripartite but severely hypoplastic. By echocardiography, there is no evidence of RV-dependent coronary circulation. You are planning an eventual biventricular repair beginning with a surgical pulmonary valvuloplasty and RVOT patch enlargement. What is the best next step in surgical planning?

    A. Go to surgery without further testing
    B. Cardiac catheterization with hemodynamic study only
    C. Catheterization with hemodynamic assessment and RV angiography
    D. MRI with RV volume quantification
    E. Biopsy of RV myocardium to evaluate for spongy myocardium and/or endocardial sclerosis

55. A newborn is found to have cyanosis shortly after birth. A holosystolic murmur is heard and PGE1 is started. An echocardiogram is performed (**Figure 2.5**):

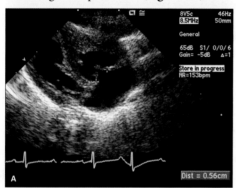

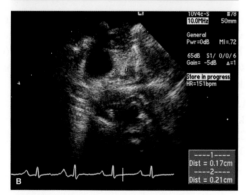

FIGURE 2.5

Color flow Doppler fails to show antegrade flow in the MPA. The ventricular septum is intact. Which of the following is true regarding neonates with this form of congenital heart disease?

    A. Coronary artery perfusion is wholly RV dependent in about 45% of cases
    B. Pulmonary blood flow most often is supplied by aortopulmonary collaterals
    C. This form of congenital heart disease is more common in males
    D. By definition, the right ventricle is always bipartite
    E. A main pulmonary trunk almost always is present

56. A 3-year-old boy has pulmonary atresia with VSD. He has a history of hypoplastic central pulmonary arteries and multiple major aortopulmonary collateral arteries (MAPCA), with multiple surgeries including a central shunt as well as right and left unifocalization surgeries. He is admitted for complete repair. Following reconstruction of the central confluence, placement of an RV-PA conduit, takedown of two MAPCAs, and VSD closure, he does not tolerate coming off bypass. His blood pressure is 84/60 mm Hg on multiple pressors. His saturation is 87% on 100% oxygen. His RV pressure is 69/15 mm Hg. TEE demonstrates patency of the conduit. What is the best course of action?

    A. Placement of ECMO until hemodynamics improve
    B. Reinstitution of bypass, takedown of RV-PA conduit, and placement of a central shunt
    C. Replacement of the RV-PA conduit with a larger conduit
    D. Treatment with nitric oxide to improve PVR
    E. Reopening the VSD

57. An 11-year-old boy with history of pulmonary atresia with VSD is status post a BT shunt early in life and is also status post multiple unifocalization procedures. He is in the operating room for a complete repair. The surgeon has completed the operation. You are performing an echocardiogram. You note that the VSD is now closed and the RV–PA conduit has laminar flow by color Doppler. The estimated RV systolic pressure is 80 mm Hg. Biventricular function appears reasonable. You see that the radial arterial pressure tracing is 100/50 mm Hg. You advise the surgeon to:

    A. Do nothing further
    B. Replace the conduit with a smaller one
    C. Replace the conduit with a larger one
    D. Reopen the VSD
    E. Place a BT shunt in addition to what has been done already

58. A 4-month-old infant with pulmonary atresia with VSD undergoes complete repair, including unifocalization, RV-PA conduit, and closure of the VSD. Before sternal closure in the operating room, she becomes hypotensive. Systemic arterial pressure is 65/45 mm Hg. She is edematous with hepatomegaly. TEE reveals RV hypertrophy and moderately decreased biventricular systolic function. She has moderate tricuspid regurgitation with a velocity of 3.5 m/s. Which of the following interventions is most urgent at this time?

    A. Milrinone
    B. Leave the chest open and return to the ICU
    C. Reopen the VSD
    D. Placement of a bidirectional Glenn
    E. ECMO

59. A neonate with pulmonary atresia (PA) with VSD undergoes heart catheterization. The angiogram in **Figure 2.6** is obtained.

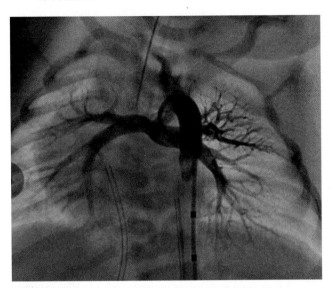

FIGURE 2.6

What is the primary source of pulmonary blood flow in this patient?

A. Ascending aorta
B. Descending aorta
C. Patent ductus arteriosus
D. BT shunt
E. Right subclavian artery

60. In a patient with pulmonary atresia with VSD, where is the proximal His bundle located relative to the VSD?

A. Along the posteroinferior rim of the VSD on the left ventricular side
B. Along the posterosuperior rim of the VSD on the right ventricular side
C. Along the anterolateral rim of the VSD on the left ventricular side
D. Along the anteromedial rim of the VSD on the right ventricular side
E. Not enough information provided

61. A 12-year-old patient with unrepaired TOF presents to clinic for preoperative evaluation before a planned complete surgical repair. Physical examination reveals severe cyanosis with marked clubbing of the fingers. Cardiac examination reveals a normal S_1, single S_2, with a grade 2/6 systolic ejection murmur at the left upper sternal border. There is also a soft continuous murmur over interscapular area. Echocardiography demonstrates severe right ventricular hypertrophy, anterocephalad malalignment of the conal septum, and a large perimembranous VSD with an overriding aorta. Owing to difficult visualization of the pulmonary artery anatomy, a cardiac catheterization is planned for the next morning at 8:30 AM. Which of the following should be done to decrease the chance of a hypercyanotic spell in the morning?

A. Make the patient NPO after midnight and start an IV at 7:00 AM
B. Use a general anesthesia-inducing agent that decreases systemic vascular resistance more than PVR
C. Make the patient NPO after midnight, perform phlebotomy to decrease Hgb to <14 before starting the IV
D. Start an esmolol drip as soon as the procedure starts
E. Make the patient NPO after midnight, start IV fluid when NPO starts, and use a topical anesthetic such as EMLA before attempting vascular access

62. A 17-year-old female with a history of tetralogy of Fallot (TOF) with a left aortic arch presents with progressive dyspnea on exertion. She describes a history of multiple operations including an RV-PA conduit revision 2 years ago. As part of her evaluation, cardiac catheterization is performed, from which the data in **Table 2.2** are obtained.

TABLE 2.2 Cardiac Catheterization Data

	Pressure	SpO$_2$
SVC	Mean 9	74
RA	Mean 8	76
RV	76/6	73
MPA	65/15, mean 46	74
RPA	27/13, mean 22	74
LPA	63/14, mean 44	74
RPCW	Mean 12	100
LPCW	Mean 12	
LV	112/10	99
Asc AO	110/68, mean 80	
Desc AO	102/67, mean 80	

SVC, superior vena cava; RA, right atrial; RV, right ventricular; MPA, main pulmonary artery; RPA, right pulmonary artery; LPA, left pulmonary artery; RPCW, right pulmonary capillary wedge pressure; LPCW, left pulmonary capillary wedge pressure; LV, left ventricular; AO, aortic.

On the basis of the information, which of the following is most likely to be true?

A. She would benefit from sildenafil
B. She would benefit from closure of her left-to-right shunt
C. She should have a conduit revision
D. Her symptoms are primarily related to diastolic dysfunction
E. She has a history of a Waterston shunt

63. A 6-day-old male infant presents with cyanosis and tachypnea. An echocardiogram confirms the diagnosis of tetralogy of Fallot (TOF) with absent pulmonary valve. He is in moderate respiratory distress. His heart rate is 190 bpm, respiratory rate is 55/min, and his ABG shows PaO$_2$ = 67, PaCO$_2$ = 68, pH = 7.25, Bicarb = 17, and an oxygen saturation of 84%. What should be done next in an attempt to alleviate his respiratory distress?

A. Inhaled albuterol
B. Intubation and mechanical ventilation
C. IV solumedrol
D. Emergent surgical repair of his congenital heart disease
E. Placement in prone position

64. A 3-day-old male infant presents to the emergency department with cyanosis. He was diagnosed prenatally with tetralogy of Fallot. He was born at home at 35 and 4/7 weeks of gestation. Over the first 48 hours of life, his color was good and he was nursing well. However, over the past 2 to 4 hours, he appeared progressively blue. At the time of presentation, his oxygen saturations are 60% to 65%, and he appears dusky. He is becoming more dusky. On examination, he has no appreciable murmur. A UVC has been placed. What is the best next step in management?

A. Echocardiogram to ascertain whether his prenatal echo had the correct diagnosis
B. Hyperoxia test to try to ascertain if he has a pulmonary component of his cyanosis
C. Emergent surgical repair
D. IV prostaglandin
E. IV morphine to encourage left-to-right shunting across his VSD

65. A 6-day-old male infant presents with a cardiac murmur and cyanosis. His saturation is 69% and his cuff blood pressure is 65/37 mm Hg. An echocardiogram reveals the following: TOF; severe infundibular obstruction (narrowest diameter 2 to 3 mm), a bicuspid pulmonary valve measuring ~5 mm at the annulus; almost entirely right-to-left shunting at the VSD with a peak Doppler VSD velocity of 2.5 m/s; accessory tricuspid valve tissue prolapsing into the VSD during systole; and a tricuspid regurgitation velocity of 4.5 m/s. He has an enlarged coronary sinus draining a left SVC. He has a large conal branch from his right coronary artery. Among the findings below, which feature is the most unusual in patients with TOF?

A. Large conal branch
B. Left SVC
C. Restrictive VSD
D. Pulmonary valve stenosis
E. Predominant right-to-left shunting through the VSD

66. A 3-week-old infant presents with tachypnea and poor feeding. Her prenatal screening ultrasound was suggestive of a severe conotruncal defect, but she was lost to follow-up and was a home delivery. Today, vital signs are as follows: P = 140 beats per minute, BP = 80/35 mm Hg, RR = 60 breaths per minute, O_2 saturation = 93% (room air). Cardiac examination reveals an active precordium, normal S_1, single S_2 with a grade 2/6 systolic murmur at left-mid sternal border. When the baby is quiet, a soft continuous murmur becomes apparent in the back. Which of the following statements is correct regarding this scenario?

A. The continuous murmur strongly suggests a diagnosis of truncus arteriosus

B. The continuous murmur is the result of truncal valve stenosis and regurgitation

C. Physical examination findings suggest a diagnosis of pulmonary atresia with VSD more than truncus arteriosus

D. Physical examination findings suggest a diagnosis of pulmonary atresia with intact ventricular septum more than truncus arteriosus

E. The presence of an apical diastolic murmur in this patient suggests anatomical mitral valve stenosis

67. Which of the following statements is correct regarding coronary artery anatomy in truncus arteriosus?

A. The posterior descending coronary artery arises from the left circumflex artery (left coronary dominance) in <3% of patients

B. The left anterior descending artery is relatively large and displaced rightward

C. The conus branch of the right coronary artery is usually small

D. The left coronary artery arises from the pulmonary trunk in ~40% of patients

E. Left coronary artery usually arises from the left posterolateral truncal surface

68. A 6-year-old girl from Mongolia presents for surgical consideration of her congenital heart disease. Echocardiogram reveals type I truncus arteriosus with a large VSD. The atrial septum is intact and there is trivial tricuspid regurgitation. Heart catheterization is performed, whereupon the data in **Table 2.3** are obtained:

TABLE 2.3 Heart Catheterization Data

	Pressure	SpO$_2$
IVC		58
SVC	Mean 9	52
RA	Mean 8	54
RV	102/12	62
Truncus	92/60, mean 72	82
RPA	83/49, mean 62	79
LPA	85/50, mean 63	79
RPCW	Mean 12	99
LPCW	Mean 13	99
LV	93/11	87
FA	96/58, mean 71	79

IVC, inferior vena cava; SVC, superior vena cava; RA, right atrial; RV, right ventricular; RPA, right pulmonary artery; LPA, left pulmonary artery; RPCW, right pulmonary capillary wedge pressure; LPCW, left pulmonary capillary wedge pressure; LV, left ventricular; FA, femoral arterial.

Her systemic cardiac index = 4.0 L/min/m^2. Which of the following is true regarding this patient?

A. No corrective intervention is indicated (palliation only)

B. She should undergo closure of her VSD and placement of an RV-PA conduit

C. Decision about whether or not to repair her lesions should be deferred until her hemodynamics are reassessed while she receives 100% oxygen

D. She should be listed for cardiac transplantation

E. She may benefit from balloon angioplasty of her pulmonary arteries

69. A neonate presents with cyanosis and a murmur. He is found to have type I truncus arteriosus with a bicuspid truncal valve and right aortic arch. He has a large secundum ASD and a left SVC draining into the coronary sinus. There is moderate RVH with normal biventricular function. Among the anatomic findings in this patient, which is most common among patients with truncus arteriosus?

A. Type I truncus

B. Bicuspid truncal valve

C. Interrupted aortic arch (IAA)

D. ASD

E. Left SVC

70. You are performing an echocardiogram on a cyanotic neonate. You note a large, thickened semilunar valve that is mildly incompetent and appears to originate from both RV and LV with a large outlet VSD. The pulmonary arteries originate separately from the ascending aorta. You also note interruption of the aortic arch. Which of the following is this baby most likely to have?

    A. Bicuspid truncal valve
    B. Right aortic arch
    C. Absent ductus arteriosus
    D. Absent left or right pulmonary artery
    E. Chromosome 22q11 deletion

71. A cardiac catheterization is performed on an 18-month-old boy with unrepaired truncus arteriosus. He has a moderate-sized ASD with no ductus arteriosus. The data in **Table 2.4** are obtained.

TABLE 2.4 Cardiac Catheterization Data

	Room Air		100% FiO$_2$	
	Pressure	SpO$_2$	Pressure	SpO$_2$
SVC	Mean 5	60	Mean 5	65
RA	Mean 4	68	Mean 4	70
RV	78/8	72	75/8	74
Truncus	85/52, mean 63	78	83/52, mean 62	89
RPA	83/49, mean 56	79	81/50, mean 58	87
LPA	82/50, mean 56	79	80/51, mean 58	87
RPCW	Mean 11	98	Mean 10	100
FA	90/51, mean 60	79	88/50, mean 60	87

SVC, superior vena cava; RA, right atrial; RV, right ventricular; RPA, right pulmonary artery; LPA, left pulmonary artery; RPCW, right pulmonary capillary wedge pressure; FA, femoral arterial.

If pulmonary blood flow is 5.0 L/min/m^2 on room air and 6.8 L/min/m^2 on 100% FiO$_2$, what course of treatment is recommended for this patient?

    A. Home oxygen therapy with repair in 1 to 2 years
    B. Pulmonary artery banding
    C. Surgical repair now
    D. Listing for heart–lung transplant
    E. Home oxygen (palliation only)

72. You are seeing a new patient in clinic with a history of truncus arteriosus. On auscultation, you hear a split second heart sound at the left sternal border. What is the most likely cause of the splitting of S$_2$?

    A. Referred tricuspid valve closure sound
    B. Ejection click after truncal valve opening
    C. Delayed closure of some of the cusps of the abnormal truncal valve
    D. Increased flow across the mitral valve
    E. Pulmonary artery ostial stenosis

73. Echocardiography of a newborn infant is performed. There is a large ventricular septal defect with an overriding semilunar valve. The pulmonary arteries are widely patent with laminar, increased flow and arise from a common trunk. The aortic arch is right sided. There is a single semilunar valve that is large in diameter, quadricuspid, and has moderate-to-severe regurgitation. There are no other complicating factors. What is the best treatment plan for this newborn infant?

    A. Perform bilateral BT shunts in first week of life, then a bidirectional Glenn at 4 to 6 months, with Fontan completion at 2 years of life
    B. Diuretics, digoxin, and afterload reduction for first 2 to 4 months if tolerated. Plan complete repair at 6 months (divide MPA from aorta, aortic valve repair, homograft conduit from RV to MPA)
    C. Band the pulmonary arteries in first 2 weeks of life, then manage medically until 4 to 6 months, when complete surgical repair can be more safely performed
    D. Complete repair by 3 weeks of age consisting of VSD closure, division of main pulmonary trunk from the aorta, aortic valve repair, placement of homograft conduit from RV to main PA
    E. Complete repair within the first 72 hours of life consisting of VSD closure, division of main pulmonary trunk from the aorta, place an aortic valve tissue prosthesis and homograft RV-MPA conduit

74. In the setting of asymmetric congenital mitral stenosis with unbalanced cord attachment, which of the following papillary muscle arrangements is the most common?

    A. Absence of both papillary muscles
    B. Absence of the anterolateral papillary muscle
    C. Absence of the posteromedial papillary muscle
    D. Presence of two separate papillary muscles
    E. Presence of two fused papillary muscles

75. A 1-month-old infant presents with tachypnea and poor feeding. A cardiac murmur is heard and an echocardiogram is performed (**Figure 2.7**).

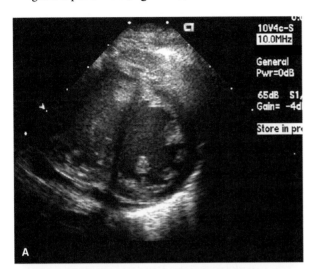

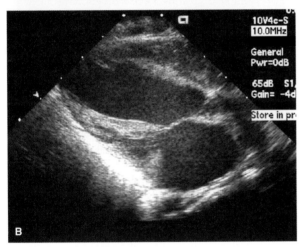

FIGURE 2.7

The echocardiogram also suggests moderate mitral inflow obstruction (mean gradient = 8 mm Hg), severe mitral regurgitation, and LA and LV enlargement. Which of the following is the most likely diagnosis?

A. Double orifice mitral valve
B. Mitral arcade
C. Supramitral ring
D. Parachute mitral valve
E. Cor triatriatum

76. A 4-year-old girl presents with tachypnea and heart failure and is found to have mitral stenosis. She undergoes a transatrial repair of her mitral valve. Attempts to extubate on post-op day 2 are unsuccessful. Her examination is significant for a soft holosystolic murmur at the apex, a loud P2, and a liver edge palpable 3 cm below the costal margin. An echocardiogram documents a mitral inflow mean gradient of 5 mm Hg and the pulmonary vein Doppler flow pattern in **Figure 2.8**.

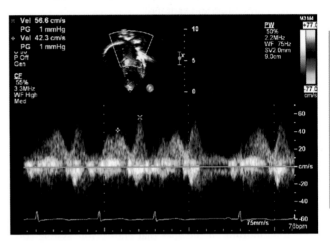

FIGURE 2.8

The RV is moderately dilated with moderately decreased systolic function, which is not significantly changed from her preoperative echocardiogram. Which of the following is the most likely cause for the patient's symptoms?

A. Pulmonary hypertension
B. Residual mitral stenosis
C. Unrecognized supramitral ring
D. Pulmonary vein stenosis
E. Right coronary infarction

77. Unlike the "cleft" in atrioventricular septal defects (AVSDs), which of the following is true about the isolated cleft of the mitral valve?

A. Is more truly a commissure as there is typically a papillary muscle associated with it
B. Causes more significant mitral regurgitation
C. Is associated with both mitral stenosis and regurgitation
D. Is directed anteriorly toward the LVOT
E. Is not associated with ASD or VSD

78. A 4-month-old infant is found to have congenital mitral insufficiency without stenosis due to a cleft in the anterior leaflet. By echocardiography, the valve appears repairable. The left ventricular end-diastolic dimension (LVEDD) is at the upper limit of normal, and left ventricular function is normal. The left atrium has mild enlargement. CXR reveals a normal cardiac silhouette. ECG is normal for age. Vital signs are normal. What is the best next step in management?

    A. Furosemide and captopril
    B. Propranolol and verapamil
    C. Propranolol and captopril
    D. Surgical referral
    E. No therapy at the present time

79. A 16-year-old female presents for clearance to participate in competitive volleyball. She has a history of vasodepressor–vasovagal syncope following a stressful event at school 2 years prior. Evaluation at that time revealed a normal physical examination and normal ECG. Now, physical examination while supine reveals a systolic click shortly after S_1 at the apex. With sitting, you note that the click moves toward S_1 and is followed by a I/VI systolic murmur at the apex that ends before systole concludes. These findings prompt an echocardiogram that reveals bileaflet mitral valve prolapse (MVP) with moderate mitral regurgitation, with a left ventricular EF of 53%. She then has a 24-hour ambulatory ECG monitor that shows frequent sustained SVT. Her resting blood pressure is 108/55 mm Hg. Along with her MVP, which of her findings would be an indication to restrict her from competitive volleyball?

    A. Degree of mitral regurgitation
    B. Left ventricular ejection fraction
    C. History of syncope
    D. Ambulatory ECG results
    E. Her blood pressure

80. An infant is diagnosed with critical aortic stenosis and resultant LV hypoplasia. According to the "Rhodes criteria" and other literature, which of the following echocardiographic criteria would indicate that the patient would benefit more from a Norwood-type palliation as opposed to a two-ventricle repair?

    A. LV long axis to heart long axis ratio of 0.9
    B. Aortic root diameter of 8 mm (4 cm/m^2)
    C. Indexed mitral valve area of 8 mm (4 cm/m^2)
    D. LV mass index of 10 g (50 g/m^2)
    E. Antegrade flow in the ascending aorta

81. A 17-year-old female immigrant presents with a 3-month history of progressive dyspnea on exertion. She had a childhood history of rheumatic fever, but she cannot remember the details of her underlying cardiac status except the painful IM antibiotic every month. On examination, she appears comfortable. Palpation reveals no thrill. Her S_1 and S_2 are normal. There is a grade 3/6 harsh systolic murmur audible along the mid-left sternal border radiating to the neck. There is no diastolic murmur or click. During auscultation, she has a few premature ventricular contractions. The systolic murmur becomes much louder in intensity following the extra beat. What is the most likely etiology of these physical examination findings?

    A. Tricuspid valve regurgitation
    B. Mitral regurgitation
    C. Pulmonary valve stenosis
    D. Subaortic stenosis
    E. Innocent murmur

82. Aortic balloon valvuloplasty is indicated in which of the following patients? All patients have bicuspid aortic valves, and all have undergone cardiac catheterization. "Peak-to-peak gradient" refers to the pressure gradient across the aortic valve.

    A. Asymptomatic 2-year-old boy with normal growth who has a peak-to-peak gradient of 45 mm Hg
    B. Asymptomatic 20-year-old female who is planning to become pregnant and whose peak-to-peak gradient is 40 mm Hg
    C. Asymptomatic 18-year-old boy who wants to play American football with a peak-to-peak gradient of 40 mm Hg
    D. A 1-day-old newborn who has an LVEF of 45% and a peak-to-peak gradient of 30 mm Hg
    E. Asymptomatic 20-year-old male with a normal ECG whose peak-to-peak gradient is 50 mm Hg

83. In assessing left ventricular myocardial function in patient with significant aortic valve stenosis, echocardiography with tissue Doppler imaging (TDI) is often used. Which of the following underlying assumptions is true in regard to the assessment of myocardial function by TDI?

    A. The echocardiographically derived ratio of early mitral inflow velocity (E) to early diastolic mitral annular velocity (E') correlates with catheter-derived LV end-diastolic pressure
    B. Measurement of mitral annular systolic velocity (S') by tissue Doppler imaging (TDI) demonstrates systolic short-axis dysfunction
    C. Longitudinally oriented fibers are present primarily in the subepicardial region
    D. The subendocardium is remarkably resilient to ischemia
    E. Transverse axis dysfunction typically precedes long-axis dysfunction

84. A 15-year-old boy with congenital aortic valve stenosis presents for interval follow-up. He underwent successful balloon dilation at age 4 years with a reduction in Doppler peak instantaneous gradient from 87 to 22 mm Hg. He has been followed annually for the past 10 years without further intervention. Blood pressure is normal. By echocardiography, his peak gradient today is 42 mm Hg (mean 26 mm Hg). There is mild LV hypertrophy without mid-cavitary obstruction. He is interested in playing hockey for his high school team. Tryouts start in 8 weeks. He is asymptomatic. What is the best recommendation?

    A. Start low-dose lisinopril, then allow participation if blood pressure remains normal
    B. Balloon dilate the valve, then allow to play after 6 weeks
    C. Replace the valve with a homograft, then allow to play
    D. Replace the valve with a mechanical valve and prohibit participation
    E. Perform an exercise ECG and reassess

85. You are asked to consult on a term neonate with a cardiac murmur. He has a harsh grade 2 to 3/6 systolic ejection murmur consistent with left ventricular outflow tract (LVOT) obstruction. He has good distal pulses and perfusion with no increased work of breathing. Echocardiography reveals a thickened bicuspid aortic valve with a velocity across the valve of 3.0 m/s and a PDA. The left ventricle has good function with no endomyocardial fibroelastosis (EFE). Which of the following is true regarding LVOT obstruction?

    A. Mild congenital subaortic stenosis, as a rule, rapidly progresses in the first few months of life
    B. The amount of EFE is independent of the degree of stenosis
    C. Significant retrograde diastolic flow in the distal arch from the PDA is consistent with severe stenosis
    D. Echo-derived pressure gradient is independent of other hemodynamic variables, such as preload and afterload
    E. Relative to balloon valvuloplasty, open surgical valvotomy results in a greater degree of aortic regurgitation

The following stem applies to questions 86 and 87:

A 10-day-old male infant presents to the emergency room with vomiting and respiratory distress. Pregnancy history was uncomplicated, and the infant was delivered at term. The patient was discharged from the hospital at day 2 of life. At day 4 of life, the patient began to have some difficulty with feeds. He was slow to feed due to fast breathing. No color changes were noted with feeds. His oral intake and urine output had been decreased over 24 hours before presentation.

Vital signs at the time of presentation are: HR = 169; respiratory rate = 70; BP (right arm) = 90/60 mm Hg, BP (right leg) = 70/30 mm Hg. On physical examination, there are no facial dysmorphic features. The skin is mottled and pale. There is a hyperactive RV impulse, normal S₁, single S₂ with S₃ gallop, and a soft systolic murmur at apex. Brachial pulses are normal, but femoral pulses are absent bilaterally. There are bilateral subcostal retractions. The liver is palpated 4 cm below the right costal margin. Extremities are cool.

*ECG and CXR are obtained (**Figure 2.9**).*

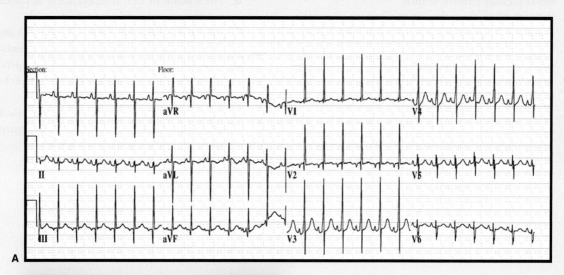

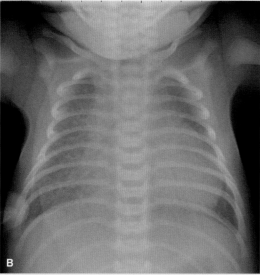

FIGURE 2.9

86. What would be the appropriate next step in management?

    A. Perform an echocardiogram
    B. IV access and give Lasix
    C. IV access and start dobutamine
    D. IV access and start PGE1
    E. IV access and give sodium bicarbonate

87. While IV access is being obtained, emergent echocardiography is performed on the baby. Pulsed wave Doppler interrogation of the abdominal aorta is performed (**Figure 2.10**).

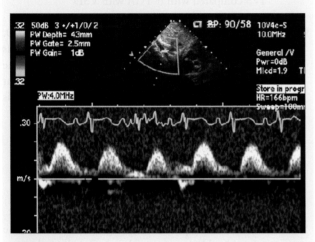

FIGURE 2.10

Which of the following statements is true?

    A. The Doppler profile suggests that surgical correction is unlikely to be necessary before 12 months of age
    B. A bicuspid aortic valve is unlikely to be associated with this defect
    C. Severe aortic regurgitation is likely to be present
    D. VSD is commonly associated with this defect
    E. Secundum atrial septal defect is the defect responsible for this clinical presentation

88. A 1-year-old child is referred for a cardiac murmur. She is asymptomatic. Her blood pressure in the right arm = 104/56 mm Hg, left leg = 84/50 mm Hg. Echocardiogram confirms isolated coarctation of the aorta. When do you recommend the patient have surgical repair?

    A. Age 2 to 3 years
    B. Age 6 to 8 years
    C. Age 12 to 14 years
    D. Only operate if systolic pressure gradient >50 mm Hg
    E. Only operate if symptoms develop, such as lower extremity claudication

The following clinical stem is used to answer Questions 89 to 91.

A 9-day-old female infant presents to the emergency department with respiratory distress. She is pale, irritable, and diaphoretic. RR 80; HR 210; 4-extremity BP: right arm 48/32 mm Hg, left arm 68/34 mm Hg, right leg 47/31 mm Hg, left leg 48/31 mm Hg. Auscultation reveals a gallop rhythm. A grade 2 to 3/6 murmur is heard at the upper left sternal border, at the base, and in the left interscapular area posteriorly. The murmur is heard throughout systole and disappears in early diastole. Moderate hepatomegaly is noted. She has widely spaced nipples and a webbed neck. She undergoes an echocardiogram.

89. What is the echocardiogram most likely to reveal?

    A. Mitral valve stenosis with moderate mitral regurgitation
    B. Anomalous left coronary artery from the pulmonary artery
    C. Isolated large outlet VSD with severe pulmonary valve stenosis
    D. Isolated severe coarctation of the aorta
    E. Coarctation of the aorta with anomalous aortic arch branching pattern

90. The above patient undergoes an echocardiogram following initiation of PGE1. The pulsed wave Doppler profile in **Figure 2.11** is obtained.

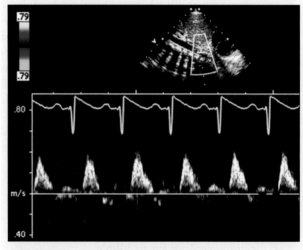

FIGURE 2.11

What is the most likely explanation for the tracing?

    A. Aortic arch is normal
    B. Ductus arteriosus is widely patent
    C. Cardiac output is extremely low
    D. Pulmonary hypertension is present
    E. Thrombus is present in the descending aorta

91. The above patient undergoes genetic testing. What is the most likely result?

    A. 45,XO genotype
    B. *JAG1* gene mutation
    C. *PTPN11* gene mutation
    D. 46,XY/47,XYY mosaicism
    E. *TBX5* gene mutation

92. A 12-year-old girl who is status post repair (end-to-end anastomosis) of coarctation of the aorta as a young child now complains of headaches with exercise. A neurologic workup including an MRI/MRA of her neck and head is negative. She is noted to have exercise hypertension on a bicycle exercise test. Further cardiology evaluation with an echocardiogram reveals no significant anatomical obstruction of the aorta. Which intervention or next step in evaluation would be beneficial to help relieve her exercise hypertension?

    A. Nothing, wait and watch
    B. Heart catheterization with possible stent placement as needed
    C. CT angiography to further evaluate aorta
    D. β-Blocker pharmacotherapy
    E. Nephrology consult

93. A 5-day-old term infant is 2 days status post a Norwood procedure with an RV-PA shunt (Sano) for hypoplastic left heart syndrome. His chest is closed and he is mechanically ventilated. Over the past 6 hours, you have noticed worsening acidosis and increasing hepatic enzymes. Creatinine has increased from 0.4 to 0.8. Urine output has been adequate. His vital signs are: HR 145, BP 60/38 mm Hg, RR 24 (all ventilator initiated). His saturation is 77% on 30% FiO_2; hemoglobin is 12 g/dL. Echocardiogram shows patent surgical connections with normal RV function. Which of the following interventions is most likely to improve this patient's clinical status?

    A. Start milrinone
    B. Increase inspired oxygen to 50%
    C. Start nitric oxide
    D. Transfuse 15 mL/kg packed RBCs
    E. Increase ventilator rate to 30/min

94. A neonate is diagnosed with d-TGA with an anterior malalignment VSD and subaortic stenosis. Which of the following is most likely to be concurrently found in this patient?

    A. Coarctation of the aorta
    B. Peripheral pulmonary stenosis
    C. Pulmonary atresia
    D. Mitral arcade
    E. Ebstein anomaly

95. Which of the following statements is correct regarding pathologic anatomy of complete d-TGA with an intact ventricular septum (IVS)?

    A. There is complete resorption of subaortic conus
    B. Ventricular septum is relatively sigmoid in shape rather than straight
    C. Functional (dynamic) subpulmonic obstruction from bulging of ventricular septum into LVOT usually occurs immediately after birth
    D. Sinus node and AV nodes are typically in their normal locations
    E. LV mass usually regresses much faster in d-TGA with IVS compared with d-TGA with VSD

96. A neonate is found to have d-TGA with VSD and ASD. There is a small patent ductus arteriosus. The VSD is nonrestrictive, but there is severe LVOT obstruction. The patient's oxygen saturation is 68% on room air. What is the most appropriate initial surgery/procedure for this patient?

    A. Jatene arterial switch with LeCompte maneuver
    B. Mustard operation
    C. BT shunt
    D. LVOT balloon arterioplasty
    E. PDA ligation

97. A 15-year-old boy presents with lightheadedness for the past 2 weeks. He has never fainted. On physical examination, he has a loud second heart sound, normal right parasternal impulse, and no cardiac murmurs. His ECG shows complete AV block, Q waves in V1, and no Q waves in V6. What is the most likely explanation for his AV dissociation?

    A. Maternal systemic lupus erythematosus
    B. Q fever
    C. Congenitally corrected transposition of the great arteries (ccTGA)
    D. Recent tick bite
    E. Myocarditis

98. Where is the AV node located in patients with congenitally corrected TGA?

    A. Along the anterior aspect of the atrioventricular ring, near the atrial septum
    B. Along the anterolateral aspect of the atrioventricular ring
    C. Along the posterior aspect of the atrioventricular ring, near the coronary sinus
    D. Along the posterior aspect of the atrioventricular ring, near the atrial septum
    E. Along the posterior aspect of the atrioventricular ring, near the IVC

99. An echocardiogram is performed on a cyanotic newborn infant in the NICU. It reveals double-outlet right ventricle (DORV) with side-by-side great arteries, a large inlet VSD with mitral valve straddle, moderate subaortic stenosis, and severe coarctation of the aorta. What is the most appropriate initial surgery for this patient?

    A. Patch VSD to aorta, repair coarctation
    B. Repair coarctation, close VSD, and repair the mitral valve
    C. Repair coarctation only
    D. Norwood palliation with Sano shunt
    E. Patch VSD to aorta, repair coarctation, resection of subaortic stenosis

100. What is the surgical procedure of choice for patients with DORV and a subpulmonary VSD without pulmonary stenosis?

    A. Pulmonary artery banding
    B. Arterial switch operation with patch closure of VSD
    C. Systemic-to-pulmonary shunt
    D. Patch closure of the VSD
    E. VSD stenting

101. You are called to the emergency department to evaluate a 6-month-old child with cyanosis. The infant is thin, frail, cyanotic, and breathing comfortably. You note oxygen saturations of 75% to 80% on room air, which do not change significantly with supplemental oxygen. His parents state that he has become gradually more blue over the past 4 months. On examination, you appreciate a gallop rhythm with a loud, harsh systolic ejection murmur. On the basis of this initial assessment, of the following diagnoses of double-outlet right ventricle (DORV), which is most likely?

    A. DORV with subpulmonic VSD and no pulmonary stenosis
    B. DORV with subpulmonic VSD and pulmonary stenosis
    C. DORV with subaortic VSD and no pulmonary stenosis
    D. DORV with subaortic VSD and pulmonary stenosis
    E. DORV with subaortic VSD and suprasystemic pulmonary hypertension

The following clinical stem refers to Questions 102 and 103.
You are called to perform an echocardiogram on a 2-day-old neonate with cyanosis. The patient is mildly tachypneic with retractions. Pulse oximetry reveals oxygen saturation of 63% to 65%. Chest x-ray demonstrates normal heart size with increased pulmonary vascular markings. On examination, you appreciate a loud S_2 with no significant murmurs.

102. Which of the following is most likely?

    A. DORV with subpulmonic VSD and no pulmonary stenosis
    B. DORV with subpulmonic VSD and pulmonary stenosis
    C. DORV with subaortic VSD and no pulmonary stenosis
    D. DORV with subaortic VSD and pulmonary stenosis
    E. DORV with subaortic VSD and suprasystemic pulmonary hypertension

103. An echocardiogram is performed and documents DORV Taussig–Bing type, with a nonrestrictive VSD, a large PDA with low-velocity bidirectional shunt, and a tiny PFO. The aortic arch appears mildly hypoplastic but unobstructed. An IV is obtained and prostaglandin is started. The patient's clinical status does not improve. Which of the following interventions is likely to be of the most immediate benefit?

    A. Increase the rate of PGE1 infusion
    B. Start nitric oxide
    C. IV furosemide
    D. Balloon atrial septostomy
    E. Surgical repair in 2 to 3 weeks

    A 3-year-old patient presents to your clinic with double-inlet left ventricle (DILV), left-sided hypoplastic subaortic right ventricle, V-A discordance, with a mildly restrictive bulboventricular foramen–type VSD. She had a pulmonary band placed at 3 months of age and is now status post bidirectional Glenn anastomosis. She is being considered for Fontan palliation.

104. Which of the following of her cardiac catheterization findings is associated with the highest mortality in patients with DILV undergoing Fontan?

    A. PVR = 2.5 Wood units
    B. Mild left AV-valve regurgitation
    C. Patent left SVC
    D. Resting subaortic gradient = 45 mm Hg
    E. Mild right atrioventricular valve regurgitation

105. A 2-year-old patient presents to your clinic for initial assessment after moving from another state. He was born with double-outlet right ventricle, multiple muscular VSDs, and normally related great arteries with no subaortic or subpulmonary stenosis. He had a prior intervention, but the parents do not recall the details. He now is found to have a resting peak subaortic gradient of 50 mm Hg by echocardiography. What prior intervention is most likely the cause of the subaortic gradient in the patient?

A. Pulmonary artery banding
B. Ligation of patent ductus arteriosus
C. Balloon atrial septostomy
D. Balloon dilation of left pulmonary artery stenosis
E. Device closure of atrial septal defect

106. A term neonate with a harsh systolic murmur at birth is found to have DILV with a hypoplastic subaortic RV, and a restrictive bulboventricular foramen and severe subaortic stenosis. A prostaglandin infusion is started. A subsequent echocardiogram documents a large PDA. Which of the following is the most appropriate initial operation for this child?

A. Enlargement of the VSD
B. Aortopulmonary anastomosis (DKS) with BT shunt
C. Pulmonary artery banding only
D. Bidirectional cavopulmonary anastomosis
E. Pulmonary artery banding with aortic arch augmentation

The following stem and angiograms apply to Questions 107 and 108.

*You are performing a cardiac catheterization on a 2-year-old girl with heterotaxy syndrome with atrial and visceral situs ambiguus, asplenia, dextrocardia, complete AV septal defect, and DORV with left anterior aorta (**Figure 2.12**).*

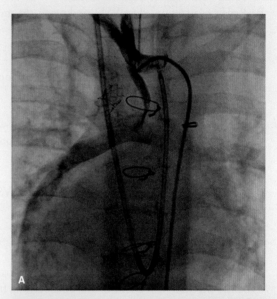

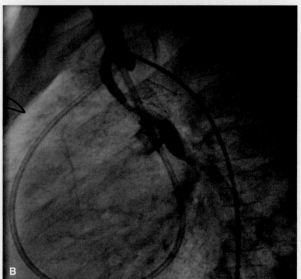

FIGURE 2.12

107. What is the course of the venous catheter?

    A. Right IJ → SVC → anomalous pulmonary vein → pleural space
    B. Right IJ → SVC → MPA → common ventricle → aorta
    C. Right IJ → SVC → common atrium → common ventricle → MPA
    D. Right IJ → SVC → common atrium → common ventricle → aorta
    E. Right IJ → SVC → azygous vein → IVC → common atrium → left SVC

108. What is the course of the arterial catheter?

    A. Femoral artery → descending aorta → aortic arch → BT shunt
    B. Femoral artery → descending aorta → left SVC → MPA
    C. Femoral artery → descending aorta → Waterston shunt → MPA
    D. Femoral artery → descending aorta → Potts shunt → MPA
    E. Femoral artery → descending aorta → aortic arch → anomalous pulmonary vein

109. A 17-year-old male has been experiencing chest pain for the past several months with exertion. One event occurred with syncope. His past medical history is negative. Physical examination revealed normal auscultation with a hyperactive impulse that is slightly displaced to the left. A chest radiograph revealed a slightly displaced cardiac silhouette to the left and prominent bulges of the aortic knob and pulmonary artery. Which diagnostic evaluation will most likely be helpful in confirming your clinical suspicion/etiology for his chest pain?

    A. Auscultation
    B. Chest x-ray
    C. Echocardiography
    D. Cardiac catheterization
    E. Magnetic resonance imaging

110. You are seeing a 14-year-old male patient for the first time. His mother died suddenly at the age of 39 and was found to have hypertrophic cardiomyopathy (HCM) on autopsy. Your patient had a negative echocardiogram performed at age 5 years due to a history of a murmur. His electrocardiogram is normal for his age. His current echocardiogram now reveals a maximal left ventricular wall thickness of 17 mm. When should the next echocardiogram and follow-up visit be performed?

    A. 6 months
    B. 1 year
    C. 3 years
    D. 5 years
    E. Only if symptoms arise

111. What is the known pattern of inheritance in HCM?

    A. Autosomal recessive
    B. X-linked recessive
    C. Autosomal dominant
    D. Sporadic
    E. X-linked dominant

112. A 17-year-old male with a family history of sudden cardiac death collapsed while watching the finale of a singing competition on television. He stood up to get something from the refrigerator and fell without warning. His girlfriend performed successful CPR. He was brought to the emergency department and subsequently admitted to the PICU. A bedside echocardiogram revealed a 28-mm interventricular septal thickness with systolic anterior motion of the mitral valve. A maximal instantaneous Doppler gradient of 100 mm Hg was demonstrated across the left ventricular outflow tract. What is your recommendation regarding management?

    A. Place ICD only
    B. Surgical septal myectomy only
    C. Perform surgical septal myectomy, then place ICD
    D. Start nadolol only
    E. Perform surgical septal myectomy, then start nadolol

113. Which of the following will increase the outflow murmur in a patient with obstructive HCM?

    A. β-Blocker
    B. Squatting
    C. Isometric handgrip
    D. Phenylephrine
    E. Amyl nitrate inhalation

114. Regarding the risk of sudden death in individuals with HCM, which of the following statements is the most correct?

    A. Most HCM-related sudden deaths occur during or just after vigorous exercise
    B. The strongest predictor of sudden death is degree of LVOT obstruction
    C. A drop in blood pressure during exercise is associated with an increased risk of sudden death
    D. Sudden death in patients with HCM is most often due to primary pulseless electrical activity
    E. For patients at high risk of sudden death, septal myectomy is a valid alternative to ICD placement

115. A 14 year old is found to have his family's genetic mutation for HCM. He has no symptoms attributable to his heart. His echocardiogram is normal. There is no family history of sudden death. According to the 36th Bethesda Conference, which of the following management strategies is most appropriate?

A. Prophylactic ICD placement

B. β-Blocker therapy alone

C. β-Blocker therapy and activity restriction

D. Activity restriction alone

E. No medical therapy or activity restriction

The following stem is used for Questions 116 and 117.

A 4-year-old boy presents to the emergency department with fever, irritability, increased work of breathing, and poor feeding. Symptoms initially began 4 weeks before presentation while visiting family in southern Mexico, but they seemed to improve over the next several days. However, he never seemed to be "back to himself" over the next several weeks. His parents report a 2- to 3-day h/o fever, vomiting, and diarrhea with progressive worsening of his condition in the hours prior to presentation.

Physical examination reveals an anxious, diaphoretic, grunting child. Vitals: T 39.2 °C, R 64 breaths per minute and labored, P 186 breaths per minute, BP 98/40 mm Hg (right arm). O₂ sat = 93% on room air. Lung examination reveals accessory muscle use and wheezing. Cardiac examination reveals a downward, laterally displaced apical impulse. S₁ is normal, S₂ is increased. An S₃ gallop rhythm is audible. There is a grade 2/6 holosystolic murmur over the left lower sternal border. His abdomen is distended. The liver edge is palpable 6 cm below the right costal margin. His extremities are somewhat cool. Capillary refill time is 4 to 5 seconds. Peripheral IV access is obtained. Labs are pending.

Chest x-ray reveals cardiomegaly. Echocardiography demonstrates a severely dilated left atrium and a dilated, poorly functioning left ventricle.

116. What drug is most likely to be of initial benefit to this patient?

A. Nebulized albuterol

B. Epinephrine

C. High-dose dobutamine

D. Milrinone

E. Digoxin

117. A Spanish translator obtains further history. It turns out that the family saw a doctor in Mexico 3 weeks before presentation who started the boy on nadolol for suspected long-QT syndrome. The patient took a dose 2 hours before arrival in the emergency department. Given this new information, what is the best therapy for the patient?

A. Nebulized albuterol

B. Dobutamine

C. Norepinephrine

D. Milrinone

E. Digoxin

118. A 10-month-old boy presents with severe respiratory distress with poor perfusion requiring admission to the pediatric ICU for mechanical ventilation and inotropic support. His history is remarkable for poor weight gain and hypotonia. He has been treated for the last 10 days with antibiotics and albuterol inhalers for a respiratory infection and reactive airway disease.

Oxygen saturation by pulse oximetry is 88% on 60% FiO₂. His CXR shows severe cardiomegaly with diffuse pulmonary infiltrates consistent with pulmonary venous congestion. An arterial blood gas reveals the following: pH 7.28, PaCO₂ 48, PaO₂ 55, HCO₃ 15, base deficit −9. A complete blood count reveals the following: WBC 2.6 (4% neutrophils, 65% monocytes, 22% lymphocytes, 6% basophils, 3% eosinophils), Hgb 14, Hct 45, platelets 220,000. This CBC is very similar to a CBC done 2 weeks ago when his illness started. His family history is significant for a maternal uncle and maternal great uncle who both died of heart disease in childhood. On general examination, he is not dysmorphic. Which of the following laboratory test results would you expect to be present in this patient?

A. Decreased acid α-glucosidase activity in skin fibroblasts

B. Elevated mucopolysaccharides in urine

C. Elevated 3-methylglutaconic acid in urine

D. Mutation in fibrillin-1 (FBN-1)

E. SCN5A mutation

119. A cardiac catheterization is performed to differentiate between restrictive cardiomyopathy (RCM) and constrictive pericarditis (CP). Which hemodynamic parameters would be more consistent with RCM rather than CP?

A. Right atrial pressure (RAP) = pulmonary wedge pressure (PWP)

B. RV systolic pressure <50 mm Hg

C. Pulmonary wedge pressure 10 mm Hg higher than RV end-diastolic pressure

D. RVEDP = LVEDP

E. Normal PVR index

120. An 18-year-old previously healthy male presents with weight loss, intermittent fever, cough, and a systemic macular rash. He has progressively worsening shortness of breath. A chest x-ray reveals vascular congestion in the lung fields. Physical examination reveals a gallop rhythm, loud P2, and a palpable liver 5 cm below the costal margin. A CT scan shows evidence of prior splenic and hepatic infarcts. Serial blood work reveals normal Hgb, WBC, and platelet counts, but shows a persistently elevated eosinophil count of >3,000 eosinophils/mm^3. Echocardiography is consistent with restrictive cardiomyopathy. Which of the following is the most appropriate initial outpatient treatment regimen for this patient?

    A. Digoxin, Lasix, Coumadin, Aspirin
    B. Digoxin, Enalapril, Aldactone
    C. Digoxin, Lasix, Diuril, Enalapril, Coumadin
    D. Digoxin, Lasix, Enalapril, Coumadin, Prednisone
    E. Lasix, Enalapril, Coumadin, Methotrexate

121. According to the WHO classification of cardiomyopathies, which of the following findings precludes the diagnosis of restrictive cardiomyopathy?

    A. Reduced RV diastolic volume
    B. LVEF 50%
    C. Normal LV wall thickness
    D. Right atrial enlargement
    E. Mildly increased LV end-diastolic volume

122. A 10-year-old patient with Duchenne muscular dystrophy is undergoing an orthopedic surgical procedure for which he will be placed under general anesthesia. Which medication should be avoided during the procedure?

    A. Fentanyl
    B. Succinylcholine
    C. Midazolam
    D. Milrinone
    E. Vecuronium

123. A 4-year-old boy is noted during a primary care evaluation to have gross motor delay. He is suspected to have Duchenne muscular dystrophy and gene testing is pending. He was referred for cardiac evaluation. What characteristic ECG findings would you most likely expect?

    A. Ventricular premature contractions
    B. Q waves in leads II, V1, V2, and V3
    C. Atrial premature contractions
    D. First-degree AV block
    E. Q waves in leads I, aVL, V5, and V6

124. You are seeing a 4-year-old boy with a waddling gait and calf pseudohypertrophy. What type of murmur do you expect to hear on cardiac examination?

    A. Systolic ejection murmur with a click
    B. No murmur
    C. Continuous murmur
    D. Diastolic murmur
    E. High-pitched holosystolic murmur

125. Which of the following is the most commonly reported arrhythmia among children with restrictive cardiomyopathy?

    A. Atrial fibrillation
    B. Atrial flutter
    C. Wolff–Parkinson–White syndrome
    D. Second-degree AV block, type II
    E. Symptomatic sinus bradycardia

126. At what point of the cardiac cycle is there maximum left-to-right shunting across an atrial septal defect?

    A. Isovolumic contraction
    B. Isovolumic relaxation
    C. End systole
    D. End diastole

127. You are examining a 5-year-old child in clinic and you note a hypoplastic right thumb. On auscultation you hear a grade 2/6 systolic ejection murmur over the left upper sternal border. The next best step/steps in the evaluation of this patient is/are:

    A. Obtain an ECG only
    B. Obtain an echocardiogram only
    C. Obtain an ECG and an echocardiogram
    D. No further testing

128. You follow a 3-month-old male infant with trisomy 21 and a complete AV septal defect in clinic. You are discussing his upcoming complete repair with his parents who ask if he will ever require another cardiac surgery in the future after his defect is repaired. You tell them that the most common reason for surgical revision is:

    A. Presence of a residual or additional muscular VSD that was not evident prior to initial repair
    B. Left AV valve regurgitation
    C. Left AV valve stenosis
    D. Subaortic stenosis

129. You see a 12-month-old infant with unrepaired complete AV septal defect who has been lost to follow-up for 8 months. You note that her 4-month checkup reported a moderate to large ASD and VSD components of the defect with a common AV valve. The baby surprisingly is not in florid heart failure. The parents report that she generally looks well but does have fast breathing occasionally. What is the most likely reason that more severe heart failure symptoms have not occurred to date?

    A. Premature pulmonary vascular obstructive disease
    B. Spontaneous closure of atrial and ventricular septal defects
    C. Severe right ventricular outflow tract obstruction
    D. Appropriately regulated diuretic use

130. Which one of these may be a usual ECG change in complete AV septal defect?

    A. Prolonged PR interval
    B. Wide QRS complex
    C. Long QTc
    D. Flattened T waves

131. You evaluated a 2-week-old infant for heart murmur in your outpatient clinic. The echocardiogram revealed a posterior malaligned VSD and a small PDA with bidirectional shunting (right to left in systole). The infant was struggling to gain weight, so you started him on 24 kcal/oz feedings and diuretic therapy. Two weeks later, he is seen in follow-up. He has persistent tachypnea and has not gained weight. What additional defect is most likely to be contributing to the clinical picture?

    A. Coarctation of the aorta
    B. Pulmonary valve stenosis
    C. Pulmonary vein stenosis
    D. Idiopathic pulmonary hypertension

132. You are seeing a 4-year-old boy in clinic who you have followed since he was 2 months old when he was found to have a small perimembranous VSD during an evaluation for a murmur. He has been growing well and has no complaints. His repeat echocardiogram today shows a persistent VSD that is partially occluded by aneurysmal tricuspid valve tissue, and there is restrictive flow across the defect. There are no other abnormal findings on his echocardiogram. His mother asks if this defect will ever require surgery. You tell his mother:

    A. The defect will require closure if it remains persistent at age 16 years
    B. The defect will require closure if he develops aortic regurgitation or RV muscle bundle hypertrophy
    C. The defect will require closure if he has a syncopal episode after standing
    D. The defect will never require closure regardless of any new findings on future echocardiograms

133. A 9-month-old infant presents to cardiology clinic. He has a known large inlet VSD with deficient posterior rim that was diagnosed by echocardiography at 3 months of age. He has been lost to follow-up for 6 months since then. On examination, he is neither tachypneic nor tachycardic and appears well. His oxygen saturations are 88% on room air. There is no significant murmur. His mother states that he has never looked better. The most likely reason for this is:

    A. The VSD has closed spontaneously
    B. The VSD was misdiagnosed initially
    C. The patient has increased pulmonary vascular resistance
    D. The patient has developed severe pulmonary valve stenosis

134. A 14-day-old neonate presents with SVT that spontaneously converts with vagal maneuvers. Baseline ECG reveals ventricular pre-excitation with suspicion for a posteroseptal accessory pathway. Which of the following venous abnormalities is most likely to be seen in this baby?

    A. Bilateral superior vena cavae, with left SVC to roof of left atrium
    B. IVC drainage to the left atrium
    C. Interrupted IVC with azygous continuation
    D. Postnatal persistence of the ductus venosus
    E. Coronary sinus diverticulum

135. When considering a bidirectional cavopulmonary anastomosis (BDCPA, or Glenn connection) in a patient with tricuspid atresia, which of the following would be of most concern (would predict a less successful outcome)?

    A. LVEDP 10 mm Hg
    B. Transpulmonary gradient 8 mm Hg
    C. Mean PA pressure 20 mm Hg
    D. LVEF 50%

136. Most cases of Ebstein anomaly are:

    A. associated with maternal benzodiazepine exposure
    B. related to NKX2.5 mutations
    C. sporadic in nature
    D. related to 10p13-p14 deletions
    E. related to mutations in the *MYH7* gene

137. Causes of a low Fontan fenestration gradient include:

    A. Pulmonary hypertension
    B. Hypovolemia
    C. Intrinsic lung disease
    D. Pulmonary venous obstruction

138. Which type of tricuspid atresia will most likely have progressive cyanosis over time?

A. Normally related great arteries; small VSD; pulmonary stenosis (Type IB)

B. Normally related great arteries; large VSD without pulmonary stenosis (Type IC)

C. Transposed great arteries; VSD; pulmonary stenosis (Type IIB)

D. Transposed great arteries; VSD; without pulmonary stenosis (Type IIC)

139. You are seeing a 17 year old with history of tetralogy of Fallot that was repaired with a transannular patch at 4 months of age. That is his only surgery to date. He complains of some mild dyspnea with exertion. Electrocardiogram demonstrates QRS duration of 175 msec with pronounced RBBB. Cardiac magnetic resonance imaging (CMR) demonstrates indexed RV volume of 173 mL/m². Which of the following treatments is the most likely to improve this patient's long-term survival?

A. Placement of an ICD/dual-chamber pacemaker

B. Surgical pulmonary valve replacement

C. Transcatheter pulmonary valve replacement

D. Starting a β-blocker to help decrease ventricular ectopy

140. You are seeing a 12 year old with a bicuspid aortic valve. He reports feeling well with no symptoms of chest pain, difficulty breathing, or syncope. He regularly plays baseball with his friends. Examination reveals a grade 3/6 systolic ejection murmur at the right upper sternal border with radiation to the neck. Left arm cuff BP is 103/67 mm Hg. ECG demonstrates normal sinus rhythm with LVH. Echocardiography reveals a mean Doppler-derived gradient of 36 mm Hg across the aortic valve trace insufficiency. The aortic root Z-score is +1.6. The LV wall thickness is normal. He wants to play baseball in a highly competitive summer league. What is the best next step in management?

A. Restrict from all sports, but no further testing or therapy indicated at this time

B. Refer for heart catheterization and balloon valvuloplasty

C. Start an ACE inhibitor

D. Arrange for exercise stress testing

141. You are following a 17 year old who underwent extended end-to-end repair of aortic coarctation as a 2 year old. By echocardiography, the site of repair appears widely patent. The ascending aorta measures normal for his BSA, and no aneurysm is evident. His resting blood pressure is 120/80 mm Hg in both upper and lower extremities. You order an exercise stress test, which demonstrates right arm BP 240/60 mm Hg and left leg BP 140/60 mm Hg in immediate postexercise period. There was a normal heart rate response. What would be the most reasonable treatment for this patient?

A. Refer for percutaneous aortic balloon angioplasty

B. Refer for transcatheter aortic stent placement

C. Start atenolol

D. Refer for surgical revision of prior coarctation repair site

142. Which of the following surgical techniques for coarctation repair is most associated with late aortic aneurysm formation?

A. End-to-end anastomosis

B. Extended end-to-end anastomosis

C. Prosthetic patch aortoplasty

D. Arch advancement

143. You have referred your 3-year-old patient for cardiac catheterization as a pre-Fontan assessment. She has tricuspid atresia with normally related great vessels and a moderate VSD. She has been palliated with primary Glenn anastomosis. Which of the following findings would designate your patient as high risk for Fontan completion?

A. Qp:Qs 0.9:1

B. Mean pulmonary artery pressure of 14 mm Hg

C. PVRi of 5.2 Wood units

D. RVEDP = 10 mm Hg

144. You are seeing a 4-week-old baby in clinic who has hypoplastic left heart syndrome s/p Norwood with right modified BT shunt. He is on aspirin and digoxin per your institution's interstage protocol. His mother reports that he is taking less feeds by mouth and requiring more supplementation with NG feeds to get adequate calories. He has gained ~18 g/day since the last visit. His oxygen saturation is 83% (baseline ~85%), heart rate 170 bpm, respiratory rate 36, BP in right arm 88/45 mm Hg, left leg 89/47 mm Hg. On his echocardiogram, there is normal ventricular function, moderate–severe tricuspid regurgitation, no neo-aortic insufficiency, patent BT shunt with flow into the bilateral pulmonary arteries. Based on this information, which outpatient therapy may be most beneficial for this patient?

A. Lasix

B. Captopril

C. Flecainide

D. Propranolol

145. Which of the following is true regarding the hemi-Fontan procedure?

   A. It involves a direct anastomosis of the superior vena cava to the right pulmonary artery with SVC disconnection from the right atrium
   B. It is less technically complex to perform compared to the bidirectional Glenn procedure
   C. It allows for later expeditious performance of the Fontan completion
   D. It can be accomplished without the use of cardiopulmonary bypass in selected cases

146. You are seeing a 4 year old with hypoplastic left heart syndrome who underwent Norwood palliation shortly after birth and Glenn palliation at 3 months. She returns to clinic today for follow-up. Her parents report that she is doing well, though she does seem more winded with exertion than prior. SpO_2 is 72% on room air. Other vital signs are normal. There is a soft systolic murmur on examination. She is taking aspirin and lisinopril daily. Echocardiogram reveals subjectively normal RV function, mild tricuspid regurgitation, trace neo-aortic insufficiency, and venophasic flow through the Glenn to the pulmonary arteries. What is the best next step in this patient's management?

   A. Refer for cardiac magnetic resonance imaging (CMR)
   B. Refer for cardiac catheterization
   C. Continue medical management
   D. Refer for surgery (Fontan completion)

147. You are participating in a case in the cardiac catheterization lab for a newborn infant with a d-transposition of the great arteries and intact ventricular septum. The prenatal fetal echocardiogram was concerning for a restrictive atrial septum (based on 2D imaging, color Doppler, and pulmonary vein Doppler profile). The postnatal echocardiogram confirmed restriction with a 2-mm atrial septal defect with left-to-right shunting and an estimated mean gradient of 8 to 10 mm Hg. The newborn is taken to the cardiac catheterization lab where a balloon atrial septostomy (BAS) is performed without echo guidance, using only fluoroscopy. At the beginning of the case, the infant's pre- and postductal saturation is 60%. Following the BAS, the infant's saturation level is unchanged. The most likely reason for this is:

   A. The atrial septum was mistakenly identified as restrictive but was in fact unrestrictive
   B. There was a small muscular VSD missed on the initial echocardiogram through which there is adequate mixing
   C. There is significant LV outflow tract obstruction
   D. The balloon was placed within a leftward juxtaposed right atrial appendage and not across the atrial septum resulting in an ineffective BAS

148. You are seeing a 14-year-old boy in clinic who was born with d-transposition of the great arteries with intact ventricular septum and underwent arterial switch procedure with LeCompte maneuver in infancy. He currently reports no symptoms and has a reassuring physical examination. He had a Holter monitor the year prior that showed no evidence of arrhythmias. He would like to try out for the varsity soccer team. What testing would be indicated to clear him for soccer?

   A. Echocardiogram and cardiac MRI
   B. Echocardiogram and cardiac catheterization
   C. Echocardiogram and exercise stress test
   D. Echocardiogram only

149. You follow an infant with congenitally corrected transposition of the great arteries (ccTGA) in outpatient clinic. After appropriate counseling with the parents, a strategy to pursue anatomic repair is decided upon. She undergoes pulmonary artery banding at 2 months of age. She presents for outpatient evaluation at 10 months of age. She is doing well without complaints. Blood pressure is 100/60 mm Hg. An echocardiogram demonstrates findings typical of ccTGA. Biventricular function is normal. There is mild tricuspid valve regurgitation. The PA band gradient measures 35 mm Hg. There is no obstruction of the systemic outflow. What is the next best step in the patient's management?

   A. Tighten the PA band and complete the double switch later
   B. Remove the pulmonary artery band and abandon plans for a double switch
   C. Perform double-switch procedure now
   D. Conservative management alone

150. Which would be the most likely expected physical examination finding for a young child with ccTGA without a large VSD or significant regurgitation of the morphologic tricuspid valve?

   A. Tachycardia
   B. Hepatomegaly
   C. Cyanosis
   D. An accentuated, palpable single second heart sound

151. Isolated dextrocardia with normal atrial situs is most commonly associated with which of the following?

   A. Congenitally corrected transposition of the great arteries
   B. Double-outlet right ventricle
   C. Double-inlet left ventricle
   D. Ebstein anomaly

Answers

1. (D) This clinical scenario is most consistent with a diagnosis of Alagille syndrome. Alagille syndrome is an autosomal dominant disorder associated with liver disease secondary to bile duct paucity, cholestasis, congenital heart disease (CHD), skeletal or ocular abnormalities, or typical facial features. Mutations in the Notch ligand, *JAG1,* are responsible for the clinical phenotype. Alagille syndrome is characterized by right-sided heart disease including peripheral pulmonary stenosis (diffuse hypoplasia of the pulmonary arterial bed as well as discrete stenosis), pulmonary valve stenosis, and tetralogy of Fallot (TOF). Left-sided lesions and septal defects have also been reported.

NOTCH1 mutations result in aortic valve pathology but not the other findings given here. *PTPN11* mutations result in Noonan syndrome (characterized by hypertelorism, ptosis, short stature, and CHD, most commonly pulmonary valve stenosis and HCM). Additional cardiac manifestations include secundum-type atrial septal defect, VSD, TOF, pulmonary artery stenosis, coarctation of the aorta, partial AVSD (primum-type atrial septal defect), and polyvalvulopathy. Other noncardiac anomalies of Noonan syndrome include webbed neck, skeletal anomalies, bleeding diathesis, lymphatic disorders, mental retardation, and cryptorchidism. *TBX1* is a gene that resides in the area of chromosome 22q11; mutations of *TBX1* lead to features of DiGeorge syndrome (hypocalcemia, immunodeficiency, and severe CHD, most commonly interruption of the aortic arch [IAA] type B, truncus arteriosus, or TOF). *GATA4* mutations appear to be involved in septation defects but are not associated with a classic syndrome as described in the vignette.

2. (E) Heart defects in congenital rubella syndrome include pulmonary stenosis (valvar, supravalvar, or peripheral) and patent ductus arteriosus. Tetralogy of Fallot has also been reported.

3. (E) Caffeine intake during pregnancy has not been shown to result in an increased risk of congenital heart disease in the fetus.

4. (C) Women with maternal phenylketonuria who have high levels of phenylalanine when pregnant have a high likelihood of having children with microcephaly and mental retardation. There is an increased risk for left-sided defects, septal defects, and tetralogy of Fallot.

5. (D) This vignette describes Williams syndrome, which is characterized in part by CHD, hypercalcemia in infancy, skeletal and renal anomalies, cognitive deficits, social personality, and so-called "elfin facies." Approximately 90% of patients with the clinical diagnosis of Williams syndrome have a deletion at chromosome 7q11.23, which is not generally apparent on a routine karyotype but can be detected by FISH. Approximately 55% to 80% of patients with Williams syndrome have CHD, which typically includes supravalvar aortic stenosis and/or supravalvar pulmonary stenosis. Therefore, a click may not be present despite a murmur and significant gradient across the involved outflow tract.

18q deletion is associated with ASD, VSD, and pulmonary stenosis and is also associated with cleft palate and GU anomalies. Tetrasomy 22p is known as "cat eye syndrome" and is associated with rectoanal anomalies, coloboma, genitourinary anomalies, and preauricular pits/tags. Deletion of 8p23 is associated with septal defects, GU anomalies, abnormally formed ears, and minor hand anomalies. Chromosome 22q11 deletion is known as DiGeorge syndrome or velocardiofacial syndrome and is characterized by hypocalcemia, immunodeficiency, and severe CHD, most commonly IAA type B, truncus arteriosus, or TOF.

6. (C) Approximately 55% to 80% of patients with Williams syndrome have congenital heart disease, which typically includes supravalvar aortic stenosis and/or supravalvar pulmonary stenosis. The degree of cardiovascular involvement varies widely. Supravalvar pulmonary stenosis tends to improve with time, while supravalvar aortic stenosis usually progresses. Sudden death has been described in Williams syndrome. Suspected etiologic factors include coronary artery stenosis and severe biventricular outflow tract obstruction. Presumably, sudden cardiac death results from myocardial ischemia, decreased cardiac output, or arrhythmias. Patients with Williams syndrome are prone to develop hypertension because of renal artery stenosis.

7. (C) This scenario describes trisomy 18. The distinctive phenotype of trisomy 18 includes growth retardation, short palpebral fissures, small mouth, and micrognathia. Specific features include a prominent occiput, short sternum, small nipples, clenched hands, disorganized or hypoplastic palmar creases, hyperconvex nails, and "rocker bottom feet." Congenital heart disease is the rule (>90% incidence). Most common associated defects include perimembranous VSD, TOF, DORV, and polyvalvular dysplasia. Approximately 90% of affected individuals die in the first year of life and usually not of their heart disease.

8. (C) The most common CHDs associated with a 22q11 deletion include tetralogy of Fallot, interrupted aortic arch type B, truncus arteriosus, perimembranous VSD, and aortic arch anomalies. A wide range of CHDs has been reported in patients with a 22q11 deletion, including pulmonary valve stenosis, atrial septal defect, heterotaxy syndrome, and hypoplastic left heart syndrome.

9. (E) This clinical scenario describes pulmonary hypertension resulting from a large unrepaired atrial septal defect. Although rare, severe irreversible hypertensive pulmonary vascular disease can develop from unrepaired ASDs. There is a female preponderance for this association. Spontaneous closure is rare for defects >8 mm in size. Although severe mitral regurgitation, nonsustained VT, and LV diastolic dysfunction can contribute to dyspnea on exertion, they are not the primary cause as indicated by this scenario.

10. (D) In general, cardiac catheterization is unnecessary for the diagnosis of sinus venosus ASD. Occasionally, however, questions about pulmonary vascular obstructive disease or associated cardiac defects arise that require catheterization. In this case, it is important to assess the presence and degree of pulmonary vascular vasoreactivity to determine appropriate treatment. It would be premature to start therapy without a thorough understanding of the pulmonary artery pressures and reactivity.

11. (B) Sinus venosus ASD accounts for 5% to 10% of ASDs and is located posterior and superior to the fossa ovalis. The sinus venosus defect commonly is associated with anomalous connection of the right pulmonary veins to either the right atrium or the superior vena cava near the caval–atrial junction. Electrocardiogram shows that about half of patients have a frontal plane P-wave axis of <30 degrees. The other types of ASDs are associated with normal P-wave axes.

12. (A) The complete form of AVSD is characterized by a large septal defect with interatrial and interventricular components and a common atrioventricular valve that spans the entire septal defect. The septal defect extends to the level of the membranous ventricular septum, which is usually deficient or absent.

The common atrioventricular valve has five leaflets. Beneath the five commissures are five papillary muscles. The two left-sided papillary muscles are oriented closer together than in a normal heart, and the lateral leaflet is smaller than usual. In addition, the two papillary muscles are often rotated counterclockwise, thus positioning the posterior muscle farther from the septum than normal and the anterior muscle closer to the septum. This papillary muscle arrangement, along with a large anterolateral muscle bundle, can contribute to progressive LVOT obstruction.

13. (A) In partial AVSD, the mitral and tricuspid annuli are separate. Partial AVSD consists of a primum ASD and a "cleft" anterior mitral valve leaflet. Although patients with partial AVSD may be asymptomatic until adulthood, symptoms of excess pulmonary blood flow typically occur in childhood. Tachypnea and poor weight gain occur most commonly when the defect is associated with moderate or severe mitral valve regurgitation or with other hemodynamically significant cardiac anomalies. Patients with a primum ASD usually have earlier and more severe symptoms, including growth failure, than patients with a secundum ASD. Repair of residual/recurrent mitral valve regurgitation or stenosis is the most common reason for reoperation.

In this clinical scenario, surgical correction was required early, suggesting a hemodynamically significant cleft mitral valve. This patient presents with progressive shortness of breath. Physical examination and chest x-ray findings suggest mitral valve regurgitation. Mitral stenosis may also be involved, but the murmur on examination suggests regurgitation is significant. The patient may indeed have pulmonary hypertension, but it would be secondary rather than primary in origin. LVOT obstruction is an important consideration for all forms of AVSD, and it is usually progressive. However, it would be characterized by a systolic ejection-type murmur. Pulmonary stenosis also would have an ejection murmur but would be heard best over the left upper sternal border.

14. (C) In the normal heart, the aortic valve is wedged between the mitral and the tricuspid annuli. In AVSD, the aortic valve is displaced or "sprung" anteriorly. This anterior displacement creates an elongated, so-called gooseneck deformity of the LVOT. LVOT obstruction may occur in all forms of AVSD. It is more frequent when two atrioventricular valve orifices are present than when there is a common orifice. Ten percent of patients with AVSD may require reoperation to relieve LVOT obstruction (while the most common indication for reoperation is left AV valve regurgitation or stenosis). Progressive LVOT obstruction is more common in partial than in complete AVSD. Mechanisms of LVOT obstruction include attachments of superior bridging leaflet to ventricular septum, extension of the anterolateral papillary muscle into the LVOT, discrete fibrous subaortic stenosis, and tissue from an aneurysm of the membranous septum bowing into the LVOT. Obstruction may develop *de novo* after initial repair of the AVSD and closure of the mitral valve cleft.

15. (D) Right bundle branch block is common and may be due to ventriculotomy or direct injury to the right bundle itself. However, right bundle branch block occurs after a transatrial repair as well. Of the other options, a residual ASD would likely not be the cause of a newly split S_2, a residual VSD would be accompanied by a murmur. Ventilation changes would not result in a newly split S_2.

16. (C) The valve closure sounds in patients with a small VSD are usually normal. Some patients, however, have wide splitting of the second sound. If there is associated pulmonary stenosis or mitral insufficiency in a patient with VSD, these lesions may be suspected when the systolic murmur is transmitted to the upper left sternal border or apex, respectively. Flow across a large (unrestrictive) VSD is limited primarily by relative resistances of the systemic and pulmonary circulations.

Minor anomalies of the tricuspid valve may be acquired secondary to left-to-right shunting across perimembranous defects. These anomalies include redundant septal leaflet tissue that can partially or completely occlude the defect. After VSD repair, the LV mass and volume decrease, but volume decreases at a much greater rate than mass. Finally, patients who develop Eisenmenger physiology typically begin manifesting cyanosis before 2 years of age.

17. (B) Prolapse of one of the aortic valve cusps may occur with outlet or perimembranous VSDs. Patients with outlet defects usually have deficiency of muscular or fibrous support below the aortic valve with herniation of the right coronary leaflet through the VSD. The aortic commissures themselves are usually normal. In contrast, patients with perimembranous VSDs and aortic insufficiency have herniation of the right or much less commonly the noncoronary cusp, have frequent abnormalities of aortic commissures (usually the right/noncoronary), and may have associated infundibular pulmonary stenosis. Echocardiography and angiography can show that the prolapsed aortic leaflet partially closes a moderate to large VSD and limits the left-to-right shunt. The associated aortic valve insufficiency is progressive.

The murmur of an incompetent tricuspid valve or mitral valve would be systolic. The patient is asymptomatic and acyanotic; hence, Eisenmenger physiology is not present. Therefore, RV and LV pressures have not equalized.

18. (B) The relationship of the atrioventricular conduction pathways to VSDs is important to surgical repair. In perimembranous defects, the bundle of His lies in a subendocardial position as it courses along the posterior-inferior margin of the defect. In inlet defects, the bundle of His passes anterosuperiorly to the defect. In muscular VSDs and outlet defects, there is little danger of heart block because the conduction tissue generally is far removed unless these defects extend into the perimembranous area.

19. (A) When signs of necrotizing enterocolitis develop in an infant with significant left-to-right shunting through a PDA, early surgical closure of the ductus arteriosus has significantly reduced mortality. Therefore, if abdominal distention is persistent, increasing residuals before feedings, blood in the stools or gastric aspirate, decreasing bowel sounds, and, particularly, intramural air occurs in association with a significant left-to-right shunt through a PDA, immediate surgical closure is recommended.

20. (A) This vignette describes a child with a hemodynamically significant PDA that has gone unrepaired and now is infected. *Streptococcus viridans* and *Staphylococcus aureus* are the most common organisms. Vegetations are almost always seen on the pulmonary artery end of the duct.

21. (B) Postnatal closure of the ductus arteriosus occurs in two phases. The first phase, "functional closure," occurs within 12 hours after birth. There is contraction and cellular migration of the medial smooth muscle in the wall of the ductus arteriosus that causes the vessel walls to become thick and protrude into the vessel lumen. The second stage usually is completed by 2 to 3 weeks and results from infolding of the endothelium, disruption and fragmentation of the internal elastic lamina, proliferation of the subintimal layers, and hemorrhage and necrosis in the subintimal region. There is connective tissue formation and replacement of muscle fibers with fibrosis with subsequent permanent sealing of the lumen, thus forming the *ligamentum arteriosum*.

22. (E) Ibuprofen has been evaluated as a possible alternative to indomethacin in preterm infants. Studies have shown a similar rate of ductal closure after ibuprofen treatment with fewer negative effects on renal function, cerebral vasculature, and cerebral blood flow than indomethacin. The risk of intraventricular hemorrhage is equivocal. Of note, using ibuprofen for prophylaxis is associated with increased risk of pulmonary hypertension.

23. (A) Surgical correction of ALCAPA involves direct reimplantation of the origin of the left coronary artery into the aorta and is considered the standard corrective surgical approach in many centers. An alternative approach is the Takeuchi procedure, in which an aortopulmonary window is created and then a tunnel fashioned that directs blood from the aorta to the left coronary ostium.

Because of papillary muscle infarction and dysfunction, significant preoperative mitral insufficiency has been found to be a risk factor for both mortality and need for late mitral valve surgery.

24. (A) A localized weakness of the wall of a sinus of Valsalva leads to aneurysmal bulging. If the aneurysm ruptures, the size of the fistula determines how large the shunt will be, and its site of entry into the heart often determines the specific features. Thus, aneurysmal rupture into the left heart does not produce signs of a left-to-right shunt, whereas rupture into the right heart produces a left-to-right shunt. With a small fistula, there may be only a continuous murmur with its maximal intensity in the third or fourth intercostal space near the sternal edge. If the fistula enters the right atrium, the murmur may be maximal to the right of the sternum. With larger fistulae, there will be a wide pulse pressure, a collapsing pulse, and left ventricular hyperactivity. If the fistula enters the right side, there will be right ventricular hyperactivity as well. A large fistula entering the left ventricle may display a to-and-fro murmur and simulate aortic incompetence. Occasionally, there is only a diastolic murmur in fistulae entering the left ventricle or the high-pressure right ventricle in a neonate.

25. (C) In this anomaly, the left coronary artery arises from the pulmonary artery, usually from the left posterior facing sinus. In fetal life, pressures and oxygen saturations are similar in the aorta and pulmonary artery, so myocardial perfusion is normal. After birth, the pulmonary arteries have low pressures and desaturated blood, which does not bode well for myocardial perfusion. Myocardial ischemia subsequently occurs. Ischemia is worsened with exertion such as feeding or crying. As time passes, infarction of the anterolateral LV free wall occurs. The mitral valve papillary muscles are affected, and mitral regurgitation develops.

Anomalous coronary artery origins from the wrong sinus of Valsalva are generally asymptomatic in infancy. The most common anomaly (a third of all major coronary arterial anomalies) is origin of the left circumflex from the right main coronary artery. This anomaly has no general clinical significance in the absence of intracardiac surgery.

The origin of the left main coronary artery from the right sinus of Valsalva is less common but more important clinically. If the anomalous vessel passes between the aorta and the RVOT, the child is at risk for sudden death during or just after vigorous exercise. In many of these cases, the ostium of the left main coronary artery is slit-like, increasing further the risk.

26. (C) A localized weakness of the wall of a sinus of Valsalva leads to aneurysmal bulging. Localized aneurysms are usually congenital, with thinning just above the annulus at the leaflet hinge. However, aneurysms can follow infective endocarditis. Approximately 75% of patients are male. Approximately 65% of aneurysms are located in the right aortic sinus, 25% in the noncoronary sinus, and 10% in the left aortic sinus. Up to 50% of cases may be associated with VSDs, especially right sinus aneurysms associated with defects of the outlet septum. Aneurysms can rupture into any cardiac chamber. Rupture is most often of the right sinus aneurysm into the right ventricle in the setting of an outlet VSD. Rupture into the pericardium is rare.

27. (E) Central nervous system AVMs manifest symptoms according to their hemodynamic effects. Infants presenting with CHF typically have large AVMs. The most common cerebral AVMs presenting with CHF are located deep (vein of Galen), superficial (pial), or dural. Affected infants have high-output CHF with dilation of all cardiac chambers, feeding arteries, and draining veins. If there is venous obstruction, flow can be restricted through the AVM, so patients may present with venous hypertension or cerebral ischemia.

The prognosis for most patients with large cerebral arterial malformations is grave. If untreated, most newborns (90%) die during the first week of life from intractable CHF or neurologic complications (seizures, intracranial hemorrhage). Those who do survive the neonatal period often suffer profound neurologic morbidity (hydrocephalus, mental retardation, hemorrhage).

28. (C) Most pulmonary AVMs are congenital or associated with HHT. Pulmonary AVMs enlarge as the child grows older. A high proportion (>85%) of patients with multiple pulmonary AVMs have HHT. Overall, 30% to 50% of patients with pulmonary AVMs have HHT.

Patients with pulmonary AVMs generally are hemodynamically stable. In contrast to systemic AVMs, cardiac output is not increased, while pulmonary blood flow and pressures are unchanged. Of note, during cardiac catheterization, the total PVR is normal. That is, resistance within the AVM is low, whereas the resistance in the other lung segments may be elevated.

29. (B) Transcatheter embolization has become the treatment of choice for pulmonary AVMs. Embolization provides persistent relief of hypoxemia, resolution of orthodeoxia, and minimal growth of small remaining AVMs. The embolization procedure is effective for preventing stroke and transient ischemic attacks but does not appear to reduce the risk of brain abscess.

To avoid device embolization (through the AVM to the systemic circulation), transcatheter occlusion of the afferent artery or fistula is usually accomplished using a coil or umbrella rather than liquid adhesive or beads. The goal is to raise the systemic arterial oxygen tension (some authors suggest to 60 mm Hg) by occluding the most significant afferent arteries (generally considered those to be >3 mm in diameter).

30. (C) Large AVMs and large patent ductus arteriosus have similar hemodynamic effects (large extracardiac left-to-right shunts) and thus are indistinguishable in terms of pulse pressure, liver span, cardiothoracic ratio on chest x-ray, and QRS axis on ECG. Diagnostic cardiac catheterization is usually unnecessary, as the diagnosis is suspected by clinical examination and confirmed by noninvasive imaging. When performed, catheterization demonstrates high cardiac output, elevated atrial and ventricular end-diastolic pressures, a widened systemic arterial pulse pressure, and a large difference in the oxygen saturation between the superior and inferior vena cava (higher saturation from the involved area).

31. (B) A barium esophagram that shows an anterior indentation is virtually pathognomonic for a pulmonary artery sling or a tumor. Origin of the left pulmonary artery from the right pulmonary artery, known as a pulmonary artery sling, is a rare anomaly in which the lower trachea is partially surrounded by vascular structures. The left pulmonary artery arises as a very proximal branch of the right and then loops around the trachea. It is the only situation in which a major vascular structure passes between the trachea and esophagus.

Pulmonary sling is frequently associated with complete cartilaginous rings in the distal trachea resulting in tracheal stenosis. It usually appears as an isolated abnormality but can be associated with other congenital cardiac defects, including tetralogy of Fallot.

32. (B) Right aortic arch with mirror-image branching describes an aortic arch that traverses the right mainstem bronchus. The first branch is a left innominate artery that divides into left carotid and left subclavian arteries. The second branch is the right carotid, and the third is the right subclavian. The ductus arteriosus (or ligamentum arteriosum) is usually on the left side and arises from the base of the innominate artery. This lesion typically does not form a vascular ring. However, this arch anomaly is frequently associated with congenital intracardiac disease. The most common association is with TOF, but other conotruncal anomalies may also be seen, as well as DORV. Therefore, an echocardiogram should be considered in this patient to evaluate the intracardiac anatomy.

The patient is asymptomatic at this time, so further workup for a vascular ring (such as swallowing study or bronchoscopy) is not necessary.

33. (A) A vascular ring is an aortic arch anomaly in which the trachea and esophagus are completely surrounded by vascular structures. The clinical picture typically includes respiratory symptoms, especially stridor. Pneumonia, bronchitis, or cough may also be present. Infants may demonstrate a posture of hyperextension of the neck. A common history is that of a 1 to 3 month old with "noisy breathing since birth" who develops more significant respiratory distress in association with an intercurrent upper respiratory infection. Less commonly (and usually in toddlers or older children), the presentation will be swallowing difficulty. Of the listed options, only a right aortic arch with retroesophageal innominate artery and a left PDA complete the ring.

34. (D) Interrupted aortic arch (IAA) is defined as a complete separation of ascending and descending aorta. Celoria and Patton classified IAA into three types: type A if the interruption was distal to the left subclavian artery, type B if between carotid and subclavian arteries, and type C if between carotid arteries. These patients typically present with acute cardiovascular collapse or heart failure after spontaneous closure of the ductus arteriosus in the first days of life.

Absence of all limb pulses suggests a type B interruption with an anomalous subclavian artery. In this situation, both carotid arteries are proximal to the interruption, while both subclavians are distal to the interruption. Strong carotid pulses help to differentiate interrupted arch from critical aortic stenosis in which all pulses are diminished.

35. (A) Right aortic arch with diverticulum of Kommerell is the second most common vascular ring after double aortic arch.

In right aortic arch with mirror-image branching, there usually is no left-sided ductus arteriosus or ligamentum arteriosum and thus no vascular ring. Left aortic arch with retroesophageal right subclavian artery is the most common aortic arch anomaly, but does not form a ring and is usually asymptomatic. Right aortic arch with retroesophageal innominate artery is a very rare abnormality of the aortic arch system. The ductus arteriosus (or ligamentum arteriosum) completes a vascular ring as it connects the left pulmonary artery with the base of the innominate artery. However, it is much less common than right aortic arch with retroesophageal diverticulum of Kommerell.

36. (C) In classic cor triatriatum, a membrane separates the more proximal chamber, which receives the pulmonary veins, from the more distal left atrium, which communicates with the mitral valve. To allow for cardiac output, typically there is a hole in the membrane that ranges from <3 mm to about 1 cm. The distal, true left atrium is in continuity with the left atrial appendage. The fossa ovalis usually is located between the distal left atrial chamber and the right atrium; occasionally, a patent foramen ovale/ASD is present in this area. Right ventricular hypertrophy and dilation are almost invariably found. Right atrial hypertrophy and dilation are present in ~25% of cases. Hypertrophy and dilation of the right atrium result in tall, broad, oftentimes peaked P waves on ECG.

The prognosis in TAPVC is influenced by the size of the interatrial communication and by the degree of obstruction in anomalous venous pathways. Overall mortality for unrepaired TAPVC is 80% or more at 1 year. Long-term prognosis depends on the state of the pulmonary vascular bed at the time of surgery as well as the patency of the pulmonary venous–left atrial anastomosis. Late arrhythmias may develop in a small number of these patients. Atrial arrhythmias are most common and include sinus bradycardia, atrial flutter, and supraventricular tachycardia. Ventricular rhythm problems are unusual.

Scimitar syndrome describes the chest x-ray findings present in anomalous connection of the right pulmonary veins to the IVC. There is a crescent-like shadow in the right lower lung field; the shape of the shadow resembles a Turkish sword, or scimitar. Frequent coexistent anomalies include hypoplasia of the right lung and chest, mesocardia or dextrocardia, and lung parenchymal abnormalities.

37. (E) A superior sinus venosus defect (also called SVC type) results from deficiency of the common wall between the SVC and the right upper pulmonary vein (RUPV). This defect "unroofs" the RUPV. The unroofed pulmonary vein then drains into the SVC, while its left atrial orifice becomes the interatrial communication. This interatrial communication is not a defect of the atrial septum.

38. (E) The correct catheter course is IVC → right atrium → SVC → innominate vein → vertical vein → anomalous pulmonary venous confluence.

39. (E) In infradiaphragmatic TAPVC, the most common site of obstruction is at the anomalous vessels' connection with the portal vein or the hepatic veins. By 2D echo, there frequently is seen a dilated venous channel proximal to the site of stenosis. If unobstructed, the anomalous vessel is characterized by a low-velocity, phasic laminar flow pattern with brief flow reversal during atrial systole. Luminal narrowing is associated with flow acceleration and turbulence by color Doppler.

Corrective surgery for the infant or child with TAPVC should be performed as soon as possible. In the sickest infants, the patient's clinical condition should be optimized, including the cardiorespiratory and metabolic states. When possible, surgery should be done on the basis of echocardiography rather than cardiac catheterization in an effort to lessen the time to operation and therefore reduce mortality.

Balloon atrial septostomy and blade atrial septostomy have been used in the past as palliative procedures. Septostomy delays the definitive procedure and is of little value when an anomalous venous channel is obstructed. Balloon dilation of obstructed anomalous venous channels is usually unsuccessful.

40. (D) The echocardiogram image demonstrates cor triatriatum. Most patients with classic cor triatriatum have onset of symptoms within the first few years of life. However, some patients present in the second or third decade of life. Frequently, these patients will present with a history of dyspnea, frequent respiratory issues including "asthma," and pneumonia. They often are considered to have primary pulmonary disease.

Untreated cor triatriatum results in pulmonary hypertension. Physical examination findings include a loud pulmonary component of the second heart sound, right ventricular heave, and pulmonary systolic ejection click. A murmur of tricuspid regurgitation may be present. Less often, a diastolic murmur is detected at the mitral area, or a continuous murmur may be heard. Right-sided heart failure is common. Pulmonary rales are heard if pulmonary edema is present.

In the patient with pulmonary edema or right heart failure, the disease frequently is progressive despite maximal medical management. Surgical intervention should be planned as soon as possible. Surgical resection of the cor triatriatum membrane under cardiopulmonary bypass is the effective treatment of choice. When pulmonary edema and right heart failure occur, survival is usually only a matter of months. However, in patients who survive operative correction, the severe pulmonary arterial changes that result in pulmonary hypertension can regress. In these patients, the prognosis seems excellent.

41. (C) Other than partial anomalous pulmonary venous connection (PAPVC) to the right SVC and to the right atrium (sinus venosus defect and malposition of the septum primum, respectively), the most common type of PAPVC is of the left pulmonary veins to the left innominate vein (LIV). The left-sided pulmonary vein(s) connect(s) to the LIV through a persistent early embryonic pathway. The connecting vein (often called a "vertical vein") between the left pulmonary veins and the LIV may incorrectly be termed a persistent left superior vena cava (LSVC). This term is incorrect both embryologically and anatomically.

Embryologically, the vertical vein represents a persistent early embryonic connection between the splanchnic plexus of the lung buds and the cardinal veins. Anatomically, it is positioned more posteriorly than the LSVC, which is located immediately behind the left atrial appendage. An LSVC usually connects with the coronary sinus, although it may connect with the left atrium when the coronary sinus is unroofed. When a left pulmonary vein drains into the LSVC, the LSVC still should connect with the coronary sinus or with the left atrium.

A secundum atrial septal defect is commonly associated with PAPVC to the LIV. A primum atrial septal defect is very uncommon. Rarely, the atrial septum is intact.

42. (D) Absence of the hepatic segment of the IVC with azygous continuation into the right or left SVC is referred to as an interrupted IVC. Pulmonary AVMs have been known to develop after a classic or bidirectional Glenn anastomosis owing to the exclusion of hepatic venous blood or "hepatic factor" to the lungs. This malformation can develop in one or both lungs if preferential blood flow is present. In the case described in this vignette, there is likely inadequate hepatic venous blood flow to the pulmonary arteries.

43. (B) Congenital malformations of the coronary sinus frequently are associated with arrhythmias. SVT and sudden cardiac death have been reported in a significant percentage of patients with diverticula of the coronary sinus. Patients with diverticula of the coronary sinus usually present with SVT associated with accessory pathways that transverse the diverticulum to form an atrioventricular connection.

44. (D) This patient is a setup for inadequate systemic blood flow, given his tricuspid valve atresia and transposition of the great arteries with a restrictive VSD. He has evidence of systemic underperfusion with acidosis. He requires a stable source of systemic blood flow. Of the given options, only a DKS procedure results in a stable systemic circulation.

45. (E) Uhl anomaly is a congenital cardiac malformation consisting of an almost total absence of the RV myocardium.

Cyanosis and hepatomegaly are often present, as is jugular venous distention. The precordium usually is quiet, and peripheral pulses are diminished. The heart tones are decreased. A pansystolic murmur of tricuspid insufficiency may be present, but patients may have no murmurs or other nonspecific murmurs present.

ECG usually shows prominent P waves and diminished QRS amplitude, especially in the right precordial leads. The chest x-ray demonstrates cardiomegaly with normal to diminished pulmonary vascularity (which can appear similar to Ebstein anomaly of the tricuspid valve).

Echocardiography demonstrates marked dilation of the right-sided cardiac chambers. An important finding is the presence of the tricuspid valve leaflets arising appropriately from the annulus, differentiating this lesion from Ebstein anomaly.

At cardiac catheterization, similar pressure wave contours are obtained from the pulmonary artery, right ventricle, and right atrium. The right atrial *a wave* is dominant. Endocardial potentials, if recorded during catheterization, show normal transition between the ventricular and atrial complexes, helping to rule out Ebstein anomaly.

Most patients die in infancy or childhood. The typical pathologic finding is the markedly dilated, "parchment-like" right ventricle. Histologically, the endocardium is thickened, and there are few if any true myocardial cells in the right ventricular free wall. The tricuspid valve arises normally from a dilated valve annulus and may be dysplastic, but is not displaced into the right ventricular cavity.

46. (C) In patients with relatively normal cardiac output, classification of severity of pulmonary stenosis routinely is based on measurements of RV pressure and valve gradient. Mild stenosis is characterized by an RV pressure less than half the LV pressure or a peak valve gradient <35 mm Hg to 40 mm Hg. In moderate stenosis, the RV pressure is ~50% to 75% of the LV pressure, or the peak gradient is ~40 mm Hg to 60 mm Hg. Severe stenosis is defined as an RV pressure ≥75% of the LV pressure or a peak gradient >60 mm Hg to 70 mm Hg.

In this case, TR velocity predicts an RV-to-RA pressure gradient of 49 mm Hg, or an RV systolic pressure of 55 mm Hg. Using the modified Bernoulli equation $4(V_2^2 - V_1^2)$, the peak gradient across the pulmonary valve is $4(16 - 4)$ or 48 mm Hg. Both of these measurements indicate moderate pulmonary valve stenosis.

47. (E) If discontinuation of prostaglandin E1 and subsequent ductal constriction are not tolerated immediately after valvuloplasty, these infants can be maintained on prostaglandin for 2 to 3 weeks while intermittently assessing whether constriction of the ductus is tolerated with O_2 saturations remaining ≥70%. Neonates who immediately remain cyanotic following valvuloplasty often demonstrate improvement over weeks to months as RV compliance improves and the atrial right-to-left shunt decreases. Ultimately, those in whom a shunt was created can undergo shunt closure either surgically or by transcatheter techniques.

48. (B) As a result of pulmonary valve stenosis, secondary changes in the RV and pulmonary arteries can occur. The infundibular region of the RV becomes hypertrophied with resultant dynamic subvalvular obstruction. This hypertrophy can persist in the immediate post-valvuloplasty period, resulting in limited pulmonary outflow. Over time, once the fixed pulmonary obstruction is removed, this hypertrophy resolves.

49. (D) In the setting of unilateral branch pulmonary artery stenosis without a significant left-to-right shunt, resting RV systolic pressure remains normal. The contralateral pulmonary artery accommodates the cardiac output without an increase in pressure. Because flow to the stenotic side is lower than normal, the severity of obstruction may be underestimated by systolic pressure difference estimations (though the diastolic pressure difference is proportional to the severity of obstruction).

The protocol for angioplasty consists of positioning a balloon dilation catheter across the stenotic segment of the pulmonary artery. In contrast to pulmonary valve dilation, the balloon diameter should be three to four times the narrowest pulmonary artery segment.

Percutaneous balloon angioplasty of peripheral pulmonary artery stenosis has a lower success rate than pulmonary valvuloplasty. The overall acute success rate for branch PA angioplasty is ~50% to 60%. The rate of recurrent stenosis has been 15% to 20% in short- to mid-term follow-up.

50. (C) It is important to confirm the coronary circulation in patients with pulmonary atresia with intact ventricular septum before proceeding with an intervention. "Right ventricular–dependent coronary artery circulation" describes the situation whereby the myocardium is supplied by blood that originates in the RV at systemic or supersystemic systolic pressure and supplies the myocardium in a retrograde fashion. Myocardial ischemia, infarction, and death may result if significant ventriculo-coronary connections are present and the right ventricular pressure is reduced secondary to an intervention.

In the normal circulation, the aortic diastolic pressure primarily drives coronary blood flow. Factors that reduce aortic diastolic pressure (or shorten diastole) will compromise coronary blood flow. The presence of ventriculo-coronary artery connections may result in coronary artery stenosis and/or interruption. In this case, aortic diastolic pressure may not be sufficient to drive coronary blood flow; elevated RV pressures are necessary. Interference with blood flow into the RV or other reduction of RV systolic pressure has deleterious effects.

51. (E) Transcatheter perforation of the atretic pulmonary valve with subsequent balloon dilation is an alternative to surgical valvotomy. The ideal patient (lowest risk) would have a tripartite right ventricle of near-normal size with valvar pulmonary atresia and a well-developed pulmonary arterial circulation. There would not be RV-depending coronary circulation.

In general, the smallest RVs are associated with the most ventriculo-coronary connections. Unipartite or bipartite ventricles are much more likely to have ventriculo-coronary communications. Using the convention of the tricuspid

Z value, data from the CHSS demonstrated a positive correlation with ventriculo-coronary connections—a more negative tricuspid Z value correlates with the presence of ventriculo-coronary connections.

52. (A) This patient demonstrates evidence of RV-dependent coronary circulation. Therefore, decompression of the RV is not warranted, eliminating an RV–PA conduit or pulmonary valvotomy.

53. (D) The angiogram demonstrates evidence of RV-dependent coronary circulation in the inferior distribution. Therefore, he would exhibit evidence of myocardial ischemia in an inferior distribution, including ST elevation in leads II, III, and aVF.

54. (C) Despite the lack of evidence of RV-dependent coronary circulation by echocardiography, cardiac catheterization is still necessary to rule out such circulation. MRI does not have a role in the preoperative management of a 4-day-old infant. Biopsy is not indicated.

55. (E) These images demonstrate pulmonary atresia with intact ventricular septum. Ventriculo-coronary connections are observed in ~45%, but <10% of patients are considered to have wholly RV-dependent coronary circulation (CHSS database). Confluent pulmonary arteries usually are supplied by a left-sided ductus arteriosus. A main pulmonary artery is almost always present. Rarely, nonconfluent pulmonary arteries are supported by bilateral ductus arteriosus or aortopulmonary collaterals. Some patients with this disease have all three RV components present; in others, the RV is extremely underdeveloped and may have an inlet only. There is no known gender predilection.

56. (E) For patients whose pulmonary artery anatomy appears amenable to reconstruction, procedures leading to complete repair are indicated. Connecting the RV to the central pulmonary artery using a conduit is performed; this may promote growth of the central pulmonary arteries. Unifocalization procedures are performed to incorporate the maximum number of pulmonary artery segments into the eventual RV outflow reconstruction. The ultimate goal is complete repair (closure of all septal defects, interruption of all extracardiac sources of pulmonary arterial blood flow, and incorporation of at least 14 pulmonary arterial segments in a connection to the right ventricle).

At the end of a full repair, the central pulmonary artery size should be at least 50% of normal size. At the end of the operation, the RV pressure should be ≤70% than that measured in the LV. If higher, the VSD should be reopened.

57. (D) At the end of the operation, the right ventricular pressure should be ≤70% of the left ventricle. If higher, the VSD should be reopened.

58. (C) This patient has an estimated RVSP of >50 mm Hg, based on the modified Bernoulli equation. Given that her systemic BP is 65 mm Hg, her VSD should be reopened. RV systolic pressure at the conclusion of the operation should be <70% of LV systolic pressure.

59. (C) In PA–VSD, the blood supply to the lungs is entirely from the systemic arterial circulation. These include the ductus arteriosus, multiple systemic-to-pulmonary collateral arteries, occasionally a coronary artery, and plexuses of bronchial or pleural arteries. Ductal and collateral sources may be present in the same patient but rarely in the same lung.

The caliber of the central pulmonary arteries appears to be directly related to the amount of blood flow present through that segment. When the ductus or collateral arteries connect proximally to the central pulmonary arteries (as in this patient), the pulmonary arteries may be mildly hypoplastic or even normal in size. When multiple collateral arteries are present more distally, the central pulmonary arteries are usually hypoplastic.

60. (A) In pulmonary atresia with VSD, the sinus node is normal. The AV node occupies its normal position within the triangle of Koch. The nonbranching proximal portion of the His bundle penetrates the central fibrous body and lies along the left ventricular aspect of the posteroinferior rim of the VSD.

61. (E) Hypercyanotic spells constitute a medical, and possibly surgical, emergency. Treatment is directed toward lowering impedance to pulmonary flow and further increasing systemic vascular resistance. Typical treatment includes administration of supplemental oxygen, volume expansion, β-blockade, and sedation with morphine or ketamine. If needed, vasopressors (such as phenylephrine) can be used to increase systemic vascular resistance and decrease the relative ratio between pulmonary and systemic resistance. Occasionally, emergent surgical palliation or repair is required.

To prevent such spells, dehydration should be avoided; hence, making the patient NPO after midnight and starting an IV at 7:00 AM or performing phlebotomy to decrease Hgb to <14 before starting the IV are incorrect. Using a general anesthesia-inducing agent that decreases systemic vascular resistance more than PVR is the inverse of what is advisable. Starting an esmolol drip as soon as the procedure starts is not a bad choice, *per se,* because β-blockade is used to treat a hypercyanotic spell. However, making the patient NPO after midnight, starting IV fluid when NPO starts, and using a topical anesthetic such as EMLA before attempting vascular access is better because such measures can help prevent a spell, rather than treat a spell once it has started.

62. (E) Waterston shunts (anastomosis of the ascending aorta to the right pulmonary artery) or Potts shunts (descending aorta to the left pulmonary artery) may result in pulmonary artery distortion with consequent inconsistent transmission of flow and pressure to the pulmonary arterial bed. Pulmonary arterial stenosis and/or pulmonary vascular disease preclude routine use of these palliative procedures.

The catheterization data demonstrate a significant gradient between the MPA and the RPA. The patient may or

may not benefit from sildenafil; further testing with inhaled NO would help make such a determination. She does not have evidence of a left-to-right shunt based upon her SpO$_2$ measurements. At this point, she does not have evidence of RV–PA conduit stenosis as the RV-to-MPA systolic gradient is <10 mm Hg. Her dyspnea on exertion more likely is due to her pulmonary vascular disease than her mild LV diastolic dysfunction (LVEDP = 10 mm Hg).

63. (E) Some newborns with TOF with absent pulmonary valve may be asymptomatic with only mild cyanosis and no findings of heart failure. Patients with TOF and absent pulmonary valve usually have some degree of RVOT obstruction, caused predominantly by a ring of tissue at the level where the pulmonary valve leaflets would be expected rather than the infundibulum. As PVR drops in early infancy, a net left-to-right shunt can develop with pathophysiology of a VSD. These patients may require minimal medical intervention and undergo elective surgical correction at a later age. Other newborns can present with respiratory failure. In the most serious cases, central bronchial compression from massively dilated pulmonary arteries can result in respiratory failure despite conventional mechanical ventilation. In this case, respiratory distress may be improved by placing the patient prone to suspend the pulmonary arteries off the airways.

64. (D) This patient demonstrates evidence of critically restricted antegrade flow to the lungs. Given a prenatal diagnosis of TOF, it is reasonable at this point to start prostaglandin to reopen the ductus arteriosus. Once he is stabilized, he can be considered for either total repair or a systemic-to-pulmonary shunt. While most newborns with TOF do not have ductal-dependent pulmonary blood flow and may be followed without specific early intervention, this patient demonstrates that he is "ductal dependent." PGE1 should be started without delay. Then other studies, such as echocardiogram, can be performed. He should not go to surgery before attempts at medical stabilization have been made.

65. (C) All patients with TOF demonstrate anterior and cephalad deviation of the outlet septum. The degree and nature of this deviation determine the severity of subpulmonic obstruction, the size of the VSD, and the degree of aortic override. In virtually all patients with severe infundibular obstruction, there is an associated large, nonrestrictive VSD and a prominent overriding aorta. In this case, it is very uncommon to have a restrictive VSD. Among other findings, a large conal branch, or accessory left anterior descending artery, is seen in ≤15% of hearts. A left SVC is found in ~10% of patients.

66. (C) A truly continuous murmur is uncommon in truncus arteriosus. When present, it usually suggests pulmonary artery ostial stenosis. Continuous murmurs are common in patients with PA/VSD. Patients with PA/VSD can have either a patent ductus arteriosus or systemic collateral arteries to the pulmonary arteries. Because the differential diagnosis of truncus arteriosus includes this lesion, a continuous murmur is strongly suggestive of pulmonary atresia rather than of truncus arteriosus.

67. (E) In truncus arteriosus, the left coronary artery tends to arise from the left posterolateral truncal surface and the right coronary artery from the right anterolateral surface. The left anterior descending coronary artery frequently is relatively small and displaced leftward. The conal branch of the right coronary artery is usually prominent and supplies several large branches to the right ventricular outflow tract.

The posterior descending coronary artery arises from the left circumflex artery (left coronary dominance) in 25% to 30% of truncus arteriosus patients. Anomalies of coronary ostial origin are common, involving 37% to 49% of patients.

68. (A) Patients with truncus arteriosus are at risk of having pulmonary vascular obstructive disease developing at an early age, and this has provided the major impetus for early surgical correction. For patients presenting beyond infancy, PVR must be assessed to select the best treatment.

Patients with truncus arteriosus who have two pulmonary arteries and a pulmonary arteriolar resistance >8 units·m^2 are at high operative risk. In most centers, corrective surgery is not offered to most of these patients. Some centers might offer repair to children who are <2 years of age and whose resistance decreases <8 units·m^2 with vasoreactivity testing. In a child of 6 years, unfortunately, pulmonary artery changes are irreversible.

Cardiac transplantation is not a good option because this patient will have irreversible obstructive pulmonary vascular disease.

69. (A) The pulmonary arteries most commonly arise from the left posterolateral aspect of the truncus arteriosus, a small distance above the truncal valve. Type I truncus arteriosus is observed in ~50% to 65% of patients, type II in 30% to 45%, and type III in 5% to 10%.

The truncal valve is tricuspid in ~70%, quadricuspid in ~20%, and bicuspid in ~10%.

A right aortic arch with mirror-image brachiocephalic branching is associated fairly commonly with truncus arteriosus, occurring in up to 35% of patients.

IAA occurs relatively frequently (~10% to 20% of patients). It is frequently associated with DiGeorge syndrome.

Among other associated anomalies, a secundum atrial septal defect has been noted in ~10% to 20% of patients, an aberrant subclavian artery in ~5% to 10%, a persistent LSVC draining into the coronary sinus in ~5% to 10%, and mild tricuspid stenosis in ~6%.

70. (E) IAA in the setting of truncus arteriosus is frequently associated with DiGeorge syndrome (chromosome 22q11 deletion).

71. (C) This child is younger than 2 years of age. His PVR decreases to <8 units·m^2 when 100% oxygen is breathed. In such young patients, surgery may still be offered if the parents are willing to accept a higher surgical risk because it is possible that the increased resistances may result from arteriolar or medial smooth muscle hypertrophy and

vasoconstriction rather than advanced intimal occlusive disease. These changes may be reversible.

72. (C) The second heart sound usually is loud and single in truncus arteriosus. The occasionally heard split second sound in these patients may be caused by delayed closure of some of the cusps of the abnormal truncal valve.

73. (D) Corrective surgery for truncus arteriosus is preferred in the first weeks of life. Delay of operation runs the risk of ischemia of the hypertrophied ventricle secondary to desaturated blood at a low diastolic perfusion pressure (caused by runoff through the pulmonary arteries as well as "aortic" insufficiency, if present). Repair of truncus at 6 to 12 months of age carries a mortality rate twice that for repair between 6 weeks and 6 months. Pulmonary vascular obstructive disease also can develop early, which provides additional impetus for correction in the first few months of life.

The preferred operation is complete repair during the neonatal period. Although techniques of repair that do not include an extracardiac conduit have been described, most prefer a valved conduit when complete repair is performed because of the presence of pulmonary hypertension.

The presence of a regurgitant truncal valve is almost always amenable to various repair techniques, and replacement is rarely required in the neonatal period. If recurrent truncal valve incompetence occurs, repair or replacement of the truncal valve can be performed at the time of reoperation for conduit replacement.

74. (D) Asymmetric congenital mitral stenosis, with unbalanced cord attachment, is often termed parachute mitral valve. In the more common type, there are two papillary muscles. However, the valve is parachute like with unbalanced chordae predominantly attached to one papillary muscle, mimicking the appearance of a classic parachute mitral valve. Less common are valves with hypoplastic, fused, or single papillary muscles and focalized cord attachments (the so-called classic parachute mitral valve).

75. (B) In this rare condition, also known as "hammock valve," the mitral valve leaflets are thickened and chordae are markedly shortened or absent. The leaflets insert directly to the papillary muscles or to the posterior ventricular wall, resulting in limited mitral valve excursion, stenosis, and insufficiency. An abnormal band of fibrous tissue often extends along the free margin of one or both valve leaflets, thus tethering the leaflets and papillary muscles.

76. (A) It is common, after surgical relief of mitral valve stenosis, for pulmonary hypertension to persist. In this vignette, physical examination findings are consistent with pulmonary hypertension and mitral valve regurgitation. The echocardiogram documents a mitral inflow gradient of 5 mm Hg, making residual mitral stenosis or an unrecognized supramitral ring unlikely. Also, the valve was repaired through an atrial approach, making an unrecognized ring very unlikely. The pulmonary vein Doppler is not suggestive of pulmonary vein stenosis.

77. (D) A cleft of the anterior mitral valve leaflet is rare and associated with significant mitral insufficiency presenting in infancy or young children. It may also occur as an isolated defect in asymptomatic individuals. In isolated cleft, the atrioventricular septum is intact, and the left ventricular outflow tract is not elongated. The valve is somewhat dysplastic, as the cleft edges usually are thickened and rolled. The cleft is directed anteriorly toward the outflow septum, as opposed to an atrioventricular canal defect where the cleft is more posteriorly directed toward the inlet septum.

In isolated cleft of the mitral valve, the papillary muscles are generally normal. In most cases, chordae attach to the papillary muscles. There may be accessory chords that attach to the membranous and muscular septum. In some cases of complete cleft, accessory chords are absent, and the anterior leaflet is usually flail and grossly insufficient. Associated left ventricular outflow tract obstruction may be caused by the accessory chords.

The mitral annulus is commonly dilated. The most commonly associated congenital heart anomalies include ASDs, VSDs, and transposition of the great arteries.

78. (A) Management of young infants and children with moderate mitral insufficiency remains primarily medical, including diuretics and afterload-reducing agents such as angiotensin-converting enzyme inhibitors. Some patients may require antiarrhythmic medication for atrial arrhythmias as well. Platelet antagonists or anticoagulation may be used in patients with atrial thrombosis (which develops secondary to severe left atrial enlargement and/or atrial fibrillation).

Patients with severe mitral insufficiency and heart failure unresponsive to medical management require surgical management.

79. (D) The physical examination findings are suggestive of MVP. While usually innocuous, there is a small subset of patients who may be at risk for sudden cardiac death. MVP patients with the following conditions are restricted to low-intensity competitive sports only (class 1A): arrhythmogenic mediated syncope; repetitive nonsustained or sustained supraventricular tachycardia or frequent/complex ventricular tachyarrhythmias on ambulatory Holter monitoring; color Doppler evidence of severe mitral regurgitation; left ventricular ejection fraction <50%. Otherwise, MVP patients are permitted participation in all competitive sports.

80. (C) In neonates with critical aortic stenosis and a small left ventricle, therapeutic direction requires a decision regarding adequacy of the left heart to support a two-ventricle circulation. Several studies have addressed methods of quantitatively assessing adequacy of the left heart to handle the entire systemic circulation. Infants with non–apex-forming left ventricle, small aortic annulus (<5 mm), and small mitral valve annulus (<9 mm) may have improved survival with Norwood-type palliation or cardiac transplant than with treatment strategies to achieve a two-ventricle circulation.

Rhodes et al. developed a predictive equation for success of two-ventricle management plan in neonates with critical aortic stenosis. The parameters that were most predictive of success or failure included aortic root dimension indexed to body surface area, the ratio of the long axis of the left ventricle to the long axis of the heart, and the indexed mitral valve area. In a prospective multicenter analysis performed by the Congenital Heart Surgeons Society, a regression equation was used to predict 5-year survival probability with Norwood-type palliation versus two-ventricle approach. Discriminating parameters included age, aortic valve *Z*-score, grade of EFE, diameter of ascending aorta, presence of significant tricuspid valve regurgitation, and left ventricular length *Z*-score. Significant retrograde flow in the distal aortic arch through the patent ductus arteriosus is also associated with lower likelihood of success with a two-ventricle approach.

81. (D) The case describes aortic stenosis or subaortic stenosis. The systolic ejection murmur is loudest at the mid-left sternal border and radiates to the upper sternal borders and into the suprasternal notch. A systolic click is rare, which helps to differentiate subvalvular aortic stenosis from valvular aortic stenosis. The left ventricular impulse may be hyperdynamic, and associated findings of aortic regurgitation and/or mitral valve regurgitation may be present.

82. (D) The American College of Cardiology/American Heart Association guidelines for management of aortic stenosis recommend the following:

- Asymptomatic children and young adults with Doppler mean gradient >40 mm Hg be considered for cardiac catheterization and possible balloon valvuloplasty.
- Patients who desire to participate in competitive sports or are contemplating pregnancy and have Doppler mean gradient >30 mm Hg should be considered for catheterization and possible valvuloplasty.
  - If the catheter-measured peak-to-peak gradient is >60 mm Hg, balloon valvuloplasty is indicated.
  - If the patient desires to play competitive sports or become pregnant, balloon valvuloplasty is indicated if the peak-to-peak gradient is >50 mm Hg.
- Patients with symptoms (angina, syncope, dyspnea on exertion) or ischemic or repolarization changes on rest or exercise ECG should have valvuloplasty if the peak-to-peak gradient is >50 mm Hg.
- Valvuloplasty is not recommended for asymptomatic patients with peak-to-peak gradients <40 mm Hg unless cardiac output is impaired.

83. (A) Tissue Doppler imaging (TDI) may be helpful in the assessment of systolic and diastolic dysfunction in patients with aortic stenosis. Doppler parameters derived from mitral or pulmonary vein flow have been used for estimation of left ventricular filling pressure, but limitations to these measurements are dependent on loading conditions and heart rate. TDI directly measures myocardial velocities, typically the systolic and diastolic mitral annular velocities. This practice allows quantification of systolic long-axis function and diastolic function.

In patients with aortic stenosis, the ratio of early mitral inflow velocity (E) to early diastolic mitral annular velocity

(E') correlates with the LV end-diastolic pressure, thereby providing a clinically useful noninvasive method of assessing diastolic dysfunction. Additionally, measurement of the mitral annular systolic velocity (S') by TDI may demonstrate systolic long-axis dysfunction in patients with aortic stenosis who have otherwise normal ejection fractions.

Because longitudinally oriented fibers are present in the subendocardial region, and the subendocardium is most susceptible to ischemia in patients with aortic stenosis, these fibers are at greater risk than the circumferentially oriented fibers. Long-axis dysfunction therefore might precede transverse axis dysfunction.

84. (E) The 36th Bethesda Conference Task Force recommendations for competitive athletics defines aortic stenosis severity as follows (peak instantaneous gradient [PIG]):

- Mild: peak-to-peak gradient <30 mm Hg, mean Doppler gradient <25 mm Hg, or PIG <40 mm Hg
- Moderate: peak-to-peak gradient 30 to 50 mm Hg, mean Doppler gradient 25 to 40 mm Hg, or PIG 40 to 70 mm Hg
- Severe: peak-to-peak gradient >50 mm Hg, mean Doppler gradient >40 mm Hg, or PIG >70 mm Hg

Patients with mild stenosis, if asymptomatic and possessing normal exercise tolerance, are permitted to participate in all competitive sports. Patients with severe aortic stenosis should not participate in any competitive sports.

Asymptomatic patients with moderate aortic stenosis, absent or mild left ventricular hypertrophy, absence of repolarization abnormality on ECG, and a normal exercise test may participate in sports with a low static component and low-to-moderate dynamic component (such as golf, bowling, baseball/softball, and volleyball).

If such patients have no history of supraventricular tachycardia or ventricular tachyarrhythmias at rest or with exercise, they may participate in sports with moderate static component and low dynamic component (such as diving, archery, equestrian, and motorcycling).

For aortic valve stenosis patients who also have aortic regurgitation, these recommendations must be considered in concert with the Task Force recommendations for aortic regurgitation.

For details regarding indications for balloon aortic valvuloplasty, please refer to **Answer 82**.

85. (C) Subaortic stenosis is a lesion that occasionally progresses rapidly. However, the rate of progression of mild subvalvular aortic stenosis is variable, and the obstruction may remain mild for many years. Factors associated with more rapid progression of obstruction include higher initial pressure gradient, short distance between the obstructive lesion and the aortic valve, and anterior mitral valve leaflet involvement.

Left ventricular hypertrophy and myocardial fibrosis are seen in patients with aortic stenosis. EFE and papillary muscle infarction can be seen in infants with severe aortic stenosis but typically are not present in mild forms of disease. Myocardial fibrosis may also be present in asymptomatic children with hemodynamically moderate congenital aortic stenosis.

Traditionally, Doppler estimates of pressure gradients across stenotic valves have been used for estimation of severity of obstruction. These measurements are dependent on loading conditions, heart rate, and other factors.

For infants with severe or critical aortic valve stenosis who are thought to be candidates for two-ventricle circulation, initial therapy usually entails balloon valvuloplasty or surgical valvotomy. For critical neonatal aortic stenosis, open surgical valvotomy or percutaneous balloon valvuloplasty procedures may be performed. Balloon valvuloplasty is the preferred procedure in most centers. Open surgical valvotomy may result in higher likelihood of residual or recurrent stenosis, whereas balloon valvuloplasty may be associated with a higher incidence of important aortic regurgitation.

86. (D) This patient has a history and physical examination concerning for a ductal-dependent lesion, most likely coarctation of the aorta. Prostaglandin E1 should be started immediately. Medical therapy and further imaging studies should not take priority until PGE1 has been started.

87. (D) This Doppler profile is suggestive of aortic arch obstruction, consistent with coarctation of the aorta. Children who present in infancy are much more likely than older children to have complex coarctation (associated lesions). Approximately 50% of patients who require surgical correction before 12 months of age have a simple coarctation. Among the remaining ~50% with complex coarctation, a large VSD is the most common associated lesion. VSDs associated with coarctation include the perimembranous, muscular, or malalignment types. A malalignment VSD may occur with posterior deviation of the conal septum and left ventricular outflow tract obstruction. Such subvalvular aortic stenosis is particularly common in the critically ill infant who presents with coarctation and VSD.

A bicuspid aortic valve occurs in up to 85% of patients with coarctation, and the valve may be stenotic or the annulus hypoplastic. Mitral stenosis also occurs in patients with coarctation and may be caused by a supravalvar mitral ring, thickening and dysplasia of the mitral leaflets, short dysplastic chordae tendineae, or the presence of a single "parachute" papillary muscle. The association of multiple left-sided obstructive lesions with coarctation has been referred to as Shone syndrome.

88. (A) Coarctation more commonly presents in an asymptomatic child as upper extremity hypertension or a heart murmur. Coarctation repair is generally recommended at 2 to 3 years of age in asymptomatic children without severe upper extremity hypertension. The risk for late recurrence of coarctation appears to be increased when repair is performed on a patient younger than 1 year of age. Studies demonstrate that the normal descending aorta has attained ~50% of its final adult diameter by 3 years of age. Because significant hemodynamic obstruction at rest occurs only if the aortic diameter is reduced by ≥50%, restenosis following coarctation repair after 3 years of age should be uncommon. Furthermore, because of an increased risk for residual hypertension and early atherosclerotic cardiovascular disease, elective repair should not be delayed into late childhood and adolescence.

89. (E) This patient has evidence of Turner syndrome and coarctation. An echocardiogram is warranted. Her left arm systolic blood pressure is 20 mm Hg higher than her right arm or lower extremities. This indicates that she likely has an anomalous right subclavian artery distal to the coarctation.

90. (B) A normal abdominal aortic Doppler profile does not rule out coarctation of the aorta. If the ductus arteriosus is patent, the pulsed wave Doppler profile can appear normal.

91. (A) Turner syndrome is associated with a 45,XO genotype.

92. (D) Exercise-induced upper extremity hypertension is usually associated with an increase in the coarctation pressure gradient during exercise. This is believed to be secondary to an increase in aortic blood flow across a relatively nondistensible coarctation repair site. Patients with exercise hypertension, but without significant anatomic stenosis following coarctation repair, may benefit from β-blocker therapy with a decrease in exercise hypertension and coarctation gradient.

The long-term prognosis following repair of coarctation may be adversely affected by systemic arterial hypertension and an associated increase in premature atherosclerotic disease. Systolic and diastolic hypertension may occur at rest, most commonly in patients whose coarctation repair is delayed beyond late childhood. The risk for late hypertension may be as high as 10% to 20%, even when the coarctation is repaired in infancy. The cause of late postoperative hypertension in patients without a residual resting coarctation gradient may relate to anatomic and functional changes in the arterial vasculature proximal to the coarctation.

93. (D) This patient is suffering from inadequate tissue delivery to end organs, as evidenced by his acidosis, elevated liver function studies, and elevated creatinine. Matching of oxygen delivery to changes in oxygen consumption is more effective through interventions in total cardiac output or hemoglobin concentration than by precise manipulation of Qp/Qs balance. In this case, the patient is relatively anemic (Hgb 12 g/dL), and therefore, transfusion is warranted.

For those patients in whom Qp/Qs is elevated and systemic perfusion is compromised, therapy with milrinone might be warranted. Milrinone, however, has also been shown to reduce PVR and carries the undesired risk of increasing Qp/Qs. Furthermore, milrinone could result in significant hypotension in a patient already at risk for decreased perfusion.

Increasing the amount of inspired oxygen or starting nitric oxide both could increase the pulmonary blood flow at the expense of systemic perfusion. Increasing the ventilator rate from 24 to 30 could drive down pCO_2, which could increase pulmonary blood flow at the expense of systemic perfusion and would not be as helpful as increasing the hemoglobin concentration.

94. (A) Anterior malalignment VSDs are associated with varying degrees of overriding of the pulmonary annulus into the right ventricle. With increasing degrees of override, the anatomy becomes more and more similar to DORV with subpulmonary defect (Taussig–Bing anomaly). The subaortic stenosis caused by the anterior malalignment of the infundibular septum is frequently associated with aortic arch hypoplasia, coarctation, or even complete interruption of the aortic arch.

95. (D) Consistent with the normal atrial anatomy, the sinus and AV nodes are in their usual locations.

The normal conus is subpulmonary, left sided, and anterior, and it prevents fibrous continuity between the pulmonary and tricuspid valve rings. In d-TGA, the infundibulum is usually subaortic, right sided, and anterior, and it prevents fibrous continuity between the aortic and tricuspid valve rings. d-TGA is hypothesized to result from the abnormal growth and development of the subaortic infundibulum with concurrent absence of growth of the subpulmonary infundibulum.

With intact ventricular septum, the entire septum is usually a relatively straight structure and does not have the sigmoid curvature typical of the normal heart.

Dynamic obstruction is rare in the neonate with elevated pulmonary artery resistance or in the presence of a nonrestrictive ductus arteriosus, as the left ventricle pumps against systemic systolic pressure and retains "normal" geometry.

Following atrial-level repair, frequently there is a small to moderate systolic pressure difference across the subpulmonary outflow tract.

96. (C) In the infant with d-TGA/large VSD and severe left ventricular outflow obstruction, there may be markedly restricted pulmonary blood flow and severe hypoxemia. In some neonates, a palliative systemic-to-pulmonary arterial shunt may be performed, with intracardiac correction carried out at a later age. Alternatively, corrective surgery can be performed in early infancy. However, none of the surgical corrections listed among the answer choices would be appropriate for this patient.

One appropriate corrective surgery in this case would be the Rastelli operation, a combination of intraventricular repair and placement of an extracardiac right ventricle-to-pulmonary artery conduit. The Rastelli repair has been considered the most appropriate operation for d-TGA with large VSD and extensive LVOTO because it achieves complete bypass of the LVOTO and an anatomic correction of the transposition pathology.

An alternative technique, termed REV (*Réparation à l'étage ventriculaire*), could potentially be used. The REV procedure appears to have some advantages over the Rastelli operation: application in younger patients, avoidance of prosthetic extracardiac conduit, and avoidance of intracardiac tunnel obstruction. This operation involves performing a high, anterior right ventricular incision and a radical excision of the outlet septum to create an unobstructed anterior right ventricular cavity; establishing a short and direct intraventricular tunnel from the LV to the aorta; closure of the pulmonary artery orifice; and reimplantation of the transected pulmonary artery directly onto the right ventricular outflow cavity without a prosthetic conduit.

Finally, posterior translocation of the aortic root and coronary arteries can be performed, with enlargement of the left ventricular outflow tract, with conduit placement from the right ventricle to the pulmonary arteries anteriorly, as originally described by Nikaidoh and advocated by others.

97. (C) In ccTGA, the interventricular septum has a sagittal position. With ventricular inversion, both its surfaces and ventricular bundle branches are inverted, and thus the sequence of initial activation is oriented from right to left and usually in a more superior and anterior direction. This results in a reversal of the normal Q-wave pattern in the precordial leads: Q waves are present in the right precordial leads but are absent in the left precordial leads. The electrocardiographic changes identified in patients with ccTGA include reversal of Q-wave distribution in the precordial leads with QS complexes in the right precordial leads, large Q waves in leads III and aVF, and left axis deviation.

98. (A) The AV node is located along the anterior aspect of the atrioventricular ring, near the atrial septum.

99. (D) Varying degrees of left ventricular outflow obstruction may be observed in patients with DORV. Subaortic stenosis appears to result from extensive hypertrophy of the aortic conus and conal septum. In addition, subaortic stenosis has resulted from marked malalignment of the conal septum. With compression of the aortic outflow tract and reduction of aortic flow, there may be secondary hypoplasia of the aortic annulus and the aorta. Thus, an association has been described with interruption of the aortic arch or coarctation of the aorta in patients with DORV and subpulmonary VSD. Coarctation of the aorta, however, has also been described in instances of subaortic, doubly committed, and remote VSD.

Complete correction of DORV depends on the complexity of the intracardiac anatomy. Because of the complexity of intracardiac repair of these anomalies, it may be necessary to palliate some infants and small children who become symptomatic in the first year of life.

In this case, mitral valve straddling indicates that complete two-ventricle repair will be impossible. To establish a stable source of systemic perfusion, aortic arch reconstruction will be necessary. Therefore, a Norwood-type palliation is indicated.

100. (B) For patients with DORV and subpulmonary VSD, physiology is that of complete transposition of the great arteries. Therefore, the arterial switch operation appears to be the procedure of choice and can be performed in the neonatal period. The VSD should be closed at the time of the arterial switch.

101. (D) Patients with subaortic VSDs and pulmonary stenosis display varying degrees of cyanosis. Their clinical presentations are similar to that in TOF. When the pulmonary stenosis is severe, early cyanosis, failure to thrive, exertional dyspnea, and polycythemia may be present. The precordium may show evidence of a right ventricular impulse at the left sternal border, and a prominent systolic thrill is often palpable over the upper left sternal border. This is associated with a grade 4 to 5/6 systolic ejection murmur, which radiates into the lung fields. The first heart sound is normal, and the second heart sound is usually single. A third heart sound may be noted at the cardiac apex. In older children, clubbing also may be evident.

102. (A) Patients with DORV with subpulmonic VSD and no pulmonary stenosis typically present clinically with features resembling those in d-TGA with VSD. Commonly, these patients present with cyanosis and heart failure in early infancy. Patients in this group who have associated coarctation of the aorta may present in infancy with heart failure, cyanosis, and diminished or absent femoral pulses.

Like patients with TGA, these patients exhibit severe failure to thrive and may have frequent respiratory tract infections. Typically, there is severe cyanosis. A precordial bulge and right ventricular impulse are present at the left sternal border. A grade 2 to 3/6 high-pitched systolic murmur may be present at the upper left sternal border. When PS is present, a systolic thrill may be present, and the murmur is loud (grade 3 to 4/6). The second heart sound is loud and single because of the proximity of the aorta to the chest wall. With increased pulmonary flow, an apical diastolic rumble may be present.

103. (D) This patient has physiology similar to d-TGA and, as such, would benefit from increased mixing at the atrial level. Increasing the rate of PGE1 would not help, as the ductus arteriosus is already patent. Nitric oxide would potentially decrease PVR and increase pulmonary blood flow, but would not have an effect on mixing such as would a septostomy. Diuresis with furosemide would not help mixing. The patient may require surgery, but it would be inappropriate to wait several weeks without first doing a septostomy.

104. (D) Systemic outflow tract obstruction in the heart with a functional single ventricle promotes myocardial hypertrophy, and this has been shown to be an unequivocal risk factor for poor outcome at the Fontan procedure.

105. (A) Pulmonary arterial banding will reduce pulmonary flow and protect the pulmonary arterioles from obstructive pulmonary arteriopathy, but may induce or aggravate subaortic stenosis due to hypertrophy of the subaortic conus. However, banding may be appropriate in the setting of DORV with multiple muscular VSDs or a remote VSD.

106. (B) DILV with a right-sided hypoplastic subaortic right ventricle is at risk for failing a two-ventricle–type surgical repair. In this case, the patient has a restrictive bulboventricular foramen and severe subaortic stenosis. Therefore, systemic perfusion is at risk and the infant needs a stable systemic blood supply. Of the choices, an aortopulmonary anastomosis (DKS) procedure is most likely to result in a stable, long-term systemic blood supply.

CHAPTER 2

Pulmonary artery banding is not the best option because it can set the stage for progressive ventricular hypertrophy and obstruction in patients who have naturally occurring mild restriction at the VSD.

PA banding with arch augmentation does not address the problem of subaortic obstruction.

107. (D) The arterial catheter is injecting the BT shunt. The venous catheter takes the course Right IJ → SVC → common atrium → common ventricle → aorta.

108. (A) The arterial catheter takes the course femoral artery → descending aorta → aortic arch → BT shunt.

109. (E) Clinical suspicion is high for a partial pericardial defect. The best way to demonstrate a defect of the pericardium is by magnetic resonance imaging.

Partial or total absence of the pericardium is a rare congenital anomaly that may be associated with significant symptoms. 80% of defects occur on the left side. They appear to be secondary to premature atrophy of the left duct of Cuvier during embryologic development. Most cases of pericardial defect are identified incidentally. Symptomatic cases are rare. Symptoms, if present, may include syncope, chest pain, arrhythmias, and death. Severe symptoms have been described secondary to herniation or incarceration of the left atrial appendage through the defect, torsion of the great arteries, or constriction of a coronary artery at the rim of the defect.

The techniques of magnetic resonance imaging and computer-assisted tomography are very useful in demonstrating the pericardial defect. By MRI, a tongue of pulmonary tissue between the aorta and the main pulmonary artery is a common finding. MRI is ideal for evaluating the pericardium and is the procedure of choice to identify this diagnosis.

Chest radiography in complete absence of the pericardium may demonstrate leftward displacement of the cardiac border with a posterior bulging of the heart. Herniation of the left atrial appendage may be apparent on the chest radiograph, where the herniated appendage resembles an enlarged main pulmonary artery.

Electrocardiography frequently may be normal, but may also show right bundle branch block or other abnormalities of conduction.

By echocardiography, the right ventricle may appear enlarged, excessive cardiac motion may be apparent, and the left atrial appendage may appear prominent. Importantly, the actual defect in the pericardium cannot be imaged by echocardiography.

Cardiac catheterization is of little diagnostic value other than to document coexisting heart disease. Thoracoscopy may be necessary to confirm the diagnosis.

110. (B) The greatest risk for sudden death in children with HCM appears to be associated with one or more of the following clinical risk markers: (a) prior cardiac arrest or sustained ventricular tachycardia; (b) family history of one or more premature HCM-related deaths, particularly if sudden and multiple; (c) syncope; and (d) massive degrees of LV hypertrophy (maximum wall thickness ≥30 mm).

In clinical practice, prospective screening of HCM family members to ascertain affected or unaffected genetic status usually takes place without access to DNA analysis and is performed primarily with 2D echocardiography and 12-lead ECG, as well as history-taking and physical examination.

The traditional recommended strategy for screening first-degree relatives calls for such evaluations on a 12- to 18-month basis, usually beginning at least by age 12. If these studies do not show evidence of LV hypertrophy by 21 years of age, echocardiographic screening can be performed every 5 years.

111. (C) HCM is an autosomal dominant trait.

112. (C) The greatest risk for sudden death in children with HCM appears to be associated with one or more of the following clinical risk markers: (a) prior cardiac arrest or sustained ventricular tachycardia; (b) family history of one or more premature HCM-related deaths, particularly if sudden and multiple; (c) syncope; and (d) massive degrees of LV hypertrophy (maximum wall thickness ≥30 mm). The risk of sudden death increases when septal thickness is >20 mm.

For any patient who has a history of aborted cardiac death, an ICD should be placed as primary prevention. Also, since the patient's septum is severely hypertrophied, and a significant gradient is present with associated symptoms, a myectomy should also be performed.

113. (E) The subaortic gradient and systolic ejection heart murmur in HCM are dynamic. They can be reduced or abolished by interventions that decrease myocardial contractility (e.g., β-blocking adrenergic drugs) or increase ventricular volume or arterial pressure (e.g., squatting, isometric handgrip, or phenylephrine administration). They can be augmented by interventions that decrease arterial pressure or ventricular volume (e.g., the Valsalva maneuver or administration of nitroglycerin) or that increase contractility, such as standing, amyl nitrite inhalation, administration of isoproterenol, or exercise.

114. (C) Sudden death due to HCM occurs most commonly during adolescence and young adulthood (12 to 35 years of age) and rarely before 10 years of age. These events are due to primary ventricular tachycardia and/or ventricular fibrillation. Most patients die while sedentary or during normal or modest physical exertion. Importantly, however, an important proportion die suddenly during or just after vigorous activity.

HCM is the most common cause of sudden cardiac death in the young, including competitive athletes. Therefore, standard recommendations are to disqualify young individuals with HCM from intense competitive sports (guidelines of the 36th Bethesda Conference).

At present, the greatest risk for sudden death in children with HCM appears to be associated with one or more of the following clinical risk markers: (a) prior cardiac arrest or sustained ventricular tachycardia; (b) family history of one or more premature HCM-related deaths, particularly if sudden and multiple; (c) syncope; and (d) massive degrees of LV hypertrophy (maximum wall thickness ≥30 mm).

Septal myectomy is performed to improve symptoms, but it is not used as a sudden death–preventative procedure. To prevent sudden death, an ICD is recommended.

115. (E) This patient is at low risk, as he is asymptomatic, has a negative family history, and a normal echocardiogram. There is at present no recommendation to limit activity or treat medically on the basis of a genetic test.

116. (D) This patient has CHF from dilated cardiomyopathy. The phosphodiesterase inhibitor milrinone increases stroke work and cardiac output. Both systemic and pulmonary vascular resistances are decreased, and the drug evokes unique lusitropic properties affecting relaxation and ventricular compliance. This drug is thought to promote increase in intracellular calcium concentration by inhibition of phosphodiesterase III.

117. (D) Nadolol is a long-acting β-blocker. Phosphodiesterase inhibitors are the treatment of choice for patients who are taking β-blocker drugs. Milrinone retains its full hemodynamic effects in the presence of β-blocker therapy. Therefore, there is no reason to change therapy.

118. (C) This vignette describes a classic presentation of Barth syndrome. Barth syndrome is an X-linked disorder characterized by skeletal myopathy, congenital dilated cardiomyopathy, short stature, and neutropenia. Affected individuals usually die early in childhood. It is diagnosed by urinalysis revealing elevated 3-methylglutaconic acid.

Typically, boys with Barth syndrome present with hypotonia and dilated cardiomyopathy, including labored breathing, poor appetite, and/or slow weight gain, typically within the first few months after birth. Another important feature of Barth syndrome is a history of bacterial infections because of neutropenia.

The gene for Barth syndrome, Tafazzin (*TAZ*), is located on chromosome Xq28. Mutations in the *TAZ* gene lead to decreased production of an enzyme required for the synthesis of cardiolipin. There is no specific treatment for Barth syndrome, but each of the individual problems can be successfully controlled, and short stature often resolves after puberty.

119. (C) Cardiac catheterization is an important part of the evaluation in patients with RCM and should be performed at the time of diagnosis. Catheterization can help differentiate between RCM and CP, although many hemodynamic features can overlap.

Both diseases typically have an early diastolic dip and subsequent plateau pattern, also called the square root sign. In classic RCM, the left ventricular end-diastolic pressure, left atrial pressure, and pulmonary capillary wedge pressure are markedly elevated and ≥4 mm Hg to 5 mm Hg (preferably 10 mm Hg) greater than the RAP and right ventricular end-diastolic pressure. In cases in which the pressures are essentially equal, volume loading may bring out the differences in pressure between the right and left sides.

120. (D) This vignette describes a classic case of Löffler endocarditis (hypereosinophilic syndrome, or HES). HES is typically seen in temperate climates and is more common in adult males. Persistent hypereosinophilia is present. HES includes persistent eosinophilia with 1,500 eosinophils/mm^3 for ≥6 months or until death with evidence of other organ involvement. Usually, in HES, various organs besides the heart are involved (lungs, bone marrow, and brain). The cause of the eosinophilia is unknown.

Cardiac histologic findings include eosinophilic myocarditis: inflammatory reaction in the small intramural coronary vessels with thrombosis and fibrinoid change, and endocardial mural thrombosis and fibrotic thickening.

The clinical picture may include weight loss, fever, cough, rash, and heart failure. Systemic embolism is frequent. Death is usually secondary to the cardiac manifestations of the disease. Therapy for the hypereosinophilia may include corticosteroids, hydroxyurea, or vincristine. Cardiac therapy has included digoxin, diuretics, afterload reduction, and anticoagulation. Surgical approaches have included mitral and/or tricuspid valve repair or replacement and excision of fibrotic endocardium.

121. (E) RCM, by definition, has small ventricular volumes with normal or near-normal systolic function. Ventricular wall thickness is usually normal. The atria are enlarged.

122. (B) It is important to realize that patients with Duchenne and Becker muscular dystrophies can have severe complications from anesthesia, including cardiac arrest. Most complications seem to be related to use of succinylcholine, a muscular relaxant that may trigger hyperkalemia. Others have been attributed to use of volatile anesthetic agents. Patients also can have a reaction similar to malignant hyperthermia, develop rhabdomyolysis, and have masseter muscle spasm.

123. (E) The characteristic electrocardiogram in Duchenne muscular dystrophy shows deep Q waves in leads I, aVL, V5, and V6, and occasionally in leads II, III, and aVF. There is often a tall right precordial R wave and an increased R/S ratio. The PR interval is shortened in many patients. Some have reported QT prolongation and QT dispersion abnormalities. Holter analysis has shown that automaticity is also affected whereby there is a resting sinus tachycardia, loss of circadian rhythm, and reduced heart rate variability in many patients with Duchenne muscular dystrophy.

There are frequent arrhythmias in older patients including ectopic atrial tachycardia, atrial fibrillation, transient second- and third-degree AV block, and more ominous ventricular tachycardias. The presence of multiform premature ventricular contractions and ventricular tachycardia on Holter monitoring portends possible sudden death owing to ventricular fibrillation.

124. (B) This vignette describes Duchenne muscular dystrophy. The cardiac examination is seldom abnormal, even in the presence of cardiomyopathy. Occasionally, third or fourth heart sound may be present. There may be neck vein distention or hepatomegaly. The examination is often distorted by chest wall deformities, especially in older patients with scoliosis.

125. (B) Of the pediatric studies reporting arrhythmias in RCM, ~15% of the patients had arrhythmias and/or conduction disturbances. Atrial flutter was the most commonly reported arrhythmia. High-grade second- and third-degree heart block were the next most commonly reported rhythm disturbances. Atrial fibrillation and atrial tachycardias, Wolff–Parkinson–White syndrome with supraventricular tachycardia, symptomatic sinus bradycardia requiring pacing, and ventricular tachycardia and torsade were also reported.

126. (D) End diastole—in the setting of interatrial communication, maximum left-to-right shunting occurs during diastole when all four cardiac chambers are in communication.

127. (C) The examination findings are highly suggestive of Holt–Oram syndrome, a rare disorder caused by mutations in the *TBX5* gene. Holt–Oram syndrome is estimated to affect 1 in 100,000 individuals, and is autosomal dominant in inheritance. *TBX5* plays a role in regulating cardiac septation as well as the development of bones in the arm and hand. This condition is characterized by upper limb anomalies, secundum atrial septal defects, and AV conduction abnormalities. About 75% of children with Holt–Oram syndrome have cardiac defects.

128. (B) Left AV valve regurgitation is the most common reason for surgical revision in partial and complete AVSD. Left AV valve regurgitation occurs in 10% to 15% of patients with repaired partial AVSD. Risk factors for reoperation include significant residual left AV valve regurgitation at the time of initial repair, the presence of a severely dysplastic valve, and failure to close the cleft in the anterior (septal) leaflet.

129. (A) Most infants with complete AV septal defect will inevitably experience heart failure symptoms, as there is significant left-to-right shunting across the atrial and ventricular septa. Pulmonary overcirculation is the rule. When patients do not develop these symptoms, often the cause is premature pulmonary vascular occlusive disease (PVOD). This limits the degree of left-to-right shunting, and affected children may appear relatively well. However, PVOD will lead to pulmonary arterial hypertension which can be irreversible, ultimately leading to hypoxemia, right heart failure, and death.

130. (A) Except for prolonged intra-atrial conduction time, other intracardiac measurements are usually normal in complete AV septal (canal) defects, including sinus node function, AV node function, His–Purkinje conduction time, and refractory periods.

131. (A) Infants with a posterior malaligned VSD are at risk for aortic valve hypoplasia and stenosis, and they frequently have aortic arch obstruction (coarctation or interrupted aortic arch). One must evaluate the subaortic region, aortic valve, ascending aorta, and aortic arch very carefully in these infants. Infants with non-critical obstruction (such as mild coarctation) will often present with earlier symptoms

of heart failure and pulmonary overcirculation, as the arch obstruction causes increased flow across the VSD. This is likely present in the infant in this vignette.

If critical arch obstruction is evident, affected infants can die after closure of the ductus arteriosus. This patient appears unlikely to be critically ill following ductal closure, but careful attention must be paid to the arch in any case.

132. (B) Indications for closure of hemodynamically insignificant but persistent perimembranous VSD in older children include the development of progressive aortic regurgitation due to prolapse of an aortic valve leaflet into the defect, development of an RV muscle bundle (double chamber RV), or recurrent bacterial endocarditis. There is no specific age by which a VSD requires closure as long as they have not developed any of the above complications.

133. (C) When a child who is expected to develop signs of congestive heart failure secondary to a large left-to-right shunt does not, one must be cognizant of pulmonary hypertension and the potential of developing early Eisenmenger syndrome. The size and location of the VSD, along with deficient posterior rim, argues against spontaneous closure. In the modern era, misdiagnosis of large VSDs is exceedingly rare. The presence of severe pulmonary valve obstruction would present with murmur, and the dysplastic/stenotic valve would have been noted at the 3-month visit.

134. (E) Coronary sinus diverticulum. A study by Guiraundon et al. (*Am J Cardiol.* 1988;62:733–735) describes an entity of coronary sinus diverticulum that is associated with Wolff–Parkinson–White syndrome and posteroseptal accessory pathways. Intraoperatively, ~10% of patients with posteroseptal accessory pathways were found to have coronary sinus diverticula in the posteroseptal region. Conduction studies indicated that the accessory pathway is closely associated with the diverticulum and that the conduction abnormality disappears only after separation or ablation of the coronary sinus diverticulum neck.

135. (C) The following parameters generally predict a successful outcome for BDCPA:

Preoperative LVEDP of <12 mm Hg
Transpulmonary gradient of <10 mm Hg
Mean PA pressure of <16 mm Hg

Though LV dysfunction can cause an increase in LVEDP, LA pressure, and PA pressure, in most patients it is feasible to perform a BDCPA even in the presence of moderate LV dysfunction (EF 35% to 40%). Therefore, in this patient, the mean PA pressure of 20 mm Hg would be of most concern.

136. (C) Most cases are sporadic, though the other genes listed may play some role.

137. (B) Hypovolemia. All others are causes of elevated Fontan fenestration gradient.

138. (A) Type IB. In the setting of tricuspid atresia with normally related great arteries, pulmonary blood flow is dependent upon the size of the VSD, and in general with time the pulmonary or subpulmonary stenosis will be progressive as the VSD becomes smaller. On the other hand, in the setting of transposed great arteries, the systemic flow is dependent upon the size of the VSD, while pulmonary flow is typically unobstructed. Pulmonary blood flow is rarely restricted in type IIB even in the setting of pulmonary stenosis, as PVR drops resulting in greater amounts of pulmonary blood flow with time.

139. (B) When to replace the pulmonary valve in the older child or adult with repaired tetralogy of Fallot remains a topic of much investigation and debate. It is evident that severe chronic pulmonary insufficiency results in adaptive RV remodeling, which ultimately proves detrimental. Beyond a certain point of RV dilation, function decreases and becomes irreversible. Most centers consider pulmonary valve replacement in patients with progressive RV dilation or when the RV end-diastolic volume approaches 160 to 180 mL/m². Other considerations when considering PVR are degree of tricuspid regurgitation, QRS duration, formally documented exercise capacity, and biventricular function.

Surgical valve replacement is indicated in a patient with significant symptoms, RV enlargement, and/or severe QRS prolongation. QRS duration ≥180 ms and/or a rate of QRS progression of >5 msec per year over a 10-year period have been shown to predict sudden cardiac death. It is likely that replacement of the valve will result in decreased RV dilation. Surgical replacement, rather than transcatheter placement, is typically needed in a native transpulmonary patch due to the degree of dilation.

140. (D) Exercise testing should be performed given that he would like to participate in organized sports. If he has ECG changes or symptoms during testing, he should be considered for intervention. If his exercise test is normal, then he should be allowed to participate in sports with low static component and low–moderate dynamic component (such as baseball). If he met criteria for intervention, balloon valvuloplasty would be reasonable. He is not hypertensive and his aortic root measures normally, so he does not require hypertensive therapy (although this should be monitored closely).

141. (C) Systolic hypertension during exercise can be seen late after coarctation repair in patients who have no anatomical evidence of recurrent coarctation. This can occur even in patients who lack resting hypertension or a coarctation gradient. These patients can demonstrate elevated upper extremity blood pressures and elevated gradients between arm and leg with exercise. Alterations of vascular physiology may play a role in this phenomenon, as exercise increases cardiac output across a relatively inelastic aortic repair site. Patients without resting coarctation gradients or clear anatomical arch obstruction who exhibit significant exercise hypertension (such as this patient) may benefit from β-blocker therapy. In the absence of definable anatomical narrowing, invasive procedures are not indicated.

142. (C) Prosthetic patch aortoplasty has the advantage of requiring less extensive aortic mobilization, preserving intercostal arteries and avoiding a circumferential suture line. Unfortunately, it has a relatively high incidence of late aortic aneurysm formation. In one study, the presence of an aortic aneurysm was documented in 24% of patients evaluated 1 to 19 years after patch aortoplasty repair of coarctation.

143. (C) The following parameters generally predict poorer outcome for Fontan completion:

Small pulmonary artery size
PVR >4 Wood units
Preoperative pulmonary artery pressure >15 mm Hg
Presence of venovenous collaterals

144. (B) Captopril. Pharmacologic therapy during the interstage period varies among institutions. Typical classes of medications include chronic afterload reducers, diuretics, and/or digoxin. Anticoagulation is also used. Though protocols may vary, afterload reduction with an ACE inhibitor such as captopril may be considered in patients who have systemic hypertension, greater than mild AV valve regurgitation, symptoms or signs of congestive heart failure, or evidence of a pulmonary-to-systemic flow ratio (Qp/Qs) >2 in the early postoperative period. Afterload reduction must be titrated with caution to avoid diastolic hypotension that could result in impaired coronary flow. Overly aggressive afterload reduction may worsen hypoxemia secondary to excessive lowering of the Qp/Qs ratio. For patients with evidence of pulmonary overcirculation or heart failure, chronic diuretic therapy such as furosemide is indicated.

145. (C) The hemi-Fontan involves a connection of the SVC to the confluent pulmonary arteries without disconnecting the SVC from the right atrium. It is a more extensive operation than the bidirectional Glenn, however, it allows for expeditious performance of completion of the Fontan. The chief advantage of the bidirectional Glenn procedure is ease of construction, as it can even be accomplished without the use of cardiopulmonary bypass (CPB) in selected cases. The hemi-Fontan requires CPB.

146. (B) The best option would be cardiac catheterization. The patient's saturations are low, while the remainder of the clinical picture is favorable. The low saturations indicate probable presence of pulmonary arteriovenous malformations (AVMs) or venovenous collaterals. These can develop in patients with delayed completion of the Fontan due to the absence of so-called "hepatic factor" reaching the pulmonary arteries. Fontan completion should be considered, and the best next step to prepare for Fontan and also investigate the low saturations is a cardiac catheterization. CMR would likely be helpful to assess anatomical reasons for the desaturation but would not provide the hemodynamic data obtainable from a catheterization.

147. (D) One rare but important associated abnormality seen in d-TGA is juxtaposition of the atrial appendages, most often left juxtaposition of the right atrial appendage.

During a BAS, it can be mistaken (particularly if using fluoroscopy only) that the balloon is in the left atrium, when in fact it is in the right atrial appendage. If not recognized, this will result in an ineffective septostomy or potentially serious/catastrophic damage to the juxtaposed right atrial appendage.

148. (C) Patients who have undergone an arterial switch procedure who have normal ventricular function, no arrhythmias, no symptoms, and a normal exercise stress test may be cleared for all sports. Echocardiography would be the first-line testing to assess this patient's ventricular function. Stress testing would be indicated to assess for ischemia and/or inducible arrhythmias. Cardiac MRI would be beneficial to assess branch pulmonary arteries following the LeCompte maneuver, but is not indicated for sports participation clearance. Catheterization would not be indicated unless there were concerning findings on stress testing, particularly with regard to coronary ischemia.

149. (A) One key component of the anatomical repair is "training" the left ventricle to handle the workload of the systemic circulation after anatomic repair. This is accomplished via placement of a band across the pulmonary arteries, which mimics systemic afterload and conditions the LV by stimulating myocardial hypertrophy. This patient's PA band gradient is only 35 mm Hg, suggesting the LV may not be adequately trained and is at risk of failure should the anatomical repair be undertaken at this point. Adequate banding usually results in LV pressure that is >70% to 80% (or more) of systemic BP. Therefore, the band should be tightened. The ideal age at which to undertake an anatomical repair is the subject of much debate, but several series describe good results when done within the first 2 to 3 years of life. The patient is not so old that the strategy should be abandoned. Conservative management could be considered as well, though the vignette indicates that an eventual anatomic repair is planned. In order to fulfill this option, the issue of the undertrained LV needs to be addressed.

150. (D) Patients with isolated ccTGA will typically be asymptomatic in childhood and may be referred for a murmur, a loud second heart sound, or bradycardia reflecting high-degree AV block. The accentuated, often palpable, single second heart sound reflects the anteriorly positioned aortic valve. On the other hand, patients with associated lesions (large VSD, pulmonary stenosis, or systemic AV valve insufficiency) will have a variable presentation including AV block, tachyarrhythmia, cyanosis, or congestive heart failure.

151. (A) While all of these other forms of congenital heart disease have been described with isolated dextrocardia and normal atrial situs, ccTGA is the most common.

Diagnosis of Congenital Heart Disease

Emily Morell, Jonathan N. Johnson, and Grace Kung

Questions

1. A 4-year-old child presents with new-onset ventricular tachycardia. Echocardiography after treatment of the arrhythmia reveals a single large mass in the wall of the left ventricle (**Figure 3.1**). Which of the following is the most likely diagnosis?

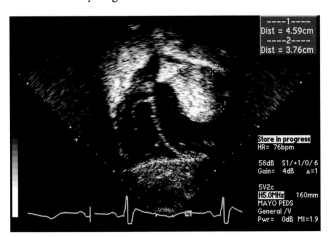

FIGURE 3.1

    A. Rhabdomyoma
    B. Fibroma
    C. Myxoma
    D. Pericardial teratoma
    E. Lymphoma

2. A 32-year-old pregnant woman undergoes fetal echocardiography due to an abnormal obstetrical scan. The echo reveals a diagnosis of tetralogy of Fallot with absent pulmonary valve. At the time of delivery, what is the most important initial step in management?

    A. Immediate sternotomy and ventricular septal defect (VSD) repair
    B. Initiation of prostaglandin drip
    C. Balloon atrial septostomy
    D. Respiratory support
    E. Initiation of epinephrine drip

3. You are seeing a 9-year-old patient in clinic who has hypertrophic cardiomyopathy (HCM). On examination, the patient has a crescendo–decrescendo systolic murmur along the left sternal border. Which of the following provocative maneuvers or medications would *decrease* the intensity of the patient's murmur?

    A. Phenylephrine
    B. Exercise
    C. Straining portion of Valsalva
    D. Nitroglycerine
    E. Isoproterenol

4. A mother with phenylketonuria (PKU) gives birth to a term male infant. The obstetricians note that she had not adhered well to her prescribed diet and likely had elevated blood phenylalanine levels during pregnancy. Which of the following defects are you most likely to see on echocardiography of the neonate?

    A. Ebstein anomaly
    B. Hypoplastic left heart syndrome
    C. Branch pulmonary stenosis
    D. Total anomalous pulmonary venous return (TAPVR)
    E. Interrupted inferior vena cava (IVC)

5. A 2-month-old infant is referred to you for evaluation of a murmur. Her weight is at the 3rd percentile for age and she has been struggling with feeding. Her parents also note that she breathes quickly. You obtain an electrocardiogram. Which of the following defects are you most likely to find on her echocardiogram (**Figure 3.2**)?

A. Secundum atrial septal defect (ASD)
B. Patent ductus arteriosus (PDA)
C. Atrioventricular (AV) canal defect
D. Tetralogy of Fallot
E. Truncus arteriosus

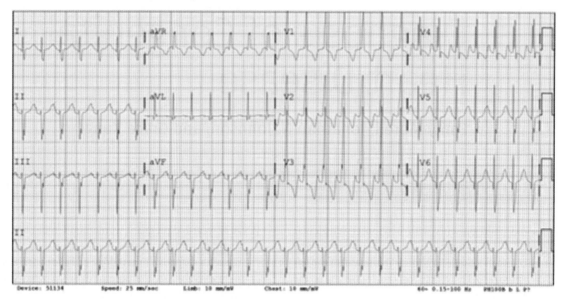

FIGURE 3.2

6. A 6-week-old infant presents to the emergency room with poor feeding, tachypnea, and wheezing. Heart rate is 169 bpm. Oxygen saturation is 93%. CXR shows cardiomegaly and mild pulmonary edema. Point of care echocardiogram reportedly shows decreased function and moderate mitral regurgitation. ECG is as follows (**Figure 3.3**).

Which of the following is the most likely diagnosis?

A. VSD
B. Anomalous left coronary artery from the pulmonary artery (ALCAPA)
C. Idiopathic dilated cardiomyopathy
D. Congenital mitral regurgitation
E. Critical pulmonary valve stenosis

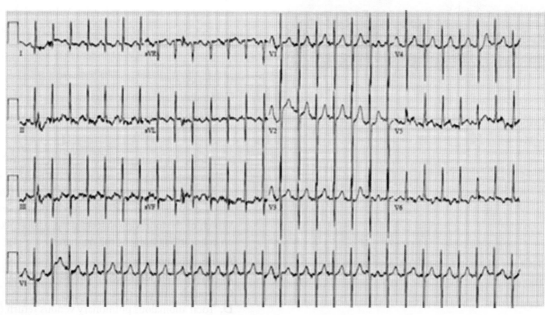

FIGURE 3.3

7. A 2-year-old girl is diagnosed with myocarditis. Her parents relate to you that she recently had a viral upper respiratory infection. Which of the following viruses are most likely implicated in this patient?

    A. Epstein–Barr virus (EBV) and respiratory syncytial virus (RSV)
    B. Parainfluenza virus and coxsackie virus
    C. Human immunodeficiency virus (HIV) and parainfluenza virus
    D. Coxsackie virus and adenovirus
    E. RSV and influenza A virus

8. While undergoing a predischarge examination in the newborn nursery, a 2-day-old term infant is noted to have poor femoral pulses. She also fails the congenital heart disease saturation screening. Electrocardiogram shows sinus tachycardia. Echocardiogram shows an interrupted aortic arch (IAA) with an intact ventricular septum. Which of the following associated findings should be looked for on the echocardiogram?

    A. Secundum ASD
    B. Left superior vena cava (SVC) to coronary sinus
    C. Atrioventricular canal defect
    D. Aortopulmonary window
    E. Cor triatriatum

9. A 14-year-old girl is referred for an unusual sound heard on auscultation by her pediatrician. There is a high-frequency "click" audible immediately after S_1 and heard best at the apex. The most likely cause of this click is:

    A. Mitral valve prolapse
    B. Subvalvar pulmonary stenosis
    C. Pulmonary valve stenosis
    D. Pericardial rub
    E. Bicuspid aortic valve

10. Prior to discharge from the newborn nursery, a neonate fails pulse oximetry screening. His saturations are 93% in both the upper and lower extremities. On examination, there is a to–fro murmur noted, systolic click, and good distal pulses. The most likely diagnosis is:

    A. Tetralogy of Fallot with pulmonary atresia and major aortopulmonary collaterals (MAPCA)
    B. Truncus arteriosus
    C. Coarctation of the aorta
    D. Pulmonary atresia with intact ventricular septum and sinusoids
    E. Friction rub

11. A 3-year-old healthy boy is referred for evaluation of a recently heard heart murmur. His peripheral pulses are normal. The first and second heart sounds are normal. There is a grade 2/6 low-to-mid frequency "vibratory" murmur along the left sternal border. One would expect this murmur to increase in intensity:

    A. When going from sitting to standing position
    B. When squatting
    C. When going from sitting to supine position
    D. With deep inhalation
    E. During the third phase of the Valsalva maneuver

12. Which of the following is the most appropriate indication for performing a pericardiocentesis?

    A. Pulsus paradoxus
    B. Presumed viral pericarditis
    C. Hypertension
    D. Asymptomatic patient with hypothyroidism
    E. Asymptomatic patient with renal failure

13. A 7-year-old patient with double-inlet left ventricle, s/p Glenn and Fontan presents with a 1-week history of abdominal pain, diarrhea, lower extremity edema, and acute weight gain. She has no respiratory distress. Heart rate is 89 bpm. Oxygen saturation is 94% in room air. Echocardiogram shows good single ventricle function and mild atrioventricular valve regurgitation. ECG is unremarkable. The most informative laboratory test is:

    A. Complete blood count (CBC)
    B. Urinalysis
    C. Fecal alpha-1-antitrypsin
    D. Thyroid function tests (TFTs)
    E. Liver function tests (LFTs)

14. You are seeing a neonate in the ICU who presented with cyanosis. The sonographer has started the echo and reports there is an aortopulmonary window with interrupted aortic arch (IAA) and intact ventricular septum. Which type of IAA is most likely for this patient?

    A. Type A (interruption distal to the left subclavian artery)
    B. Type B (interruption between the left carotid and left subclavian arteries)
    C. Type C (interruption between the carotid arteries)
    D. Type D (interruption proximal to the innominate artery)
    E. All types occur with equal frequency

CHAPTER 3

15. A neonate fails the pulse oximetry screen. On ECG, they have evidence of left axis deviation. Which of the following is the most likely diagnostic cause of the left axis deviation?

A. Total anomalous pulmonary venous connection
B. Concentric left ventricular hypertrophy (LVH)
C. Tricuspid atresia
D. Secundum atrial septal defect
E. Double outlet right ventricle (DORV)

16. A 13-year-old girl presents to the clinic complaining of a rapid heart rate, which she has noticed for the past month. She denies any chest pain, syncope, or presyncope. Heart rate is 120 bpm while sitting on the examination table. Blood pressure is 115/72 mm Hg. Body mass index is 15. A faint systolic ejection murmur is heard. Of the following, the most appropriate laboratory test to order would be:

A. Electrolyte panel
B. Chromosome panel (karyotype)
C. Hemoglobin A1C
D. Thyroid-stimulating hormone (TSH)
E. Serum cortisol

17. A 2-year-old boy presents with poor weight gain and difficulty feeding. When he gets agitated during the examination, you note inspiratory stridor. CXR is unremarkable and ECG shows normal sinus rhythm. Barium esophagram shows an anterior indentation (**Figure 3.4**).

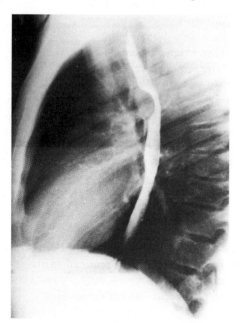

FIGURE 3.4

The most likely diagnosis is:

A. Double aortic arch
B. Left arch with aberrant right subclavian artery
C. Right arch with aberrant left subclavian artery
D. Pulmonary artery sling
E. Right arch with left-sided descending aorta

18. An outreach echocardiogram performed on a 2-day-old female infant reveals ventricular hypertrophy and an abnormal aortic arch. The baby is transported to your institution, and on arrival, the nurse performs four-extremity blood pressure measurements. The findings are as follows:

Right leg: 40/25

Left leg: 42/22

Right arm: 73/36

Left arm: 72/35

Which of the following is the most likely diagnosis?

A. Coarctation of the aorta
B. Complete AV canal defect
C. Truncus arteriosus with pulmonary artery ostial stenosis
D. Tetralogy of Fallot
E. Coarctation of the aorta with aberrant right subclavian artery

19. A 38-week-old term infant with congenital heart disease is diagnosed with necrotizing enterocolitis (NEC). Which of the following diagnoses is associated with the highest risk of developing NEC in a term neonate?

A. Tetralogy of Fallot
B. Patent ductus arteriosus
C. Tricuspid atresia
D. Complete AV canal
E. Hypoplastic left heart syndrome

20. A 5-year-old boy presents to the emergency department following a motor vehicle accident. The attending physician notes that his blood pressure is now 70/40 mm Hg and that his heart sounds are distant. Which of the following physical examination findings would be consistent with traumatic cardiac tamponade?

A. A third heart sound
B. A precordial rub
C. A precordial knock
D. Neck vein distention
E. Bradycardia

21. You are seeing a 12-year-old girl in clinic, who was referred to you for cardiomegaly. On examination, you hear distant breath sounds as well as pulsus paradoxus. Her heart rate is 65 bpm. She has complained of progressively worsening fatigue over the last 2 months, which she attributes to her recent 20 lb weight gain. Which of the following is the most likely cause of her pericardial effusion?

A. Rheumatic fever
B. Hypothyroidism
C. Recent isoniazid administration
D. Renal failure
E. Purulent pericarditis

22. A 6-month-old infant with a known history of atrial septal defect and ventricular septal defect presents with poor weight gain, feeding difficulty, and tachypnea. Respiratory rate is 60 and saturation is 96% in room air. Which examination finding is consistent with a large left-to-right shunt as an etiology of the failure to thrive?

    A. Increased precordial activity, 2/6 low-frequency holosystolic murmur, diastolic rumble
    B. Normal precordial activity, 2/6 high-frequency holosystolic murmur
    C. Increased precordial activity, prominent single S$_2$, no murmur
    D. Normal precordial activity, wide split S$_2$, 1/6 low-frequency systolic ejection murmur
    E. Increased precordial activity, 3/6 systolic ejection murmur

23. A 5-year-old boy presents to your office with exercise intolerance. You note a 3/6 systolic ejection murmur at the left upper sternal border with a widely fixed split S$_2$ and a soft middiastolic rumble. Which of the following would you most likely find on further investigation?

    A. Right atrial enlargement on ECG
    B. Evidence of LVH on ECG
    C. $Q_p{:}Q_s = 1.2$
    D. Accessory left anterior descending coronary artery
    E. Spontaneous closure of the defect by age 10

24. You are consulted on a 1-day-old neonate in the NICU for a heart murmur. On examination, you note a loud systolic ejection murmur radiating throughout the precordium, with a prominent left ventricular (LV) impulse. The neonate has poor peripheral perfusion and weak femoral pulses. On echocardiography, you obtain a right parasternal image with the following velocity in the ascending aorta (**Figure 3.5**). Of the following, which is the most appropriate next intervention to perform?

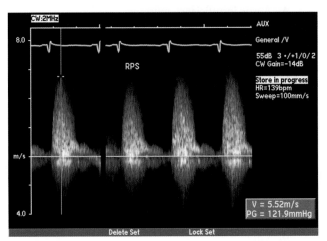

FIGURE 3.5

A. Initiation of IV milrinone
B. Pericardiocentesis
C. Urgent aortic valvuloplasty
D. Urgent atrial balloon septostomy
E. Initiation of extracorporeal membrane oxygenation

25. A murmur is heard at a 1-week well-child examination. The infant is referred for an echocardiogram, which reveals several well-circumscribed masses in the left and right ventricular walls (**Figure 3.6**). What is the most likely diagnosis?

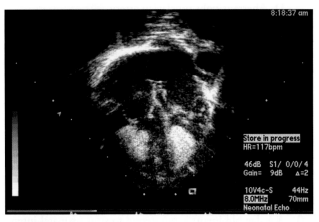

FIGURE 3.6

A. Fibroma
B. Myxoma
C. Blood cyst
D. Hemangioma
E. Rhabdomyoma

26. A 30-year-old woman presents for a fetal echocardiogram. You note in her history that she was treated with retinoic acid during early pregnancy. Which of the following categories of congenital heart anomalies is of particular concern for this fetus?

A. Coarctation of the aorta
B. Hypoplastic left heart syndrome
C. Ebstein anomaly
D. Laterality defects
E. Conotruncal defects

27. A 14-year-old male patient is referred to you for a murmur. On history, the patient reports recurrent low-grade fevers, malaise, and a 20 lb weight loss in the last 2 months. On the echocardiogram, you find a pedunculated mass (2 cm × 2 cm) attached to the fossa ovalis in the left atrium. What is the most likely diagnosis?

A. Rhabdomyoma
B. Myxoma
C. Teratoma
D. Fibroma
E. IVC extension of Wilms tumor

28. A neonate fails their pulse oximetry screen with saturation of 89% in the right arm. Saturation is 94% in the right leg. CXR shows a narrow mediastinum and no significant pulmonary edema. Cardiac examination is notable for a prominent S₂, no murmur, and good distal pulses. Echocardiogram shows d-transposition of the great arteries. What other finding must also be present?

    A. Wide open PDA with pulmonary hypertension
    B. Wide open PDA with dropping pulmonary vascular resistance (PVR)
    C. Intact atrial septum
    D. Aberrant right subclavian artery
    E. VSD

29. A 12-year-old boy with congenital heart disease is noted to have complete AV block. Which of the following is the most likely structural cardiac diagnosis for this patient?

    A. VSD
    B. d-Transposition of the great arteries
    C. Asplenia with tetralogy of Fallot
    D. Maternal lupus
    E. Congenitally corrected transposition of the great arteries (CCTGA)

30. A 4-day-old infant is transferred to your neonatal intensive care unit due to concern for an "abnormal rhythm." You are told that the heart rate is 110 bpm. Echocardiogram shows a common atrium, complete atrioventricular canal defect, interrupted IVC with azygos continuation, and right aortic arch. Abdominal ultrasound shows a midline liver. Electrocardiogram is most likely to show which of the following:

    A. Two QRS morphologies consistent with twin AV nodes
    B. Alternating P-wave axis
    C. Sinus node dysfunction with junctional escape rhythm
    D. Multifocal atrial tachycardia
    E. Wolff–Parkinson–White (WPW) pattern

31. A 6-week-old infant is referred to your clinic for evaluation of a murmur. She was born at 36-week gestational age. On examination, you hear a II/VI systolic ejection murmur that radiates from the left upper sternal border over the lung fields to both axillae and the back. Saturation is 99% in room air. Which of the following is most likely true?

    A. This is most consistent with an innocent murmur that will be heard best when the baby is supine
    B. This is likely a pathologic murmur and echocardiogram is warranted for further evaluation
    C. This is most consistent with an innocent murmur that will likely disappear by 6 months of age
    D. This is most consistent with an innocent murmur that will decrease in intensity if you have the baby turn their head to look over the contralateral shoulder
    E. The baby needs referral for cardiac catheterization

32. A 5-year-old boy is diagnosed with Wolff–Parkinson–White (WPW) syndrome. He is found to have an abnormal echocardiogram. Which of the following forms of congenital heart disease is most commonly associated with WPW?

    A. Hypertrophic cardiomyopathy (HCM)
    B. VSD
    C. Bicuspid aortic valve
    D. Tetralogy of Fallot
    E. Atrial septal defect

33. You have been following a 2-year-old boy with pulmonary stenosis. Which of the following would be a clinical clue that the degree of stenosis has worsened?

    A. The murmur peaks earlier
    B. The ejection click occurs later
    C. The "a" wave becomes less prominent
    D. S₁ becomes more prominent
    E. The split of S₂ becomes wider

34. A 3-month-old presents with tachypnea and failure to thrive. CXR shows right lung hypoplasia and cardiac dextroposition. Which of the following associated findings is most likely?

    A. Transposition of the great arteries
    B. Large patent ductus arteriosus
    C. Partial anomalous pulmonary venous return with the right pulmonary veins draining into the IVC
    D. VSD
    E. Kartagener syndrome

35. A 19-month-old female infant presents for evaluation due to a cardiac murmur. On examination, a high-frequency continuous murmur is present at the right upper sternal border. The murmur is maximal in the upright position and is softer when the neck is turned. This murmur is most likely:

    A. Aortic insufficiency murmur
    B. Patent ductus arteriosus
    C. Peripheral pulmonary branch stenosis
    D. Venous hum
    E. Carotid bruit

36. A 15-year-old boy is referred for dyspnea on exertion. On examination, his S₁ and S₂ sounds are normal, but there is a harsh 3/6 systolic murmur with a musical quality heard from the sternal border down to the apex. There are no clicks, thrills, or rubs, and diastole is quiet. Just after a PVC that you note on his cardiac monitor, the murmur increases in intensity. What is the most likely cause of the murmur?

    A. Aortic stenosis
    B. VSD
    C. Mitral regurgitation
    D. Pulmonary stenosis
    E. Innocent murmur

37. A 15-month-old girl presents with dyspnea, fatigue, and cyanosis on exertion. On examination, she has a widely split S_1 and S_2, and a II/VI holosystolic murmur heard best at the left lower sternal border. Her CXR is shown below (**Figure 3.7**).

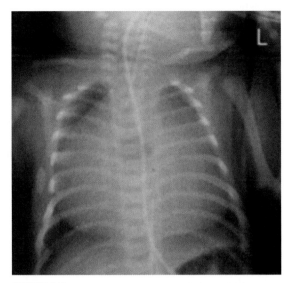

FIGURE 3.7

Which of the following are you least likely to find on her ECG?

A. Right bundle branch block
B. Left axis deviation
C. Ventricular preexcitation
D. First-degree AV block
E. Sinus rhythm

38. A 17-year-old boy is referred to you for a murmur heard over the left scapula. Basic laboratory studies are normal. The patient is noted to be hypertensive, and an abdominal ultrasound with renal Doppler is normal. An echocardiogram is performed and thought to be normal, but images are difficult secondary to the patient's size (particularly subcostal images). The following chest x-ray is taken (**Figure 3.8**). Which of the following is the next best diagnostic test to order?

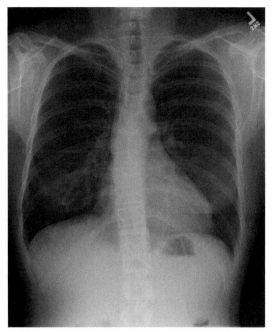

FIGURE 3.8

A. Left and right heart catheterization
B. Further imaging with computed tomography (CT) or magnetic resonance imaging (MRI) of the chest
C. Stress echocardiogram
D. Treadmill exercise test using the Bruce protocol
E. Urine metanephrines

39. You diagnose a 2-month-old male infant with congenitally corrected transposition of the great arteries (CCTGA or L-TGA). What is this patient most likely to also have on echocardiography?

A. Atrial septal defect
B. Left ventricular outflow tract obstruction
C. Ventricular septal defect (VSD)
D. Tricuspid valve dysplasia
E. Mitral valve dysplasia

40. A 3 day old with cyanosis is found to have transposition of the great arteries with a ventricular septal defect (VSD). Which of the following additional findings is most likely to be found on echocardiogram?

A. Partial anomalous pulmonary venous return
B. Left ventricular outflow tract obstruction
C. Discontinuous pulmonary arteries
D. Moderate tricuspid regurgitation
E. Coarctation

CHAPTER **3**

41. You are called to perform an echocardiogram on a 5-day-old female infant with cyanosis. The patient is mildly tachypneic with retractions. Pulse oximetry reveals an oxygen saturation of 70%. Chest x-ray shows a normal heart size with mildly increased pulmonary vascular markings. On examination, you appreciate a loud S_2 with no significant murmurs. Echocardiography shows side-by-side great arteries. Which of the following diagnoses is most likely?

    A. DORV with subpulmonic VSD and no pulmonary stenosis
    B. DORV with subpulmonic VSD and pulmonary stenosis
    C. DORV with subaortic VSD and no pulmonary stenosis
    D. DORV with subaortic VSD and pulmonary stenosis
    E. DORV with subaortic VSD and coarctation of the aorta

42. A 2-day-old infant born at term with the assistance of a midwife at home presents to the emergency room with respiratory distress and poor feeding. Oxygen saturation is 90% in room air. CXR shows cardiomegaly and pulmonary edema. On examination, the infant has delayed capillary refill and poor distal pulses. Auscultation reveals a single S_2 and no murmur. Which of the following is the most likely diagnosis?

    A. Pulmonary atresia with intact ventricular septum
    B. TAPVR
    C. Hypoplastic left heart syndrome
    D. Ebstein anomaly
    E. Truncus arteriosus

43. A 15-year-old patient with hypertrophic cardiomyopathy (HCM) is referred to your clinic. You hear a murmur consistent with LV outflow obstruction. Which of the following maneuvers will increase the outflow murmur in this patient?

    A. Beta blocker
    B. Squatting
    C. Exercise
    D. Isometric handgrip
    E. Phenylephrine

44. A 17-year-old athlete is found to have thickened LV myocardium. Which of the following characteristics supports a diagnosis of hypertrophic cardiomyopathy over "athlete's heart"?

    A. Increased LV end diastolic volume
    B. Symmetric ventricular hypertrophy
    C. Male gender
    D. T-wave inversions in the lateral leads
    E. Mitral inflow E/A = 1.5

45. A 3-year-old child presents with dilated cardiomyopathy (DCM). The child was adopted 2 weeks ago from Chile, but birth records report no family history of congenital heart disease, cardiomyopathy, or HIV. Which of the following is the most likely infectious cause of DCM in this patient?

    A. Human papillomavirus
    B. HIV
    C. Chagas disease
    D. Lymphocytic choriomeningitis
    E. West Nile virus

46. A series of studies are undertaken to differentiate between restrictive cardiomyopathy and constrictive pericarditis in a 14-year-old boy. Which of the following findings would be more consistent with restrictive cardiomyopathy?

    A. "Septal bounce" on echocardiography
    B. Right ventricular systolic pressure <30 mm Hg on catheterization
    C. Increased atrial size on echocardiography
    D. Right ventricular end-diastolic pressure (RVEDP) = Left ventricular end-diastolic pressure (LVEDP) on catheterization
    E. Normal PVR index on catheterization

47. You are seeing a 7-year-old boy in clinic with mitral valve regurgitation from a prior episode of rheumatic fever. How would you ask the patient to be positioned in order to best hear his murmur?

    A. Sitting
    B. Left lateral decubitus
    C. Sitting up and leaning forward
    D. Standing
    E. Right lateral decubitus

48. A neonate is being evaluated in the newborn nursery. Fetal echocardiography had indicated a concern for tetralogy of Fallot, which is confirmed on postnatal echocardiography. An ECG is performed and shows left axis deviation. In addition to tetralogy of Fallot, what additional finding should be looked for on the echocardiogram?

    A. Coarctation of the aorta
    B. Interrupted aortic arch
    C. AV septal defect
    D. Aortopulmonary window
    E. Absent pulmonary valve

49. A 16-year-old male is diagnosed with a bicuspid aortic valve on echocardiography. The echo was performed after his father was also diagnosed with a bicuspid aortic valve. The patient plays American football, and lifts weights daily. His history is unremarkable, without recent hospitalizations or surgeries, and he is asymptomatic. He has a normal resting blood pressure in the office (116/72 mm Hg). Which potential associated echocardiographic finding is important to evaluate in this patient?

    A. Aortic root size
    B. Ascending aorta size
    C. Descending thoracic aorta size
    D. Abdominal aorta size
    E. Main pulmonary artery size

50. A 2-month-old infant is referred to you for a murmur. The saturations in both upper and lower extremities are 86%. Initial echocardiographic imaging shows a large ASD with right-to-left shunting, and the sonographer is unable to show pulmonary veins entering the left atrium. Further echocardiographic imaging reveals the following image from a leftward-directed suprasternal notch view (**Figure 3.9**).

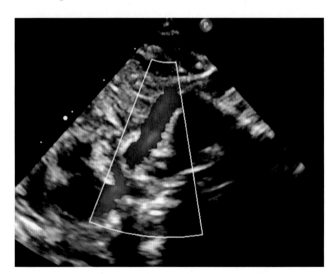

FIGURE 3.9

    Which of the following is the most likely diagnosis?
    A. Infradiaphragmatic total anomalous pulmonary venous return (TAPVR)
    B. Obstructed supracardiac TAPVR
    C. Unobstructed supracardiac TAPVR
    D. TAPVR with drainage to the coronary sinus
    E. Left SVC to coronary sinus

51. A 16-year-old football player presents with an episode of syncope while singing in church. His pediatrician obtained an ECG and referred him to you for sports clearance. Which of the following findings on the ECG are most concerning for an underlying pathology (i.e., not related to training)?

    A. Left bundle branch block
    B. Incomplete right bundle branch block
    C. First-degree AV block
    D. Early repolarization
    E. Isolated QRS voltage for LVH

52. A 2 month old with tuberous sclerosis is referred to your practice. On echocardiography, you find several moderate-sized cardiac tumors, all located within the walls of the LV and RV without obstruction of the LVOT or RVOT. The patient is asymptomatic. What is the most likely future course for this patient?

    A. The patient will eventually have to undergo surgical resection
    B. Around 50% chance of requiring surgical resection
    C. Complete resolution of the tumors
    D. The tumors will resolve after an interventional procedure
    E. The tumors will not resolve, but the patient will remain asymptomatic

53. A 2-month-old infant has hypotonia, and undergoes echocardiography as part of a genetic workup. Initial echocardiographic images reveal the following (**Figure 3.10**).

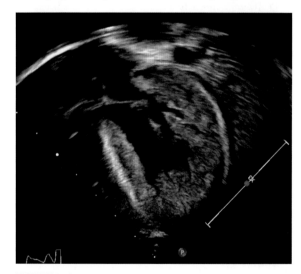

FIGURE 3.10

    Which of the following ECG findings would you see in this patient?
    A. Right axis deviation
    B. Right ventricular hypertrophy
    C. Complete heart block
    D. Normal ECG
    E. Short PR interval with prominent precordial voltages

54. A 6-month-old infant presents with recurrent respiratory infections and stridor. A vascular ring is found on echocardiography. Which type of vascular anomaly is most likely to be found in this patient?

A. Retroesophageal right subclavian artery with left aortic arch

B. Retroesophageal left subclavian artery with right aortic arch

C. Left pulmonary artery sling

D. Double aortic arch

E. Persistent fifth aortic arch

55. A 10-year-old girl presents with chest pain and diffuse ST-segment elevation. You diagnose her with acute pericarditis. On examination, you hear a typical friction rub. Which of the following maneuvers will cause the rub to become louder on auscultation?

A. Have the patient blow out as much air as possible

B. Have the patient lie on their side

C. Have the patient stand up straight

D. Have the patient lean forward

E. Have the patient lie supine

56. A 2-year-old female presents for evaluation of bradycardia. On examination, the patient has an accentuated, single second heart sound. CXR demonstrates mesocardia. The following four-chamber view is obtained on echocardiography (**Figure 3.11**).

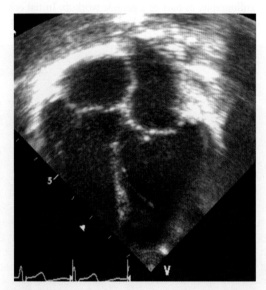

FIGURE 3.11

In addition to the findings demonstrated on the echo image, which of the following will most commonly also be found in this patient?

A. Ventricular septal defect (VSD)

B. Pulmonary stenosis

C. Moderate tricuspid valve regurgitation

D. Ventricular tachycardia

E. Q-waves in the left precordial leads on ECG

57. A neonate is admitted with concerns for congenital rubella infection. Which of the following congenital heart defects is mostly likely to be found on echocardiography?

A. Pulmonary stenosis

B. Coarctation of the aorta

C. Transposition of the great arteries

D. Hypoplastic left heart syndrome

E. Ectopia cordis

58. A 12-year-old boy is referred for evaluation of a murmur by his pediatrician. On examination, there is a systolic click heard in early to midsystole with the patient standing; however, the click moves later in systole with the patient in the squatting and supine positions. There is also a late systolic murmur heard best at the apex. Which of the following is the most likely diagnosis?

A. Bicuspid aortic valve

B. Subvalvar pulmonary stenosis

C. Mitral valve prolapse

D. Pulmonary valve stenosis

E. Pericardial rub

59. You are caring for a 16-year-old boy who had a cardiac arrest during a football game. Which of the following is the most likely underlying diagnosis?

A. Short QT syndrome

B. Long QT syndrome

C. Hypertrophic cardiomyopathy

D. Mitral valve prolapse

E. Aortic dissection

60. An outreach echocardiogram performed on a critically ill 3-day-old male infant reveals ventricular hypertrophy and an abnormal aortic arch. The baby is transported to your institution, and on arrival, the nurse performs four-extremity blood pressure measurements. The findings are as follows:

Right leg: 40/25

Left leg: 42/22

Right arm: 48/27

Left arm: 72/35

Which of the following is the most likely diagnosis?

A. Coarctation of the aorta

B. Coarctation of the aorta with VSD

C. Truncus arteriosus with pulmonary artery ostial stenosis

D. Coarctation of the aorta with supravalvar mitral ring

E. Coarctation of the aorta with aberrant right subclavian artery

61. A 6-year-old boy presents with prolonged malaise and fever. A new murmur is noted on examination. He denies any chest pain or cough. His past medical history is otherwise unremarkable. While performing an echocardiogram, you note the following Doppler flow pattern in the descending aorta (**Figure 3.12**).

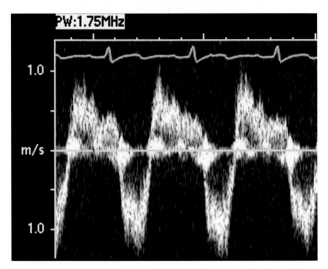

FIGURE 3.12

Which of the following is the most likely diagnosis?

A. Ascending aorta dilation
B. Mitral regurgitation
C. Aberrant right subclavian artery from the descending aorta
D. Ruptured sinus of Valsalva
E. Coarctation

62. An 18-month-old girl with hypoplastic left heart syndrome palliated to a bidirectional Glenn is noted to have serial saturations in the low 70s. She is breathing comfortably without any signs of respiratory distress. You place her on 2L NC 100% FiO_2 in clinic and there is no improvement in her saturations. Her hematocrit is 45%. Echocardiogram shows good function, unrestrictive atrial septum, unobstructed aortic arch, and patent Glenn and branch pulmonary arteries (PAs). Which of the following is the next best step?

A. Cardiac catheterization
B. Contrast echocardiogram
C. Cardiac MRI
D. Cardiac CT angiography
E. Blood transfusion

63. Contrast echo in the above patient with injection into the right upper extremity shows contrast from the inferior vena cava (IVC) to the right atrium. The most likely diagnosis is:

A. Pulmonary arteriovenous malformations
B. Interrupted IVC with azygos continuation
C. Venovenous collaterals
D. Normal study
E. Left SVC draining directly into an unroofed coronary sinus

CHAPTER 3

Answers

1. (B) Fibromas are typically single, firm, intramural tumors involving the ventricular free wall or septum. Clinical manifestations depend largely on the location of the tumor; however, ventricular arrhythmias are frequently seen in these patients and may be the presenting symptom. The presence of ventricular arrhythmias in the vignette should prompt one to think about fibroma as the answer. Successful surgical excision has occurred in some patients, while patients with extensive involvement of critical structures have occasionally been treated with transplantation.

2. (D) Tetralogy of Fallot with absent pulmonary valve is associated with aneurysmal pulmonary artery dilatation. This may cause compression of the bronchi. Up to 40% to 50% of patients may have respiratory distress at birth, some with lobar emphysema. In the acute setting, prone positioning may help by allowing the aneurysmal pulmonary arteries to fall forward and away from the bronchi. Patients with significant respiratory distress requiring surgery at birth

have a worse outcome compared to those who do not need respiratory intervention early after birth.

3. (A) The murmur described is that of dynamic outflow tract obstruction. This murmur is typically increased by anything that increases the gradient. Thus, it will be louder with exercise, standing (particularly after squatting), and with the straining portion of the Valsalva maneuver. Systemic vasodilation with nitroglycerin or administration of isoproterenol will also increase the gradient. Administration of phenylephrine, or stimulation of the alpha-adrenergic system, will increase the afterload pressure, decreasing the gradient and thus the intensity of the dynamic outflow murmur.

4. (B) Specific heart defects associated with maternal PKU include left-sided heart defects (coarctation, hypoplastic left heart syndrome), tetralogy of Fallot, and sepal defects. The other defects listed are not commonly seen in maternal

PKU. The degree of elevation of the maternal serum phenyl-alanine level has been shown to be predictive of congenital heart disease in the fetus.

5. (C) The timing of presentation would be most consistent with a diagnosis of AV canal defect, PDA, or tetralogy of Fallot with minimal pulmonary obstruction. The ECG shows a superior QRS axis which is seen with AV canal defects due to the conduction around the inlet VSD. None of the other choices would have a superior QRS axis.

6. (B) The ECG finding of "q" waves in leads I and AVL are typical for ALCAPA. ALCAPA typically presents at 4 to 6 weeks of age when the PVR has dropped significantly causing a steal phenomenon from the coronary arteries affected. This results in ischemia of the LV and can affect the mitral valve papillary muscles resulting in poor LV function, abnormal coaptation of the mitral valve, and mitral regurgitation. VSD would not give you these findings. Idiopathic cardiomyop-athy and congenital mitral regurgitation are diagnoses of exclusion after ALCAPA has been ruled out.

7. (D) The most common viral causes of myocarditis are adenovirus and enterovirus—most commonly the Coxsackie virus. Cytomegalovirus, parvovirus, influenza A, herpes sim-plex virus, EBV, HIV, and RSV are other rare viral causes of myocarditis.

8. (D) In the setting of IAA without a VSD, an aortopulmonary window can be associated and needs to be ruled out. The others are not common associations that are significant.

9. (E) The click described is an aortic ejection click, heard commonly in patients with bicuspid aortic valves. If accom-panied by a suprasternal notch thrill, the stenosis is more likely to be valvular than subvalvar or supravalvular. A pul-monary valve ejection click may present similarly but with respiratory variation (louder with expiration). A nonejection systolic click may be heard in early systole in mitral valve prolapse with the patient standing, but will occur later in systole with squatting or supine position.

10. (B) This neonate has decreased saturations and a to–fro murmur. Tetralogy of Fallot/MAPCAs would have a continu-ous murmur from the MAPCAs. A significant coarctation with right-to-left PDA shunting would have a saturation differ-ential with higher saturations in the upper extremities, and there is typically no to–fro murmur. Pulmonary atresia with intact ventricular septum may have a PDA murmur but no to–fro murmur. Truncus arteriosus commonly has an abnor-mal truncal valve with some degree of insufficiency and stenosis, causing the characteristic murmur in question.

11. (C) The murmur described is a Still murmur, a common innocent systolic murmur of childhood. Chest x-ray and electrocardiography are normal. The murmur is best heard when the patient is supine.

12. (A) Pericardiocentesis should be performed in patients with clinical tamponade (hypotension, low cardiac output,

or pulsus paradoxus >10 mm Hg) and patients with bac-terial pericarditis, with immunocompromised hosts, or for diagnosis when the etiology of an effusion is unclear. Asymptomatic effusions in patients with known diagnoses do not require pericardiocentesis unless in hemodynamic compromise. The diagnosis of viral pericarditis is not by itself an indication. In patients with bacterial pericarditis, the fluid may often be too thick to drain or may be loculated within the pericardium. In this case, a surgical intervention (pericardial window, pericardiectomy) should be consid-ered. Pulsus paradoxus is defined as a decrease in systolic blood pressure of greater than 10 mm Hg during inspira-tion. Normally during inspiration, systolic blood pressure decreases by 4 to 6 mm Hg due to decreased intrathoracic pressure and increased capacity of the pulmonary venous bed. With tamponade, the left ventricular diastolic volume is restricted by increased pericardial pressure, decreased pulmonary venous return, and shifting of the ventricular septum.

13. (C) This patient is presenting with symptoms of protein losing enteropathy. Although lymphopenia can be seen on CBC, it is not specific and neither are abnormal LFTs or UA. TFTs are usually not affected. The most informative and diagnostic test is fecal alpha-1-antitrypsin.

14. (A) Type A IAA occurs more commonly in patients with aortopulmonary septation defects and accounts for around one-third of patients with IAA. Type B interruptions occur more commonly in patients with DiGeorge syndrome. Type C is much more rare than types A and B, accounting for <1% of patients with IAA. The so-called type D is incompatible with life. See **Figure 3.13**.

Interrupted Aortic Arch

Three Types

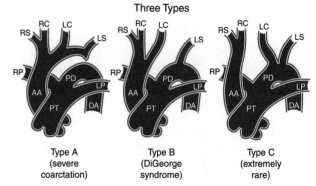

Type A
(severe
coarctation)

Type B
(DiGeorge
syndrome)

Type C
(extremely
rare)

FIGURE 3.13 AA, ascending aorta; DA, descending aorta; LC, left carotid; LP, left pulmonary artery; LS, left subclavian; PD, patent ductus; PT, pulmonary trunk; RC, right carotid; RP, right pulmonary artery; RS, right subclavian. (Image courtesy of Dr. William Edwards, Mayo Clinic.)

15. (C) Common causes of left axis deviation in infants include the AV canal defects (complete or partial) and tri-cuspid atresia, with or without transposition of the great vessels. Many patients with AV canal defects may have a more superior axis (–60 degrees to –100 degrees). Right axis deviation may be indicative of right ventricular hypertrophy in certain patients.

16. (D) When presented with a teenage patient with a persistent sinus tachycardia, common things to consider may include hyperthyroidism, substance abuse, pheochromocytoma, autonomic dysfunction, and tachyarrhythmias. Patients with eating disorders more commonly present with bradycardia. Hyperthyroidism is an important cause of resting tachycardia in a teenager and may present with heat intolerance, sweating, palpitations, weight loss, insomnia, and irritability. Pheochromocytoma will present with episodic symptoms of sweating hypertension, and tachycardia. If any dysmorphisms are present, consideration should be given for ordering a karyotype. Diabetes can produce an autonomic neuropathy which may involve an inappropriate tachycardia.

17. (D) With pulmonary artery sling, the left pulmonary artery courses in between the esophagus and trachea causing an anterior indentation on a barium swallow study. All other options may either be normal or show a posterior indentation.

18. (A) With coarctation, the blood pressures in the legs are typically lower than those in the upper extremities. The similar blood pressures in the right and left arm imply that the right and left subclavian arteries originate proximal to the coarctation. If there were a low blood pressure in the right arm (but not the left arm), there could be an aberrant right subclavian artery. Patients with AV canal defects and tetralogy of Fallot do not typically present with blood pressure discrepancies between the upper and lower extremities.

19. (E) There is a higher risk of developing NEC in patients with truncus arteriosus and hypoplastic left heart syndrome. This is thought to be secondary to the relatively tenuous balance between systemic and pulmonary blood flow in these patients prior to surgical palliation or repair. Changes in physiology can markedly reduce the amount of systemic flow (due to preferential pulmonary flow) and cause gut ischemia and NEC.

20. (D) The patient is presenting with Beck triad, including hypotension, muffled or distant heart sounds, and jugular venous distension, indicative of cardiac tamponade. Patients will be tachycardic and will show evidence of pulsus paradoxus.

21. (B) Pericardial effusions can result as a secondary process of many diseases, including rheumatic fever, lupus, and renal failure, or secondary to a lupus-like reaction to a medication like isoniazid or hydralazine. With this clinical vignette, the patient has a significant effusion with tamponade physiology (pulsus paradoxus is present), but has an unexpected bradycardia. In addition to the recent weight gain and fatigue, this is highly suggestive of hypothyroidism.

22. (A) If the cause of the failure to thrive is due to a large shunt, there would be evidence of increased precordial activity and a diastolic rumble. Choice B reflect a pressure restrictive VSD and unlikely significant pulmonary overcirculation; choice C is indicative of pulmonary hypertension, and this would not have a large shunt; and choice D can be found with a large ASD, but unlike a large enough shunt to cause failure to thrive. A systolic ejection murmur suggests right ventricular or left ventricular outflow tract obstruction and would not result in pulmonary overcirculation as the cause of the failure to thrive.

23. (A) The physical examination findings are consistent with an atrial septal defect with a large left-to-right shunt (as indicated by the diastolic flow rumble). In the presence of a diastolic rumble, $Q_p:Q_s$ is at least 1.5:1 and likely higher. This type of large atrial septal defect will present more commonly with right-sided enlargement and is unlikely to close spontaneously. The expected right atrial enlargement may cause peaked p-waves seen on ECG.

24. (C) The patient is presenting with critical aortic stenosis, with a systolic ejection murmur, a prominent LV impulse, and poor peripheral perfusion. The current standard of care for these patients is a balloon aortic valvuloplasty to be performed in the cath lab. Use of an afterload reducer such as milrinone will result in worsening of the gradient.

25. (E) The most common type of cardiac tumor in children, and especially infants, is rhabdomyomas. Rhabdomyomas are well-circumscribed, noncapsulated, intramural, or intracavitary nodules that can occur in any location in the heart, most typically the ventricles. They may occur singly, but often several are found in the same patient. They have a characteristic "bright" appearance on echo.

26. (E) Retinoic acid, including other forms such as isotretinoin and etretinate, is commonly used in adolescents and young adults with acne and other skin conditions. Strict guidelines have been enacted due to the high risk of complex congenital heart anomalies (particularly conotruncal defects) in exposed fetuses. Extracardiac defects are also common.

27. (B) Patients with myxomas often present with a classic triad of symptoms: cardiac obstruction (80% of patients), embolism (~70% of patients), and systemic illness (~60% of patients). The masses are most often pedunculated and friable, and occur most commonly in the left atrium. Myxomas can be found attached to the foramen ovale or either ventricle.

28. (A) There is a finding of differential cyanosis and in order for that to exist, there must be a PDA with right-to-left shunting. Choice B would have left-to-right shunting. Choices C and E would not cause differential cyanosis. Choice D would not show differential cyanosis due to the aberrant subclavian artery often coming off distal to the PDA.

29. (E) Patients with CCTGA and those with polysplenia are most at risk for developing high-grade AV block. Patients with CCTGA should be monitored closely over follow-up with regular ECGs and Holter monitors. Patients with polysplenia, or bilateral left sidedness, often have other anatomical findings including dextrocardia, ventricular inversion, and an interrupted IVC. Due to underdevelopment of right-sided structures in polysplenia, nodal and conduction tissue is often affected in these patients, placing them at a high risk for complete AV block. This occurs more commonly in patients with polysplenia than patients with asplenia.

30. (C) The infant described has features consistent with heterotaxy syndrome. Specifically, the presence of an interrupted IVC with azygos continuation indicates left atrial isomerism. Because the sinus node is a right-sided structure, in left atrial isomerism, sinus nodes are either absent or hypoplastic and displaced, resulting in sinus node dysfunction. As a result, junctional escape or ectopic atrial rhythms are common. Twin AV nodes are seen in asplenia syndrome. WPW is not more associated with either type of heterotaxy and does not necessarily go with an AV canal defect.

31. (C) The murmur described is most consistent with a peripheral pulmonary flow murmur, which is commonly heard in the newborn period, especially in infants born prematurely. It is thought to be related to turbulence in the branch pulmonary arteries. It classically radiates to the axillae and back. This murmur usually disappears by 6 months of age. If the murmur persists beyond this time period, further evaluation is warranted. An innocent "Still's" murmur typically does not radiate to the back and neither does a venous hum as suggested by answer D. There is no indication for further assessment with a catheterization.

32. (A) Depending on the study, up to 10% of patients with HCM may have evidence of pre-excitation. The other form of congenital heart disease with an increased incidence of WPW is Ebstein anomaly. Between 20% and 30% of patients with Ebstein anomaly will have WPW, with left axis deviation and pre-excitation, suggesting a right-sided accessory pathway.

33. (E) With worsening of pulmonary stenosis, the systolic murmur peaks later in systole and the split of the S_2 sound widens (the P_2 sound is delayed). Once there is severe stenosis, the murmur spills over into diastole and the S_2 sound may become inaudible.

34. (C) The triad of respiratory distress, cardiac dextroposition, and right lung hypoplasia should raise concern for Scimitar syndrome. Scimitar syndrome is a malformation consisting of anomalous pulmonary venous return from the right lung to the inferior vena cava and right lung hypoplasia. Other associated anomalies include bronchial abnormalities, horseshoe lung, dextroposition, right pulmonary artery hypoplasia, anomalous connection between right pulmonary artery and aorta, and pulmonary sequestration. CXR classically shows a rightward shift of the cardiac silhouette with the appearance of a Turkish sword called a scimitar.

35. (D) Venous murmurs are more often benign and heard best over the upper chest. They change with head position or compression of the jugular vein and vary with respiration. The murmur is often heard loudest in the standing position.

36. (A) The murmur of aortic stenosis increases after a premature ventricular contraction. This is secondary to an increased gradient across the aortic valve, produced by enhanced diastolic filling during the compensatory pause of the premature ventricular contraction.

37. (B) The patient described has features most consistent with Ebstein anomaly of the tricuspid valve, which is characterized by apical displacement of the septal leaflet of the tricuspid valve. This results in varying degrees of atrialization of the right ventricle. In severe cases, cyanosis and heart failure manifest in the first few days of life; while in milder cases, the diagnosis is made late into adulthood. Characteristic ECG findings include right bundle branch block, right atrial enlargement, and prolonged PR interval. These patients are also at risk for Wolff–Parkinson–White syndrome and may demonstrate ventricular preexcitation on baseline ECG or present with episodes of supraventricular tachycardia.

38. (B) The chest radiograph displays rib notching bilaterally, as well as the "figure of 3" sign in the upper chest. These are relatively specific for the diagnosis of coarctation of the aorta. Urine metanephrines may be ordered if one is concerned for a pheochromocytoma, which may present with intermittent hypertensive, flushing, tachycardic, sweating episodes. If the arch is unable to be adequately visualized by transthoracic echo, then a stress echocardiogram is unlikely to provide further information.

39. (C) Around 80% of patients with congenitally corrected transposition will have a VSD. These defects are typically perimembranous and subpulmonary and are due to atrial and septal malalignment. Left ventricular outflow tract (subpulmonary ventricular outflow tract) obstruction occurs in 30% to 50% of patients. Morphologic tricuspid valve dysplasia is common as well in CCTGA.

40. (B) Left ventricular outflow tract obstruction (i.e., subpulmonary stenosis) occurs in about one-third of patients with d-transposition of the great arteries with a ventricular septal defect. This is important to identify as it plays a significant role in preoperative planning. Those with VSD and severe subpulmonary stenosis cannot undergo a simple arterial switch operation and instead consideration should be given to a Nikaidoh or *REV* procedure.

41. (A) Due to variations in the location of the VSD and great arteries, DORV can present in several different ways. This patient is presenting with cyanosis but mildly increased pulmonary vascular markings. If the VSD were subaortic, there typically will not be cyanosis. If there were pulmonary stenosis, the pulmonary vascular markings should be normal or decreased. This patient therefore most likely has the Taussig–Bing anomaly, DORV with side-by-side great arteries, and a subpulmonary VSD.

42. (C) Postnatally diagnosed hypoplastic left heart syndrome typically presents in the first several hours to days of life. If the atrial septum is restrictive, presentation will be earlier (within hours) with signs of pulmonary congestion, tachypnea, and cyanosis. If the atrial septum is widely patent, the infant may appear normal until the ductus arterious begins to close (between 1 and 3 days of life). Because systemic perfusion is ductal-dependent, the infant will present with signs of inadequate systemic perfusion, ultimately progressing to cardiogenic shock.

43. (C) The murmur of obstruction heard in HCM will typically be increased with exercise, standing, and Valsalva maneuver. Increasing the systemic afterload pressure (handgrip, phenylephrine) will decrease the gradient and thus the intensity of the dynamic outflow murmur. Amyl nitrate is a potent vasodilator that can decrease afterload and increase the gradient, increasing the intensity of the murmur.

44. (D) The differentiation between HCM and "athlete's heart" can be difficult. Factors that favor the diagnosis of HCM include the presence of irregular hypertrophy (as opposed to pure concentric hypertrophy), normal-sized LV diastolic dimensions, left atrial enlargement, abnormal ECG, abnormal LV diastolic function, family history of HCM, and female gender. A test of deconditioning can be performed, after which the LV thickness will resolve in those with the diagnosis of "athlete's heart."

45. (C) A severe form of myocarditis can be a complication of Chagas disease, caused by *Trypanosoma cruzi*. Chagas is endemic throughout much of Latin and South America, but is rarely seen in the United States except in recent immigrants.

46. (C) In restrictive cardiomyopathy, the atria are markedly enlarged. RVSP is often greater than 50 mm Hg, as opposed to constrictive pericarditis, where it is typically less than 50 mm Hg. The other options—including the presence of a septal bounce, equal RVEDP and LVEDP, and normal PVR index—are more typical of constriction. Patients with restrictive cardiomyopathy will rarely show changes in Doppler flow velocities with inspiration and expiration.

47. (B) The murmur of rheumatic heart involvement of the mitral valve is typically high pitched, holosystolic, heard best at the apex, and radiating to the left axilla. The murmur will be heard best at the end of expiration while the patient is lying in the left lateral decubitus position.

48. (C) 2% of patients with tetralogy of Fallot will also have an associated atrioventricular septal defect. A specific finding in these patients is that they will have left axis deviation on ECG, as opposed to patients with isolated tetralogy of Fallot who typically have normal or right axis deviation.

49. (B) Patients with bicuspid aortic valve are at risk of having an enlarged ascending aorta. Patients with connective tissue disorders including Marfan syndrome or Loeys–Dietz Syndrome more commonly have aortic root (sinus of Valsalva) dilatation. There can be overlap, however, with some patients with connective tissue disorders also having ascending aorta or aortic arch dilatation. For this patient, if the ascending aorta is unable to be visualized on

echocardiography, other imaging such as CT or MRI should be performed. The role of pharmacologic treatment in this clinical situation remains controversial.

50. (C) The image is showing flow through a vertical vein in a neonate with TAPVR of the supracardiac type. This patient had unobstructed flow to the innominate vein and was clinically stable. In this situation, surgery is not emergent, and can even be delayed for several months if appropriate mixing is present. In the infradiaphragmatic type, flow typically drains inferiorly, ultimately draining into the portal or hepatic veins. In the cardiac type, pulmonary venous flow will drain into the coronary sinus. There can also be mixed types, with different pulmonary veins draining to different locations rather than a single confluence. If the image was of a left SVC, the flow would have been blue in color, heading away from the echo probe (draining into the coronary sinus).

51. (A) Common training-related ECG findings include sinus bradycardia, first-degree AV block, incomplete right bundle branch block, early repolarization, and isolated QRS voltage criteria for LVH. Studies have reported that up to 10% to 40% of high school or college athletes may meet voltage criteria for LVH, despite having normal echoes. Left bundle branch block is uncommon and mandates further evaluation.

52. (C) The characteristic cardiac tumor in patients with tuberous sclerosis is rhabdomyoma. These patients are often asymptomatic, but may present with symptoms of obstruction if the tumors are large. The vast majority of these tumors will resolve without intervention. Surgical excision can be performed in patients with hemodynamic compromise or arrhythmia secondary to their rhabdomyomas.

53. (E) The image demonstrates ventricular hypertrophy which is global in nature. In a patient with hypotonia, Pompe Disease is high on the list of differential diagnoses. Board examiners may also show you an ECG which has a short PR interval and very high voltages in the precordial leads.

54. (D) The double aortic arch commonly presents in infancy or in the first few months of life. Patients with a retroesophageal left subclavian artery with right aortic arch do not have a technical vascular ring and rarely require treatment in the absence of other concerns. A retroesophageal right subclavian artery with a left aortic arch is the most common arch anomaly, occurring in 0.5% of the general population, but does not commonly cause symptoms in infancy. Left pulmonary artery slings will result in anterior indentation of the esophagus on barium swallow, but typically present with respiratory distress and stridor in the first few years of life. Persistent fifth aortic arch is extremely rare and may present incidentally on an imaging study, incidentally in conjunction with other congenital heart disease or a pattern similar to coarctation.

55. (D) The typical friction rub is loudest when the heart is closest to the chest wall; this occurs when the patient leans forward, kneels, and inspires. The absence of a rub does not exclude pericarditis, especially in the presence of a large effusion.

56. (A) The patient has congenitally corrected transposition of the great arteries, demonstrated by the left-sided AV valve arising more apically compared to the right-sided AV valve. These patients commonly have VSDs (80%), pulmonary/LV outflow obstruction (30% to 50%), and tricuspid regurgitation due to an abnormal tricuspid valve architecture. A VSD and PS would both cause a systolic murmur. The tricuspid valve can have varying degrees of regurgitation, which may or may not be audible on examination. Heart block is common, and may be the cause of the "bradycardia" on the referral. On ECG, patients with CCTGA often have Q-waves in the right precordial leads instead of the left precordial leads as seen in normal patients.

57. (A) Pulmonary stenosis and patent ductus arteriosus are the two most common cardiac defects diagnosed in patients with congenital rubella syndrome. Patients may also present with ventricular septal defects or tetralogy of Fallot.

58. (C) The question is describing the click and murmur of mitral valve prolapse. In this setting, the murmur is typically preceded by the click. The click is heard in early or midsystole with the patient in the standing position, but moves later in systole with squatting or supine position. The aortic ejection click of a patient with a bicuspid valve is heard most often early in systole after S_1. A pulmonary valve ejection click may present similarly but with respiratory variation (louder with expiration). A rub is typically present in both systole and diastole.

59. (C) Hypertrophic cardiomyopathy is the most common cause of sudden death in athletes in the United States, affecting up to 44% of patients. Coronary artery anomalies are implicated in a further 17%, with myocarditis affecting

6% of patients. The ion channelopathies are implicated in 3% of cases.

60. (E) With coarctation, the blood pressures in the legs are typically lower than those in the upper extremities. A low blood pressure in the right arm (but not the left arm) suggests that the right subclavian artery originates distal to the coarctation, as occurs with an aberrant right subclavian artery.

61. (D) The diagram above shows evidence of large flow reversals in the descending aorta. This can be caused by a large ductus arteriosus, severe aortic insufficiency, or an intracranial arteriovenous malformation such as a vein of Galen malformation. Another potential cause of this is a direct communication from the aorta to the LV through a ruptured sinus of Valsalva due to endocarditis. Mitral regurgitant flow would be at a much higher velocity than is shown here and would not affect diastolic aortic flow. None of the other answer choices would cause diastolic flow reversal.

62. (B) This patient has had a Glenn with persistently low saturations and patent appearing Glenn and branch PAs. Differential diagnosis included venovenous collaterals and pulmonary AVMs. Although these can be diagnosed by catheterization, the simplest way to entertain the diagnosis is with contrast echocardiography. MRI and CT may not necessarily show the collaterals unless they are significant.

63. (C) Contrast returning to the heart is not a normal study. Pulmonary arteriovenous malformations would have contrast returning to the left atrium; an interrupted IVC would not have connection to the right atrium and with the Glenn, would have essentially been a Kawashima, but neither would show return to the heart. Venovenous collaterals decompress from the Glenn commonly to the IVC and thus is the answer.

Cardiac Catheterization and Angiography

Jason H. Anderson and Nathaniel W. Taggart

Questions

The following clinical scenario applies to Questions 1 to 3.

An 8-year-old boy was referred for a hemodynamic catheterization due to concern for pulmonary hypertension. The patient is sedated and intubated prior to the case on mechanical ventilation.

1. Based upon the data in **Table 4.1**, which of the following best represents this patient's cardiac output?
   A. 2.2 L/min/m^2
   B. 2.6 L/min/m^2
   C. 3.2 L/min/m^2
   D. 3.6 L/min/m^2
   E. Unable to determine

TABLE 4.1 Cardiac Catheterization Data

Location	Pressure (mm Hg)	SpO$_2$ (%)
Superior vena cava		72
Inferior vena cava		70
Right atrium	Mean 5	70
Right ventricle	33/8	70
Left pulmonary artery	52/26/35	70
Pulmonary capillary wedge	Mean 10	
Left ventricle	80/10	99
Descending aorta	84/50/68	99
VO$_2$ (assumed) = 150 mL/min/m^2		
ABG (femoral) = pH 7.35; pCO$_2$ 36; pO$_2$ 37		
Hemoglobin = 12 g/dL		

Ventricular pressures are shown as systolic/end-diastolic.
Arterial pressures are shown as systolic/diastolic/mean.

2. Which of the following best represents this patient's pulmonary vascular resistance (PVR)?
   A. 5.0 Woods units $\times$ m^2
   B. 7.8 Woods units $\times$ m^2
   C. 8.1 Woods units $\times$ m^2
   D. 10.9 Woods units $\times$ m^2
   E. Unable to determine

3. Which of the following best represents the ratio of PVR:SVR?
   A. 0.2
   B. 0.3
   C. 0.4
   D. 0.5
   E. 0.7

4. A 6-month-old infant is referred for cardiac catheterization due to an inability to visualize the left pulmonary artery on transthoracic echocardiography. The angiograms in **Figure 4.1** were obtained. What is the most likely diagnosis for this patient?

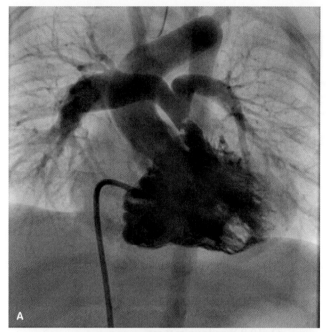

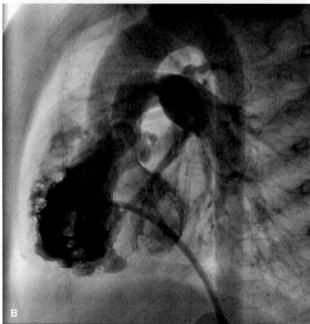

FIGURE 4.1

A. Pulmonary atresia with VSD
B. Tetralogy of Fallot
C. Transposition of the great arteries
D. Isolated ventricular septal defect
E. Isolated branch pulmonary artery stenosis

5. A 6-year-old boy with complex congenital heart disease (atrial situs solitus, visceral situs ambiguous, polysplenia, dextrocardia, single left SVC, partial AV canal defect) has undergone surgical baffling of the left SVC to the right atrium and subsequent stent implantation due to baffle stenosis. He is referred for catheterization. Based on the catheter course demonstrated in **Figure 4.2**, what additional diagnosis is likely present in this patient?

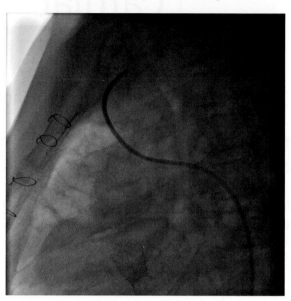

FIGURE 4.2

A. Interrupted aortic arch type A
B. Interrupted aortic arch type B
C. Interrupted aortic arch type C
D. Interrupted inferior vena cava
E. Fontan procedure

6. Which of the following abnormalities would most likely result in a prominent V wave on right atrial pressure tracing?

A. Tricuspid valve stenosis
B. Hypertrophic cardiomyopathy with severe septal hypertrophy
C. Atrial septal defect
D. Pulmonary valve regurgitation
E. Gerbode defect

7. A 17-year-old boy is undergoing an interventional cardiac catheterization when he manifests a change in the arterial pressure waveform (**Figure 4.3**) and marked jugular venous distention. Which of the following interventions is most likely indicated at this time?

A. Removal of the guidewire
B. Repositioning of the endotracheal tube
C. Pericardiocentesis
D. External defibrillation
E. Lidocaine administration

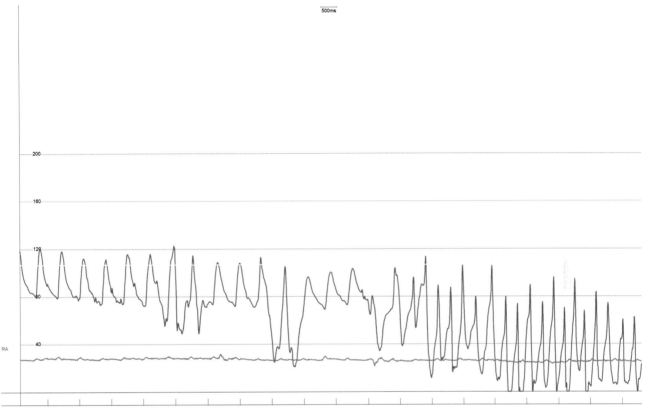

FIGURE 4.3

8. An 18-year-old woman experiences headaches and urticaria 72 hours after implantation of an Amplatzer septal occluder device for closure of a moderate ASD. The only medication recommended postoperatively was aspirin, which she has tolerated without complication in the past. An allergic reaction to which of the following compounds would best explain her symptoms?

A. Titanium
B. Selenium
C. Copper
D. Stainless steel
E. Nickel

9. A 13-year-old boy undergoes ASD device closure utilizing a 22-mm Amplatzer septal occluder device with subsequent atrial tachycardia to 280 bpm with 2:1 AV conduction block. Which of the following statements is true regarding conduction abnormalities following ASD device closure?

A. Most resolve within the first 24 hours of device placement
B. Most resolve 2 weeks after device placement
C. Complete heart block occurs in approximately 5% of patients
D. Aspirin therapy should be continued indefinitely for any device-induced conduction abnormality
E. Friction from the device can cause extranodal AV pathways to develop

The following clinical scenario applies to Questions 10 to 14.

Cardiac catheterization is performed on a 4-month-old infant from South America with an unrepaired congenital heart defect; hemodynamic data are shown in **Table 4.2.**

TABLE 4.2 Cardiac Catheterization Data

Location	Pressure (mm Hg)	SpO$_2$ (%)
Superior vena cava		64
Right atrium	12/14/10	68
Right ventricle	77/12	72
Left pulmonary artery	70/28/42	83
Right pulmonary artery	69/28/42	83
Left ventricle	69/12	95
Left atrium	12/13/11	99
Ascending aorta	76/34/49	83
Femoral artery	82/33/48	83

VO$_2$ (assumed) = 150 mL/min/m^2

ABG (femoral) = pH 7.35; pCO$_2$ 36; pO$_2$ 51

Hemoglobin = 17.4 g/dL

Atrial and pulmonary capillary wedge pressures are shown as a-wave/v-wave/mean. Ventricular pressures are shown as systolic/end-diastolic. Arterial pressures are shown as systolic/diastolic/mean.

10. Based upon the hemodynamic data in **Table 4.2**, what is this patient's Q_p/Q_s?

   A. 0.8
   B. 1.2
   C. 1.6
   D. 2.0
   E. Unable to calculate

11. Based upon the hemodynamic data in **Table 4.2**, which of the following most closely represents the volume of this patient's *left-to-right* shunt?

   A. 0.8 L/min/m^2
   B. 1.5 L/min/m^2
   C. 2.2 L/min/m^2
   D. 2.8 L/min/m^2
   E. Unable to calculate

12. Based upon the hemodynamic data in **Table 4.2**, which of the following most closely represents the volume of this patient's *right-to-left* shunt?

   A. 0.8 L/min/m^2
   B. 1.5 L/min/m^2
   C. 2.2 L/min/m^2
   D. 2.8 L/min/m^2
   E. Unable to calculate

13. Based upon the hemodynamic data in **Table 4.2**, what is this patient's pulmonary vascular resistance?

   A. 4.2 Woods units × m^2
   B. 7.8 Woods units × m^2
   C. 9.1 Woods units × m^2
   D. 14.1 Woods units × m^2
   E. Unable to calculate

14. Which of the following diagnoses is most consistent with this clinical scenario?

   A. Truncus arteriosus
   B. Tetralogy of Fallot
   C. Patent ductus arteriosus (PDA) with Eisenmenger syndrome
   D. Interrupted aortic arch with PDA
   E. D-transposition of the great arteries with large atrial septal defect (ASD)

15. An 8-year-old patient with history of congenital heart disease undergoes cardiac catheterization. The angiogram in **Figure 4.4** is obtained. Which of the following disorders is most commonly associated with the defect shown?

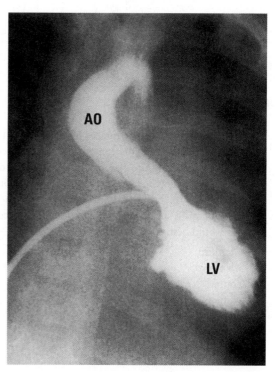

FIGURE 4.4 Ao, aorta; LV, left ventricle.

   A. Marfan syndrome
   B. Loeys–Dietz syndrome
   C. Williams syndrome
   D. Down syndrome
   E. Ellis–van Creveld

16. A cyanotic newborn was emergently taken for cardiac catheterization. Angiography was performed (**Figure 4.5**). Which of the following was the most likely indication for catheterization?

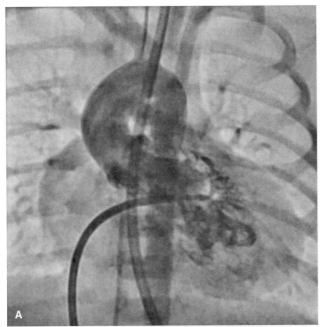

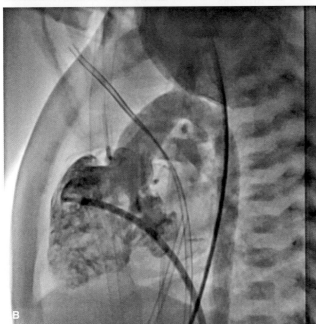

FIGURE 4.5

A. Balloon angioplasty of the aortic coarctation
B. Balloon atrial septostomy
C. Balloon valvuloplasty of the aortic valve
D. Balloon valvuloplasty of the pulmonary valve
E. Delineation of the source of pulmonary blood flow

17. A 19-year-old man with dyspnea on exertion is referred for hemodynamic cardiac catheterization. Because of some abnormal hemodynamic findings, the angiogram in **Figure 4.6** was obtained. Which of the following is demonstrated in the angiogram?

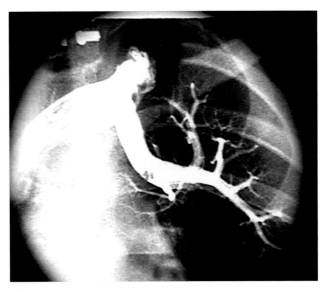

FIGURE 4.6

A. Left SVC connecting to the coronary sinus
B. PAPVC of the left upper pulmonary vein to the left SVC
C. PAPVC of the left upper pulmonary vein to the innominate vein
D. PAPVC of the left upper pulmonary vein to the coronary sinus
E. MAPCA from the aortic arch to the left upper pulmonary artery

The following clinical scenario applies to Questions 18 to 21.

*A 17-year-old girl presents with syncope during exertion. Physical examination is significant for a right ventricular lift and a single, loud S_2. Echocardiogram demonstrates a small ASD with small right-to-left shunt and a dilated, hypertrophied right ventricle with moderately decreased systolic function. Cardiac catheterization is performed, and the data are shown in **Table 4.3**.*

TABLE 4.3 Cardiac Catheterization Data

Location	Room Air Pressure (mm Hg)	SpO$_2$ (%)	pO$_2$ (mm Hg)	100% FiO$_2$ Pressure (mm Hg)	SpO$_2$ (%)	pO$_2$ (mm Hg)
IVC		68			74	
SVC		76			84	
RA	15/17/13	74		16/17/14	81	
RV	130/14	73		124/15	82	
MPA	126/88/107	72	35	120/82/100	78	44
LPA	125/87/106	72	35	119/80/99	78	44
RPA	127/86/106	72	35	121/77/99	78	44
LA	12/14/10	94		13/14/11	99	
LUPV		99	97		100	394
RUPV		99			100	
LV	114/11	96		106/11	98	
Asc Ao	110/76/88	96	83	102/71/83	98	93
Desc Ao	108/74/87	84		101/72/83	92	
VO$_2$ (assumed)	125 mL/min/m^2			125 mL/min/m^2		
Blood gas (pulm vein)	pH 7.38; pCO$_2$ 38; pO$_2$ 98; hemoglobin 12.5 g/dL			pH 7.40; pCO$_2$ 41; pO$_2$ 394; hemoglobin 12.5 g/dL		

18. Which of the following defects best explains the clinical and hemodynamic findings?

   A. Primary (idiopathic) pulmonary hypertension
   B. Anomalous pulmonary venous connections
   C. Ventricular septal defect
   D. Patent ductus arteriosus
   E. Anomalous right pulmonary artery from the ascending aorta

19. Based upon the hemodynamic data in **Table 4.3**, which of the following most closely represents Q_p/Q_s on room air?

   A. 0.3
   B. 0.5
   C. 0.7
   D. 0.9
   E. Unable to calculate

20. Based upon the hemodynamic data in **Table 4.3**, which of the following most closely represents pulmonary vascular resistance on *room air*?

   A. 28 Woods units × m^2
   B. 31 Woods units × m^2
   C. 35 Woods units × m^2
   D. 42 Woods units × m^2
   E. Unable to calculate

21. Based upon the hemodynamic data in **Table 4.3**, which of the following most closely represents pulmonary vascular resistance on *100% FiO$_2$*?

   A. 19 Woods units × m^2
   B. 26 Woods units × m^2
   C. 31 Woods units × m^2
   D. 34 Woods units × m^2
   E. Unable to calculate

22. A child is referred for preoperative cardiac catheterization. The angiogram in **Figure 4.7** is obtained. Which of the following connections is demonstrated in this angiogram?

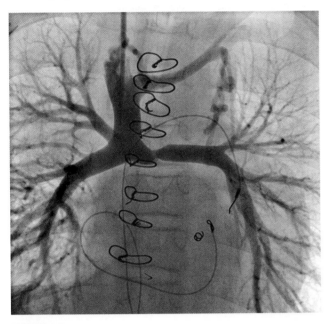

FIGURE 4.7

    A. Classic Blalock–Taussig–Thomas (BTT) shunt
    B. Modified BTT shunt
    C. Classic Glenn shunt
    D. Bidirectional Glenn shunt
    E. Damus–Kaye–Stansel anastomosis

23. A 12-month-old boy undergoes cardiac catheterization. The angiogram shown in **Figure 4.8** is obtained. Which of the following is shown in the angiogram?

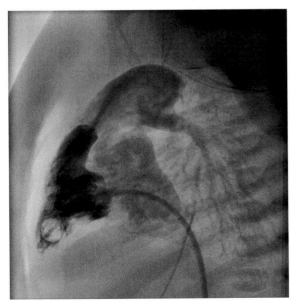

FIGURE 4.8

    A. Severe dynamic infundibular obstruction
    B. Poststenotic pulmonary artery dilation
    C. Right ventricular apical diverticulum
    D. Right ventricular outflow tract pseudoaneurysm
    E. Diverticulum of Kommerell

24. The angiogram shown in **Figure 4.9** is obtained in an otherwise healthy, asymptomatic 8-month-old girl with an enlarged cardiac silhouette on chest x-ray. Based on these findings, which of the following is recommended for the patient?

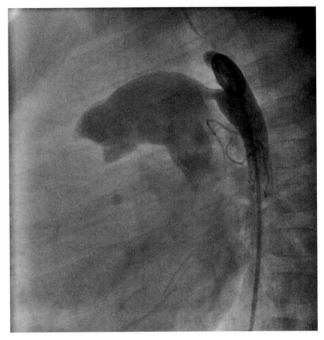

FIGURE 4.9

    A. No further cardiology follow-up is necessary
    B. Repeat catheterization in 6 to 12 months
    C. Transcatheter intervention
    D. Oral diuretic therapy
    E. Surgical referral for operative management

CHAPTER 4

The following clinical scenario applies to Questions 25 and 26.

A 4-year-old boy with a history of surgical repair of anomalous origin of the right pulmonary artery from the ascending aorta developed proximal right pulmonary artery stenosis. Mean Doppler gradient across the stenosis is 13 mm Hg. Lung perfusion scan demonstrates 60% flow to the left lung and 40% to the right lung.

He undergoes cardiac catheterization. Hemodynamic catheterization performed prior to intervention produces the data shown in Table 4.4.

TABLE 4.4 Hemodynamic Cardiac Catheterization Data

Location	Pressure[a] (mm Hg)	SpO$_2$ (%)
SVC		75
RA	7/6/5	78
RV	32/6	72
MPA	31/14/20	73
LPA	30/15/20	73
RPA	16/10/12	73
PCWP	10/12/8	
Femoral artery	108/74/87	99
VO$_2$ (assumed)	140 mL/min/m^2	
Blood gas (pulm vein)	pH 7.40; pCO$_2$ 40; pO$_2$ 100; hemoglobin 10.8 g/dL	

[a]Pressures shown are a/v/mean for atrial and pulmonary capillary wedge pressures, systolic/end-diastolic for ventricular pressures, and systolic/diastolic/mean for arterial pressures.

25. Based upon the hemodynamic data in **Table 4.4**, which of the following most closely represents this patient's cardiac index?
    A. 3.2 L/min/m^2
    B. 3.7 L/min/m^2
    C. 4.0 L/min/m^2
    D. 4.6 L/min/m^2
    E. Unable to calculate

26. Based upon the hemodynamic data in **Table 4.4**, which of the following most closely represents this patient's pulmonary vascular resistance?
    A. 1.8 Woods units × m^2
    B. 2.2 Woods units × m^2
    C. 2.7 Woods units × m^2
    D. 3.2 Woods units × m^2
    E. Unable to calculate

27. After assisting with an ASD closure utilizing a Gore Cardioform septal occluder in an adult patient, the primary team asks for follow-up recommendations prior to discharge. A chest x-ray was obtained on the morning of discharge (**Figure 4.10**). Which of the following would you advise?

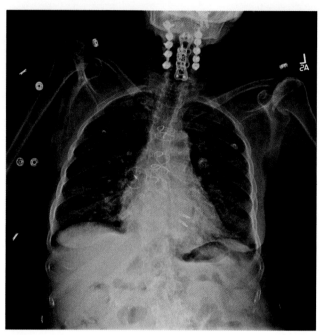

FIGURE 4.10

    A. Continue aspirin therapy for 6 months
    B. Continue aspirin therapy for 6 months and clopidogrel for 1 month
    C. Initiate warfarin therapy
    D. Device retrieval
    E. Perform emergent pericardiocentesis

28. A newborn with Williams syndrome is referred for catheterization with angiography due to an inability to visualize the LPA on echocardiography. The patient is known to have severe supravalvar aortic stenosis and severe supravalvar pulmonary stenosis. This patient has an elevated risk over the general population for which of the following complications?
    A. Access site complications
    B. Cardiac perforation
    C. Supraventricular tachycardia
    D. Sudden death
    E. None of the above

29. An adult patient with congenital heart disease is referred for preoperative right and left heart catheterization. Prior to beginning the case, the patient is noted to be taking NPH insulin for diabetes. Which of the following agents should be avoided in this patient?

    A. Fentanyl
    B. Heparin
    C. Lorazepam
    D. Papaverine
    E. Protamine

The following scenario applies to Questions 30 and 31.

*A 12-year-old boy undergoes hemodynamic cardiac catheterization. Hemodynamic data obtained are shown in **Table 4.5**.*

TABLE 4.5 Hemodynamic Cardiac Catheterization Data

Location	Pressure (mm Hg)	SpO₂ (%)
Inferior vena cava		70
Left innominate vein		92
Superior vena cava		80
Right atrium	8/6/4	74
Right ventricle	24/7	76
Main pulmonary artery	24/13/18	75
Left pulmonary artery	23/12/17	75
Right pulmonary artery	24/14/18	75
Left pulmonary capillary wedge	7/7/6	
Right pulmonary capillary wedge	12/11/10	
Left ventricle	97/11	99
Femoral artery	108/68/76	99

Atrial and pulmonary capillary wedge pressures are shown as a/v/mean. Ventricular pressures are shown as systolic/end-diastolic. Arterial pressures are shown as systolic/diastolic/mean.

30. Which of the following defects best explains the discrepancy between right and left pulmonary capillary wedge pressures?

    A. Anomalous pulmonary venous connection
    B. Right pulmonary vein stenosis
    C. Left pulmonary vein stenosis
    D. Increased flow through the right pulmonary artery
    E. Technical or equipment error

31. Which of the following additional findings is most likely based upon these hemodynamic data?

    A. Sinus venosus defect
    B. Pulmonary sequestration
    C. Left vertical vein
    D. Unroofed coronary sinus
    E. Right ventricular enlargement

32. A 12-year-old boy is referred for device closure of a secundum atrial septal defect. The preliminary plan is to close the lesion utilizing an Amplatzer septal occluder device in the cath lab. As part of the consent process, what is the appropriate incidence to cite for the complication of device erosion as a complication of the procedure?

    A. 1 in 1,000,000
    B. 1 in 100,000
    C. 1 in 10,000
    D. 1 in 1,000
    E. 1 in 100

33. A 10-year-old boy is referred for coarctation of the aorta. In considering the treatment options, which of the following early- to midterm complications is more likely to occur from balloon angioplasty than aortic stent implantation or surgical repair?

    A. Acute aortic wall injury
    B. Arrhythmias
    C. Access site arterial injury
    D. Need for planned re-intervention
    E. Need for unplanned re-intervention

34. An 18-year-old woman undergoes cardiac catheterization secondary to severe right ventricular enlargement with findings consistent with pulmonary hypertension on echocardiography. **Figure 4.11** was obtained. What is the most commonly associated defect with this finding?

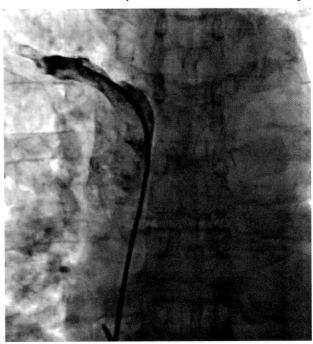

FIGURE 4.11

    A. Scimitar syndrome
    B. Secundum atrial septal defect
    C. Sinus venosus defect
    D. Membranous ventricular septal defect
    E. Partial atrioventricular canal defect

35. A 3-day-old male infant with d-TGA is referred for atrial septostomy. Following completion of the procedure, the aortic root angiogram in **Figure 4.12** was obtained to define the coronary artery anatomy. Which of the following coronary artery arrangements is present?

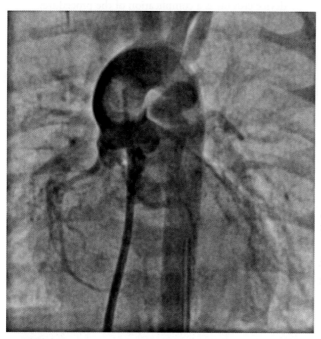

FIGURE 4.12

A. Anomalous left coronary artery from the pulmonary artery

B. Circumflex arising from the RCA

C. LAD arising from the RCA

D. Single origin of the coronary arteries

E. Normal branching pattern of d-TGA

The following scenario applies to Questions 36 and 37.

A 5-month-old girl with tricuspid atresia and normally related great arteries undergoes cardiac catheterization prior to bidirectional cavopulmonary anastomosis. Hemodynamic data are shown in **Table 4.6**.

TABLE 4.6 Hemodynamic Cardiac Catheterization Data

Location	Pressure (mm Hg)	SpO$_2$ (%)
Superior vena cava		53
Right atrium	11/10/8	57
Left pulmonary vein	10/8/7	100
Left pulmonary vein wedge	Mean 14	
Right pulmonary vein	9/9/7	100
Right pulmonary vein wedge	Mean 14	
Left atrium	10/9/7	94
Left ventricle	84/9	82
Femoral artery	89/58/68	82

VO$_2$ (assumed) = 150 mL/min/m^2

ABG (femoral) = pH 7.37; pCO$_2$ 35; pO$_2$ 50

Hemoglobin = 16.2 g/dL

Atrial and pulmonary capillary wedge pressures are shown as a/v/mean. Ventricular pressures are shown as systolic/end-diastolic. Arterial pressures are shown as systolic/diastolic/mean.

36. Based upon the hemodynamics above, what is the Q_p/Q_s?

A. 0.6

B. 1.0

C. 1.6

D. 2.0

E. Unable to calculate

37. What is this patient's pulmonary vascular resistance?

A. 1.1 Woods units $\times$ m^2

B. 1.4 Woods units $\times$ m^2

C. 1.6 Woods units $\times$ m^2

D. 1.8 Woods units $\times$ m^2

E. Unable to calculate

38. A 3-year-old girl with tricuspid atresia and normally related great arteries had a bidirectional cavopulmonary anastomosis and ligation of the main pulmonary artery. She undergoes cardiac catheterization prior to total cavopulmonary anastomosis. Hemodynamic data are shown in **Table 4.7**. Which of the following most closely represents this patient's Q_p/Q_s?

TABLE 4.7 Hemodynamic Cardiac Catheterization Data

Location	Pressure (mm Hg)	SpO$_2$ (%)
Superior vena cava	Mean 12	53
Left pulmonary artery	Mean 12	53
Right pulmonary artery	Mean 12	53
Right atrium	11/10/8	57
Left pulmonary vein	10/9/8	100
Right pulmonary vein	9/9/8	100
Left atrium	10/9/8	94
Left ventricle	84/9	82
Femoral artery	89/58/68	82
VO$_2$ (assumed) = 150 mL/min/m^2		
ABG (femoral) = pH 7.37; pCO$_2$ 35; pO$_2$ 50		
Hemoglobin = 16.2 g/dL		

Atrial and pulmonary capillary wedge pressures are shown as a/v/ mean. Ventricular pressures are shown as systolic/end-diastolic. Arterial pressures are shown as systolic/diastolic/mean.

A. 0.6
B. 0.8
C. 1.2
D. 1.6
E. Unable to calculate

39. An infant is referred for preoperative cardiac catheterization and the angiogram in **Figure 4.13** is obtained. What finding is demonstrated in this angiogram?

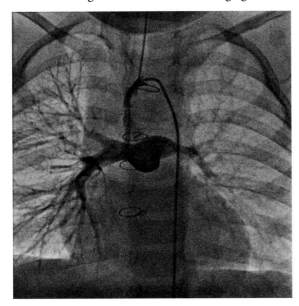

FIGURE 4.13

A. Modified BTT shunt
B. Sano shunt
C. Bidirectional Glenn
D. Extracardiac Fontan
E. Damus–Kaye–Stansel anastomosis

40. A 4-month-old male infant is referred for preoperative cardiac catheterization and the angiogram in **Figure 4.14** is obtained. This angiogram demonstrates which of the following?

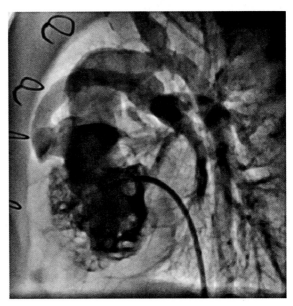

FIGURE 4.14

A. Classic BTT shunt
B. Modified BTT shunt
C. Sano shunt
D. Potts shunt
E. Waterston shunt

41. A 4-year-old boy with a history of repaired complete AV canal has severe left AV valve regurgitation. Accentuation of which of the following would be expected on the pulmonary capillary wedge tracing?

A. A wave
B. C wave
C. V wave
D. X descent
E. Y descent

CHAPTER 4

42. On the RA waveform, the C wave corresponds to which of the following cardiac event?

    A. Tricuspid valve closure with bowing of the valve into the atrium
    B. Opening of tricuspid valve
    C. Atrial filling with closed AV valve
    D. Atrial contraction
    E. Descent of AV valve ring into the ventricle

43. Which of the following events will decrease the hemoglobin affinity for oxygen?

    A. Decrease in temperature
    B. Decrease in 2,3-biphosphoglycerate levels
    C. Decrease in pH
    D. Decrease in pCO_2
    E. Decrease in serum glucose concentration

44. During a routine right heart catheterization, the hemodynamic data in **Table 4.8** are obtained. What is the most likely cause for the abnormal results obtained?

TABLE 4.8 Routine Right Heart Catheterization: Hemodynamic Data

Location	Pressure (mm Hg)	SpO$_2$ (%)
Superior vena cava	Mean 5	74
Inferior vena cava	Mean 5	78
Right atrium	Mean 6	45
Right ventricle	37/13	75
Left pulmonary artery	Mean 12	75
Right pulmonary artery	Mean 12	75
Right pulmonary capillary wedge	Mean 6	99
VO_2 (assumed) = 150 mL/min/m^2		

Ventricular pressures are shown as systolic/end-diastolic.

    A. Improper catheter position
    B. Anemia
    C. Acidosis
    D. Right-to-left shunt at the atrial level
    E. Arteriovenous malformation

45. During a routine right heart catheterization, the hemodynamic data in **Table 4.9** are obtained. What is the most likely cause for the abnormal results obtained?

TABLE 4.9 Routine Right Heart Catheterization: Hemodynamic Data

Location	Pressure (mm Hg)	SpO$_2$ (%)
Superior vena cava	Mean 5	64
Inferior vena cava	Mean 5	68
Right atrium	Mean 6	85
Right ventricle	37/13	85
Left pulmonary artery	Mean 12	85
Right pulmonary capillary wedge	Mean 6	99
Femoral artery	89/58/68	99
VO_2 (assumed) = 150 mL/min/m^2		
Cardiac output by thermodilution = 3 L/min/m^2		
Cardiac output by Fick = 2 L/min/m^2		

Ventricular pressures are shown as systolic/end-diastolic. Arterial pressures are shown as systolic/diastolic/mean.

    A. Technical error
    B. Anemia
    C. Acidosis
    D. Left-to-right shunt at the atrial level
    E. Nonsteady hemodynamic state

46. A 13-year-old boy from South America with pulmonary atresia and VSD with hypoplastic, confluent pulmonary arteries and multiple major aortopulmonary collateral arteries (MAPCAs) is referred for preoperative cardiac catheterization and angiography. Preprocedure laboratory data demonstrate a hematocrit of 75%. Which of the following is the next best step to pursue?

    A. Cancel the procedure due to a high risk of stroke
    B. Give the patient a dose of warfarin the evening prior to procedure
    C. Admit the patient for IV fluid hydration the evening before procedure
    D. No special precautions need to be taken
    E. Perform the entire procedure on 100% FiO_2

The following scenario applies to Questions 47 and 48:

*A 22-year-old with tetralogy of Fallot had a complete repair at 5 years of age. The native pulmonary valve was initially preserved, but subsequently (age 14 years) he developed significant valvular stenosis and regurgitation, and the valve was replaced with a 27-mm porcine bioprosthesis. That valve has now developed severe regurgitation, and he undergoes cardiac catheterization with the plan to insert a transcatheter valve within the pulmonary bioprosthesis. The data in **Table 4.10** are obtained during the study. No residual shunts were identified during the study.*

TABLE 4.10 Cardiac Catheterization Data

Position	Pressure (mm Hg)
RA	Mean = 5
RV	60/8
MPA	60/8
PCWP	Mean = 20
LV	120/24

RA, right atrium; RV, right ventricle; MPA, main pulmonary artery; PCWP, pulmonary capillary wedge pressure; LV, left ventricle.

47. The data presented in **Table 4.11** are most consistent with which of the following?

TABLE 4.11 Cardiac Data

Location	Pressure (mm Hg)	SpO$_2$ (%)
Superior vena cava		72
Right atrium	Mean 13	70
Right ventricle	60/16	70
Left pulmonary artery	60/12/34	70
Left pulmonary capillary wedge	Mean 18	99
Left ventricle	120/22	98
Ascending aorta	122/64/84	98
Femoral artery	124/64/86	98

VO$_2$ (assumed) = 150 mL/min/m^2

ABG (femoral) = pH 7.35; pCO$_2$ 36; pO$_2$ 51

Hemoglobin = 13 g/dL

Atrial and pulmonary capillary wedge pressures are shown as mean. Ventricular pressures are shown as systolic/end-diastolic. Arterial pressures are shown as systolic/diastolic/mean.

  A. Mild pulmonary regurgitation
  B. Moderate pulmonary valve stenosis
  C. Restrictive physiology
  D. Cardiac tamponade
  E. Severe tricuspid regurgitation

48. Which of the following findings on the RA waveform would be consistent with a diagnosis of restrictive cardiomyopathy rather than constrictive pericarditis (CP)?

  A. Presence of M waves
  B. Inspiratory rise in RA pressure
  C. Normal respiratory variation in mean RA pressure
  D. Equalization of mean RA pressure with RVEDP, PA diastolic, PCWP, and LVEDP
  E. Absence of the A wave

49. A 6-year-old boy is referred for a hemodynamic right heart catheterization secondary to progressive right atrial and right ventricular enlargement with no identifiable cause on echocardiography. An arterial blood gas was performed at the start of the case demonstrating hemoglobin of 12.5 g/dL and pO$_2$ of 74 mL/dL. The oximetry data in **Table 4.12** were obtained during the study. What is the ratio of pulmonary blood flow to systemic blood flow?

TABLE 4.12 Blood Oximetry Data

Site	Sat (%)
High right SVC	63
Low right SVC	88
Right atrium	73
Right ventricle	73
MPA	73
RPA	73
Femoral artery	98

  A. 0.4
  B. 0.7
  C. 1.0
  D. 1.4
  E. 2.5

CHAPTER 4

50. A 16-year-old patient from Africa has the chest radiograph in **Figure 4.15**. Which of the following pressure measurements would you expect to find during cardiac catheterization?

A. Mean RA pressure 10 mm Hg
B. RVSP 70 mm Hg
C. Mean PA pressure 20 mm Hg
D. PCWP 18 mm Hg
E. Ascending aorta 152/84 mm Hg

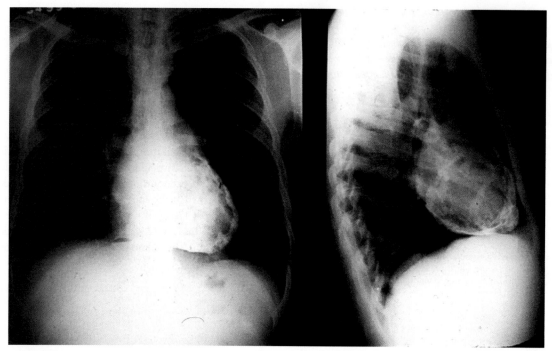

FIGURE 4.15

51. The following oxygen saturation data were obtained during a baseline hemodynamic study in an intubated 5-year-old patient: SVC 72%; RA 85%; RV 83%; MPA 83%; RPA 84%; LA 92%; RPV 99%; LPV 83%. Which of the following is the best next step?

A. Perform an LV angio to look for a VSD
B. Perform a PA angiogram to evaluate for a pulmonary AV fistula
C. Reevaluate the endotracheal tube position
D. Continue with the ASD device closure
E. Reverse his sedation

52. A 30-year-old woman with a history of tricuspid atresia and nonfenestrated Fontan procedure at age 5 presents with a 2-year history of dyspnea on exertion and cyanosis that is worse when in the standing position. Which of the following is the most likely cause of her symptoms?

A. Hepatic arteriovenous malformation (AVM)
B. Vein of Galen malformation
C. Lower extremity AVM
D. Upper extremity AVM
E. Pulmonary AVM

53. Which of the following patients has the strongest indication for catheter-based intervention?

A. 20-year-old patient, asymptomatic, pulmonary valve mean Doppler gradient = 24 mm Hg
B. 30-year-old patient with refractory migraines and a PFO
C. 40-year-old patient, asymptomatic, pulmonary valve peak-to-peak gradient = 54 mm Hg
D. 25-year-old patient, asymptomatic, with a continuous murmur and small PDA on echo
E. 28-year-old patient with a small membranous VSD and recurrent endocarditis

54. A 6-month-old infant with severe aortic valve stenosis is undergoing cardiac catheterization with consideration of aortic valvuloplasty. His aortic valve annulus diameter is 9 mm. Which of the following balloon diameters is most appropriate for initial valvuloplasty?

A. 6 mm
B. 8 mm
C. 10 mm
D. 12 mm
E. 14 mm

55. A 6-month-old infant with severe pulmonary valve stenosis is undergoing cardiac catheterization with consideration of pulmonary valvuloplasty. Her pulmonary valve annulus diameter is 9 mm. Which of the following balloon diameters is most appropriate for initial valvuloplasty?

    A. 8 mm
    B. 9 mm
    C. 10 mm
    D. 12 mm
    E. 15 mm

56. A full-term infant with complete TGA and a pH of 7.1 is in the cath lab for balloon atrial septostomy. After vascular access is obtained, which of the following is the best management of this situation?

    A. Balloon atrial septostomy should be performed promptly
    B. Obtain mixed venous saturation in the RA
    C. Perform RV angiography to evaluate coronary anatomy
    D. Perform RA angiography to assess right-to-left shunt
    E. The procedure is not required when patients have a coexistent VSD

57. In an asymptomatic 6-year-old girl, the transthoracic echocardiographic images in **Figure 4.16** were obtained.

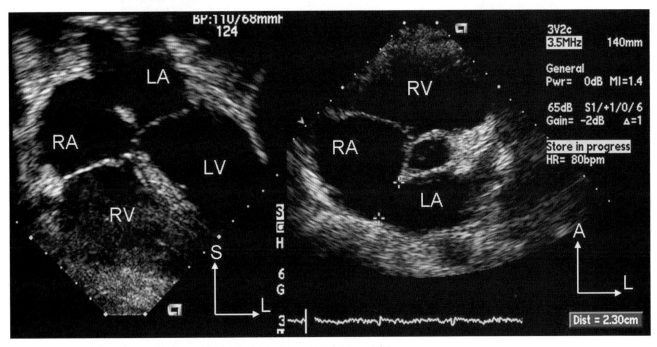

FIGURE 4.16 LA, left atrium; LV, left ventricle; RA, right atrium; RV, right ventricle.

You are counseling the parent regarding type and timing of intervention. Based upon the images shown, what would you say to the patient?

A. This is a sinus venosus defect and therefore not amenable to device closure
B. The defect is well centered and should be easily closed with a device
C. Closure is not indicated at this time due to the absence of significant right ventricular enlargement
D. The defect is large and some rims are deficient preventing device closure
E. Surgery is indicated to repair the anomalous pulmonary vein(s)

58. You are assessing a 5-year-old girl for possible PDA closure. Echocardiogram shows a large PDA with bidirectional shunting. There is no murmur on examination. Her echo is otherwise normal with no tricuspid regurgitation and no chamber enlargement. Her parents report she is a quiet child but does not seem to be limited in any way. What is the next best step?

    A. Surgical closure of her PDA
    B. Transcatheter closure of her PDA
    C. Return in 3 years for follow-up echo evaluation
    D. Return in 6 to 12 months for follow-up echo
    E. Hemodynamic cardiac catheterization

CHAPTER 4

59. A newborn with an in utero diagnosis of pulmonary atresia with intact ventricular septum is admitted to the NICU. An echocardiogram confirms the diagnosis. The infundibulum appears unobstructed. There is a mild pulmonary valve hypoplasia with no systolic or diastolic flow across the annulus. The RV is small with systolic pressure. The tricuspid valve is hypoplastic with a Z score = −2.5 with moderate regurgitation. The left ventricle has normal size and function. The coronary arteries were not well identified. A large ASD with right-to-left shunting is noted. The patient has a cardiac catheterization to perform radiofrequency perforation and balloon valvuloplasty. The angiogram in **Figure 4.17** was obtained. What should be the next step for this patient?

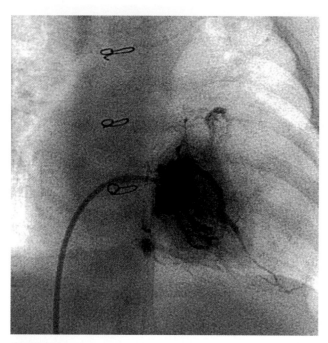

FIGURE 4.17

  A. Dilation of the right coronary artery
  B. Balloon atrial septostomy
  C. Abort perforation and balloon valvuloplasty
  D. Refer for surgical pulmonary valvotomy
  E. Perform pulmonary valvuloplasty with MPA stent placement

60. A 17-year-old patient with no significant past medical history presents with a transient ischemic attack. She had a similar episode 2 years prior but failed to report that event. During the workup, she is found to have a 5-mm secundum atrial septal defect (ASD) with predominant left-to-right shunt but does have transient right-to-left shunt. Tests for hypercoagulable disorders were negative. The patient is a Jehovah Witness. According to the AHA guidelines, what would you recommend for management of the ASD?

  A. Recommend device closure of the ASD
  B. Recommend observation and treatment with aspirin
  C. Recommend observation alone
  D. Recommend observation and treatment with warfarin
  E. Recommend surgical closure

61. Which of the following lesions with a restrictive atrial communication would be at highest risk of complication with balloon atrial septostomy (BAS)?

  A. Hypoplastic left heart syndrome
  B. d-TGA with intact ventricular septum
  C. Tricuspid atresia
  D. d-TGA with VSD
  E. Total anomalous pulmonary venous connection

62. A 45-year-old man presents with exertional cyanosis. He has a history of heart block following Mustard palliation of d-TGA and had transvenous pacemaker lead placement. He has an echo which reveals a SVC baffle leak with bidirectional shunting. Which of the following is the most appropriate next step for this patient?

  A. Initiate aspirin therapy only
  B. Closure of the baffle leak
  C. Initiate warfarin therapy and reassess in 6 months
  D. Pacemaker externalization
  E. No additional treatment is necessary

63. During cardiac catheterization, a child with coarctation of the aorta is found to have a systolic gradient <20 mm Hg, meeting criteria for a mild coarctation. Which of the following findings is most likely to result in underestimation of the severity of coarctation by gradient alone?

  A. CI = 1.5 L/min/m² by thermodilution
  B. Right pulmonary capillary wedge pressure of 8 mm Hg
  C. Right pulmonary artery stenosis with inability to pass a wire to the distal RPA
  D. LV end-diastolic pressure of 12 mm Hg
  E. ABG demonstrating pCO_2 of 68 mm Hg at the start of the case

64. A colleague requests a cardiac catheterization on an infant with diastolic heart failure due to dilated cardiomyopathy in association with 3-methylglutaconic aciduria type II. Prior to proceeding with cardiac catheterization, which of the following laboratory abnormalities should be ruled out?
  A. Thrombocytopenia
  B. Thrombocytosis
  C. Anemia
  D. Neutropenia
  E. Hyperglycemia

The following clinical scenario applies to Questions 65 and 66.

A 2-week-old infant undergoes cardiac catheterization. He has a diagnosis of pulmonary atresia with VSD and confluent pulmonary arteries supplied by a tortuous ductus arteriosus. Hemodynamic measurements are shown in **Table 4.13**.

TABLE 4.13 Cardiac Data

Location	Pressure (mm Hg)	SpO_2 (%)
Superior vena cava		58
Right atrium	Mean 8	63
Right ventricle	72/9	68
Left atrium	Mean 10	98
Left ventricle	75/11	93
Descending aorta	75/36/49	82

VO_2 (assumed) = 160 mL/min/m^2

ABG (descending aorta) = pH 7.35; pCO_2 36; pO_2 60

ABG (left atrium) = pH 7.39; pCO_2 39; pO_2 100

Hemoglobin = 14 g/dL

65. Which of the following most closely represents this patient's effective pulmonary blood flow (Q_{ep})?
  A. 1.6 L/min/m^2
  B. 2.1 L/min/m^2
  C. 3.5 L/min/m^2
  D. 5.1 L/min/m^2
  E. Unable to determine

66. Which of the following most closely represents this patient's effective systemic blood flow (Q_{es})?
  A. 1.6 L/min/m^2
  B. 2.1 L/min/m^2
  C. 3.5 L/min/m^2
  D. 5.1 L/min/m^2
  E. Unable to determine

Answers

Note: For all questions regarding shunt calculations use Figure 4.18 as a reference.

$$Q_p = \frac{VO_2}{[(PV_{sat} - PA_{sat}) \times Hgb \times 1.36 + \text{A-V dissolved } O_2] \times 10}$$

$$Q_s = \frac{VO_2}{[(SA_{sat} - MV_{sat}) \times Hgb \times 1.36 + \text{A-V dissolved } O_2] \times 10}$$

$$Q_{es} = Q_{ep} = \frac{VO_2}{[(PV_{sat} - MV_{sat}) \times Hgb \times 1.36 + \text{A-V dissolved } O_2] \times 10}$$

$$\text{Shunt}_{L-R} = \frac{Q_p - Q_{ep}}{Q_p} = 1 - \frac{(PV_{sat} - PA_{sat})}{(PV_{sat} - MV_{sat})}$$

$$\text{Shunt}_{R-L} = \frac{Q_s - Q_{es}}{Q_s} = 1 - \frac{(SA_{sat} - MV_{sat})}{(PV_{sat} - MV_{sat})}$$

FIGURE 4.18 Formulas for shunt calculations.

1. (C) In order to solve this problem, the Fick principle must be incorporated. It is absolutely vital to know this equation.

The scenarios to follow throughout the chapter will continue to expand on the utility of this principle. This equation is listed above for systemic flow but can be adapted to pulmonary blood flow in the presence of a shunt by interchanging pulmonary vein (PV) – pulmonary artery (PA) for systemic artery (SA) – mixed venous (MV).

$$\text{Systemic flow (indexed)} = \frac{O_2 \text{ consumption (VO}_2)}{\text{oxygen content}_A - \text{oxygen content}_V}$$

$$\text{Systemic flow (indexed)} = \frac{O_2 \text{ consumption (VO}_2)}{(SA - MV)O_2 \times O_2 \text{ bound to Hgb} + \text{dissolved } O_2}$$

$$\text{Systemic flow (indexed)} = \frac{O_2 \text{ consumption (VO}_2)}{(SA - MV)O_2 \times Hgb \times 1.36 \times 10}$$

$$\text{Systemic flow (indexed)} = \frac{150 \text{ mL/min/m}^2}{(0.99 - 0.70)O_2 \times 12 \text{ g/dL} \times 1.36 \times 10 \text{ dL/L}}$$

$$\text{Systemic flow (indexed)} = \frac{150 \text{ mL/min/m}^2}{46.6 \text{ mL } O_2/L}$$

Systemic flow

(indexed) = 3.2 L/min/m^2

If the patient is not on supplemental oxygen, the dissolved pO_2 can be ignored as it will be negligible to the final result. The value 1.36 represents the Hüfner factor (oxygen-binding capacity of human hemoglobin). By utilizing the given VO_2 and hemoglobin, along with the systemic arterial sat (LV of 99%; SA = 0.99) and mixed venous sat (RPA of 70%; MV = 0.70), the systemic flow is calculated as 3.2 L/min/m^2.

2. (B) PVR is calculated by dividing the mean pressure gradient through the pulmonary bed (PA$_{mean}$ – LA$_{mean}$) by Q_p. In this case, the transpulmonary gradient is 35 – 10 = 25 mm Hg and Q_p = 3.2 L/min/m^2, so PVR = 7.8 Woods units × m^2.

3. (C) When Q_p = Q_s, as in this scenario, the ratio of PVR to SVR is the same as the ratio of transpulmonary gradient (PA$_{mean}$ × LA$_{mean}$) to transsystemic gradient (AO$_{mean}$ – RA$_{mean}$). In this case, transpulmonary gradient is 25 mm Hg and transsystemic gradient is 63 mm Hg. Thus, PVR:SVR is 0.4.

4. (B) The catheter course from the IVC to the RA and to the anterior ventricle is consistent with a right ventricular angiogram. There is moderate enlargement of the RV with severe RV outflow tract obstruction at the subpulmonary and pulmonary valve levels with hypoplasia of the main and branch pulmonary arteries. There is right-to-left shunting through the VSD with opacification of the aorta. These findings in constellation are consistent with a diagnosis of tetralogy of Fallot.

5. (D) Figure 4.2 is taken from a straight lateral projection. The catheter in this image is located quite posterior (well over the vertebral bodies) and courses cranially, eventually taking an anterior turn. This position is posterior to the descending aorta, which is located along the anterior aspect of the vertebral bodies, as demonstrated on an LV angiogram from the same case (**Figure 4.19**). The catheter

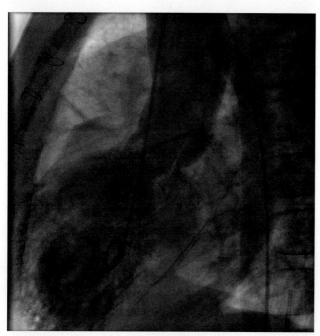

FIGURE 4.19

is coursing through an azygos vein with the anterior turn located at the anastomosis with the superior vena cava. Azygos continuation into the right or left SVC is seen with an interrupted IVC. This is due to failure to form the right subcardinal-hepatic anastomosis. This venous malformation does not result in clinical manifestations but can complicate interventional cath and EP procedures.

6. (E) The congenital left ventricle to right atrial shunt (Gerbode defect) would result in enhanced right atrial filling during AV valve closure through ventricular systole. The same finding would be expected in the presence of severe tricuspid valve regurgitation. A prominent A wave would be expected for lesions causing RV diastolic dysfunction or obstruction to RV inflow, such as tricuspid valve stenosis.

7. (C) This waveform demonstrates rapid onset hypotension and tachycardia consistent with impaired cardiac output due to cardiac tamponade. The cause is likely hemopericardium due to a complication from catheterization. Sudden circulatory collapse warrants immediate pericardiocentesis and may necessitate drain placement.

8. (E) The metal frame of the Amplatzer® device is made from nitinol, a nickel–titanium alloy. Detectable levels of nickel have been identified in the bloodstream after successful Amplatzer device placement, and allergic reactions have been reported, albeit rarely. The estimated rate for nickel hypersensitivity in the general population is 15%.

9. (A) ECG abnormalities after ASD closure device placement have been reported in 5% to 10% of patients. The incidence appears higher in older patients as compared to children and the vast majority of these abnormalities resolve, especially in children, typically within 24 hours of the procedure. Heart block is a very rare complication from ASD device closure.

10. (B) In room air, Q_p/Q_s can be calculated if you know the mixed venous (MV) saturation, systemic arterial (SA) saturation, pulmonary venous (PV) saturation, and pulmonary arterial (PA) saturation by using the following equation: Q_p/Q_s = (SA – MV)/(PV – PA). For this patient, superior vena cava is the best choice for MV (right atrium is not a mixed chamber), and left atrium can be used at PV because the saturation is near 100%. If left atrial saturation is low (e.g., less than 96%), then one must consider the possibility of a right-to-left shunt at the atrial level. Using these values, Q_p/Q_s = (0.83 – 0.64)/(0.99 – 0.83) = 1.18.

11. (C) To calculate shunt volume or shunt percentage, you need to know the *effective pulmonary blood flow* (Q_{ep}), which is the volume of systemic venous blood that goes to the lungs. Left-to-right shunt volume (Q_{L-R}) is then calculated by subtracting Q_{ep} from Q_p. Q_{ep} is calculated by dividing VO_2 by the difference in pulmonary venous (PV) and mixed systemic venous (MV) oxygen content. For this patient, VO_2 is 150 mL/min/m^2. Ignoring dissolved oxygen, the PV – MV oxygen content difference is 1.36 × 10 × 17.4 × (0.99 – 0.64) = 83 mL/L. Therefore, Q_{ep} = 150/83 = 1.8 L/min/m^2. Q_p is 150/[1.36 × 10 × 17.4 × (0.99 – 0.83)] = 4.0 L/min/m^2. Q_{L-R} is the difference between Q_p and Q_{ep}, or 2.2 L/min/m^2.

12. (B) Since effective pulmonary blood flow (Q_{ep}) = effective systemic blood flow (Q_{es}) = 1.8 L/min/m², right-to-left shunt volume (Q_{R-L}) can be calculated in a similar manner to that described in the previous answer. Using the superior vena cava as mixed venous saturation and ignoring dissolved oxygen, Q_s = 150/[1.36 × 10 × 17.4 × (0.83 − 0.64)] = 3.3 L/min/m². Q_{R-L} is the difference between Q_s and Q_{es}, or 1.5 L/min/m².

13. (B) Pulmonary vascular resistance is calculated by dividing the mean pressure gradient through the pulmonary bed ($PA_{mean} − LA_{mean}$) by Q_p. In this case, the transpulmonary gradient is 42 − 11 = 31 mm Hg and Q_p = 4.0 L/min/m², so PVR = 7.8 Woods units × m².

14. (A) There are four main hemodynamic abnormalities present—pulmonary hypertension, increased pulmonary artery saturation (left-to-right shunting), systemic arterial desaturation (right-to-left shunting), and a widened pulse pressure. The fact that right ventricular and left ventricular saturations are significantly different, but pulmonary artery and aorta saturations are the same, tells us that most of the mixing is occurring at the level of the great arteries, as is seen with truncus arteriosus. Tetralogy of Fallot will have differential systemic and pulmonary artery saturations due to preferential streaming of blood in the ventricles to the ipsilateral great artery. PDA with Eisenmenger syndrome can produce right-to-left shunting, but ascending aorta saturation would be expected to be higher than descending aorta. Interrupted aortic arch with PDA can cause pulmonary hypertension and descending aorta desaturation, but ascending aorta saturation should be relatively normal in the absence of other defects. Transposition of the great arteries with a large ASD can cause mixing of systemic and pulmonary venous blood, but not typically enough that aortic and pulmonary artery saturations are the same.

15. (D) The catheter is advanced from the RA across an ASD to the LA and subsequently the LV. The angiogram demonstrates elongation of the LV outflow tract (the "goose neck" deformity). This finding is present in patients with an AVSD due to the anterior displacement of the aortic valve, creating an elongated LVOT and predisposing the patient to progressive subaortic obstruction. Roughly 40% to 45% of children with Down syndrome will have congenital heart disease, with approximately 45% having an AVSD. The other answer choices reference primary aortic disease (Marfan and Loeys–Dietz), supravalvar AS and branch PA stenoses (Williams), and large ASD that commonly causes a common atrium (Ellis–van Crevald).

16. (B) The catheter traverses from the IVC to the RA and to the anterior ventricle. The angiogram demonstrates that the anterior ventricle gives rise to the aortic outflow tract, consistent with transposition of the great arteries and the question stem is consistent with TGA with intact ventricular septum and inadequate intercirculatory mixing. Catheterization is not indicated for a newborn with TGA, unless there is severe hypoxia with an inability to provide oxygenation via the native atrial communication or a patent ductus arteriosus with PGE1 administration. In this clinical scenario, balloon atrial septostomy precedes early arterial switch procedure.

17. (C) The left upper pulmonary vein was injected demonstrating a PAPVC with drainage of the LUPV via a vertical vein to the left innominate vein. The innominate vein is the usual site for connection of an anomalous left pulmonary vein. The vertical vein demonstrated in this angiogram is separate embryologically from a left-sided SVC, with a LSVC located directly posterior to the left atrial appendage and draining to the coronary sinus. Much less common sites of PAPVC of the left pulmonary veins would include the coronary sinus, right SVC, left SVC, and azygos vein.

18. (D) This patient has severe pulmonary hypertension both clinically and hemodynamically. While there is a small atrial level shunt (demonstrated echocardiographically and by a small "step-down" in saturation from pulmonary vein to left atrium and left ventricle), the striking hemodynamic abnormalities are suprasystemic pulmonary artery pressure and a significant "step-down" in saturation from ascending aorta to descending aorta. The most likely explanation for this finding is a right-to-left shunt between the ascending and descending aorta, such as a PDA or aortopulmonary window. Primary (idiopathic) pulmonary hypertension would be a consideration in the absence of a significant shunt lesion. The saturation step-down occurs at the level of the great arteries, making anomalous pulmonary veins (an "atrial" level shunt) and ventricular septal defect less likely. Anomalous origin of the right pulmonary artery from the aorta (so-called "hemitruncus") can result in pulmonary hypertension/Eisenmenger syndrome, but invasive hemodynamics would demonstrate right pulmonary artery saturation equal to aortic, and a lower left pulmonary artery saturation.

19. (E) While there are sufficient data to calculate Q_p, the available data are inadequate to calculate Q_s. Similarly, the Fick principle cannot be used to calculate pulmonary blood flow in situations where there are multiple sources of pulmonary blood flow, each with different oxygen content (e.g., tetralogy of Fallot with a surgical aortopulmonary shunt). In this patient, systemic arterial blood flow is derived from both the ascending aorta (higher oxygen content) and the ductus arteriosus (lower oxygen content). Without knowing the proportion of blood flowing to the brachiocephalic arteries relative to the proportion flowing to the descending aorta, we cannot account for this difference in oxygen content by the Fick equation alone.

20. (C) Pulmonary arteriolar resistance is calculated by dividing the pressure difference through the pulmonary bed by pulmonary blood flow (Q_p). The pressure difference through the pulmonary bed (96 mm Hg) is calculated by subtracting the mean left atrial (10 mm Hg) or pulmonary capillary wedge pressure from the *mean* pulmonary artery pressure (in this case RPA = LPA = 106 mm Hg). Q_p is calculated using the Fick equation, where oxygen consumption (VO₂) is divided by the change in blood oxygen content across the pulmonary capillary bed. The change in oxygen content is calculated by multiplying Hüfner factor for the oxygen-binding capacity of hemoglobin (1.36 mL O₂/g hemoglobin) by the hemoglobin concentration in blood (12.5 g/dL), multiplied by a factor of 10 (to convert dL to L), multiplied again by the difference in hemoglobin saturation before (pulmonary artery = 72% or 0.72) and after (pulmonary vein = 99% or 0.99) the capillary bed. On room air, a small amount of oxygen is dissolved in blood (pO_2); this can be disregarded. In the presence of a higher concentration of inhaled oxygen, pO_2 can be significantly greater and should be included in the calculation. For this patient, the denominator of the Fick equation is $1.36 \times 12.5 \times 10 \times (0.99 - 0.72) = 45.9$. Dividing 125 ($VO_2$) by 45.9 results in an indexed $Q_p = 2.72$ L/min/m^2. Pulmonary vascular resistance is then calculated by dividing 96 mm Hg by 2.72 L/min/m^2 = 35.2 Woods units × m^2.

21. (D) When inhaled oxygen is increased, the relative contribution of dissolved oxygen to total blood oxygen content likewise increases and should be factored into the Fick equation for calculating Q_p. Dissolved oxygen is calculated as $0.003 \times pO_2$. For this patient, pulmonary vein oxygen content is $1.36 \times 12.5 \times 10 \times (100\%) + 0.03 \times 394 = 182$ mL O_2/L blood. Pulmonary artery oxygen content is $1.36 \times 12.5 \times 10 \times (78\%) + 0.03 \times 44 = 134$ mL O_2/L blood. Dividing VO_2 by the difference in oxygen content $= 125/(182 - 134) = 2.60$ L/min/m^2. Pulmonary vascular resistance is then calculated by dividing the pressure difference (99 mm Hg − 11 mm Hg) by Q_p; $88/2.60 = 34$ Woods units × m^2.

22. (D) The angiogram demonstrates an injection of the right SVC with a cavopulmonary anastomosis communicating with the right and left pulmonary arteries, consistent with a bidirectional Glenn shunt. There is also stenosis along the left side of the PA insertion of the SVC, a common complication encountered following this procedure. The other options are incorrect and include the classic BTT shunt (right subclavian to RPA anastomosis with native vessel), modified BT shunt (right subclavian to RPA anastomosis with artificial material), classic Glenn shunt (RSVC to distal RPA anastomosis supplying a single lung), and DKS anastomosis (transected MPA anastomosed with the ascending aorta).

23. (B) This lateral projection demonstrates an RV injection with pulmonary valve stenosis causing a small, anteriorly directed jet streaming to the MPA with poststenotic dilation of the MPA. The exact mechanism for poststenotic dilation remains controversial, but is likely a result of multiple hemodynamic factors including high velocity and turbulent blood flow accompanied by remodeling of the vascular wall. The other options (A, C, D) address RV pathology, with a normal appearing RV on this angiogram. The diverticulum of Kommerell is a term referencing the bulbous configuration of the origin of an aberrant left subclavian artery in a right-sided aortic arch or aberrant right subclavian artery in the setting of a left-sided aortic arch.

24. (C) The angiogram is a lateral projection demonstrating retrograde access for a left heart catheterization with an angiogram performed in the proximal descending aorta. There is left-to-right shunting through a patent ductus arteriosus to the left pulmonary artery. All symptomatic PDAs with left-to-right shunting and asymptomatic PDAs with LA or LV enlargement should be closed, regardless of age. In the current era, transcatheter device closure is the standard of care.

25. (B) As described previously, cardiac output (index) is calculated using the Fick equation. Oxygen consumption (VO_2) is divided by the difference in blood oxygen concentration across the capillary bed. In this case, cardiac index is $140/1.36 \times 10.8 \times 10 \times (0.99 - 0.73) = 3.7$ L/min/m^2.

26. (A) In the presence of unequal branch pulmonary artery pressures, the Fick equation can still be used to calculate Q_p, but consideration of the proportion of flow going to one lung or the other is needed to calculate an accurate pulmonary arteriolar resistance. To accomplish this, we use the data from the lung perfusion scan (40% flow to the right lung; 60% to the left) and calculate the resistance for each lung individually. The flow to the right lung is 40% of 3.7 L/min/m^2 or 1.5 L/min/m^2. The arteriolar resistance of the right lung (R_{right}) is 2.7 Woods units × m^2. Similarly, the flow to the left lung is 2.2 L/min/m^2 and the resistance (R_{left}) is 5.5 Woods units × m^2. Because the lungs form a parallel circuit, total pulmonary arteriolar resistance is calculated by the following equation: $1/R_{total} = 1/R_{right} + 1/R_{left}$. Thus the total resistance is $(1/2.7 + 1/5.5)^{-1} = 1.8$ Woods units × m^2.

27. (D) The ASD closure device has embolized to the right pulmonary artery. This is demonstrated by the device borders extending beyond the borders of the cardiac silhouette. Emergency retrieval is indicated and may be performed percutaneously or via an open surgical approach.

28. (D) A thorough preoperative evaluation is recommended for patients with Williams syndrome to identify those with anatomical abnormalities which may result in coronary artery involvement. Even without evidence of coronary abnormalities on preoperative imaging, these patients remain at risk for sudden cardiac arrest and death, which must be considered when discussing the risk–benefit ratio of cardiac catheterization or any procedure that requires sedation. During sedation or anesthetic induction, patients with supravalvar aortic stenosis can experience coronary artery malperfusion and ischemia, leading to ventricular dysfunction and impaired cardiac output. If not promptly recognized and treated, death can occur.

29. (E) Patients taking NPH insulin are at an increased risk of hypersensitivity reaction to protamine, with an incidence of a reaction in 27% of patients compared to 0.5% in patients with no history of taking insulin. Reactions to protamine can range from back/flank pain, flushing, and peripheral vasodilation to vasomotor collapse, which may be fatal.

30. (A) This patient has an anomalous left pulmonary vein draining to the left innominate vein. This manifests as elevated left innominate vein saturation, representing drainage of the anomalous vein(s) to the innominate vein via a vertical vein. Because the right pulmonary veins drain to the left atrium, the right capillary wedge pressure will reflect left atrial pressure. The left pulmonary vein(s), on the other hand, ultimately drain to the right atrium. Therefore, left capillary wedge pressure will reflect right atrial pressure (in the absence of vertical vein obstruction). Right or left pulmonary vein stenosis would manifest as a gradient between ipsilateral pulmonary capillary wedge pressure and left atrial pressure or left ventricular diastolic pressure. In addition, pulmonary vein stenosis would not explain the elevated innominate vein saturation. There is no evidence to suggest increased right pulmonary artery flow or technical error.

31. (C) As explained in the answer to the previous question, this patient has evidence of anomalous pulmonary vein drainage to the left innominate vein. Therefore, the patient is almost certain to have a draining left vertical vein. Sinus venosus defect is much more common with anomalous right pulmonary veins draining directly to the superior vena cava or right atrium. Pulmonary sequestration is often seen in Scimitar syndrome, in which the anomalous pulmonary vein typically drains inferiorly to the inferior vena cava. An unroofed coronary sinus is rare and is more commonly associated with a persistent left superior vena cava. Right ventricular enlargement may occur as a result of significant left-to-right shunt over time, but this patient's overall shunt volume is relatively small, as evidenced by the minimal elevation in pulmonary pressures.

32. (D) Device erosion with the Amplatzer® device occurs in approximately 0.1% of implants. Speculation regarding oversizing and impingement on the wall of the aorta has been debated. However, erosions have still been reported with smaller devices (20 mm). The newer Gore Helex™ has not, to date, been associated with erosions.

33. (A) Forbes et al. (*J Am Coll Cardiol*. 2011 Dec 13;58(25):2664–74.) reported a multivariate analysis comparing surgical, stent, and balloon angioplasty treatment of coarctation of the aorta. This study demonstrated that in a select age range of patients (6 to 12 years), balloon angioplasty is more likely to result in an acute aortic wall injury of any type in comparison to stent implantation or surgical repair. Stent patients reported the lowest rate for acute complications, but there are several limitations to the study, including the overrepresentation of surgical patients necessitating a tube graft interposition or patch reconstruction rather than an isolated end-to-end anastomosis.

34. (C) This angiogram demonstrates an injection in an anomalous right upper pulmonary vein with contrast entering the right SVC and returning to the right atrium. Right upper PAPVC is most commonly associated with a superior sinus venosus defect (deficiency of the common wall between the right SVC and the RUPV resulting in the LA orifice of the RUPV with an unroofed pulmonary vein). Occasionally, a secundum ASD and/or left SVC are present. Scimitar syndrome was first described by Neill et al. in 1960 and results from anomalous drainage of the RPVs to the IVC, just above or below the diaphragm.

35. (B) A fundamental component to the success of surgical correction of TGA involves the identification of the origin and course of the coronary arteries. This AP projection demonstrates the circumflex arising from the region of the right-facing sinus and coursing leftward. The LAD arises from the left-facing sinus. The lateral projection would further assist in defining the anterior–posterior course. Based on the information provided, the only answer consistent with this angiogram is the circumflex arising from the RCA.

36. (C) The available data are adequate to calculate Q_p/Q_s. With this anatomy, aortic and pulmonary artery saturations will be the same. Using SVC as mixed venous (the right atrium is not a well-mixed chamber), $Q_p/Q_s = (0.82 − 0.53)/(1.00 − 0.82) = 1.6$.

37. (D) For this patient, Q_p can be calculated using femoral artery saturation since it equals pulmonary artery saturation (see answer above). Dividing VO_2 by the pulmonary venous and pulmonary arterial oxygen content difference results in $Q_p = 150/[1.36 × 16.2 × 10 × (1.00 × 0.82)] = 3.8$ L/min/m^2. The pulmonary vein wedge pressure can be used as a surrogate of mean pulmonary artery pressure; thus, the transpulmonary gradient is $14 − 7 = 7$ mm Hg. PVR = 7 mm Hg/3.8 L/min/m^2 = 1.8 Woods units × m^2.

38. (A) Even though this patient has the same mixed venous, systemic arterial and pulmonary venous saturation and the same hemoglobin as the patient in the previous scenario, her pulmonary arterial saturation is lower, reflecting a lower, but more efficient rate of pulmonary blood flow. For her, $Q_p/Q_s = (0.82 − 0.53)/(1.00 − 0.53) = 0.6$.

39. (A) The catheter is coursing from the aorta to the first brachiocephalic branch allowing for a hand injection in a right-sided BTT shunt. Also demonstrated is LPA stenosis with preferential flow through the RPA. The alternative answer choices have been previously described.

40. (C) This RV angiogram was performed in a patient with HLHS following a Norwood procedure and demonstrates a Sano shunt arising from the anterior wall of the RV providing an RV-PA shunt. The other options are incorrect and include the classic BTT shunt (right subclavian to RPA anastomosis with native vessel), modified BTT shunt (right subclavian to RPA anastomosis with artificial material), Potts shunt (direct descending aorta to LPA anastomosis), and Waterston shunt (direct ascending aorta to RPA anastomosis).

41. (C) Usually the A wave in the RA is slightly higher than the V wave, with the opposite true for the LA (V wave is slightly higher than the A wave). The V wave is due to atrial filling with a closed AV valve during LV contraction. In the setting of left AV valve regurgitation, the V wave will be increased when blood flows back to the LA through the regurgitant orifice. An increased A wave would be expected in mitral valve stenosis or LV diastolic dysfunction.

42. (A) There are five key components to the RA waveform which should be well understood. These include:

A wave—atrial contraction

C wave—closure of the AV valve with bowing of the AV valve into the atrium during the start of the ventricular contraction

X descent—descent in pressure as the AV valve ring is pulled into the ventricle

V wave—passive filling of the atrium with a closed AV valve

Y descent—descent due to AV valve opening and passive atrial emptying

43. (C) The oxygen–hemoglobin dissociation curve plots hemoglobin saturation (*y*-axis) against oxygen tension (*x*-axis). A decrease in the hemoglobin affinity for oxygen would be represented by a rightward shift of the oxyhemoglobin curve, resulting in an increased partial pressure of oxygen in the tissue. The events that result in a rightward shift would include an increase in pCO_2, 2,3-BPG, hydrogen ion production (decreased pH = acidosis), and body temperature. Glucose is not a factor in this calculation.

44. (A) The hemodynamic data demonstrate a clear discrepancy between the RA sat and the upstream/downstream sat trend. This sample was most likely obtained from the coronary sinus, consistent with improper catheter position. Coronary artery O_2 extraction is the highest in order to supply the myocardial oxygen demands. Hence, venous saturation from the coronary sinus (coronary venous drainage) is the lowest of any systemic venous structure entering the right atrium. Coronary sinus return makes up ~5% to 7% of systemic venous return. A typical oxygen saturation in the coronary sinus is between 25% and 45%; and if oversampled, can misrepresent mixed venous saturation when there is no shunt lesion.

45. (D) Thermodilution, introduced in 1950, utilizes a temperature indicator and fixed volume of fluid to measure a downstream change in temperature. The area under the temperature–time curve is used to determine cardiac output. There are multiple advantages to this method including accurate and reproducible results, short steady-state time requirement, and only the need for venous access. There are several sources of error, however, with discrepancies occurring in the presence of low cardiac output, AV valve regurgitation, and intracardiac shunting. Thermodilution does not accurately reflect systemic cardiac output in shunt physiology ($Q_p \neq Q_s$), as is present in this patient with an ASD and left-to-right shunt.

46. (C) Erythrocytosis is defined as a hematocrit over 65% and is commonly encountered in patients with cyanotic heart disease. Secondary erythrocytosis increases the O_2-carrying capacity while decreasing the cardiac output and O_2 delivery to tissues. It also significantly increases the risk of thrombosis and emboli and warrants hydration 24 hours prior to the procedure with consideration of phlebotomy in the cath lab. Prehydration is further prudent in this patient as renal insufficiency may be further exacerbated by prolonged NPO status and angiography.

47. (C) The data demonstrate a markedly elevated RVEDP and LVEDP, not an unexpected finding in a patient with two prior cardiopulmonary bypass exposures. The pulmonary pulse pressure is wide and consistent with severe pulmonary regurgitation. The RA pressure is similar to the RVEDP, making severe tricuspid regurgitation unlikely. The final issue to address is whether this patient is experiencing restrictive filling or constrictive physiology (typically observed in patients with cardiac tamponade or constrictive pericarditis). The following features are more suggestive of restriction rather than constrictive pericarditis or tamponade: RVSP >50 mm Hg, LVEDP – RVEDP >4 mm Hg, PCWP – mean RAP >4 mm Hg, and RVEDP/RVSP <0.3.

48. (C) There will continue to be respiratory variation in the mean RA pressure in restrictive cardiomyopathy rather than constrictive pericarditis (CP). CP will result in an inspiratory rise or lack of a decline in RA pressure, which is a Kussmaul sign. M waves can be seen in both CP and RCM. Equalization of pressures as listed in option (D) is diagnostic for CP. Absence of A waves should raise concerns for an arrhythmia, specifically atrial fibrillation or flutter.

49. (D) This question expands on the prior information related to calculating Q_p/Q_s and demonstrates the importance of utilizing a proper mixed venous saturation. This patient has PAPVR with a step-up at the low right SVC. Therefore, the appropriate selection for the mixed venous sat is the high right SVC (63%). $Q_p/Q_s = (98\% - 63\%)/(98\% - 73\%) = 35/25 = 1.4$.

50. (D) The chest radiograph demonstrates a heavily calcified pericardium. One would expect this person to have constrictive physiology with elevated LVEDP, mean PCWP, RVEDP, and mean RA pressure. The only answer choice consistent with elevated intracardiac filling pressures is an elevated PCWP. Systemic hypertension is not necessarily a part of constriction; in fact, patients frequently are hypotensive.

51. (C) The left pulmonary venous saturations are unexpectedly low. The right pulmonary veins are fully saturated. If the ET tube is in the right mainstem bronchus, the left lung may be ineffectively ventilated and oxygenated. Pulmonary venous desaturation may be caused by other things, such as pulmonary arteriovenous malformation, but the first step in this situation would be to confirm correct positioning of the endotracheal tube.

52. (E) Pulmonary arteriovenous malformations occur commonly in patients following Fontan procedure. Dyspnea on exertion and orthostatic or exertional cyanosis in Fontan patients can occur due to right-to-left shunting at a widely patent fenestration or can be due to right-to-left shunting from pulmonary AVM. These most commonly occur in the basal region of the lung.

53. (C) Interventional catheterization in adult congenital heart disease. *Circulation.* 2007;115:1622–1633 is an excellent review of indications for catheter-based therapy in adults with congenital heart disease. The 40-year-old patient, asymptomatic, pulmonary valve catheter gradient = 54 mm Hg is the only class I indication listed. Asymptomatic adults with mean Doppler or catheter peak-to-peak gradient >40 mm Hg should undergo pulmonary balloon valvuloplasty. Interventions have been recommended for the other answers but they are class II indications.

54. (B) During balloon aortic valvuloplasty, the balloon size should not exceed the annulus dimension. The risk of significant postprocedure valve regurgitation may occur if the balloon exceeds 100% of the aortic annulus diameter.

55. (D) The general recommendation is that pulmonary balloon valvuloplasty should be performed with a balloon that is 120% of the annulus diameter and should not exceed 140% of the annulus diameter. The risk of significant postprocedure valve regurgitation is increased when the balloon size exceeds 140% of the pulmonary annulus diameter.

56. (A) The patient is acidotic; hence, balloon septostomy should be performed promptly. RV angiography and other diagnostic procedures may be performed later if the patient's systemic arterial oxygen saturations improve dramatically. Mixing primarily occurs at atrial level in patients with complete TGA, and those with a VSD may still be profoundly cyanotic and acidotic requiring a septostomy.

57. (D) The defect is large (23 mm) particularly for a small child. The anterior-superior and the posterior rim are small or deficient making device closure unlikely, and this patient likely is best treated with surgical closure.

58. (E) AHA Pediatric Catheterization Guidelines—In patients with a large PDA and bidirectional flow due to pulmonary vascular disease, occlusion may be beneficial only if the pulmonary lung bed shows some reactivity to pulmonary vasodilator therapy. These patients should undergo hemodynamic assessment and pulmonary vasoreactivity testing before consideration for ductal occlusion. However, data on this group of patients are scant, and long-term follow-up data are unknown. Should pulmonary vascular disease continue to progress, the ductus will no longer be available to prevent the RV pressures from becoming supersystemic. Class III transcatheter PDA occlusion should not be attempted in a patient with a PDA with severe pulmonary hypertension associated with bidirectional or right-to-left shunting that is unresponsive to pulmonary vasodilator therapy (level of evidence: C).

59. (C) Patients with pulmonary atresia and intact ventricular septum (PA-IVS) have increased risk of coronary abnormalities such as right ventricular sinusoids, coronary-cameral fistulae, and coronary stenosis or atresia. RV-to-coronary artery fistulae and RV-dependent coronary circulation (significant portion of LV is supplied by fistulae fed by hypertensive RV) are present in 5% to 35% of PA-IVS patients. Decompression of the RV in the setting of significant RV-dependent myocardial circulation can result in irreversible myocardial ischemia and is usually fatal. See **Table 4.14** for recommendations for pulmonary valvuloplasty.

60. (A) Recommendations for device closure of secundum ASDs are listed in **Table 4.15**. Given that the patient has experienced recurrent TIAs, she meets criteria for closure as a Class IIa indication.

61. (A) BAS is performed to improve atrial mixing (simple d-TGA or d-TGA with VSD) or to treat atrial septal defect restriction in the setting of significant obstruction or stenosis of an atrioventricular valve (HLHS being the most common). It is rarely needed in right heart obstructive lesions, that is, tricuspid atresia (one must be aware that performing a balloon septostomy in a redundant atrial septum, such as in tricuspid atresia, is challenging and one may disrupt the RA/IVC junction with aggressive techniques). It is not performed in patients with TAPVR. This is a lesion that will be surgically corrected at the time of diagnosis and the atrial septum is not typically the location of "obstruction" of the venous return pathway. The procedure is usually straightforward in patients with d-TGA where the flap of the fossa ovalis is thin and easy to tear with the balloon catheter. BAS

TABLE 4.14 Recommendations for Pulmonary Valvuloplasty

Class I

1. Pulmonary valvuloplasty is indicated for a patient with critical valvar pulmonary stenosis (defined as pulmonary stenosis present at birth with cyanosis and evidence of patent ductus arteriosus dependency), valvar pulmonic stenosis, and a peak-to-peak catheter gradient or echocardiographic peak instantaneous gradient of ≥40 mm Hg or clinically significant pulmonary valvar obstruction in the presence of RV dysfunction (*level of evidence: A*)

Class IIa

1. It is reasonable to perform pulmonary valvuloplasty on a patient with valvar pulmonic stenosis who meets the above criteria in the setting of a dysplastic pulmonary valve (*level of evidence: C*)
2. It is reasonable to perform pulmonary valvuloplasty in newborns with pulmonary valve atresia and intact ventricular septum who have favorable anatomy that includes the exclusion of RV-dependent coronary circulation (*level of evidence: C*)

Class IIb

1. Pulmonary valvuloplasty may be considered as a palliative procedure in a patient with complex cyanotic CHD, including some rare cases of tetralogy of Fallot (*level of evidence: C*)

Class III

1. Pulmonary valvuloplasty should not be performed in patients with pulmonary atresia and RV-dependent coronary circulation (*level of evidence: B*)

can be performed up to a few weeks of age; after this time, the atrial septum may be too thick to balloon successfully in any lesion without significant risk of disruption of normal tissue. A blade septostomy will then be needed. The exception to this is the neonate with HLHS and restrictive atrial septum, where the tissue may be very thick, with minimal or no opening at the time of delivery. This procedure is usually performed emergently and immediately after delivery. It may require various techniques, including transseptal or radiofrequency access to the left atrium, the use of dilation balloon (cutting balloon), and stent placement for complete relief of obstruction. A simple balloon septostomy in HLHS with thick, restrictive atrial septum may avulse the pulmonary veins (i.e., the tissue with the least resistance will give way) during the BAS.

62. (B) Patients with a history of Mustard palliation may present with either SVC or IVC baffle obstruction, or with baffle leaks. These can cause significant right-to-left shunt with exercise and produce exertional cyanosis. The most appropriate treatment of a symptomatic baffle leak is an attempted closure, either by surgery or catheterization. Recent advances in septal occluding devices have allowed for many of these patients to have their leaks closed in

TABLE 4.15 Recommendations for Transcatheter Device Closure of Secundum ASD

Class I

1. Transcatheter secundum ASD closure is indicated in patients with hemodynamically significant ASD with suitable anatomic features (*level of evidence: B*)

Class IIa

1. It is reasonable to perform transcatheter secundum ASD closure in patients with transient right-to-left shunting at the atrial level who have experienced sequelae of paradoxical emboli such as stroke or recurrent transient ischemic attack (*level of evidence: B*)

2. It is reasonable to perform transcatheter secundum ASD closure in patients with transient right-to-left shunting at the atrial level who are symptomatic because of cyanosis and who do not require such a communication to maintain adequate cardiac output (*level of evidence: B*)

Class IIb

1. Transcatheter closure may be considered in patients with a small secundum ASD who are believed to be at risk of thromboembolic events (e.g., patients with a transvenous pacing system or chronically indwelling intravenous catheters, patients with hypercoagulable states) (*level of evidence: C*)

the cath lab with success. Stent placement is indicated in patients with baffle obstruction.

63. (A) Several factors may affect the pressure gradient across the coarctation site. These include LV dysfunction with low cardiac output, a large PDA, or multiple collaterals decompressing the aorta.

64. (D) The patient in this stem has 3-methylglutaconic aciduria type II (Barth syndrome), which is an X-linked disease characterized by DCM, endocardial fibroelastosis, proximal skeletal myopathy, growth failure, neutropenia, and organic aciduria. Prior to catheterization, documentation of the patient's leukocyte count with consideration for G-CSF administration and appropriate antibiotic prophylaxis is indicated.

65. (B) Effective pulmonary blood flow (Q_{ep}) is a measure of the amount of *deoxygenated* blood that flows to the lungs, simply put—the amount of blood going to the lungs that *should* go to the lungs. In the setting of left-to-right shunting, Q_{ep} will necessarily be lower than Q_p (i.e., both deoxygenated and oxygenated blood are flowing to the lungs). As with Q_p and Q_s, the Fick equation can be used to calculate Q_{ep}. The only change to the equation is that in the denominator, the saturation difference ($S_aO_2 - S_vO_2$) will be the difference between the most oxygenated blood (pulmonary venous; $S_{pv}O_2$) and least oxygenated blood (mixed venous, $S_{mv}O_2$). In this clinical scenario, pulmonary venous saturation is left atrial saturation (98%) and mixed venous saturation is SVC saturation (58%). Plugging those numbers into the Fick equation produces a $Q_{ep} = 2.1$ L/min/m^2.

66. (B) Effective systemic blood flow (Q_{es}) is the amount of *oxygenated* blood that goes to the body—that is, the amount of blood going to the body that *should* go to the body. As with Q_{ep}, Q_{es} can be calculated using the Fick equation, subtracting the saturation of the most oxygenated blood from the least oxygenated blood. Thus, the calculation for Q_{es} is identical to that for Q_{ep}, which is to say that at steady-state, Q_{es} *always* equals Q_{ep}. So, in this scenario, $Q_{es} = 2.1$ L/min/m^2.

CHAPTER 5

Noninvasive Cardiac Imaging

Benjamin W. Eidem, M. Yasir Qureshi, and Talha Niaz

Questions

1. Which statement is correct regarding the Doppler examination?

   A. Pulsed-wave (PW) Doppler requires one crystal to transmit the sound wave and another crystal to receive the reflected sound wave
   B. The maximum frequency shift that can be measured accurately by PW Doppler is termed pulse repetition frequency (PRF)
   C. Nyquist limit = PRF/2
   D. Nyquist limit can be extended by using higher frequency transducer
   E. High PRF is a technique to increase Nyquist limit without range ambiguity

2. In which of the following scenarios is it most appropriate to use the simplified Bernoulli equation to estimate a change in pressure?

   A. Severe pulmonary valve stenosis
   B. Aortic coarctation with bicuspid aortic valve
   C. Patent ductus arteriosus
   D. Subaortic stenosis and aortic stenosis
   E. Blalock–Taussig shunt

3. The Doppler pattern in **Figure 5.1** is consistent with which of the following?

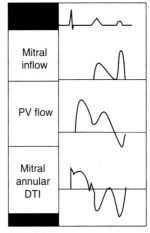

FIGURE 5.1

   A. Normal pattern
   B. Grade 1 diastolic dysfunction (impaired relaxation)
   C. Grade 2 diastolic dysfunction (pseudonormalization)
   D. Grade 3 diastolic dysfunction (restrictive physiology)
   E. Grade 4 diastolic dysfunction (severe irreversible restrictive physiology)

4. A patient has coarctation of the aorta. PW Doppler reveals a peak velocity of 2.0 m/s proximal to the coarctation. A continuous wave (CW) Doppler across the coarctation reveals a peak Doppler velocity of 4.0 m/s. What is the pressure gradient across the coarctation?

   A. 8 mm Hg
   B. 9 mm Hg
   C. 36 mm Hg
   D. 48 mm Hg
   E. 64 mm Hg

5. The Doppler tracing of the descending aorta in **Figure 5.2** was obtained in a patient with suspected aortic regurgitation. What is the degree of regurgitation?

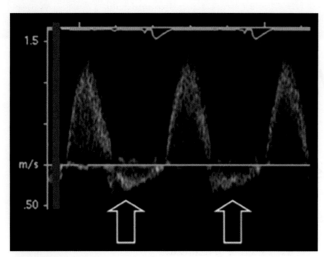

FIGURE 5.2

A. Unable to determine degree of regurgitation
B. Trivial
C. Mild
D. Moderate
E. Severe

6. Which of the following statements is correct concerning contrast echocardiography?

A. Contrast agents utilize microbubbles that are 50 to 100 microns in size
B. In the normal heart, contrast agents should opacify the right heart but not the left heart
C. Contrast agents can pass through the pulmonary circulation to opacify the left atrium and left ventricle
D. Acoustic impedance of contrast agents is higher than that of the blood pool
E. Contrast effect persists for 10 to 15 seconds in the normal heart

7. Which of the following is correct concerning echocardiographic use of agitated saline injections?

A. Microbubbles are 1 to 10 microns in size and easily traverse the pulmonary bed to the left heart
B. In the presence of an intrapulmonary shunt, the majority of these bubbles appear in the left atrium within one to two cardiac cycles.
C. A negative bubble study (i.e., no bubbles imaged within the left heart) with agitated saline rules out a right-to-left shunt
D. Indications for agitated saline studies include unexplained cyanosis and stroke
E. Bubbles cannot be present in the left heart in the normal circulation without the presence of a left-to-right shunt

8. Which of the following is *most* helpful to diagnose the severity of aortic insufficiency?

A. Degree of left ventricular (LV) dilatation
B. Length of the color Doppler regurgitant jet into the LV
C. Amount of diastolic Doppler flow reversal in the ascending aorta
D. Vena contracta width of the regurgitant jet
E. Comparison of the forward flow Doppler time velocity integral (TVI) to reverse flow TVI in the abdominal aorta

9. Which of the following formulas is correct for the myocardial performance index (MPI) (i.e., Tei index)?

A. [ICT + IRT]/ET
B. PEP/ET
C. E/E_a
D. Pulmonary venous atrial reversal duration − mitral inflow atrial duration
E. [LVEDD − LVESD]/LVET

10. Which echocardiographic scan plane is *most* optimal to define a *secundum atrial septal defect*?

A. Suprasternal long-axis view
B. Parasternal long-axis view
C. Parasternal short-axis view
D. Subcostal four-chamber view
E. Apical four-chamber view

11. Which of the following is the *most* common associated cardiac defect found with a *sinus venosus atrial septal defect*?

A. Anomalous right pulmonary venous connection
B. Inlet ventricular septal defect
C. Bicuspid aortic valve
D. Persistent left superior vena cava
E. Coarctation of the aorta

12. Which of the following findings on echocardiography is consistent with constriction?

A. E/A ratio of mitral Doppler inflow <1.0
B. Decreased E_a velocity on tissue Doppler of the lateral mitral annulus
C. Increased respiratory variation in mitral inflow E-wave velocity >30%
D. Increased hepatic venous atrial systolic Doppler flow reversals during inspiration
E. Increased E-wave deceleration time on mitral inflow Doppler

13. Which of the following parameters is consistent with restrictive LV physiology?

    A. Mitral inflow E/A Doppler ratio <1
    B. Increased lateral mitral annular E_a velocity
    C. Mitral inflow deceleration time <80 ms
    D. Increased systolic/diastolic ratio of pulmonary venous Doppler
    E. Lateral mitral annular E/E_a ratio <10

14. A newborn male born at 38-week gestation was found to be cyanotic at birth. He was started on prostaglandin infusion until an echocardiogram could be performed. VIDEOS 5.1A,B show subcostal views of the left and right ventricular outflow tracts. His oxygen saturation at the time of echocardiogram was 71% and initial arterial blood gas was: pH 7.3, pCO_2 45 mm Hg, pO_2 28 mm Hg, and base of −1. Infant is currently stable with adequate hemodynamics and supported by nasal cannula for mild respiratory distress. Which of the following is the next best step in the management of the patient?

    A. Discontinue PGE and plan for neonatal repair
    B. Patient should undergo emergent surgical intervention
    C. Ductal stenting and complete repair at 6 months of age
    D. Patient should undergo balloon atrial septostomy
    E. Continue PGE followed by complete surgical repair in 1 week

15. Which of the following is the *most* common *anatomic finding* in a *complete AVSD*?

    A. Cleft in posterior leaflet of mitral component of AV valve
    B. Medial rotation of left ventricular papillary muscles
    C. Ratio of left ventricular inlet to outlet distance >1.0
    D. Left ventricular outflow tract (LVOT) is "sprung" anteriorly
    E. Left and right atrioventricular valve attachments are present at different levels

16. Which of the following statements is *true* regarding *M-mode*?

    A. Has a low PRF
    B. Has excellent temporal resolution
    C. *X*-axis represents distance from transducer
    D. *Y*-axis represents time
    E. Utilizes two imaging crystals to transmit and receive impulses

17. Which of the following statements regarding *spatial resolution* in echocardiography is *correct*?

    A. Spatial resolution is defined as the smallest distance between two points distinguishable as separate points
    B. Axial resolution is the ability to differentiate points perpendicular to the ultrasound beam path
    C. Lateral resolution is the ability to differentiate between points along the path of the ultrasound beam
    D. Lateral resolution is better than axial resolution
    E. Image resolution is best where the ultrasound beam is widest

18. Which of the following is the most likely *source of error* in calculation of Doppler flow velocity?

    A. Angle of incidence of the ultrasound beam
    B. Depth of the vascular structure
    C. Frequency of the transducer
    D. Presence and degree of imaging artifact
    E. Variation in heart rate

19. Which of the following is true regarding *CW Doppler*?

    A. Utilizes a single ultrasound crystal that continuously transmits and receives
    B. No limit to maximal velocity measured
    C. Excellent range resolution
    D. Less dependent on angle of incidence compared to PW Doppler
    E. Lower Nyquist limit compared to PW Doppler

20. Which of the following statements regarding *PW Doppler* is *correct*?

    A. Utilizes two ultrasound crystals that continuously transmit and receive
    B. No limit to maximal velocity measured
    C. Excellent range resolution
    D. Lower PRF than color Doppler
    E. PRF is fixed

21. Which of the following is a *correct* statement regarding the *Nyquist limit*?

    A. Represents the highest frequency shift that can be unambiguously detected and displayed
    B. Is equal to the PRF
    C. Is higher with PW Doppler versus CW Doppler
    D. Remains the same with all transducer frequencies
    E. Is lower at more shallow depths of interrogation

22. Which of the following is a *true* statement regarding *color Doppler*?

    A. Color Doppler represents the mean velocity of blood flow

    B. Intensity of color represents peak Doppler flow velocity

    C. 2D image content is unchanged with color Doppler imaging

    D. Nyquist limit is increased with color Doppler imaging

    E. Utilizes a single ultrasound beam with multiple sampling sites along that beam

23. Which of the following is the *optimal* echocardiographic view to delineate a *subpulmonary ventricular septal defect (VSD)*?

    A. Parasternal long-axis view

    B. Apical four-chamber view

    C. Suprasternal long-axis view

    D. Parasternal short-axis view

    E. Apical five-chamber view

24. A 4-month-old male with tetralogy of Fallot (TOF) is undergoing surgical repair. Which of the following is the most common coronary artery abnormality among patients with TOF?

    A. Single coronary artery

    B. Left circumflex artery from the right coronary artery

    C. Anomalous left coronary artery from the pulmonary artery

    D. Left anterior descending artery from the right coronary artery

    E. Right coronary artery from the left main coronary artery

25. Which of the following is the most characteristic physiologic effect of a large ventricular septal defect?

    A. Right ventricular volume overload

    B. Low pulmonary arterial pressure

    C. Equal right ventricular and left ventricular systolic pressure

    D. Increased systemic blood flow

    E. Decreased pulmonary blood flow

26. Which of the following is the *best* morphologic marker of the *right atrium*?

    A. Broad-based triangular appendage

    B. Receives superior vena cava (SVC)

    C. Chamber is connected to morphologic RV

    D. Presence of the valve of the fossa ovalis

    E. Connected to tricuspid valve

27. The *atrial septum* is *best* imaged in which scan plane?

    A. Suprasternal

    B. Subcostal

    C. Parasternal long axis

    D. Parasternal short axis

    E. Apical four chamber

28. Which of the following is a typical echocardiographic feature of the *morphologic right ventricle*?

    A. Ellipsoid shape

    B. More apical insertion point of atrioventricular valve

    C. Smooth superior septal surface

    D. Finely trabeculated apical portion

    E. Lack of atrioventricular valve septal attachments

29. Which of the following is a typical echocardiographic feature of the *morphologic left ventricle (LV)*?

    A. Heavily trabeculated inflow portion

    B. Triangular shape

    C. Trabeculated septal surface

    D. Lack of atrioventricular valve septal chordal attachments

    E. More apical insertion of atrioventricular valve

30. A neonate with *pulmonary valve stenosis* has a peak Doppler velocity by CW Doppler of 4.0 m/s. Which of the following is the estimated maximum instantaneous Doppler gradient?

    A. 64 mm Hg

    B. 77 mm Hg

    C. 72 mm Hg

    D. 50 mm Hg

    E. Cannot be calculated

31. Which of the following is the *most* common anatomic type of *subaortic stenosis*?

    A. Tunnel type

    B. Discrete membrane

    C. Asymmetric septal hypertrophy

    D. Systolic anterior motion of mitral valve

    E. Anomalous mitral chordal insertion within the LVOT

32. The *most* common associated cardiac abnormality in the patient with *coarctation of the aorta* is:

    A. Bicuspid aortic valve

    B. Ventricular septal defect

    C. Atrial septal defect

    D. Pulmonary valve stenosis

    E. Coronary artery anomaly

33. A newborn female born at 38-week gestation had mild–moderate respiratory distress at birth requiring continuous positive airway pressure (CPAP). She has lower extremity cyanosis with saturations of 80% in the right lower extremity and 95% in the right upper extremity due to which an echocardiogram was obtained. **Figure 5.3** shows the pulsed-wave spectral Doppler pattern obtained within the patent ductus arteriosus. Which of the following is the most likely diagnosis?

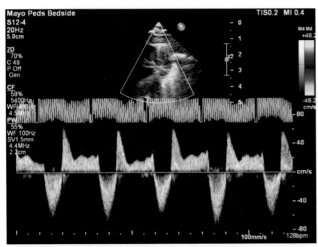

FIGURE 5.3

A. Transposition of the great arteries with coarctation of the aorta
B. Persistent pulmonary hypertension
C. Tausig–Bing anomaly
D. Tricuspid atresia with transposed great arteries
E. None of the above

34. Which of the following is the most diagnostic echo finding in *pericardial effusion with cardiac tamponade*?

A. Diastolic right atrial wall collapse
B. 10% variation in mitral inflow Doppler velocities with respiration
C. Diastolic right ventricular wall collapse
D. Effusion >25 mm circumferentially
E. 15% variation in tricuspid inflow Doppler velocities with respiration

35. Which of the following methods of assessing LV systolic function is *most independent of loading conditions*?

A. Ejection fraction
B. Shortening fraction
C. Myocardial performance index
D. Rate-corrected velocity of circumferential fiber shortening
E. Stress–velocity index

36. A 2-month-old female with tricuspid atresia and normally related great arteries presents for follow-up. Her oxygen saturations on the current visit are 87%, blood pressure is 78/55 mm Hg, and a heart rate of 125 bpm. On physical examination she has a grade 2/6 systolic ejection murmur, liver is 3 inches below the subcostal margin and she has pedal edema with prominent lower extremity veins. Which of the following echocardiographic findings will likely explain the current clinical scenario?

A. Narrowing of the bulboventricular foramen
B. Coarctation of the aorta
C. Severe subpulmonary stenosis
D. Restricted atrial septal communication
E. Unrestricted pulmonary flow

37. Holodiastolic *Doppler flow reversal* in the abdominal aorta can be attributed to which of the following?

A. Bidirectional cavopulmonary anastomosis
B. Large patent ductus arteriosus
C. Moderate aortic insufficiency
D. Sano shunt
E. High output state

38. Which of the following is the *most* common type of *ventricular septal defect (VSD)* that is associated with *coarctation of the aorta*?

A. Apical muscular
B. Anterior malalignment
C. Perimembranous
D. Inlet
E. Subpulmonary

39. The Doppler finding often seen in patients with supravalvar aortic stenosis has been demonstrated to be a high-velocity poststenotic jet that hugs the aortic wall and preferentially transfers kinetic energy into the right innominate artery. Which of the following best describes this Doppler finding?

A. Coanda effect
B. Ohm's law
C. Continuity equation
D. Poiseuille's law
E. Bernoulli equation

40. In the simplified Bernoulli equation, which *component* of the complete equation is *not* ignored?

A. Flow acceleration
B. Convective acceleration
C. Viscous friction
D. Proximal Doppler velocity
E. Vessel length

41. Which of the following is true about an *overriding* atrioventricular valve?

  A. Has chordal attachments into both ventricles
  B. Must have chordal attachments to the ventricular septal crest
  C. Empties into two ventricles
  D. Cannot coexist with straddling
  E. Is never associated with malalignment type of VSD

42. Which of the following is true about a *straddling* cardiac valve?

  A. Cannot coexist with overriding
  B. Is always associated with malalignment type of ventricular septal defect (VSD)
  C. Frequently involves the aortic valve
  D. Is a common component of tetralogy of Fallot
  E. Involves anomalous insertion of chordae tendineae

43. Which statement is correct regarding *polysplenia syndrome*?

  A. The situs of abdominal viscera is always ambiguous
  B. The spleen are multiple and located on both left and right sides
  C. Inferior vena cava (IVC) fails to join the heart directly with azygos continuation
  D. Multiple gallbladders common
  E. Biliary atresia never occurs

44. A 5-year-old female with a vascular ring underwent division of the ligamentum arteriosum due to progressive dysphagia. After surgery, she had slight improvement in her symptoms but continues to have persistent dysphagia. **Figure 5.4** shows the CT angiogram of the patient at the level of the aortic arch. Which of the following structures could be a potential cause of residual compression on the esophagus?

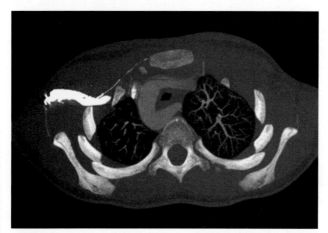

FIGURE 5.4

  A. Aberrant right subclavian artery
  B. Right-sided aortic arch
  C. Innominate artery
  D. Left-sided aortic arch
  E. Aberrant left subclavian artery

45. *Tricuspid atresia* is an example of which of the following?

  A. Common inlet
  B. Double inlet
  C. Single inlet
  D. Absent inlet
  E. Ambiguous AV connection

46. A 13-year-old male presents to your clinic with a concern for an intracardiac mass diagnosed during evaluation for a murmur. He is completely asymptomatic from clinical standpoint. A transesophageal echocardiogram was obtained to assess the characteristics of the mass as shown in **Figure 5.5**. There is no significant mitral valve obstruction or regurgitation on the echocardiogram. Which of the following is *true* regarding the management of this cardiac mass?

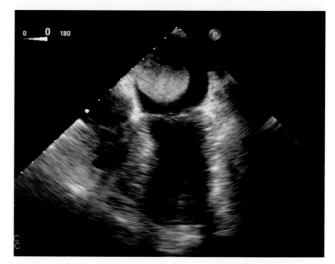

FIGURE 5.5

  A. Patient should be evaluated for tuberous sclerosis
  B. No treatment is necessary as tumor will regress spontaneously
  C. Lesion will resolve with chemotherapy
  D. Lesion will resolve with radiotherapy
  E. Surgical resection of mass is indicated

47. Which of the following statements is correct concerning *venous return* to the normal heart?

    A. When the IVC is interrupted, venous return to the SVC is from the thebesian veins

    B. When a persistent left SVC drains to a severely dilated coronary sinus, the brachiocephalic vein is typically small or absent

    C. The connection of the right SVC to the right atrium confidently identifies the morphologic right atrium

    D. It is more common for the right pulmonary veins than the left pulmonary veins to merge into a single vein that enters the left atrium

    E. Interruption of the IVC is more common in asplenia versus polysplenia syndrome

48. Which of the following is the most reliable feature that distinguishes the mitral valve from the tricuspid valve?

    A. Shape of the orifice
    B. Atrioventricular valve—semilunar valve continuity
    C. Presence of septal chordal attachments
    D. Level of attachment of atrioventricular valve at cardiac crux
    E. Number of leaflets

49. A 12-year-old male with history of systemic lupus erythematous presents with chest pain, dyspnea, and exercise intolerance. On physical examination, he has no murmurs, rubs, or gallops. His ECG showed diffuse ST segment elevation primarily in the inferolateral leads. An echocardiogram was obtained that demonstrated a small posterior pericardial effusion and normal biventricular systolic function. Pulsed-wave spectral Doppler tracings obtained at the mitral inflow level and hepatic vein are shown in **Figures 5.6A,B**, respectively. Which of the following is the most likely diagnosis based on the Doppler tracings?

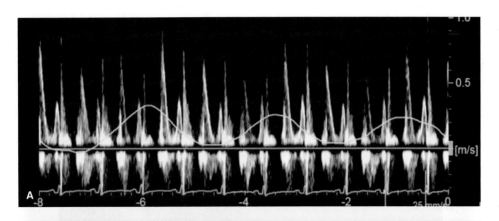

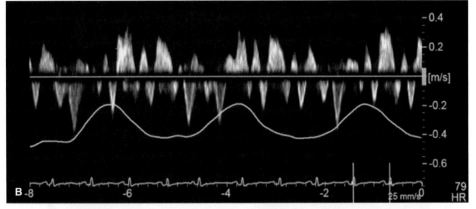

FIGURE 5.6 A: Mitral inflow pulsed-wave Doppler. **B:** Hepatic vein pulsed-wave Doppler.

    A. Acute pericarditis without tamponade
    B. Acute pericarditis with tamponade physiology
    C. Constrictive pericarditis
    D. Restrictive cardiomyopathy
    E. Effusive pericarditis

50. A 9-year-old patient presents with decreased exercise tolerance and cardiomegaly on chest x-ray. An echocardiogram was subsequently performed. What is the defect designated by the asterisk in **Figure 5.7**?

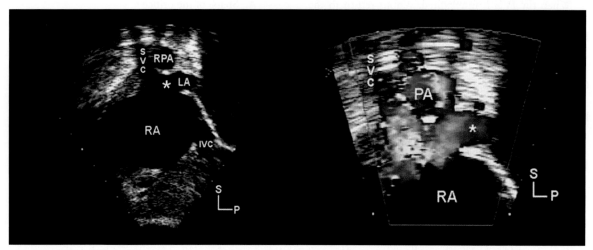

FIGURE 5.7 IVC, inferior vena cava; RA, right atrium; RPA, right pulmonary artery; SVC, superior vena cava.

A. Secundum atrial septal defect
B. Coronary sinus atrial septal defect
C. Sinus venosus atrial septal defect

D. Persistent left superior vena cava to unroofed coronary sinus
E. Primum atrial septal defect

51. Which of the following congenital heart defects is demonstrated in **Figure 5.8**?

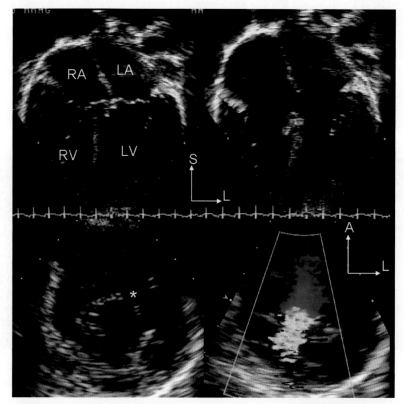

FIGURE 5.8 LA, left atrium; LV, left ventricle; RA, right atrium; RV, right ventricle.

A. Partial AVSD
B. Unroofed coronary sinus
C. Complete AVSD

D. Total anomalous pulmonary venous connection
E. Large inlet ventricular septal defect

52. A 4-year-old male was admitted to the pediatric intensive care unit in cardiogenic shock. On initial evaluation, he had elevated transaminases, laboratory evidence of acute kidney injury, and elevated troponins. His initial echocardiogram revealed mildly depressed left ventricular systolic function with an estimated ejection fraction of 40% and otherwise normal intracardiac anatomy. A nasopharyngeal PCR for SARS-CoV-2 was negative but a SARS-CoV-2 serology was positive. Which of the following should be carefully evaluated during follow-up with pediatric cardiology?

    A. Mitral valve regurgitation
    B. Coronary arteries
    C. Ascending aortic dimensions
    D. Right ventricular hypertrophy
    E. Left ventricular mass

53. A 6-month-old child presents with failure to thrive and the echocardiographic image (**Figure 5.9**) is obtained. What is the congenital heart defect demonstrated?

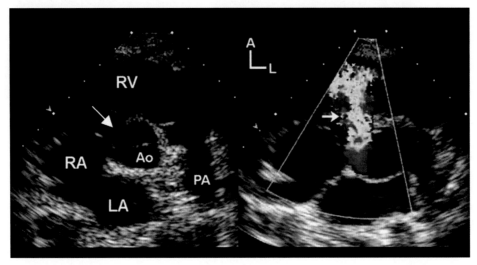

FIGURE 5.9 Ao, aorta; LA, left atrium; PA, pulmonary artery; RA, right atrium; RV, right ventricle.

    A. Muscular VSD
    B. Membranous VSD
    C. Infundibular VSD
    D. Inlet VSD
    E. Doubly committed VSD

54. Which of the following diagnoses is most consistent with the echocardiographic image in **Figure 5.10**?

    A. Down syndrome
    B. DiGeorge syndrome
    C. Marfan syndrome
    D. Noonan syndrome
    E. Williams syndrome

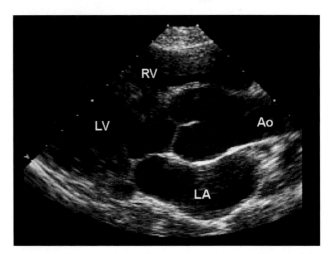

FIGURE 5.10 Ao, aorta; LA, left atrium; LV, left ventricle; RV, right ventricle.

55. What is the most likely etiology of the echocardiographic image in **Figure 5.11**?

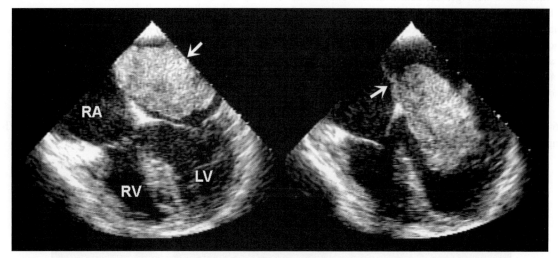

FIGURE 5.11 LV, left ventricle; RA, right atrium; RV, right ventricle.

A. Thrombus
B. Myxoma
C. Fibroma
D. Rhabdomyoma
E. Secondary metastasis

56. An 8-year-old patient has a resuscitated sudden cardiac death event while playing soccer. An echocardiogram performed in the emergency room displays the image in **Figure 5.12**. What is the most likely diagnosis?

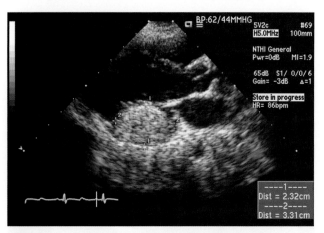

FIGURE 5.12

A. Rhabdomyoma
B. Myxoma
C. Fibroma
D. Fibroelastoma
E. Sarcoma

57. A 15-year-old male was recently diagnosed with hypertrophic cardiomyopathy due to an abnormal ECG. His echocardiogram reveals a septal thickness of 30 mm, normal left ventricular size and systolic function, and a normal mitral valve. **Figure 5.13** shows the continuous wave Doppler across the left ventricular outflow tract (LVOT). Based on the Doppler profile, which of the following is the most important echocardiographic parameter for surgical decision making?

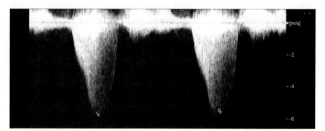

FIGURE 5.13

A. Mean systolic Doppler gradient
B. Maximum instantaneous Doppler gradient
C. Cardiac output
D. Velocity time integral
E. Ejection time

58. A 16-year-old male with hypertrophic cardiomyopathy is referred to you for further management. An echocardiogram is obtained which shows severe reverse curve configuration of the septum with septal thickness of 25 mm. He had systolic anterior motion of the anterior leaflet of the mitral valve with moderate mitral valve regurgitation. A left ventricular outflow tract (LVOT) gradient was unable to be obtained due to contamination from mitral valve regurgitation signal. **Figure 5.14** shows the continuous wave Doppler across the mitral valve. If the left atrial pressure is 10 mm Hg and blood pressure in right upper extremity is 100/55 mm Hg, what is the estimated peak LVOT gradient?

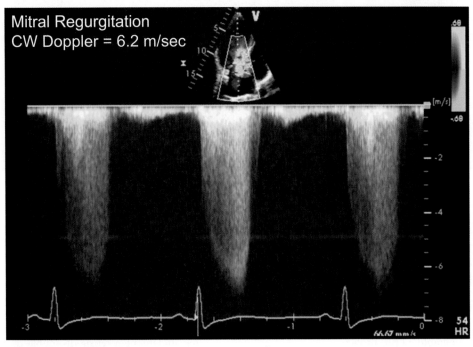

FIGURE 5.14 Mitral regurgitation. CW Doppler = 6.2 m/s.

A. 44 mm Hg
B. 64 mm Hg
C. 154 mm Hg
D. 164 mm Hg
E. 100 mm Hg

59. Which of the following cardiac interventions or cardiac surgeries would benefit most from transesophageal echocardiography (TEE) imaging?

A. Left pulmonary artery unifocalization
B. Jump graft from ascending to descending aorta in a patient with interrupted aortic arch
C. Mechanical mitral valve prosthesis (bileaflet tilting disk)
D. Melody valve implantation in the pulmonary valve position
E. Innominate vein stent

60. Which of the following is the most likely complication of transesophageal echocardiography (TEE) performed in pediatric patients?

A. Gastric perforation
B. Laceration of pharynx
C. Airway compromise
D. Infective endocarditis
E. Esophageal hemorrhage

61. You are evaluating a patient with double-chambered right ventricle (DCRV). The best transesophageal echocardiography (TEE) window/position from which to obtain an accurate spectral Doppler gradient across the area of right ventricle (RV) obstruction is which of the following (**Figure 5.15**)?

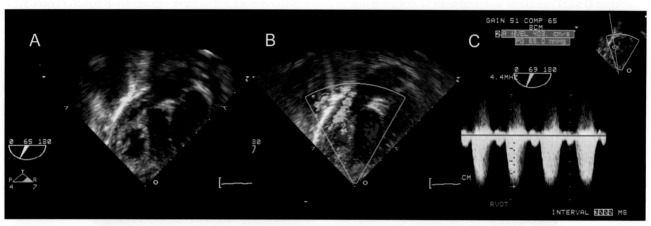

FIGURE 5.15

    A. Deep transgastric
    B. Upper esophageal
    C. Midesophageal
    D. Transgastric
    E. Descending aorta

62. Which of the following maneuvers is specifically utilized during imaging using a pediatric multiplane transesophageal echocardiography (TEE) probe?

    A. Rocking the probe toward or away from a particular transducer orientation
    B. Tilting the probe right/left
    C. Sliding the probe to a new position
    D. Rotating the probe transducer angle forward/backward between 0 degrees and 180 degrees
    E. Angling the probe tip to visualize a certain structure

63. You are performing a transesophageal echocardiogram (TEE) on a 5-year-old patient. What does the TEE (**VIDEO 5.2**) demonstrate?

    A. Eccentric aortic regurgitation
    B. Coronary arteriovenous fistula into the right atrium
    C. Tricuspid regurgitation
    D. Ventricular septal defect with left ventricle to right atrial shunt (Gerbode defect)
    E. Primum atrial septal defect

64. You are performing a postoperative transesophageal echocardiogram (TEE) on a 16-month-old patient who has undergone a repair of double outlet right ventricle (DORV), including patch closure of a ventricular septal defect (VSD). What does the postoperative TEE (**VIDEO 5.3**) show?

    A. Residual VSD: peri-patch leak
    B. Intramural VSD
    C. Aortic valve regurgitation
    D. Aortic left ventricle tunnel
    E. Ruptured sinus of Valsalva aneurysm to the right ventricle (RV)

65. The presence of which of the following devices is a relative contraindication to performing a cardiac magnetic resonance (MR) imaging study?

    A. Stainless steel vascular occluding coil
    B. Hemostatic vascular clip
    C. Temporary pacemaker lead without a generator
    D. Atrial septal occluder device
    E. AICD

66. Which of the following devices would generate the most prominent imaging artifact with cardiac magnetic resonance imaging?

    A. Atrial septal occluder device
    B. Permanent pacemaker lead
    C. Stainless steel PDA coil
    D. Nonferromagnetic stent
    E. PDA clip

67. Blood appears *black* on which cardiac magnetic resonance imaging technique?
    A. Spin echo
    B. Gradient echo cine images
    C. Isotropic 3D steady-state free precession (SSFP) images
    D. Cardiac-triggered, navigator-gated free-breathing 3D SSFP
    E. Contrast-enhanced MRA

68. Which of the following would be the optimal technique to calculate Q_p:Q_s by cardiac magnetic resonance imaging in a patient with a large secundum atrial septal defect?
    A. Spatial modulation of magnetization (SPAMM)
    B. Contrast-enhanced MR angiogram
    C. Velocity-encoded cine (VEC) images
    D. Myocardial perfusion study
    E. Spin echo images

69. Which of the following is correct regarding the *spin echo* cardiac magnetic resonance (MR) imaging technique?
    A. Produces bright-blood images
    B. Low tissue contrast
    C. Images acquired during a single cardiac cycle
    D. Facilitates tissue characterization of myocardial walls and cardiac tumors
    E. Increased imaging artifact with metallic implants compared to other CMR techniques

70. Which of the following is characteristic of the "gradient echo" cardiac magnetic resonance (MR) imaging technique?
    A. Produces bright-blood images
    B. Images take longer to acquire than "spin echo" technique
    C. High tissue contrast
    D. Relatively slow imaging speed compared to spin echo technique
    E. Less imaging artifact with metallic implants compared to other CMR techniques

71. Which of the following is the best cardiac magnetic resonance (MR) technique to assess *myocardial viability*?
    A. Myocardial delayed enhancement (MDE)
    B. First-pass myocardial perfusion
    C. Dobutamine stress CMR
    D. ECG-gated VEC MRI sequence
    E. SPAMM

72. Which of the following sequences of cardiac MRI can be done without intravenous administration of contrast agent?
    A. Conventional MR angiogram
    B. Phase-contrast (velocity-encoded) cine imaging
    C. Delayed myocardial enhancement
    D. Myocardial perfusion imaging
    E. Time-resolved imaging of contrast kinetics (TRICKS)

73. Which of the following sequences allows best assessment of myocardial edema?
    A. MR angiogram
    B. T1-weighted black-blood imaging
    C. T2-weighted black-blood imaging
    D. Myocardial perfusion imaging
    E. Steady-state free precession imaging

74. Which of the following tests is best to establish a diagnosis of anomalous origin of left coronary artery from right sinus of Valsalva with intramural course?
    A. Contrast-enhanced MR angiogram
    B. Computed tomography angiography (CTA) without ECG gating
    C. CTA with ECG gating
    D. Invasive coronary angiography
    E. Thallium scan

75. Which advanced imaging modality is best to assess coarctation of aorta?
    A. Retrospective ECG-gated CTA
    B. Conventional MRA
    C. Transesophageal echocardiogram
    D. Stress echocardiogram
    E. Thallium scan

76. Which of the following statements is *true* regarding MRI scanners?
    A. The magnet is always on
    B. The magnet is only on during bright-blood imaging
    C. The magnet is only on during black-blood imaging
    D. The magnet is only on when any imaging is being performed
    E. It makes a noise when the magnet is on

77. Which of the following is true for cardiac MRI performed on a patient with acute myocarditis?
    A. Myocardial edema is best seen on SSFP cine images
    B. T2-weighted sequences can show fatty infiltrate of myocardial wall
    C. Early myocardial enhancement is due to impaired perfusion
    D. Distribution of delayed myocardial enhancement can help in distinguishing infarction from myocarditis
    E. MR angiogram can show filling defect in myocardium

78. Which of the following allows best assessment of pericardial calcification in a patient with pericardial constriction?

    A. Noncontrast CT

    B. Non–ECG-gated CTA

    C. MRA

    D. Delayed enhancement on MRI

    E. Transthoracic echocardiography

79. Which of the following MRI sequence allows assessment of myocardial iron overload in patients with thalassemia?

    A. Myocardial T2* quantification

    B. T1-weighted sequences of myocardium

    C. T2-weighted sequences of myocardium

    D. Delayed myocardial enhancement

    E. T1 mapping

80. What is the likely diagnosis on the MRI (**Figure 5.16**) of this 17 year old who presented to emergency room with a 2-day history of chest pain?

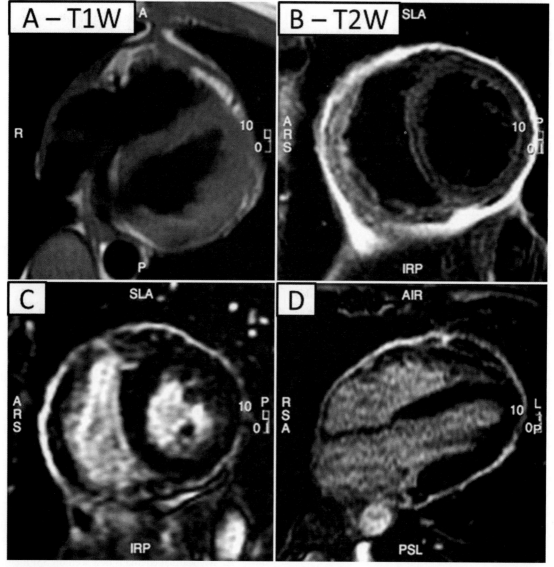

FIGURE 5.16

    A. Cocaine abuse

    B. Myocardial infarction

    C. Myocarditis

    D. Pericarditis

    E. Musculoskeletal chest pain

81. What is the likely diagnosis on this coronal reformat of CT angiogram (**Figure 5.17**) in a 27-year-old acyanotic man presenting with easy fatigability?

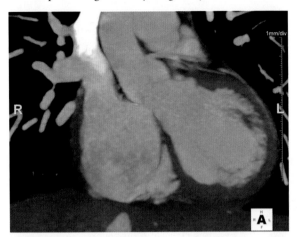

FIGURE 5.17

  A. Total anomalous pulmonary venous connection
  B. Partial anomalous pulmonary venous connection
  C. Anomalous origin of right coronary artery
  D. Anomalous origin of left coronary artery
  E. Tricuspid atresia

82. Which was the most likely surgery performed on this patient (**Figure 5.18**)?

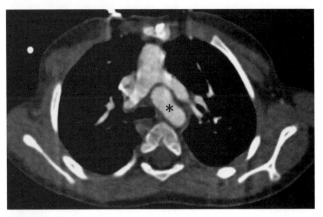

FIGURE 5.18

  A. Norwood procedure
  B. Glenn procedure
  C. Fontan procedure
  D. Atrial switch operation
  E. Arterial switch operation

83. What is an additional imaging finding in this patient with tetralogy of Fallot (**Figure 5.19**)?

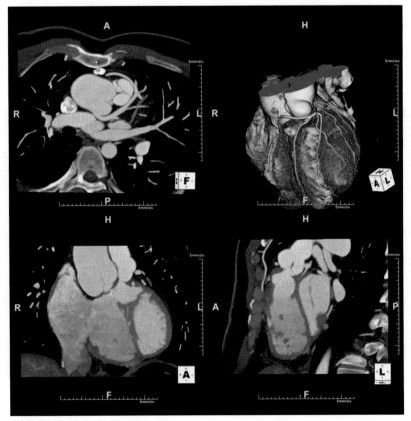

FIGURE 5.19

  A. Anomalous origin of left coronary artery from pulmonary artery
  B. Single left coronary artery
  C. Single right coronary artery
  D. Coronary atherosclerosis
  E. Prominent conal branch of right coronary artery anterior to the pulmonary valve

CHAPTER 5

84. What is the name of the surgical shunt shown on this MR angiogram (**Figure 5.20**)?

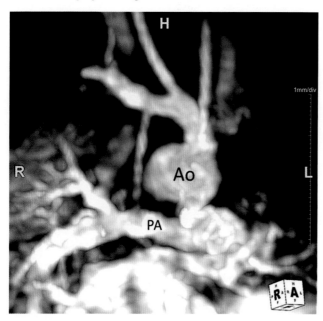

FIGURE 5.20 Ao, aorta; PA, pulmonary artery.

    A. Waterston shunt
    B. Potts shunt
    C. Classic Blalock–Taussig shunt
    D. Modified Blalock–Taussig shunt
    E. Central shunt

85. What is the likely diagnosis in this 32-year-old patient (**Figure 5.21**)?

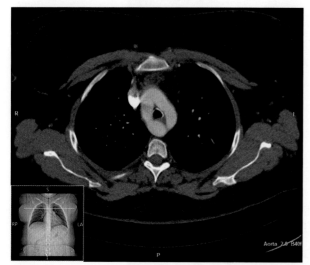

FIGURE 5.21

    A. Left aortic arch with normal branching pattern
    B. Left aortic arch with aberrant left subclavian artery origin
    C. Right aortic arch with mirror image branching pattern
    D. Right aortic arch with aberrant left subclavian artery origin
    E. Double aortic arch

86. What is the likely diagnosis in this 47-year-old patient (**Figure 5.22**) with reduced exercise tolerance?

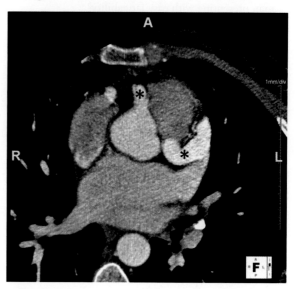

FIGURE 5.22

    A. Anomalous origin of right coronary artery (RCA) from left aortic sinus
    B. Anomalous origin of left coronary artery (LCA) from right aortic sinus
    C. Anomalous origin of LCA from pulmonary artery
    D. Coronary artery fistula
    E. Long-term complication of Kawasaki disease

87. What is the likely diagnosis in this 12 year old (**Figure 5.23**) who had Fontan procedure?

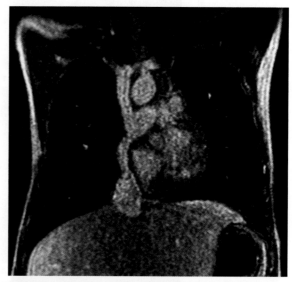

FIGURE 5.23

    A. Stenosis of superior cavopulmonary anastomosis
    B. Stenosis of inferior cavopulmonary anastomosis
    C. Stenosis of IVC–Fontan conduit anastomosis
    D. Stenosis of Fontan conduit
    E. Thrombosis in Fontan circuit

88. What is the most common additional coexisting diagnosis in the patient with this CTA finding (**Figure 5.24**)?

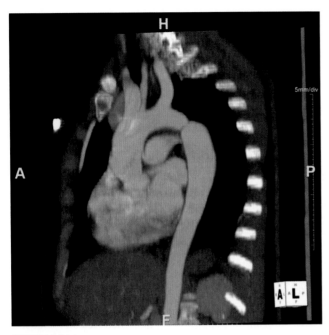

FIGURE 5.24

A. Atrial septal defect
B. Ventricular septal defect (VSD)
C. Common AV valve
D. Tetralogy of Fallot
E. Anomalous pulmonary vein connection

Answers

1. (C) PW Doppler utilizes one crystal that both emits and receives the sound pulses. The maximal frequency shift that can be determined by PW Doppler is equal to one-half the PRF and is termed the Nyquist limit. This Nyquist limit can be extended by using lower frequency transducers. High PRF lacks range gating resulting in range ambiguity.

2. (A) The simplified Bernoulli equation ignores the components of flow acceleration and viscous friction. Doppler velocities across a patent ductus arteriosus or Blalock–Taussig shunt will likely be underestimated due to viscous friction in these tortuous connections and difficulties with proper ultrasound beam alignment. Multiple obstructions in series, such as multiple sites of LVOT obstruction (subvalvar, valvar, coarctation), will need to account for flow acceleration proximal to the distal site(s) of obstruction. Isolated valvar stenoses would be an appropriate use of the simplified Bernoulli equation.

3. (B) These Doppler patterns are consistent with impaired relaxation. Mitral inflow Doppler demonstrates an *E:A* ratio <1, while mitral annular tissue Doppler imaging also demonstrates a decreased early annular velocity and abnormal *E′/A′* ratio <1. Pulmonary venous Doppler shows a systolic dominance and a prominent atrial reversal wave, consistent with grade 1 diastolic dysfunction (**Figure 5.25**).

4. (D) The pressure gradient can be predicted by using the "expanded" Bernoulli equation, $P_1 - P_2 = 4(V_2^2 - V_1^2)$, utilizing

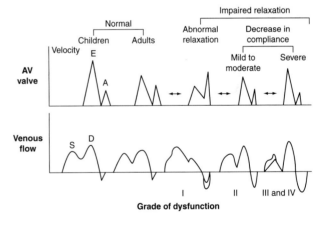

FIGURE 5.25

the Doppler velocities proximal and distal to the coarctation: $4([4.0]^2 - [2.0]^2) = 48$ mm Hg.

5. (E) The presence of holodiastolic flow reversal in the abdominal aorta is consistent with severe aortic regurgitation.

6. (C) Contrast agents are designed to pass through the pulmonary capillary bed to opacify the left heart structures. The typical size of these microspheres is 1 to 10 microns. The acoustic impedance of contrast agents is much lower than that of the blood pool. The contrast effect persists for 3 to 5 minutes with most contrast agents.

7. (D) Microbubbles created with agitated saline range in size from 10 to 100 microns and do not pass through the pulmonary capillary bed. These microbubbles opacify the right atrium and right ventricle but not left heart structures in the absence of an intracardiac or intrapulmonary shunt (**VIDEO 5.4A**). They can be helpful to identify an intracardiac right-to-left shunt that may be an etiology in stroke or unexplained cyanosis (**VIDEO 5.4B**). In the presence of an intrapulmonary shunt, the microbubbles typically appear in the left heart in three to five cardiac cycles compared to one to two cardiac cycles for an intracardiac shunt (**VIDEO 5.4C**). A negative bubble study does not definitively exclude the presence of an intermittent right-to-left shunt.

8. (D) The width of the regurgitant jet (vena contracta) and the ratio of the vena contracta dimension to the aortic annulus dimension are quantitative measures to grade aortic regurgitation. The degree of LV dilatation is a semiquantitative measure and is most consistent with the duration of aortic regurgitation in addition to its severity. The length of the regurgitant jet into the left ventricle is influenced by many factors in addition to regurgitant severity including LV end-diastolic pressure and eccentricity of the jet. The degree of Doppler flow reversal in the abdominal aorta is an excellent predictor of regurgitation degree as is the forward to reverse flow TVI ratio in the distal transverse aortic arch.

9. (A) The MPI is the ratio of the total time spent in isovolumic activity (isovolumic contraction and isovolumic relaxation times) divided by the time spent in ventricular ejection (**Figure 5.26**).

10. (D) The subcostal imaging window is optimal to demonstrate the atrial septum and any associated atrial septal defects that may be present. To visualize the atrial septum without potential drop-out, the imaging plane of sound should be perpendicular to the cardiac structure of interest. With respect to the atrial septum, the imaging plane that is optimally perpendicular is the subcostal four-chamber and sagittal views. Atrial septal defects can be demonstrated in other imaging windows including the parasternal short-axis, apical four-chamber, and high right parasternal views but care must be taken not to diagnose an atrial septal defect when the plane of sound is more parallel to the atrial septum creating the potential for false drop-out in the 2D image. The addition of color Doppler and spectral Doppler interrogation in these views will also facilitate the diagnosis of an atrial septal defect (**Figure 5.27**).

11. (A) Sinus venosus atrial septal defects are most commonly associated with anomalous connection of the right pulmonary veins. Either a single right upper pulmonary vein or the right upper and middle pulmonary veins insert anomalously to the superior vena cava or the SVC–right atrial junction. Sinus venosus defects are found most commonly in the superior portion of the atrial septum creating a "biatrial" insertion of the superior vena cava. These defects can also be located inferiorly near the entrance of the inferior vena cava into the right atrium.

12. (C) Constrictive pericarditis is characterized by increased respiratory variation in mitral inflow Doppler velocities by >25%. Transmitral Doppler often demonstrates an increased *E:A* ratio and a shortened E-wave deceleration time. Lateral mitral tissue Doppler velocities are usually normal. Hepatic venous Doppler will demonstrate increased atrial systolic flow reversals during expiration.

13. (C) Echocardiographic hallmarks of restrictive LV physiology in adults include an increased mitral inflow Doppler *E:A* ratio >2.0, shortened mitral E-wave deceleration time <160 ms, decreased lateral mitral E_a velocity, and an increased *E/E'* ratio >15. Pulmonary venous Doppler demonstrates decreased systolic to diastolic pulmonary venous filling wave ratio with significantly increased atrial reversal wave velocity and duration.

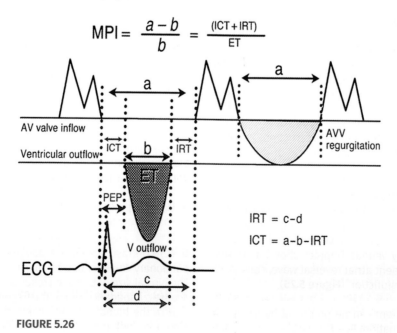

$$MPI = \frac{a-b}{b} = \frac{(ICT+IRT)}{ET}$$

IRT = c–d

ICT = a–b–IRT

FIGURE 5.26

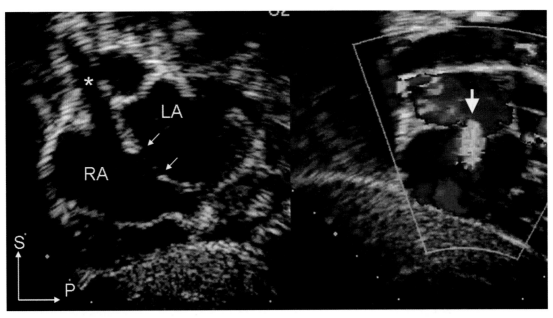

FIGURE 5.27 LA, left atrium; RA, right atrium.

14. (D) The newborn male has D-transposition of the great arteries (D-TGA) as evident from the **VIDEOS 5.1A,B** demonstrating pulmonary artery arising from the left ventricle and aorta arising from the right ventricle. Neonates with D-TGA can have a variable degree of desaturation depending primarily on the atrial and also on ventricular level shunts. The initial blood gas in the patient revealed a low arterial PaO_2 of 29 mm Hg in addition to low oxygen saturations, which suggest restricted atrial level shunt. All of these will be prominent indications for balloon atrial septostomy as the next best step in the management of the current patient.

15. (D) Anatomic hallmarks of AVSD include a cleft in the anterior leaflet of the left atrioventricular valve, lateral rotation of the left ventricular papillary muscles, and attachments of the left and right atrioventricular valves at the same level at the cardiac crux. In addition, due to the absence of the atrioventricular septum in these defects, the left ventricular inflow is shortened and the left ventricular outflow is elongated ("goose-neck deformity") creating a ratio of LV inlet to LV outlet ratio <1. Owing to the presence of a common atrioventricular valve, the aortic valve is no longer "wedged" between the tricuspid and the mitral valves and is pushed anteriorly ("sprung").

16. (B) M-mode has excellent temporal resolution and a high fixed PRF. The *x*-axis represents time while the *y*-axis represents distance from the transducer. M-mode utilizes a single imaging crystal.

17. (A) Spatial resolution is defined as the smallest distance between two points that are distinguishable from one another. Axial resolution is the ability to differentiate points along the ultrasound beam and is equal to its wavelength. Lateral resolution is the ability to resolve points perpendicular to the ultrasound beam and is dependent on beam width, with the best resolution found where the beam is the narrowest. Axial resolution is better than lateral resolution.

18. (A) Doppler velocity is calculated as follows: $V = [c(f_d)]/[2f_o \cos \theta]$. The speed of sound (*c*) and the transmitted ultrasound frequency (f_o) are constant while the frequency shift (f_d) can be measured very accurately. Therefore, the main source of error in velocity calculation is the angle of incidence (θ) between the ultrasound beam and the moving structure or blood. When the angle of incidence is <20 degrees, the Doppler velocity is not significantly underestimated (**Figure 5.28**).

19. (B) CW Doppler utilizes two crystals, one that is continuously transmitting and one that is continuously receiving, making the sampling rate infinite so that there is no limit to the detection of the maximal frequency shift. A disadvantage is that there is no range gating resulting in lack of range resolution (the maximal Doppler velocity can be anywhere along the ultrasound beam path). Both CW and PW Dopplers are equally dependent on the angle of incidence for accurate velocity determination (**Figure 5.29**).

20. (C) PW Doppler utilizes one crystal that intermittently transmits and receives. The time between transmission and reception allows the determination of the depth of the signal providing excellent range resolution. However, the maximal detectable frequency shift is limited resulting in a lower Nyquist limit than CW Doppler. Spectral Doppler has a higher PRF than color Doppler. PRF varies with the depth of the sample volume with PW Doppler, with a higher PRF with more shallow sample volumes.

21. (A) The Nyquist limit is the maximal frequency shift detectable by PW Doppler and is equal to one-half of the PRF. The Nyquist limit is lower with PW Doppler and is

CHAPTER 5

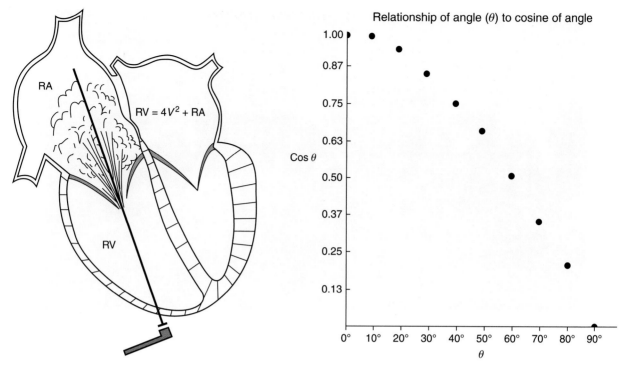

FIGURE 5.28 RA, right atrium; RV, right ventricle.

increased with lower frequency transducers and at shallow depths of interrogation.

22. (A) Color Doppler utilizes multiple sampling sites along multiple ultrasound beams to generate frequency shifts that are converted into a digital format and autocorrelated into a color scheme. Color Doppler is a mean velocity of blood flow with the intensity of color representing mean Doppler flow velocities. The Nyquist limit is lower with color Doppler compared to spectral Doppler. Color Doppler is superimposed on 2D images resulting in less resolution.

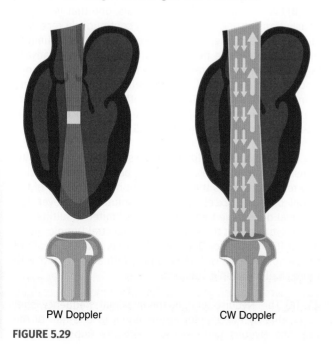

PW Doppler   CW Doppler

FIGURE 5.29

23. (D) Subpulmonary VSDs are located adjacent to the pulmonary valve and aortic valve. These VSDs have been termed subpulmonary, supracristal, or doubly committed defects. These defects can be best demonstrated in the parasternal short-axis scan plane but can also be demonstrated from the subcostal and apical windows with appropriate angulation into the right ventricular outflow tract.

24. (C) Coronary artery anomalies have been reported in approximately up to 10% of the patients with TOF. It is critical to delineate the coronary artery anatomy preoperatively as they can potentially affect the surgical management. The most common coronary artery anomaly is origin of left anterior descending (LAD) from the right coronary artery (RCA) or accessory LAD from the RCA. A single coronary artery (more often from the left coronary sinus) is the next most frequent variant and occurs in up to 1% of patients. Although a prominent conal branch can be commonly seen in many patients with significant right ventricular hypertrophy, it is not considered as anomalous anatomy.

25. (C) Large ventricular septal defects result in equalization of right and left ventricular pressures as well as elevated pulmonary arterial pressure. Left-to-right shunting at ventricular level results in a substantial increase in pulmonary blood flow with left atrial and left ventricular volume overload. Overall systemic blood flow is not significantly increased in this setting.

26. (A) (Figure 5.30) The best morphologic hallmarks of the right atrium are the broad-based right atrial appendage and the connections of the inferior vena cava and coronary sinus. Superior vena caval connection(s) have significant anatomic variability. Atrioventricular relationships

Echo Correlates of Atrial Morphology

RA Findings
- Pectinate muscles
- Broad appendage
- Thick septal limbus
- Coronary sinus
- Supra-hepatic IVC

LA Findings
- Smooth walls
- Finger-like appendage
- Thin valve of the atrial septum

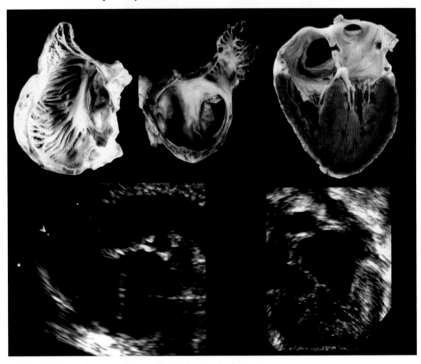

FIGURE 5.30 Echo correlates of atrial morphology.

can also vary and are not hallmarks of right atrial morphology. The valve of the fossa ovalis is septum primum and is a left atrial structure. The atrioventricular valve is a hallmark of ventricular morphology, with the morphologic tricuspid valve being the anatomic hallmark of the right ventricle.

27. (B) The best imaging plane to define the entire atrial septum is the subcostal imaging plane because it is perpendicular to this anatomic structure. (**VIDEOS 5.5A,B**) False drop-out can occur in imaging planes that are more parallel to the atrial septum.

28. (B) The best anatomic hallmark of the morphologic right ventricle is the connection of the tricuspid valve with a more apical insertion at the cardiac crux compared to the morphologic mitral valve. The tricuspid valve is "septophilic" with attachments to the ventricular septum. The right ventricle is more crescent in shape with prominent trabeculations (**Figure 5.31**).

29. (D) A higher insertion of the morphologic mitral valve at the cardiac crux and lack of atrioventricular valve chordal attachments to the ventricular septum ("septophobic") are excellent anatomic hallmarks of the morphologic LV. The LV

is elliptical in shape with fine trabeculations, mainly toward the cardiac apex (**Figure 5.31**).

30. (A) Utilizing the modified Bernoulli equation to obtain the peak instantaneous gradient across the pulmonary valve, $4 \times (velocity)^2$, then $4 \times (4.0)^2 = 64$ mm Hg.

31. (B) The most common type of subaortic stenosis is related to a discrete membrane proximal to the aortic valve within the LVOT (**Fig. 5.32**) (**VIDEOS 5.6A,B**). This membrane is most often circumferential and can be adherent to both the aortic valve and the anterior leaflet of the mitral valve. LVOT obstruction in the setting of hypertrophic cardiomyopathy (HCM) is often related to asymmetric septal hypertrophy in combination with systolic anterior motion of the mitral valve chordal and leaflet tissue. Anomalous mitral chordal insertions within the LVOT can be isolated or found in association with congenital heart disease and may result in obstruction but are not as common as discrete membranes.

32. (A) Bicuspid aortic valve is the most commonly associated cardiac finding in patients with simple coarctation, with some studies showing as high as an 80% occurrence in patients with coarctation. Atrial and ventricular septal defects are also common in patients with coarctation.

CHAPTER 5

**AV Connection, the Internal Crux
& Ventricular Morphology**

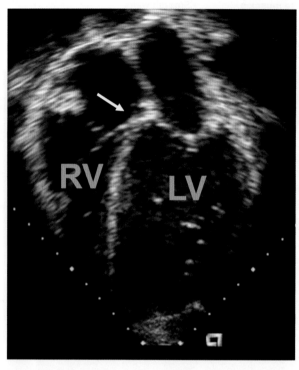

- AV Valve morphology
  is directly correlated
  with ventricular type

  - TV ⇒ RV
  - MV ⇒ LV
- Internal Cardiac Crux
  - Septal TV leaflet
    always inserts
    slightly apical to
    anterior MV leaflet

MAYO CLINIC

FIGURE 5.31 AV connection, the internal crux, and ventricular morphology.

Pulmonary valve stenosis and coronary arterial anomalies are much less frequent in this cohort.

33. (B) Newborn baby is demonstrating persistent pulmonary hypertension evident by the bidirectional flow at the level of patent ductus arteriosus (PDA) demonstrated by the spectral Doppler pattern in the PDA. There is >10% split between pre- and postductal oxygen saturation with lower postductal saturation due to the right-to-left shunting at the

level of PDA. However, in patients with transposition of great arteries and coarctation of the aorta, a reverse differential cyanosis is seen with lower preductal and higher postductal oxygen saturation due to the shunting of oxygenated blood from the pulmonary artery to the aorta.

34. (C) Cardiac tamponade occurs when increasing fluid in the pericardial space causes a rise in intrapericardial pressure (typically greater than intracardiac pressure)

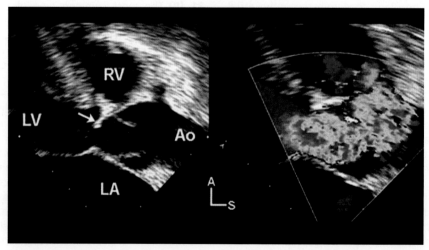

FIGURE 5.32 Ao, aorta; LA, left atrium; LV, left ventricle; RV, right ventricle.

compromising systemic venous return to the right atrium. Diastolic right atrial and right ventricular wall collapse occurs when intrapericardial pressure exceeds intracardiac pressure, with collapse of the right ventricle more sensitive to identify tamponade physiology. Pulsed-wave Doppler is more sensitive to identify cardiac tamponade with respiratory changes in Doppler flow across the tricuspid valve (>30%) and mitral valve (>25%) being most characteristic due to ventricular interdependence. While the overall size of the pericardial effusion is important, how quickly the fluid accumulates has more of an effect on intrapericardial pressure due to the relative compliance of the pericardium in the acute and chronic settings.

35. (E) The relationship between velocity of circumferential fiber shortening and end-systolic wall stress is independent of heart rate and preload and incorporates afterload making it a quantitative measure of ventricular contractility. Ejection fraction, shortening fraction, and the myocardial performance index are all significantly impacted by both preload and afterload.

36. (D) Patients with tricuspid atresia can develop restriction at the level of atrial septum with varying clinical presentation ranging from asymptomatic to severe right-sided congestion or poor perfusion. Elevated right atrial pressure, hepatomegaly, peripheral edema, hypotension, and poor perfusion may be some of the presenting clinical symptoms. Patients with atrial septal aneurysm on their initial echocardiogram have been shown to be at increased risk for developing atrial septal restrictions. On the other hand, restriction of the ventricular septal defect or increase in the pulmonary/subpulmonary obstruction generally manifest with declining oxygen saturations as the initial presentation without evidence of right-sided congestion.

37. (B) The presence of holodiastolic Doppler flow reversal is consistent with a significant run-off from the descending aorta including a large patent ductus arteriosus, severe aortic valve regurgitation, systemic-to-pulmonary artery shunts, and large arteriovenous fistula.

38. (C) The most common VSD associated with coarctation is a perimembranous defect. While less common, a posterior malalignment VSD often results in severe coarctation or interruption of the aortic arch. Muscular VSD as well as inlet VSD can also occur in the setting of coarctation, in particular with an unbalanced RV-dominant AVSD.

39. (A) The systolic jet in patients with supravalvar aortic stenosis propagates further than the jet originating with aortic valvar stenosis and has a tendency to be entrained along the aortic wall thereby transferring its kinetic energy into the right innominate artery. This physical principle, termed the Coanda effect, often is expressed clinically in these patients by marked discrepancy in upper arm blood pressures, with the right arm pressure higher than the left arm blood pressure.

40. (B) In the simplified Bernoulli equation, convective acceleration is calculated while flow acceleration and viscous friction are ignored. To accurately utilize the simplified equation, the proximal Doppler velocity must be negligible (**Figure 5.33**).

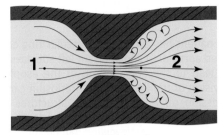

Bernoulli equation

$$P_1 - P_2 = 1/2\,\rho\,(V_2^2 - V_1^2) + \rho \int_1^2 \frac{dv}{dt}\,\vec{ds} + R\,(\vec{V})$$

Convection   +   Flow   +   Viscous
acceleration   acceleration   friction

P_1 = pressure at location 1
P_2 = pressure at location 2
ρ = mass density of the blood (1.06×10^3 kg/m^3)
V_1 = velocity at location 1
V_2 = velocity at location 2

FIGURE 5.33

41. (C) An overriding atrioventricular valve empties into two ventricles. It is committed to the ventricle to which >50% of its orifice is directed (**Figure 5.34**). This connection is always associated with a malalignment VSD. Valves that override can also straddle by having chordal attachments to the contralateral ventricle (**Figure 5.34**).

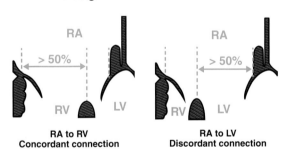

50% Rule
Assignment of AV connection

RA   RA

> 50%   > 50%

RV   LV   RV   LV

RA to RV   **RA to LV**
Concordant connection   **Discordant connection**

FIGURE 5.34 AV, atrioventricular; LV, left ventricle; RA, right atrium; RV, right ventricle.

42. (E) A straddling atrioventricular valve has anomalous chordal insertions or papillary muscles in the contralateral ventricle. Straddling and override often coexist. Straddling is associated with the presence of a VSD but does not require a malalignment type of defect. Semilunar valves do not have chordae or papillary muscles so they do not straddle. Straddling is not a common feature of tetralogy of Fallot.

43. (C) Interruption of the intrahepatic portion of the IVC with azygos vein continuation to the superior vena cava is a common feature of polysplenia syndrome (left atrial isomerism). The abdominal situs is variable and can be ambiguous, inversus, or solitus. The spleens are usually multiple and are characteristically located on the same side. A single gallbladder is most typical but biliary atresia can and does occur.

44. (E) The patient has a complete vascular ring consisting of right-sided aortic arch and aberrant left subclavian artery which can lead to the compression of the esophagus or trachea. Division of the ligamentum arteriosum can release the compression on the surrounding structures in most cases, while some patients may require translocation of the aberrant subclavian artery traversing behind the esophagus or trachea.

45. (C) Tricuspid atresia is an example of a single-inlet atrioventricular valve connection (**Figure 5.35**).

46. (E) Atrial myxoma is the second most common form of cardiac mass in children, second to rhabdomyomas. The most common location of atrial myxomas is left atrium in 75% of the cases. They are commonly friable, pedunculated, red lobular tumors typically attached to the atrial septum. Myxomas can be associated with the triad of (a) valvular obstruction, (b) embolic events, and (c) systemic illness. Once a diagnosis of atrial myxoma has been made on imaging studies, prompt resection is indicated due to the risk of embolization or cardiovascular complications, including sudden death.

47. (B) When a persistent left superior vena cava drains to the coronary sinus, the size of the coronary sinus is inversely proportional to the size of the bridging innominate vein. When the coronary sinus is severely dilated, the innominate vein is most commonly very small or absent.

When the inferior vena cava is interrupted, venous return is directed from the azygos vein to the superior vena cava. Interruption of the IVC is more common in polysplenia syndrome versus asplenia syndrome. Superior vena caval connections are variable and are not an anatomic hallmark of the morphologic right atrium. The left pulmonary veins more commonly merge than the right veins as they connect to the left atrium.

48. (D) While all these are features that distinguish the morphologic tricuspid valve from the mitral valve, the most reliable anatomic hallmark is the level of attachment of the atrioventricular valve at the cardiac crux. The atrioventricular valves are invariably associated with their appropriate morphologic ventricle (tricuspid valve with the right ventricle and mitral valve with the left ventricle) and are the best marker for atrioventricular connection and ventricular morphology.

49. (C) Constrictive pericarditis is caused by thickened, inflamed, or calcific pericardium that limits the diastolic filling of the heart causing heart failure. Risk factors for constriction include previous cardiac surgery, recurrent pericarditis, episodes of pericardial effusion, and radiation therapy. Due to the fixed cardiac volume within the thickened pericardium, diastolic filling of right and left ventricles rely on each other. On echocardiography, it is characterized by increased respiratory variation in mitral inflow Doppler velocities by >25% and increased diastolic flow reversal with expiration in the hepatic vein. Other features of constriction may include an increased E:A ratio and a shortened E-wave deceleration time.

50. (C) Subcostal images demonstrate a sinus venosus atrial septal defect with partial anomalous pulmonary venous connection to the superior vena cava. The defect is located in the superior/posterior portion of the atrial septum adjacent to the superior vena cava. The right upper and middle

Univentricular AV connections

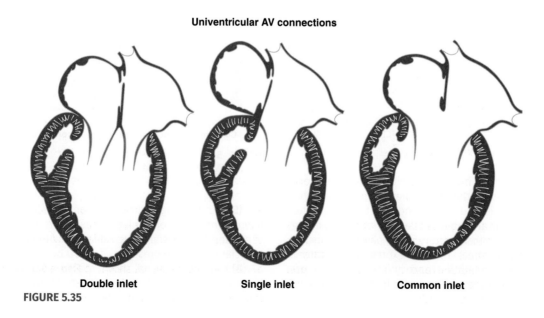

Double inlet Single inlet Common inlet

FIGURE 5.35

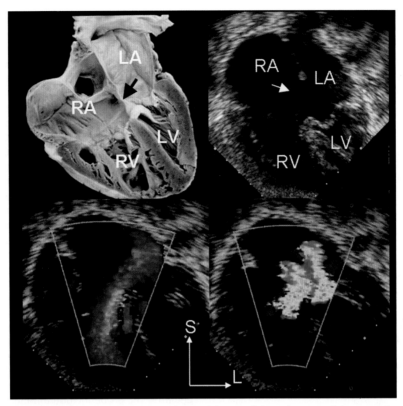

FIGURE 5.36 LA, left atrium; LV, left ventricle; RA, right atrium; RV, right ventricle.

pulmonary veins are often anomalous and most commonly connect to the superior vena cava.

51. (A) These images demonstrate the classic features of a partial AVSD (**Figure 5.36**). There is a large primum atrial septal defect with a large left-to-right atrial level shunt. Owing to lack of the atrioventricular septum, both atrioventricular valves are inserted at the same level at the cardiac crux. The inlet ventricular septum is intact. Color Doppler also demonstrates significant mitral regurgitation, most likely related to a cleft in the anterior leaflet.

52. (B) Patient in the current scenario fulfills the criteria for multisystem inflammatory syndrome in children (MIS-C) due to SARS-CoV-2 infection. Patients with MIS-C may present with acute cardiogenic shock and ventricular dysfunction. Generally, the ventricular dysfunction resolves promptly. However, patients diagnosed with MIS-C should have adequate follow-up to evaluate coronary arteries due to risk for development of coronary ectasia and aneurysms similar to patients with Kawasaki disease.

53. (B) This parasternal short-axis scan demonstrates a large membranous VSD with a large left-to-right shunt.

54. (C) This parasternal long-axis scan demonstrates significant aortic root dilatation consistent with Marfan syndrome. Classic echocardiographic features of Marfan syndrome include aortic root dilatation and mitral valve prolapse. Hallmark cardiac findings in Down syndrome include AVSD and VSDs. Most common cardiac lesions in DiGeorge

syndrome include aortic arch anomalies and conotruncal defects. Noonan syndrome typically has right ventricular outflow and pulmonary artery anomalies as well as atrial septal defects and HCM. Williams syndrome classically presents with supravalvar aortic stenosis and supravalvar/branch pulmonary arterial stenoses.

55. (B) Cardiac myxomas are the most common adult cardiac tumor and the second most common childhood cardiac tumor. The majority (75%) are located in the left atrium and are typically attached to the fossa ovalis. When large, they can obstruct atrioventricular valve inflow leading to symptoms including positional dyspnea, syncope, and even death. Constitutional symptoms include weight loss, malaise, arthralgias, and myalgias. Carney syndrome is a familial form of myxoma and is associated with lentigines and endocrine abnormalities.

56. (C) This parasternal long-axis scan shows a large homogeneous echogenic mass in the posterior wall of the left ventricle consistent with a cardiac fibroma. Fibromas are firm, white, nonencapsulated tumors. They are typically located in the left ventricle within the posterior wall or septum and commonly at the cardiac apex. They are often large and can result in cavitary obstruction or impair atrioventricular valve function. These tumors also have a significant risk of sudden death due to ventricular arrhythmias.

57. (B) The Doppler signal shown in **Figure 5.5** shows a "dagger-shape" profile which is characteristic for dynamic left ventricular outflow obstruction. Due to the late-peaking nature of the obstruction, the maximum instantaneous Doppler gradient has the best correlation with the peak-to-peak gradient measured during cardiac catheterization. Therefore, maximum instantaneous Doppler gradient is generally considered among other factors for clinical and surgical decision making. This is distinctly different from fixed obstructions, like aortic valve stenosis where mean Doppler gradient best reflects the pressure drop across the stenotic aortic valve.

58. (B) In some patients with hypertrophic cardiomyopathy, the LVOT Doppler signal can be difficult to separate from the mitral regurgitation profile. In such cases, the LVOT gradient can be estimated from the maximum mitral regurgitant velocity. Mitral regurgitation peak velocity is converted to the left ventricle (LV) to left atrial (LA) pressure difference using simplified Bernoulli equation ($4V^2$). The patient's systolic blood pressure can then be subtracted from the gradient to calculate the estimated left ventricular to aortic gradient. In the example given in this question using a mitral regurgitant velocity of 6.2 m/sec, the LV to LA pressure difference would be 154 mm Hg. Left atrial pressure of 10 mm Hg can be added to the LV to LA pressure difference to accurately assess the LV maximal systolic pressure of 164 mm Hg. The patient's blood pressure was 100 mm Hg which can be subtracted from the LV maximal systolic pressure to obtain an estimated peak LVOT gradient of 64 mm Hg.

59. (C) It is well-known that mechanical mitral valve prostheses can interfere with optimal transthoracic echocardiographic imaging of mechanical valves due to the significant acoustic shadowing produced by the polycarbonate composition of the valve. At times, echocardiographic imaging of the more distal portions of the valve is inhibited by acoustic shadowing produced by the more proximal portions. Because of this, transthoracic echocardiographic imaging of a mechanical mitral valve can be difficult from standard precordial windows. In contrast, the position of the esophagus—situated posterior and close to the left atrium—locates the TEE probe in an optimal position to visualize a mechanical mitral valve prosthesis, free of acoustic shadowing from the valve itself or other intervening structures that might interfere with ultrasonic imaging. The other choices in this question are interventions located in areas that can sometimes be more difficult to visualize clearly and consistently by TEE imaging. These areas include the innominate vein, aortic arch, and left pulmonary artery. A Melody valve in the pulmonary position can be seen by TEE, but in general, Melody valve implantation does not require TEE imaging.

60. (C) In several published studies on pediatric TEE (see references below), there is a low incidence of complications, in the range of 1% to 3%. The most common complication is airway compromise, with a rate of 1% to 2.6% in these studies. Except for infective endocarditis, all of the other complications listed in this question can potentially occur with pediatric TEE, but they are much less common. Infective endocarditis is not a generally recognized complication of TEE, and endocarditis prophylaxis is not routinely recommended prior to a TEE procedure.

61. (A) The deep transgastric position provides the best angle of insonation for the area of obstruction in the mid-portion of the RV that typifies DCRV. **Figure 1A** shows a deep transgastric right ventricular outflow tract view (transducer angle 65 to 70 degrees) of the muscle bundles; **Figure 1B** shows the same view with color flow Doppler across the area of obstruction. **Figure 1C** shows the measured gradient across the RV outflow tract obstruction (~4.0 m/s). While the RV muscle bundles and the anatomic narrowing of DCRV can also be well-seen using the midesophageal views, such as the midesophageal right ventricular inflow–outflow view, the angle of insonation for Doppler evaluation tends to be perpendicular to the flow, producing a measured spectral Doppler velocity that will significantly underestimate the actual flow velocity across the area. The other esophageal and gastric positions will not adequately visualize DCRV.

62. (D) The pediatric multiplane TEE transducer consists of an array of elements mounted on a small circular platform located at the tip of the TEE probe. Using a control on the TEE probe handle, the platform can be rotated either electronically or mechanically to achieve a beam orientation between 0 degrees and 180 degrees. The other options given in this question—tilting, rocking, sliding, and angling the probe tip—all represent *transthoracic* echocardiography probe maneuvers, and do not apply to TEE. The other basic maneuvers for a pediatric TEE probe include anteflexion/retroflexion, advancing and withdrawal, and clockwise/counterclockwise rotation.

63. (D) This video, taken from the midesophageal four-chamber view and modified midesophageal right ventricular inflow–outflow view (transducer angle 36 degrees), demonstrates a perimembranous ventricular septal defect with direct left ventricle to right atrial shunting, often through perforations in the septal leaflet of tricuspid valve (the jet bypasses the right ventricular chamber). This defect is also known as a Gerbode defect. As shown in the video, the jet is systolic—as evidenced by the closed tricuspid valve and open pulmonary valve—therefore it is not an eccentric aortic regurgitant jet, which would be diastolic, nor is it likely to be a coronary arteriovenous fistula to the right atrium, which would be a continuous flow pattern seen both in systole and diastole. The jet is not seen to cross the atrial septum, nor is a septal defect seen on the midesophageal four-chamber view, therefore this is not a primum atrial septal defect. In some instances of a Gerbode defect, the jet can appear to be a medial jet of tricuspid regurgitation. However, in this case, the jet appears to arise from the left ventricular outflow tract, not from the right ventricle.

64. (B) This TEE video, taken from a modified midesophageal long axis view followed by a deep transgastric right ventricular outflow tract view, demonstrates an intramural VSD. This is an interventricular communication that can occur following repair of a conotruncal defect such as DORV. The surgically placed VSD patch is anchored to RV free wall trabeculations; these trabeculations communicate with the RV cavity in multiple locations. When attached to the trabeculations, the VSD patch effectively separates the "new" left ventricular outflow tract (LVOT) above the patch from the RV cavity below the patch (i.e., the physiologic RV). If the intramural trabeculations interconnect the new LVOT with the physiologic RV, a pressure gradient exists between the two chambers that leads to a left-to-right shunt through the trabeculations. The intramural VSD is often confused with a residual VSD adjacent to the VSD patch, but in this patient the VSD patch is intact. Close inspection shows no flow around the edge of the patch itself, as would be expected with a residual peri-patch leak. Rather, the interventricular shunting begins through a large opening below the aortic valve (above the VSD patch), through multiple trabeculations in the RV free wall, exiting below the VSD patch into the RV cavity. Regarding the other options: aortic left ventricle tunnel is a channel that arises from the ascending aorta (generally above the right and left aortic cusps), tunnels through the aortic wall and ventricular septum, and empties into the left ventricular outflow tract; and it results in diastolic flow from aorta to left ventricle (physiology similar to aortic regurgitation). Similarly, a ruptured sinus of Valsalva aneurysm would also be expected to originate above the level of the aortic valve, with communication directly into the RV, and continuous shunting seen from aorta to RV. However, in the video, the abnormal flow is systolic and begins below the level of the aortic valve. The systolic nature of the flow also rules out aortic valve regurgitation; furthermore, the origin of the flow below the aortic valve is not consistent with aortic valve pathology.

65. (E) Most implanted metallic objects, including coils, clips, pacemaker leads, and occluder devices, are weakly ferromagnetic and are relatively immobile after implantation. Pacemakers and AICDs are a relative contraindication to a cardiac MR examination, but recent reports suggest that even these devices may be safe for the MR examination.

66. (C) Stainless steel objects, such as PDA coils, cause the most imaging artifact with MR imaging. Occluder devices including the Amplatzer ASD device also cause significant imaging artifact. Pacemaker leads, PDA vascular clips, and nonferromagnetic stents cause less artifact with MR imaging.

67. (A) With spin echo, there is a relatively long time period between spin excitation and data sampling resulting in blood flow leaving the imaging plane when the signal is sampled. This produces an image where blood appears black and surrounding cardiac tissue is encoded in shades of gray or white. Spin echo sequences provide still images for anatomy and tissue characterization. Blood appears bright in gradient echo, SSFP, and contrast-enhanced images.

68. (C) VEC MRI is a gradient echo sequence that can measure blood flow velocity and quantify blood flow. The other sequences do not provide any quantifiable flow or velocity information.

69. (D) Spin echo cardiac magnetic resonance imaging is a black-blood technique where the blood pool is black and the surrounding cardiac tissue is encoded in shades of gray or white. Signal acquisition is performed over several cardiac cycles. This technique produces high tissue contrast and has less imaging artifact with metallic implants compared to other cardiac MR techniques. Spin echo applications include imaging myocardial and blood vessel walls, cardiac masses and tumors, and the pericardium. T1- and T2-weighted sequences in spin echo imaging can help in tissue characterization.

70. (A) Gradient echo sequences have less time between spin excitation and signal detection resulting in a faster acquisition than spin echo sequences. Therefore, the gradient echo technique results in high imaging speed with multiple images acquired during each cardiac cycle. The signal from slower moving tissue is gray and has less contrast compared to spin echo images and is more susceptible to imaging artifacts. Faster moving blood has a stronger signal resulting in bright-blood images.

71. (A) MDE has become the primary cardiac MR technique to assess myocardial viability. Washout of gadolinium contrast agents is delayed in necrotic myocardium as well as areas of fibrotic tissue. Nonviable myocardium therefore appears bright when compared to viable myocardium. MDE has been shown to be very effective in determining the presence, size, and transmurality of myocardial infarctions as well as in the identification of the presence and extent of myocardial fibrosis in patients with HCM.

72. (B) Phase-contrast (or velocity-encoded) cine imaging is used for flow quantification and does not require any contrast administration. Conventional MRA is performed with contrast; however, newer noncontrast MRA sequences do not require contrast agents. Intravenous contrast administration is needed for myocardial perfusion, delayed enhancement, and TRICKS.

73. (C) T2-weighted sequences are fluid-sensitive and can best detect myocardial edema such as in a patient with acute myocarditis. First-pass perfusion imaging may or may not show a hypoattenuated filling defect in the area of myocardial edema. Other sequences do not help in assessment of myocardial edema.

74. (C) ECG-gated CTA is the best test to assess intramural course of anomalous coronary artery origin. MRA does not have the spatial resolution to confirm this diagnosis. CTA without ECG gating does not allow assessment of coronary arteries. Invasive coronary angiography cannot assess the intramural course of anomalous coronary artery. Thallium scan can only show myocardial areas of hypoperfusion.

75. (B) Conventional MRA can assess the coarctation of aorta. CTA can also do the assessment; however, ECG gating is not needed for this purpose. Retrospective ECG-gated CTA has highest dose of radiation. TEE, stress echo, and thallium scan are not optimal tests for coarctation assessment.

76. (A) *The magnet is always on!* This is an important fact for MRI safety. Ferromagnetic objects brought into the room can act as projectiles and may cause injury to patient or personnel. The magnet is always on, even when not in use.

77. (D) Delayed myocardial enhancement is typically subepicardial or midmyocardial and patchy in myocarditis. In infarction, the delayed enhancement is typically suben-docardial or transmural. Myocardial edema is best seen on T2-weighted black-blood images. Fatty infiltrates can be seen on T1-weighted images and are not a hallmark of myocarditis. Early myocardial enhancement is due to hyper-emia of the inflamed areas. MR angiogram does not help in myocardial assessment.

78. (A) Noncontrast CT is the best test to assess pericardial calcification. Contrast enhancement and ECG gating are not needed for this purpose. The other imaging modalities do not help in this assessment.

79. (A) T2* quantification is required for measurement of iron in myocardial tissue in patients with thalassemia or other chronic blood transfusion recipients. Other sequences cannot be used to quantify tissue iron load.

80. (D) MR images show typical features of pericarditis. Panel A shows thickened pericardium on T1-weighted double-inversion recovery sequence. Panel B shows pericardial edema and a small effusion on T2-weighted sequence. Panels C and D show diffuse postcontrast delayed enhance-ment of the pericardium. Myocardium has normal appear-ance in all these images.

81. (B) CTA shows anomalous drainage of right upper and right middle pulmonary veins draining to superior vena cava. The left coronary artery seems to be originating nor-mally in this view, whereas the right coronary is not seen. This single coronal plane does not show the tricuspid valve, right ventricle, and the left pulmonary veins but the clinical history of acyanosis precludes the diagnoses of TAPVC and tricuspid atresia.

82. (E) Asterisk marks the aortic arch. The image shows the main pulmonary artery anterior to the aorta with the branch pulmonary arteries "draped-over" the aorta. This is consistent with the LeCompte maneuver performed with an arterial switch operation in patients with D-TGA. In atrial switch procedures, the great arterial relationship remains transposed.

83. (B) The images show single left coronary artery with the right coronary branch traveling anterior to the pulmonary valve. This is important if transannular patch augmentation of pulmonary valve is intended. To avoid trauma to RCA, a RV-PA conduit may be needed to relieve the RV-PA gradient.

84. (D) The image shows a shunt placed between the right subclavian artery and the pulmonary artery, which is consistent with a modified BT shunt. Classic BT shunt is direct end-to-side anastomosis of subclavian artery to the PA. Waterston shunt is direct side-to-side anastomosis of ascending aorta to the right pulmonary artery. Potts shunt is direct side-to-side anastomosis of descending aorta to the left pulmonary artery. Central shunt is a small conduit from aorta to pulmonary artery.

85. (E) The single axial image of this CT angiogram shows aortic arches on both sides of trachea, consistent with double aortic arch. The branching pattern is not seen in this image. Typical branching pattern for double aortic arch is separate origin of four aortic arch branches. The right common carotid and right subclavian arteries arise from the right aortic arch, whereas the left common carotid and the left subclavian arteries arise from the left aortic arch.

86. (C) The CT angiogram shows anomalous origin of LCA from the pulmonary artery. Asterisks mark the RCAs and LCAs. With chronic run-off of blood from the LCA into the pulmonary artery, the main coronary arteries become dilat-ed over time due to increased flow from RCA to LCA via collaterals.

87. (D) The MR angiogram shows a coronal plane with Fontan conduit stenosis. This is a common finding in patients who received a conduit made of biologic material such as aortic homograft. The anastomotic sites appear patent without any thrombi in the Fontan circuit.

88. (B) The CTA shows coarctation of aorta. VSD and bicuspid aortic valve are common coexisting diagnoses in patients with coarctation of aorta.

ACKNOWLEDGMENT

Figures 5.5, 5.6, 5.11, 5.9, 5.12, 5.24, 5.26, 5.27, 5.28, and 5.36 are from Eidem BW, Cetta F, O'Leary PW. *Echocardiography in Pediatric and Adult Congenital Heart Disease.* Lippincott Williams & Wilkins; 2010. © Mayo Foundation for Medical Education and Research. All rights Reserved.

SUGGESTED READINGS

Allen HD, Driscoll DJ, Shaddy RE, et al. *Moss and Adams' Heart Disease in Infants, Children, and Adolescents.* 7th ed. Lippincott Williams & Wilkins; 2008.

Didier D, Ratib O, Beghetti M, et al. Morphologic and functional evaluation of congenital heart disease by magnetic resonance imaging. *J Magn Reson Imaging.* 1999;10:639–655.

Drose JA. *Fetal Echocardiography.* 2nd ed. Saunders Elsevier; 2010.

Eidem BW, Cetta F, O'Leary PW. *Echocardiography in Pediatric and Adult Congenital Heart Disease.* Lippincott Williams & Wilkins; 2010.

Hance-Miller W, Fyfe DA, Stevenson JG, et al. Indications and guidelines for performance of transesophageal echocardiography in the patient with pediatric acquired or congenital heart disease. A report from the Task Force of the Pediatric Council of the American Society of Echocardiography. *J Am Soc Echocardiogr.* 2005;18:91–98.

Kilner PJ, Geva T, Kaemmerer H, et al. Recommendations for cardiovascular magnetic resonance in adults with congenital heart disease from the respective working groups of the European Society of Cardiology. *Eur Heart J.* 2010;31:794–805.

Lai WW, Geva T, Shirali GS, et al.; Task Force of the Pediatric Council of the American Society of Echocardiography, Pediatric Council of the American Society of Echocardiography. Guidelines and standards for performance of a pediatric echocardiogram: a report from the Task Force of the Pediatric Council of the American Society of Echocardiography. *J Am Soc Echocardiogr.* 2006;19: 1413–1430.

Lang RM, Bierig M, Devereux RB, et al. Recommendations for chamber quantification: a report from the American Society of Echocardiography's Guidelines and Standards Committee and the Chamber Quantification Writing Group, developed in conjunction with the European Association of Echocardiography, a branch of the European Society of Cardiology. *J Am Soc Echocardiogr.* 2005;18:1440–1463.

Lopez L, Colan SD, Frommelt PC, et al. Recommendations for quantification methods during the performance of a pediatric echocardiogram: a report from the Pediatric Measurements Writing Group of the American Society of Echocardiography Pediatric and Congenital Heart Disease Council. *J Am Soc Echocardiogr.* 2010;23:465–495.

Oh JK, Seward JB, Tajik AJ. *The Echo Manual.* 3rd ed. Lippincott Williams & Wilkins; 2006.

Prakash A, Powell AJ, Geva T. Multimodality noninvasive imaging for assessment of congenital heart disease. *Circ Cardiovasc Imaging.* 2010;3:112–125.

Prakash A, Powell AJ, Krishnamurthy R, et al. Magnetic resonance imaging evaluation of myocardial perfusion and viability in congenital and acquired pediatric heart disease. *Am J Cardiol.* 2004;93:657–661.

Rychik J, Ayres N, Cunco B, et al. American Society of Echocardiography guidelines and standards for performance of the fetal echocardiogram. *J Am Soc Echocardiogr.* 2004;17:803–810.

CHAPTER 5

Cardiac Electrophysiology

Bryan C. Cannon, Philip L. Wackel, Mark Shwayder, and Yaniv Bar-Cohen

Questions

1. A fetal ultrasound performed at 32-week gestation reveals fetal SVT at a rate of 250 beats per minute (bpm) with 1:1 AV relationship. There is no evidence of hydrops fetalis and the ventricular function is good. Over the next 24 hours, the fetus is observed, and tachycardia persists. You would advise which of the following:

   A. Adenosine administration via cordocentesis through umbilical vein
   B. Continued observation
   C. Atenolol
   D. Digoxin
   E. Immediate delivery

2. A patient presents after an irregular heartbeat was noted on a preparticipation sports physical. The electrocardiogram (ECG) is shown in **Figure 6.1**. There is no murmur and he has an otherwise normal examination. He is asymptomatic. What would you advise?

   A. He can participate in all sports
   B. No competitive sports
   C. He may participate in all sports if the rhythm can be normalized by an antiarrhythmic medication
   D. He may participate in all sports if he undergoes a successful ablation procedure
   E. He may participate in low-impact sports such as golf

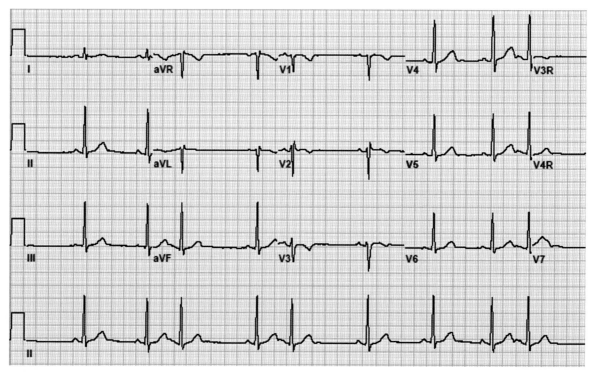

FIGURE 6.1

3. A 3-year-old asymptomatic boy is referred to you after an ECG is obtained on preoperative screening prior to a tonsillectomy. There is no family history of sudden death. The ECG is shown in **Figure 6.2**. What would be the most appropriate therapy?

A. Implant an ICD
B. Begin β-blocker therapy
C. Perform an electrophysiology study
D. Start amiodarone
E. Direct current cardioversion

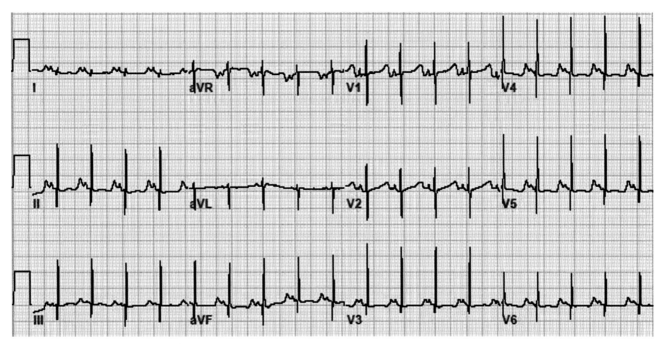

FIGURE 6.2

4. An 8-year-old patient with a repaired VSD presents with a new-onset seizure. The rhythm strip shown in **Figure 6.3** was obtained during the seizure episode and sent to you for review. Which of the following therapies is most appropriate?

A. Direct current cardioversion
B. IV lidocaine drip
C. Oral β-blocker
D. No therapy
E. IV amiodarone

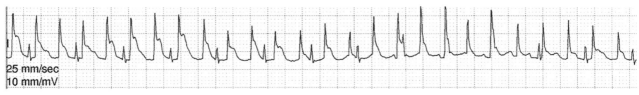

25 mm/sec
10 mm/mV

FIGURE 6.3

5. A 14-year-old boy presents for evaluation of a murmur and is noted to have left ventricular septal hypertrophy on his echocardiogram consistent with hypertrophic cardiomyopathy. Which of the following additional factors most increases the risk of sudden death?

A. Marked left ventricular hypertrophy on the ECG (R wave 50 mm in V6)
B. Left ventricular septal wall thickness of 3.2 cm in diastole
C. Presence of systolic anterior motion of the mitral valve
D. Presence of a mid-cavitary LV gradient
E. Chest pain with exercise

6. A 14-year-old patient with dilated cardiomyopathy is on digoxin, furosemide, and enalapril for his heart failure. He is now starting to have frequent episodes of supraventricular tachycardia (SVT) and you would like to start him on amiodarone. Which medication adjustment will most likely be required?

A. Decrease the dose of digoxin
B. Increase the dose of digoxin
C. Increase the dose of furosemide
D. Decrease the dose of enalapril
E. Make no changes in any of the medications

7. An 8-year-old boy has been complaining of episodes of fast heart rates lasting 15 to 20 minutes. These typically occur with exercise. He has an episode every 3 months. A 24-hour Holter monitor shows variability in the QRS morphology as shown in **Figure 6.4**. The etiology of his symptoms is most likely to be which of the following?

A. Ventricular tachycardia
B. Junctional tachycardia
C. Reentrant supraventricular tachycardia
D. Atrial flutter
E. Automatic focus atrial tachycardia

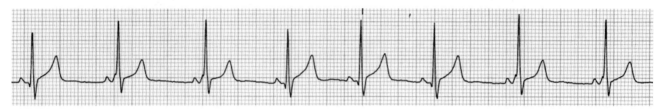

FIGURE 6.4

8. A 14-year-old girl presents with a rash with central clearing, nonspecific joint pain, and the ECG shown in **Figure 6.5**. The treatment of choice would be:

A. Gentamicin
B. Doxycycline
C. Vancomycin
D. Intravenous immuno globulin (IVIG)
E. β-Blocker

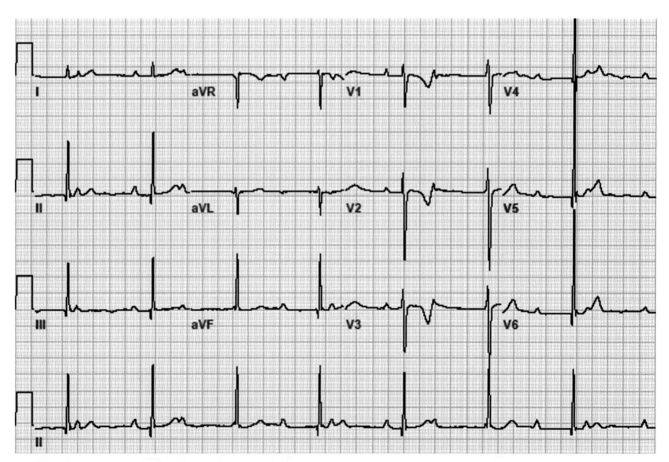

FIGURE 6.5

CHAPTER 6

9. A 15-year-old girl presents following a syncopal episode. Upon further investigation you find out that she had been standing on a hot day in church and felt lightheaded before passing out. The event was witnessed, and her parents describe a brief episode of jerking of her arms following her syncope. She awoke within 10 seconds and was oriented to time and place but did have a headache. Her ECG and physical examination were normal. What is the next most appropriate step?

A. Implantable loop recorder placement
B. 24-Hour ambulatory monitoring
C. Recommend increased fluid intake
D. EP study
E. Neurology referral

10. A 16-year-old football player comes to you for evaluation of palpitations and dizziness. The ECG shown in **Figure 6.6** is obtained. What would you do?

A. Perform a 24-hour Holter monitor. If there are no arrhythmias, let him play
B. Permanently disqualify him from all competitive sports based on the ECG
C. Let him play as the ECG findings are a normal variant
D. Not let him play until evaluation including an echocardiogram is performed
E. Let him play and repeat the ECG in 6 months

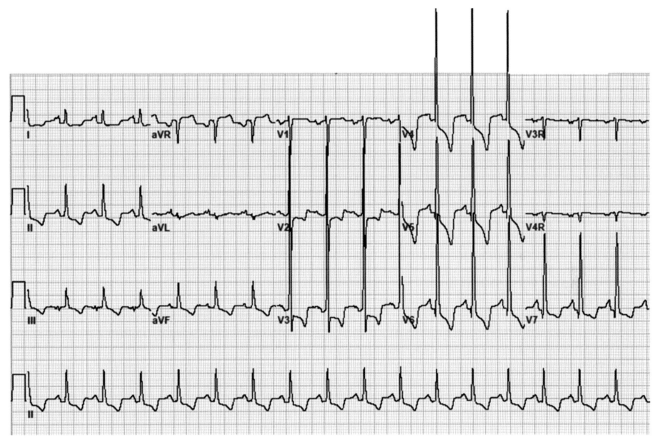

FIGURE 6.6

11. A 14-year-old girl is referred to your office after she was noted to have a first-degree AV block, a right bundle branch block, and a left anterior fascicular block on a 12-lead ECG. On your examination, you also note drooping eyelids and ataxia. What would be the most logical next step?

A. Implant a pacemaker
B. IV steroid administration
C. Perform an electrophysiologic study
D. Initiate medical therapy with theophylline
E. Watchful waiting with plan for repeat evaluation in 6 months

12. A 1-week-old male child gets a 12-lead ECG for bradycardia. The ECG (**Figure 6.7**) shows which of the following:

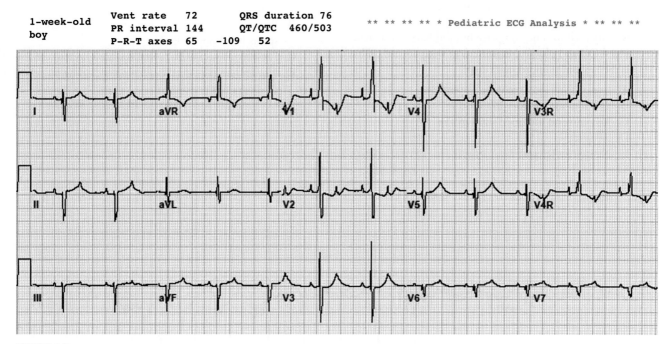

1-week-old boy	Vent rate	72	QRS duration 76	
	PR interval	144	QT/QTC	460/503
	P-R-T axes	65	-109	52

** ** ** ** * Pediatric ECG Analysis * ** ** ** **

FIGURE 6.7

A. Sinus node dysfunction
B. Complete heart block
C. Ectopic atrial tachycardia
D. Long QT syndrome
E. Wenckebach block (Mobitz I block)

13. What is the relationship of the conduction system to the ventricular septal defect in a patient with an AV canal?

A. Posterior and superior to the ventricular septal defect
B. Posterior and inferior to the ventricular septal defect
C. Anterior and superior to the ventricular septal defect
D. Anterior and inferior to the ventricular septal defect
E. On the left side of the heart

14. Risk of sudden death in patients who have had repair of tetralogy of Fallot is highest in those with which of the following?

A. QRS duration of 190 ms with residual right ventricular hypertension
B. Frequent premature ventricular contractions
C. Sinus bradycardia on 24-hour Holter monitoring
D. Neonatal primary repair with right ventricular outflow tract patch
E. Bifascicular block with a QRS duration of 140 ms

15. A 13-year-old child with polyarthritis has the ECG shown in **Figure 6.8**. Which of the following may the patient also have?

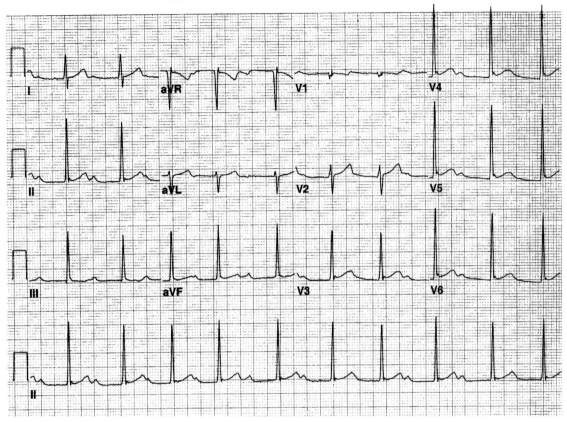

13-year-old girl

Vent. rate	75	bmp
PR interval	439	msec
QRS duration	96	msec
QT/QTc	384/429	msec
P–R–T axes	* 76	28

FIGURE 6.8

A. Choreiform movements of the hands
B. Coronary artery aneurysms
C. A dilated ascending aorta
D. Glomerulonephritis
E. Bifid uvula

16. Irregular fetal heart sounds are heard during a routine prenatal visit at 32-week gestation. Results of fetal ultrasonography suggest appropriate fetal size and development, normal ventricular function, and no evidence of hydrops. A fetal echocardiographic M-mode tracing shows frequent premature atrial beats, some of which are not conducted to the ventricle with the heart rate intermittently dropping into the 60s. The most appropriate management is:

A. Maternal digoxin therapy
B. Maternal sotalol therapy
C. Maternal flecainide therapy
D. Immediate delivery
E. Observation only

17. A 7-year-old boy has had three episodes of SVT in the past month. Apart from some palpitations and mild dizziness, he does not have any symptoms. He has a documented heart rate of 240 bpm. The tachycardia is able to be terminated by one dose of adenosine, intravenously. An ECG is obtained following conversion to sinus rhythm and is shown in **Figure 6.9**. Which of the following drugs should be recommended to decrease the chance of a recurrence of SVT?

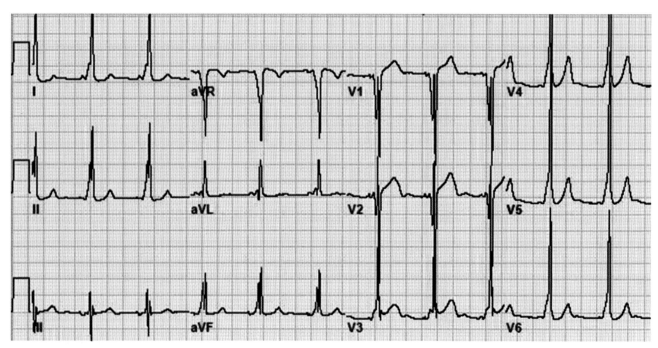

FIGURE 6.9

    A. Verapamil
    B. Oral amiodarone to be taken only after tachycardia starts
    C. Digoxin
    D. Mexiletine
    E. Propranolol

18. Which of the following statements most accurately describes the normal change in the ECG during the first week after birth?

    A. An increase in the size of the R wave in lead V1
    B. A shift in the QRS frontal plane axis from greater than +135 degrees to less than +30 degrees
    C. A change in T-wave polarity from positive to negative in lead V1
    D. Development of a Q wave in lead V1
    E. Shortening of the PR interval

19. In an 8-year-old girl who has permanent junctional reciprocating tachycardia, electrocardiography during an episode of tachycardia would most likely show:

    A. Deeply negative P waves in leads II, III, and aVF
    B. No visible P waves
    C. Two P waves for every QRS complex
    D. P waves that are positive in lead aVF and negative in lead I
    E. A P-wave axis identical to sinus rhythm

20. A 5-year-old child with diabetic ketoacidosis has a heart rate of 140 bpm. Serum potassium concentration is 8.5 mEq/L. The ECG rhythm strip would be expected to demonstrate which of the following?

    A. Low-amplitude T wave
    B. Prominent Q wave
    C. Prolonged QRS duration
    D. Short PR interval
    E. High-amplitude P wave

21. A 6 month old presents with tachycardia immediately following complete repair for tetralogy of Fallot. The ECG is shown in **Figure 6.10**. The most likely diagnosis is:

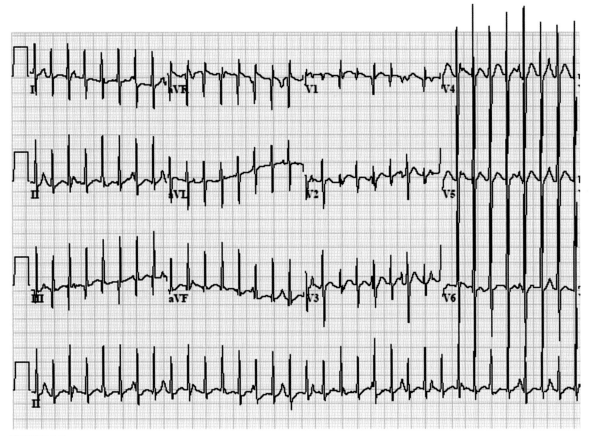

FIGURE 6.10

A. Atrial flutter with variable AV conduction
B. Ventricular tachycardia
C. Reentry supraventricular tachycardia using an accessory pathway
D. Ectopic atrial tachycardia
E. Junctional ectopic tachycardia

22. Which of the following is most likely a result of maternal treatment with amiodarone during pregnancy?

A. Neonatal hypothyroidism
B. Neonatal jaundice
C. Neonatal pulmonary fibrosis
D. Neonatal cataracts
E. Neonatal renal dysfunction

23. A 4 year old is noted to have a murmur and an ECG is obtained and shown in **Figure 6.11**. Which of the following diagnoses is most likely?

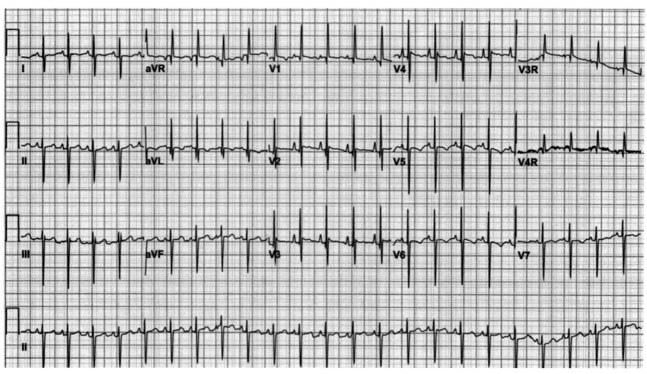

FIGURE 6.11

    A. Primum atrial septal defect
    B. Secundum atrial septal defect
    C. Sinus venosus atrial septal defect
    D. Unroofed coronary sinus
    E. Patent foramen ovale

24. Which of the following drugs is relatively contraindicated in a patient with congenital long QT syndrome?

    A. Lidocaine
    B. Amoxicillin with clavulanate
    C. Verapamil
    D. Erythromycin
    E. Metoprolol

25. On a routine physical examination, a 1-month-old infant has a heart rate of 240 bpm. There is no murmur and the heart size is normal. There is no tachypnea, and blood pressure and perfusion are normal. ECG documents tachycardia with a normal QRS duration and an unvarying RR interval. Ice is applied to the infant's face without change in the cardiac rhythm. The next most appropriate step in management would be:

    A. IV amiodarone
    B. IV verapamil
    C. IV adenosine
    D. IV propranolol
    E. IV digoxin

26. A 3-hour-old infant weighing 4 kg is noted to be in atrial flutter. The blood pressure is 75/40 mm Hg and perfusion to the extremities is good. A synchronized direct current cardioversion is attempted with 4 J. The patient remains in atrial flutter following delivery of energy. Which of the following is the next most appropriate treatment for this patient?

    A. Attempt unsynchronized cardioversion with 4 J
    B. Attempt synchronized cardioversion with 8 J
    C. Wait 1 hour, then repeat cardioversion with 4 J
    D. IV adenosine
    E. IV amiodarone

27. Which of the following ECG findings constitutes a class I indication for cardiac pacemaker implantation in a 1-day-old male infant with complete AV block, no structural heart disease, and normal cardiac function?

    A. Ventricular rate of 60 bpm and QRS duration of 60 ms
    B. Atrial rate of 70 bpm and ventricular rate of 70 bpm
    C. Atrial rate of 140 bpm and ventricular rate of 80 bpm
    D. Ventricular rate of 70 bpm and rare uniform premature ventricular contractions (PVCs)
    E. Ventricular rate of 75 bpm and a QRS duration of 130 ms

28. A 14-year-old previously healthy girl collapses while playing soccer. Following successful cardiopulmonary resuscitation, the ECG in **Figure 6.12** was obtained. Which of the following is the most likely test to define her diagnosis?

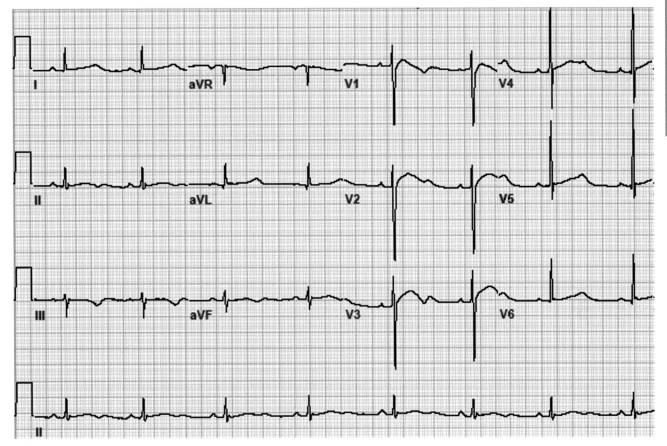

FIGURE 6.12

    A. Cardiac MRI
    B. Measurement of AH and HV intervals on intracardiac electrophysiology study
    C. Echocardiogram
    D. Genetic testing for KCNQ1 mutation
    E. Procainamide challenge

29. In order for reentry to occur in cardiac muscle and to result in dysrhythmia, which of the following must also be present?

    A. An area of conduction delay
    B. Delayed repolarization
    C. Entrainment
    D. Triggered activity
    E. Increased automaticity

30. A 16-year-old girl underwent closure of a VSD at 8 months of age. She did well until the present examination when a slow irregular heart rate was noted. The patient has had no symptoms. An ECG shows Mobitz type II block and a heart rate of 70 bpm. Which of the following is the most appropriate management for this patient's condition?

    A. Theophylline therapy
    B. Amiodarone therapy
    C. Digoxin therapy
    D. Permanent pacemaker placement
    E. Observation

31. A 13-year-old boy currently postoperative day #1 from atrial septal defect repair goes into an arrhythmia (**Figure 6.13**). His blood pressure is 90/56 mm Hg. Which of the following will most likely terminate this arrhythmia?

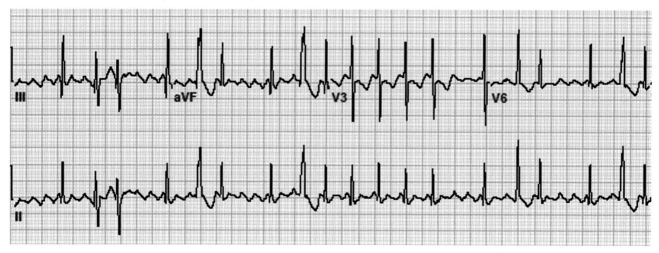

FIGURE 6.13

    A. IV adenosine
    B. IV labetalol
    C. Rapid atrial pacing through atrial pacing wires
    D. Oral propranolol
    E. Correction of hypokalemia

32. Cardiovascular manifestations of hyperthyroidism include which of the following?

    A. Heart block
    B. Atrial fibrillation
    C. Narrow pulse pressures
    D. Decreased ejection fraction
    E. Low voltage on ECG

33. In pediatric patients, sick sinus syndrome is most likely to be associated with which of the following?

    A. Surgery for congenital heart disease
    B. Lyme disease
    C. Maternal systemic lupus erythematosus (SLE)
    D. Cardiomyopathy
    E. Myocarditis

34. A 12-year-old patient presents for follow-up several years after a sinus venosus atrial septal defect (SVASD) that was repaired surgically. The patient has signs and symptoms of intermittent dizziness. An ECG during symptoms will most likely show:

    A. Complete AV block
    B. Sinus bradycardia
    C. Ventricular tachycardia
    D. Junctional tachycardia
    E. Mobitz type II second-degree AV block

35. A 7 year old has a pacemaker implanted for complete heart block following his surgery. A dual-chamber pacemaker is implanted with the lower rate set at 60. On examination, you note the patient's heart rate to be 85 bpm and regular. What is the most likely mode of this pacemaker at this time?

    A. AAI
    B. VVI
    C. DDI
    D. DDD
    E. DOO

36. Which of the following is the most likely side effect of β-blocker therapy in children?

    A. Hypothyroidism
    B. Behavioral changes
    C. Rash
    D. Headache
    E. Weight loss

37. An 8-month-old patient has the ECG shown in **Figure 6.14**. Which of the following is the most likely metabolic disorder?

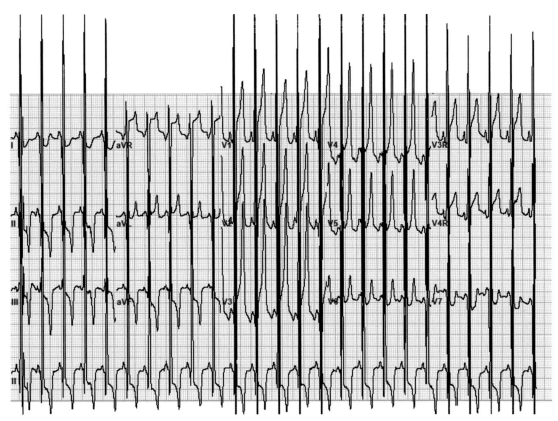

FIGURE 6.14

A. Hunter
B. Hurler
C. Pompe disease
D. Phenylketonuria
E. Maple syrup urine disease

38. A 12-year-old patient has congenitally corrected transposition of the great arteries (ccTGA) but has not undergone any surgical intervention. This patient is at most risk for which of the following?

A. Sinus node dysfunction
B. Complete AV block
C. Junctional ectopic tachycardia
D. Atrial flutter
E. Torsades de pointes (TdP)

39. During an electrophysiology study, an atrial extrastimulus protocol is performed where a train of 8 paced beats in the atrium at 600 ms (S_1) is followed by a premature beat (S_2) at sequentially decreasing intervals. The AH interval is measured after each prematurely paced (S_2) beat. This sequence in **Figure 6.15** demonstrates:

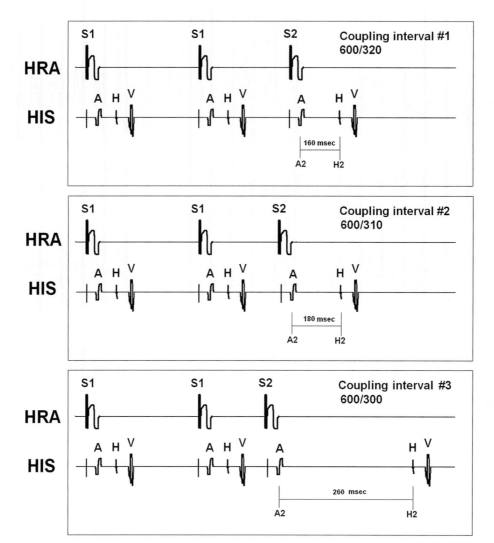

FIGURE 6.15

A. AV node effective refractory period (ERP)
B. A jump in the AH interval indicating dual AV nodal physiology
C. Atrial muscle effective refractory period
D. Wenckebach
E. AV node conduction disease

40. In **Figure 6.16**, a single ventricular extrastimulus protocol is being performed as described in Question 39. The drive train (S_1) and premature ventricular beat (S_2) are labeled. This tracing shows:

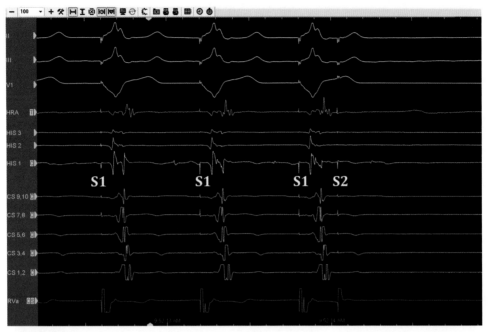

FIGURE 6.16

A. VA Wenckebach

B. Failure of ventricular output

C. Retrograde effective refractory period (ERP) of an accessory pathway

D. Ventricular muscle ERP

E. Retrograde ERP of AV node

41. The ECG in **Figure 6.17** was obtained from a patient with a permanent pacemaker. Based on the ECG, the pacemaker is working in what mode?

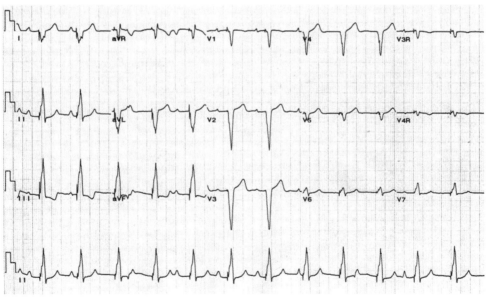

FIGURE 6.17

A. AAI

B. DDD

C. VVI

D. DOO

E. VDD

42. A 12-year-old boy has had a documented heart rate of 250 bpm. He is brought to the EP lab where a tachycardia is induced with cardiac stimulation. The catheters are in the following positions: RVa, right ventricular apex; CS, proximal coronary sinus (CS) with CS 9–10 in the right atrium outside the mouth of the CS; His, bundle of His. The intracardiac tracings in **Figure 6.18** are recorded. These are most consistent with which of the following?

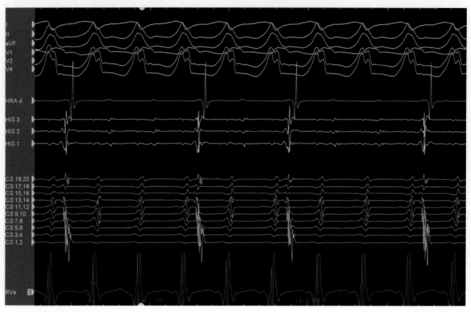

FIGURE 6.18

A. Ventricular tachycardia
B. AV reentry tachycardia using an accessory pathway
C. AV nodal reentry tachycardia

D. Ectopic atrial tachycardia
E. Complete AV block

43. A 3-day-old baby presents with saturations of 76% on 100% oxygen. An ECG is obtained and shown in **Figure 6.19**. The ECG is most suggestive of:

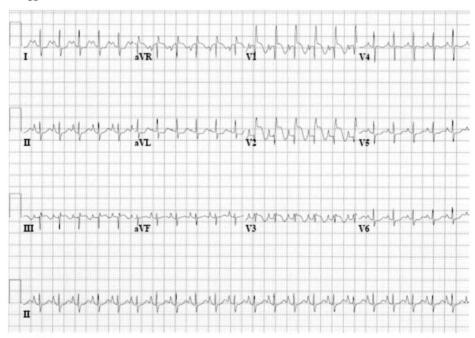

FIGURE 6.19

A. Tetralogy of Fallot
B. Pulmonary atresia with intact ventricular septum
C. Truncus arteriosus

D. Total anomalous pulmonary venous return
E. Large patent ductus arteriosus

44. A 12-lead ECG is obtained on a patient with a permanent pacemaker (**Figure 6.20**). The lower rate limit is set at 60, but no information is available on the pacemaker. You conclude that the pacemaker is most likely programmed in which of the following modes?

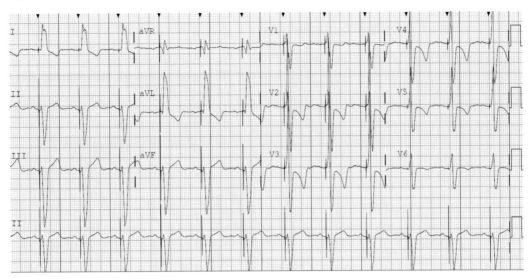

FIGURE 6.20

A. DDD
B. VVI
C. AAI

D. VOO
E. DOO

45. A 3-year-old boy is noted to be bradycardic in the immediate postoperative period after a VSD repair. He is otherwise stable, and his blood pressure is within the normal range. The ECG in **Figure 6.21** is obtained. You would advise which of the following?

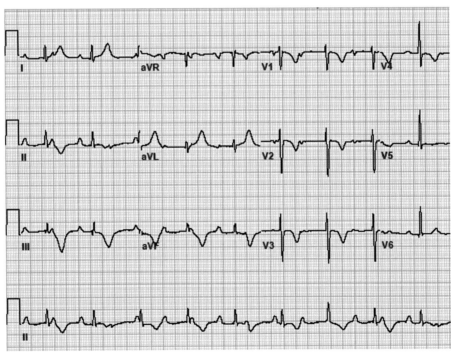

FIGURE 6.21

A. Start epinephrine
B. Start isoproterenol
C. Implant a permanent epicardial pacemaker

D. Use the temporary epicardial pacemaker and observe for at least 7 days
E. Discharge home with follow-up in 2 weeks

46. Which of the following is an indication for placement of a permanent pacemaker in an asymptomatic patient with a structurally normal heart?

A. PR interval of 300 ms
B. Progressive prolongation of the PR interval followed by a dropped beat
C. No change in the PR interval followed by a dropped beat
D. Sinus rate of 30 bpm
E. Left bundle branch block with a QRS duration of 200 ms

47. A 12-year-old boy has a cardiac arrest while riding his bicycle. He is appropriately resuscitated and brought to the intensive care unit. You notice the rhythm in **Figure 6.22** when he becomes very upset and agitated. His diagnosis is most consistent with which of the following?

A. Long QT syndrome
B. Catecholaminergic polymorphic ventricular tachy-cardia (CPVT)
C. Arrhythmogenic right ventricular dysplasia
D. Brugada syndrome
E. Hypertrophic cardiomyopathy

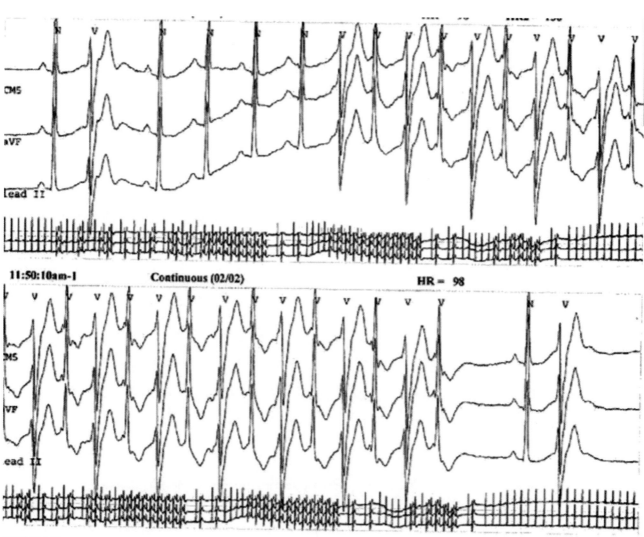

FIGURE 6.22

48. A 4-year-old child with Down syndrome had repair of a VSD at 6 months of age and subsequently developed complete heart block. A permanent epicardial pacemaker was implanted. He now presents with irritability and decreased oral intake for 1 day. You obtain the ECG in **Figure 6.23**. This ECG is most consistent with which of the following?

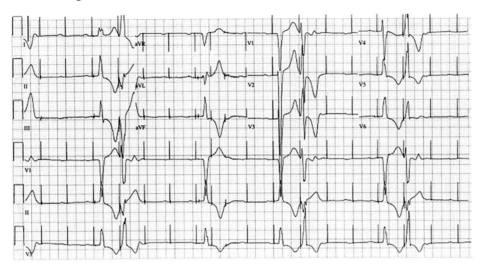

FIGURE 6.23

- **A.** Oversensing
- **B.** Magnet placement over the pacemaker
- **C.** Pacemaker at elective replacement indicator (ERI)
- **D.** Pacemaker self-test
- **E.** Intermittent capture of ventricular lead

49. A 16-year-old patient is being started on amiodarone. The family asks you about potential side effects with this medicine. You would advise them that potential adverse effects of amiodarone include all of the following *EXCEPT*:

- **A.** Photosensitivity
- **B.** Thyroid dysfunction
- **C.** Peripheral neuropathy
- **D.** Corneal microdeposits
- **E.** Renal dysfunction

50. A 6-month-old child has SVT at a rate of 240 bpm and a grade 3/6 pansystolic murmur best heard at the right lower sternal border. She has had no previous cardiac operations. The resting ECG is shown in **Figure 6.24**. What is the most likely underlying heart disease?

- **A.** Ventricular septal defect
- **B.** Ebstein anomaly
- **C.** Pulmonary stenosis
- **D.** Corrected transposition of the great arteries
- **E.** Dilated cardiomyopathy

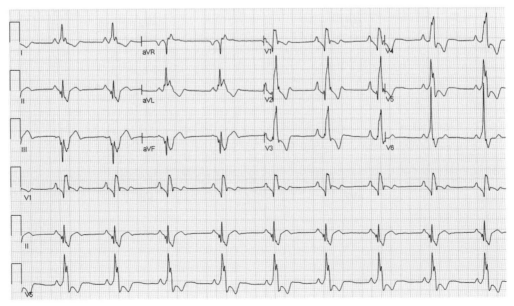

FIGURE 6.24

51. A 16-year-old girl presents with dizziness with postural changes, but no syncope. On Holter monitoring, you document a 3.5-second pause during a documented episode of dizziness. The rest of her evaluation including echocardiography and baseline ECG is normal. What do you do next?

    A. Electrophysiology study
    B. Tilt table testing
    C. Liberalize fluid intake in addition to regular exercise
    D. Recommend pacemaker implantation
    E. Recommend ICD implantation

52. A 4-year-old child presents with digoxin toxicity, 2:1 heart block, and periods of complete heart block. You would consider all the following management options in this patient *EXCEPT*:

    A. Administration of oxygen
    B. Place a temporary transvenous pacemaker
    C. Digoxin immune Fab
    D. Lidocaine for ventricular arrhythmias
    E. Induce hypokalemia

53. A 14-year-old boy en route to the hospital by ambulance following his collapse in the street has the rhythm in **Figure 6.25**. In addition to defibrillation, what would you consider?

    A. Digoxin IV
    B. Atropine IV
    C. Magnesium sulfate IV
    D. Potassium IV
    E. Adenosine IV

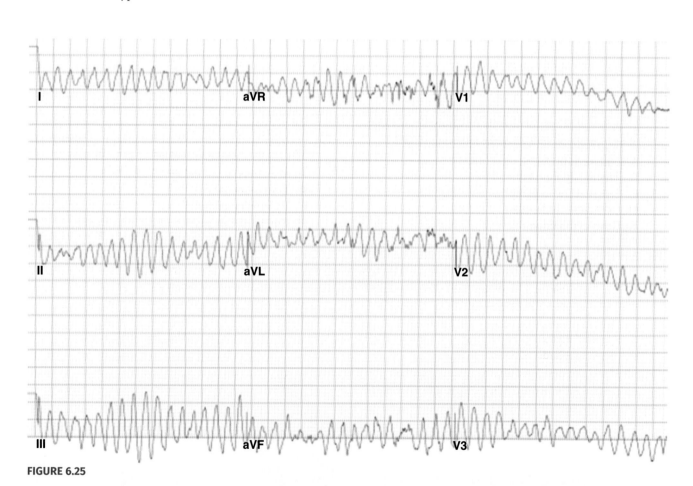

FIGURE 6.25

54. You are called down to the emergency department (ED) to help manage a hemodynamically stable 10 year old with a known history of AV node reentry tachycardia who presented with palpitations and a narrow complex tachycardia at a rate of 240 bpm. His palpitations began 4 hours prior to presenting to the ED. The patient's weight is 30 kg. The ED physician has already attempted, unsuccessfully, to terminate the tachycardia via vagal maneuvers. He gave two separate doses of adenosine (3 and 6 mg, respectively), administered through a 24-gauge IV in the left hand followed by a 5-cc saline flush. The IV appears to be functioning well. There is no change in the tachycardia with the administration of adenosine. The most likely reason that the adenosine was not effective is due to:

   A. The mechanism of tachycardia
   B. The size and position of the IV
   C. The dose of adenosine
   D. The duration of his tachycardia
   E. The rate of the tachycardia

55. What does the "R" in DDDR, VVIR, or AAIR represent?

   A. Automatic reprogram
   B. Biventricular pacing
   C. Reverse polarity
   D. Rate response
   E. Rapid pacing

56. What would be an appropriate indication for programming a pacemaker AAIR?

   A. Third-degree (complete) heart block
   B. Type I second-degree heart block
   C. Type II second-degree heart block
   D. Sinus node dysfunction
   E. Intermittent third-degree heart block

57. A patient's implantable cardioverter-defibrillator (ICD) is programmed at VVI with a lower rate limit of 80 bpm with a ventricular fibrillation zone of 180 bpm. Under what circumstance will the patient receive a shock?

   A. The heart rate drops below 80 bpm
   B. A wide complex rhythm is detected at a rate >80 bpm
   C. Sinus tachycardia occurs at 190 bpm
   D. Ventricular tachycardia occurs at a rate of 160 bpm
   E. Atrial flutter occurs with an atrial rate of 220 bpm with 2:1 AV conduction

58. A 13-year-old patient with a pacemaker for complete heart block and no underlying escape rhythm is undergoing surgery for resection of a mass in the abdomen. The surgeon anticipates use of electrocautery during the procedure. A recommendation is made to place a magnet over the pacemaker during the procedure. Which of the following is the reason for making this recommendation?

   A. Improves sensing during the procedure
   B. Avoids inappropriate pacemaker inhibition due to oversensing from electrocautery during surgery
   C. Makes the pacemaker more rate responsive during surgery
   D. Deflects the electrical energy from entering the pacemaker generator
   E. Prevents overheating of the pacemaker generator

59. A 16-year-old patient has an ICD for hypertrophic cardiomyopathy and cardiac arrest. When asked about the effects of placement of a magnet over an ICD, you would advise that all of the following are correct *EXCEPT*:

   A. Disables all shock therapy
   B. Enables asynchronous pacing in programmed mode
   C. Avoids inappropriate shocks due to oversensing from electrocautery during surgery
   D. Stops appropriate shock delivery due to ventricular tachycardias
   E. The effects are temporary and present only as long as the magnet is placed over the ICD

60. A 15-year-old boy collapses while playing basketball. An AED is placed and he is in ventricular fibrillation and receives an appropriate shock that converts him into normal sinus rhythm. His ECG, EST, echo, cardiac MRI, and neurologic examination are normal. His drug screen is negative as is the rest of his evaluation. Which of the following is the MOST appropriate next step?

   A. Discharge on amiodarone
   B. Discharge on β-blocker therapy
   C. Hemodynamic catheterization
   D. Placement of an implantable loop recorder
   E. ICD implantation

61. A newborn is suspected of having congenital heart disease and an ECG is performed and shown in **Figure 6.26**. The ECG shown is most closely associated with:

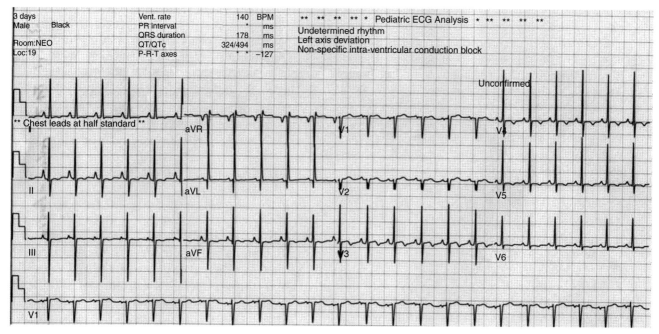

FIGURE 6.26

- **A.** Hypoplastic left heart syndrome
- **B.** Tricuspid atresia
- **C.** Truncus arteriosus
- **D.** Transposition of the great arteries
- **E.** Tetralogy of Fallot

62. A newborn baby presents with complete AV block with a narrow complex junctional escape rhythm. Which of the following is the most likely finding in the mother?

- **A.** Serum potassium of 8
- **B.** Ventricular septal defect
- **C.** Low platelet count
- **D.** 22q11 deletion
- **E.** Anti-Ro (SSA) and anti-La (SSB) antibodies

63. The most likely electrolyte abnormality with the ECG in **Figure 6.27** is:

- **A.** Sodium
- **B.** Potassium
- **C.** Calcium
- **D.** Magnesium
- **E.** Chloride

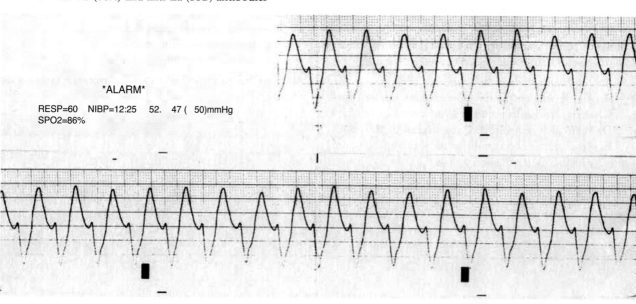

FIGURE 6.27

64. The intracardiac electrogram in **Figure 6.28** shows an HV interval of −9 ms (measured from the His deflection to the earliest ventricular deflection on the ECG). What does this indicate?

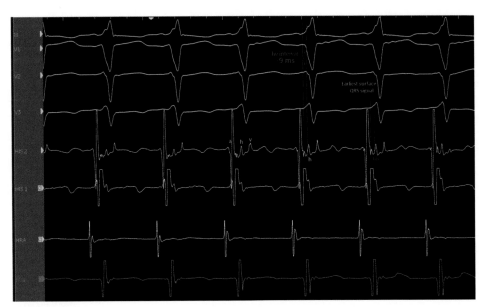

FIGURE 6.28

   A. First-degree AV block
   B. Dual AV node physiology
   C. Infra-Hisian conduction delay
   D. Preexcitation
   E. Bundle branch block

65. The neonate with the ECG in **Figure 6.29** most likely has:

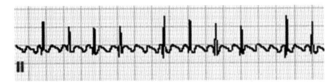

FIGURE 6.29

   A. Complete AV canal
   B. Ventricular septal defect
   C. Electrolyte abnormality
   D. No structural heart disease
   E. Absence of the radius on radiograph

66. The patient with the ECG in **Figure 6.30** is most at risk for which of the following?

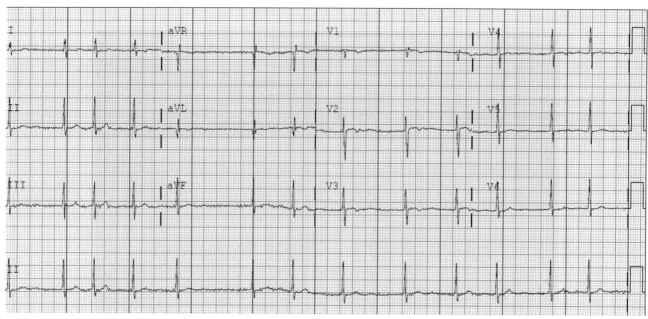

FIGURE 6.30

    A. Stroke
    B. Torsade de pointes
    C. Liver failure
    D. Complete AV block
    E. Pulmonary fibrosis

67. An asymptomatic 14-year-old patient with a normal examination and resting ECG has a 24-hour Holter showing the finding in **Figure 6.31** while sleeping. The rest of the Holter is normal. Which of the following is the next most appropriate step?

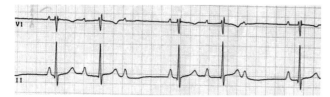

FIGURE 6.31

    A. EP study
    B. Exercise treadmill test
    C. Reassurance and future monitoring
    D. Cardiac MRI
    E. Pacemaker implantation

68. An asymptomatic 10-year-old patient has the ECG shown in **Figure 6.32** during an exercise treadmill test. His resting ECG shows preexcitation. What does this tracing indicate when compared to other asymptomatic children with preexcitation?

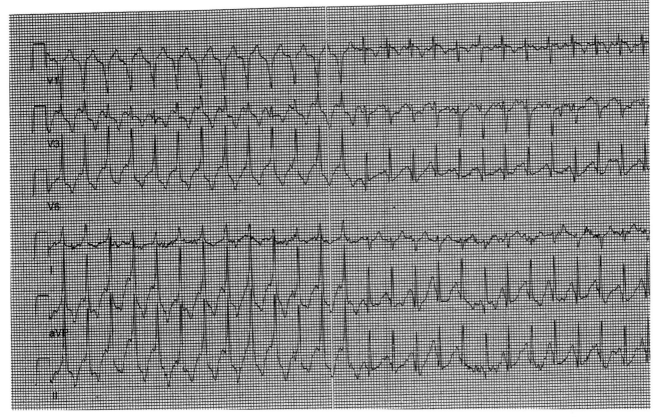

| 172bpm | EXERCISE
STAGE 4
10:06 | BRUCE
4.2 mph
16.0 % | 25mm/s
10mm/mV
20hz |

FIGURE 6.32

A. The patient is at lower risk for sudden death
B. The patient is at higher risk for sudden death
C. The patient is at lower risk for supraventricular tachycardia
D. The patient is at higher risk for supraventricular tachycardia
E. The patient has ventricular tachycardia rather than preexcitation

69. The patient with the tracing in **Figure 6.33** likely has which of the following?

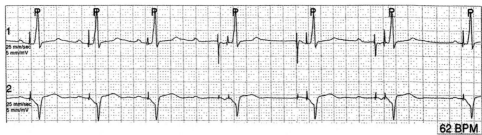

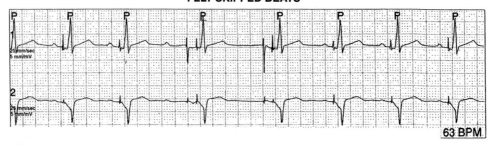

FIGURE 6.33

A. Normally functioning DDD pacemaker
B. Atrial lead dysfunction
C. Ventricular lead dysfunction
D. Atrial and ventricular lead dysfunction
E. Biventricular pacemaker

70. The underlying diagnosis in the patient in **Figure 6.34** is most likely to be which of the following?

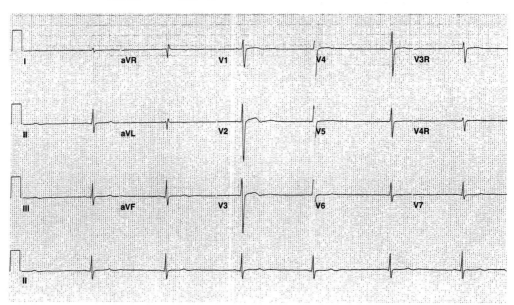

FIGURE 6.34

A. Wolff–Parkinson–White
B. Renal failure
C. Atrial septal defect
D. Thyroid storm
E. Anorexia nervosa

71. The intracardiac tracing in **Figure 6.35** shows which of the following?

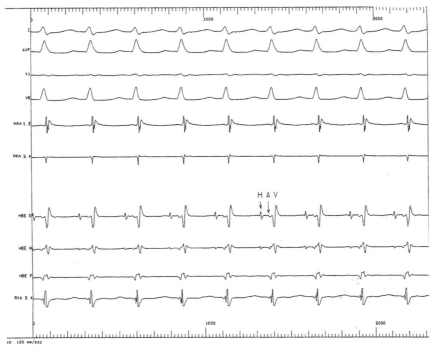

FIGURE 6.35

A. Atrial flutter with 2:1 conduction
B. SVT using an accessory pathway
C. Atypical AV node reentry tachycardia
D. Typical AV node reentry tachycardia
E. Normal sinus rhythm

72. The patient with the ECG in **Figure 6.36** is most at risk for which of the following?

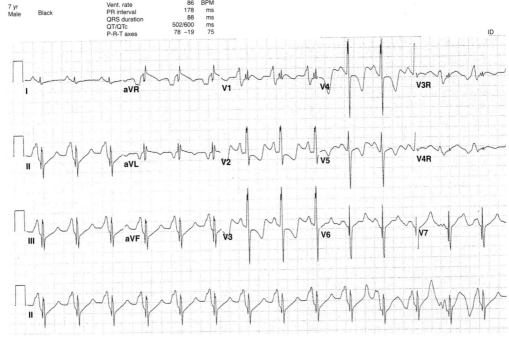

FIGURE 6.36

A. Pulmonary hypertension
B. AV node reentry tachycardia
C. Intracranial tumor
D. Polysplenia
E. Aortic regurgitation

73. The patient with the ECG in **Figure 6.37** most likely will have which of the following?

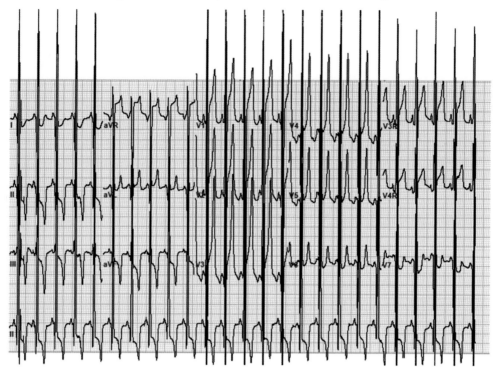

FIGURE 6.37

A. Hypertonia
B. Hepatomegaly
C. Widely spaced nipples

D. Aniridia
E. Hematuria

74. A 16-year-old patient presents with two episodes of syncope with no warning signs and no underlying discernible cause. He has the ECG shown in **Figure 6.38**. What is the next most appropriate step?

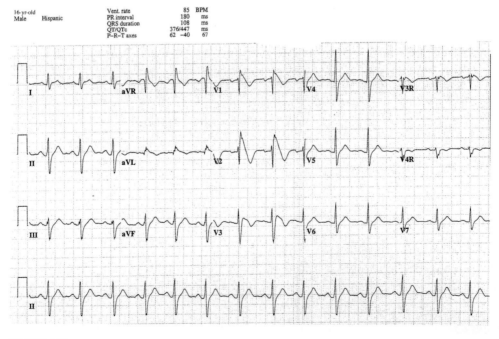

FIGURE 6.38

A. Cardiac catheterization with coronary angiography
B. Initiation of atenolol
C. ICD

D. Initiation of amiodarone
E. Reassurance and discharge from clinic

75. The most likely genetic defect with the ECG in **Figure 6.38** is which of the following?

    A. HERG mutation

    B. KCNQ1 mutation

    C. 22q11.2 deletion

    D. Trisomy 21

    E. SCN5A mutation

76. Which of the following is the drug most likely to bring out this finding on ECG (**Figure 6.38**)?

    A. Epinephrine

    B. Lidocaine

    C. Esmolol

    D. Adenosine

    E. Procainamide

77. The intracardiac tracing in **Figure 6.39**, performed during atrial pacing in the high right atrium (HRA), shows which of the following?

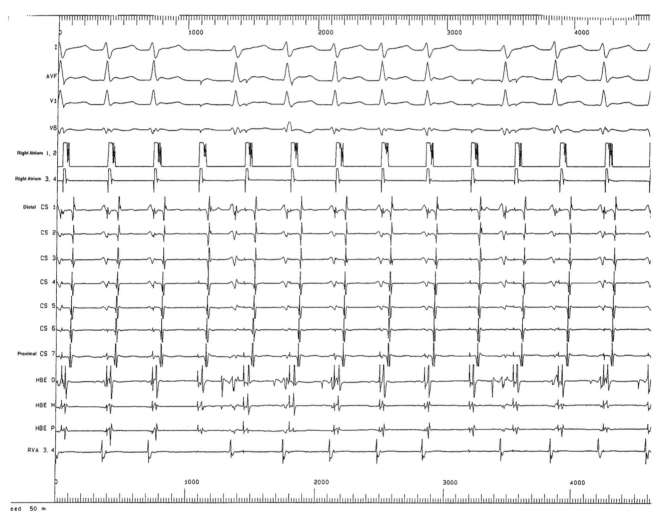

FIGURE 6.39

    A. Wenckebach (Mobitz type I second-degree AV block)

    B. Initiation of supraventricular tachycardia

    C. AH jump (ERP of the fast pathway of the AV node)

    D. Loss of preexcitation

    E. Initiation of atrial fibrillation

78. A 17-year-old boy presents with chest pain and the ECG tracing in **Figure 6.40**. The most likely etiology of the ECG findings is:

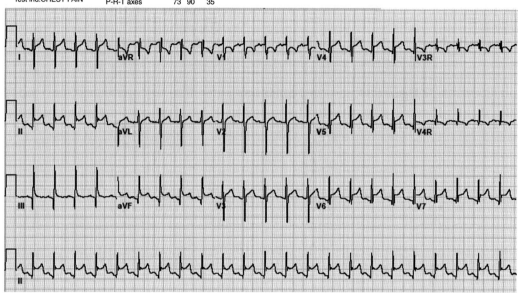

FIGURE 6.40

A. Cocaine

B. Myosin heavy chain mutation

C. Increased intracranial pressure

D. Coxsackievirus

E. Erythromycin

79. A previously asymptomatic patient presents with the ECG shown in **Figure 6.41**. The patient most likely has an underlying diagnosis of which of the following?

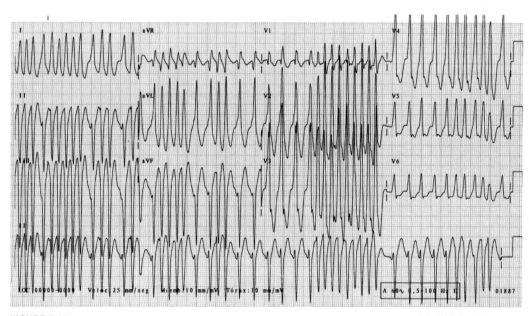

FIGURE 6.41

A. Ebstein anomaly

B. Atrial septal defect

C. LQTS

D. Arrhythmogenic right ventricular dysplasia

E. Truncus arteriosus

80. Which drug is relatively contraindicated with this ECG
    (**Figure 6.41**)?

    A. Amiodarone
    B. Adenosine
    C. Flecainide
    D. Fentanyl
    E. Diphenhydramine

81. A 13-year-old patient presents with fatigue and exercise intolerance with a normal echocardiogram. The presenting ECG is
    shown in **Figure 6.42**. This patient will most likely require which of the following?

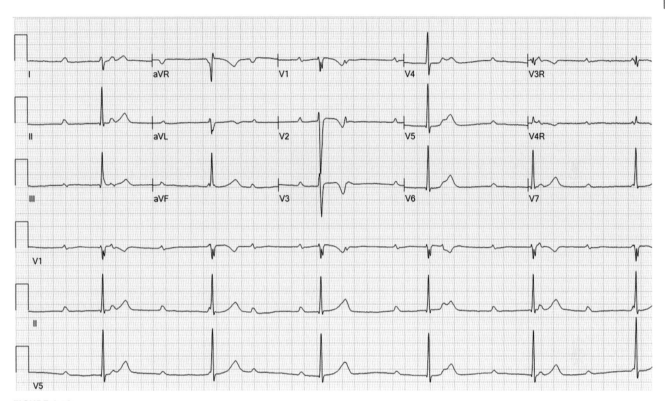

FIGURE 6.42

A. Pacemaker
B. ICD
C. β-Blocker therapy
D. Left stellate ganglionectomy
E. Cardiac transplantation

82. Which of the following is NOT associated with the ECG
    in **Figure 6.42**?

    A. Chagas disease
    B. Congenitally corrected transposition of the great
       arteries
    C. Maternal Ro and La antibodies
    D. Hypertrophic cardiomyopathy
    E. Endocarditis with abscess formation

83. With adenosine, the tachycardia in the ECG (**Figure 6.43**) will likely:

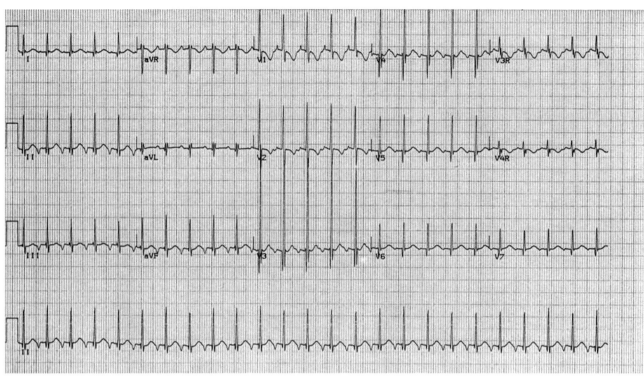

FIGURE 6.43

A. Continue with only P waves in a saw-tooth configuration
B. Terminate followed by several sinus beats, then restart
C. Slow transiently, then speed up
D. Have no changes
E. Widen transiently, then narrow

84. Which of the following is NOT in the differential diagnosis for a long RP tachycardia with a narrow QRS complex?

A. Atypical AV node reentry tachycardia
B. Atrial tachycardia
C. Mahaim fiber tachycardia
D. Permanent junctional reciprocating tachycardia (PJRT)
E. Sinus tachycardia

85. The intracardiac tracing in **Figure 6.44** was obtained in a patient after placement of catheters. The proximal coronary sinus (CS) catheter is placed 2 mm inside the mouth of the CS. The tracing shows which of the following?

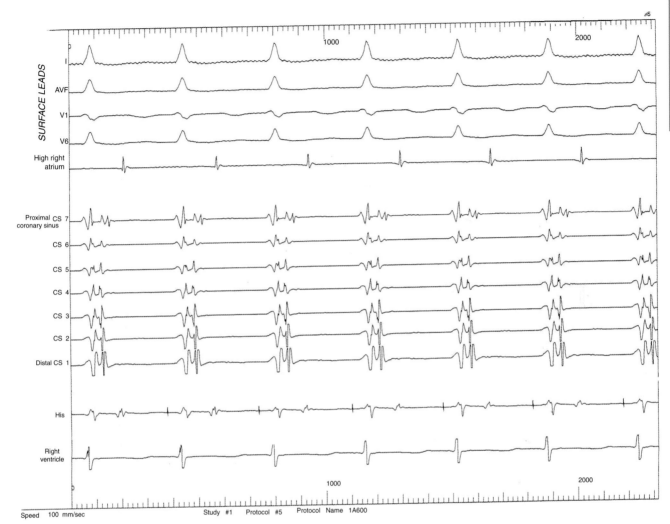

FIGURE 6.44

A. Supraventricular tachycardia due to a right-sided accessory pathway

B. Supraventricular tachycardia due to a left-sided accessory pathway

C. Atypical AV node reentry tachycardia

D. Normal sinus rhythm

E. Wenckebach

86. Which of the following is NOT true in the patient with the ECG in **Figure 6.45**?

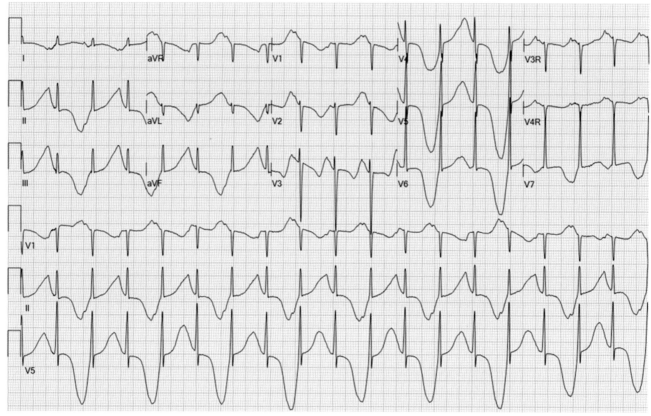

FIGURE 6.45

A. Patient is at risk for sudden death
B. Patient should avoid methadone
C. Family members should be screened for the same condition

D. The underlying problem is likely due to a mutation in a calcium channel
E. The patient is at risk for 2:1 AV block (pseudo 2:1 AV block)

87. An 18-year-old man underwent repair of a sinus venosus atrial septal defect at the age of 12. He developed sinus node dysfunction and underwent implantation of a single-chamber atrial pacemaker set AAIR at a rate of 60. He also has a history of atrial ectopic tachycardia and atrial fibrillation requiring cardioversion. He notices that every day when driving on the bumpy road to his job on a farm, his heart rate steadily increases and he feels uncomfortable. He has an old truck and carries multiple electronic devices in the back seat. The most likely source of his increased heart rate is:

A. The rate-responsive feature of the pacemaker
B. An atrial arrhythmia
C. Electromagnetic interference to the pacemaker
D. Pacemaker oversensing
E. Magnet response of the pacemaker

88. A 5-year-old boy is diagnosed with Brugada syndrome by genetic testing after his father was diagnosed with Brugada syndrome. His initial ECG is normal, but you tell the family that the classic ECG findings in Brugada syndrome will most likely become evident during:

A. Emotional stress
B. Fever
C. Hypertension
D. Dehydration
E. Sleep

89. Which of the following is a class I indication for chronic resynchronization therapy (CRT or biventricular pacing)?

- **A.** Left bundle branch block pattern, ejection fraction 25%, QRS duration 140 ms
- **B.** Left bundle branch block pattern, ejection fraction 40%, QRS duration 200 ms
- **C.** Left bundle branch block pattern, ejection fraction 30%, QRS duration 170 ms
- **D.** Right bundle branch block pattern, ejection fraction 25%, QRS duration 190 ms
- **E.** Right bundle branch block pattern, ejection fraction 30%, QRS duration 180 ms

90. A 4 year old presents for evaluation of a murmur. An echocardiogram reveals a large secundum ASD. The patient's ECG is shown in **Figure 6.46**. Of the following, a mutation in which gene is most likely present in this patient?

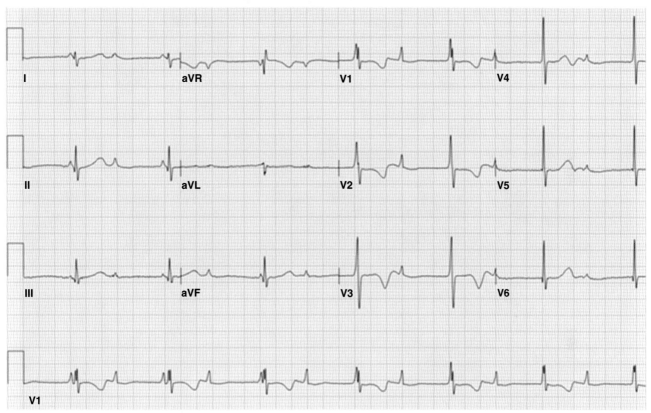

FIGURE 6.46

- **A.** KCNH2
- **B.** PKP2
- **C.** NOTCH1
- **D.** NKX2.5
- **E.** PTPN11

91. A 17-year-old female undergoing a workup for ptosis, ataxia, and mild muscle weakness has an echocardiogram showing normal biventricular size and function. Which of the following is the ECG most likely to show?

- **A.** Complete heart block
- **B.** Prolonged QT interval
- **C.** Epsilon waves
- **D.** ST depression and T-wave inversion in the inferolateral leads
- **E.** Delta wave

92. A 10-year-old female is scheduled for an electrophysiology study to further investigate symptoms of recurrent palpitations. Catheters are positioned in the high right atrium (HRA), overlying the His bundle (HIS), in the coronary sinus (CS 9,10 is proximal and CS 1,2 is distal), and the right ventricular apex (RVa). The ablation catheter is positioned at 12:00 on the tricuspid valve annulus (ABL) when there is a sudden change in the electrograms shown in **Figure 6.47**. What is the most likely cause of this patient's palpitations?

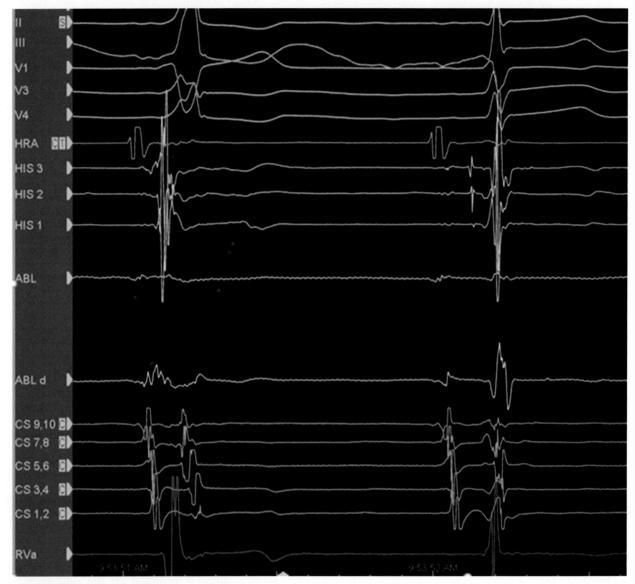

FIGURE 6.47

    A. Ventricular tachycardia
    B. Ectopic atrial tachycardia
    C. AV nodal reentrant tachycardia
    D. Atrial flutter
    E. AV reentrant tachycardia

93. A 14-year-old male has a history of syncope while running laps. There was no prodrome, and the patient sustained several significant skin abrasions. An ECG demonstrates a QTc of 485 ms. Genetic testing is performed and demonstrates a pathologic mutation in KCNQ1. The patient has no other medical problems. Which of the following are appropriate?

    A. Initiation of nadolol
    B. Discussion regarding avoiding QT-prolonging medications and potential exercise restrictions
    C. Implantation of an ICD
    D. A and B
    E. A, B, and C

94. A 7-year-old female (34 kg) with single ventricle physiology and {S,L,L} anatomy who has undergone a Fontan procedure was discovered to have complete AV block with narrow complex escape at 40 bpm during a routine follow-up examination. A Holter monitor demonstrates persistent complete AV block with an average rate of 42 bpm. The patient does not have clear symptomatology and no other medical problems. Which of the following is appropriate?

A. Implantation of a single-chamber (ventricular lead only) transvenous pacemaker system

B. Implantation of a dual-chamber (atrial and ventricular lead) transvenous pacemaker system

C. Implantation of a single-chamber (ventricular lead only) epicardial pacemaker system

D. Implantation of a dual-chamber (atrial and ventricular lead) epicardial pacemaker system

E. Continued monitoring for symptoms with plan to repeat the Holter monitor in 6 months

95. In which of the following patients is implantation of an ICD NOT appropriate?

A. A 15-year-old male with tetralogy of Fallot and syncope as well as sustained, hemodynamically significant VT induced during an electrophysiology study

B. A 14-year-old male with hypertrophic cardiomyopathy that survived a cardiac arrest

C. A 5-month-old infant with incessant VT due to a cardiac fibroma

D. A 12 year old with catecholaminergic polymorphic VT who has a single episode of syncope while on nadolol

E. A 17-year-old male with Brugada syndrome who survived a cardiac arrest that occurred while running

96. Which of the following pacemaker abnormalities is seen in this patient (pacemaker setting is = DDD 60) (**Figure 6.48**)?

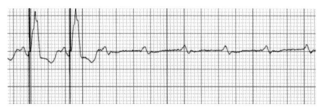

FIGURE 6.48

A. Loss of ventricular sensing
B. Loss of atrial sensing
C. Ventricular oversensing
D. Loss of ventricular capture
E. Normal pacemaker function

97. Which of the following is the most common cause of sudden cardiac death in young athletes?

A. Coronary artery anomalies
B. Dilated cardiomyopathy
C. Commotio cordis
D. Catecholaminergic polymorphic ventricular tachycardia (CPVT)
E. Hypertrophic cardiomyopathy (HCM)

98. All of the following are important components of the initial outpatient workup for syncope *EXCEPT*:

A. Electrocardiogram
B. Echocardiogram
C. History
D. Physical examination
E. Family history

Answers

1. (D) Fetal arrhythmias occur in 1% to 2% of pregnancies and account for 10% to 20% of referrals to pediatric cardiologists. Of these arrhythmias, 80% to 90% are premature atrial contractions with only around 10% of the arrhythmias being sustained. SVT may limit diastolic filling time and result in hydrops or decreased ventricular function. Treatment is recommended for sustained arrhythmia (typically >50% SVT burden) or evidence of hydrops. Digoxin is usually first-line agent if no hydrops is present, with case series reports of 60% to 80% positive responders. It takes a relatively high digoxin level (typically around 2) to achieve adequate fetal transfer (0.6 fetal transfer rate). The fetal transfer rate decreases by around 50% in the presence of hydrops. Other agents used in the treatment of atrial flutter include flecainide, sotalol, and amiodarone. Both flecainide and sotalol have an excellent fetal transfer (0.8 to 1). These medications are used when SVT is refractory to digoxin or in the presence of hydrops. Amiodarone can also be used and may have a role in very hydropic infants, but the maternal transfer is poor (0.1 to 0.3). In the patient described, continued observation is not the best option as the fetus will likely develop hydrops (usually within 48 hours) if the tachycardia is sustained. At 32-week gestation on no therapy, immediate delivery is not indicated. Atenolol is very poorly transported across the placenta and is not typically used in the treatment of fetal SVT. Adenosine has a half-life of 3 to 5 seconds and would be metabolized prior to reaching the fetus. Administration of adenosine to the fetus via direct injection in the umbilical vein has been reported, but carries some risk to the fetus performing the injection and would only be used in extreme cases if medical management fails.

2. (A) Premature atrial contractions (PACs) are a benign finding and are present in many otherwise healthy adolescents.

Although a very small percentage may have an atrial tachycardia, the finding of isolated premature atrial contractions does not require any restriction for athletic participation in a patient who is asymptomatic. In general, minimal workup is required for asymptomatic PACs and an echo is not typically required if the examination is normal. No treatment is required and the patient may participate in competitive sports without restrictions.

3. (B) The ECG shows a prolonged corrected QT interval (around 520 ms) consistent with a diagnosis of long QT syndrome (LQTS). β-Blockers are the first-line therapy for LQTS. β-Blockers have been shown to decrease the incidence of sudden cardiac death and syncope in LQTS, particularly in long QT syndrome type 1. Risk factors for sudden cardiac death in LQTS are length of the QT interval (with QT intervals over 500 being the highest risk) and previous episodes of syncope. A prophylactic ICD is not indicated in most cases of LQTS. In this 3 year old, placement of an ICD would be technically challenging and would have a high incidence of long-term complications. Given the lack of symptoms, a β-blocker would be a better first line of therapy. There is no indication for a routine electrophysiology study in LQTS as the diagnosis can be made based on the ECG. Amiodarone would be relatively contraindicated in LQTS as it prolongs the QT interval. A cardioversion is not indicated as the patient is in sinus rhythm.

4. (D) The rhythm strip (**Figure 6.49**) shows artifact mimicking a wide complex tachycardia. Any motion of the ECG leads during recording may create an artifact that may initially appear to be supraventricular or ventricular tachycardia. However, in this tracing, the narrow QRS complexes can be marched through the tracing (shown by the *red arrows*) and show an underlying sinus rhythm. The *red star* shows two very closely spaced deflections as the artifact fuses with the true QRS. It would not be physiologically possible to have two QRS complexes that are so closely coupled together as the ventricular myocardium needs time to repolarize prior to contracting again. With all of the evidence showing artifact, no therapy is necessary.

5. (B) A number of risk markers are used to assess the risk for sudden death in patients with hypertrophic cardiomyopathy, but these have changed over time and risk factors in children and adults are not always the same. Septal hypertrophy is a generally agreed-on risk factor for dangerous events (especially septal thickness >30 mm). While a family history of premature sudden death has been suggested as a risk factor, in a recent study in children, family history had no association with sudden cardiac death. Other risk factors include nonsustained ventricular tachycardia, unexplained

(not neurally mediated) syncope, and a blood pressure decrease or inadequate increase during exercise testing. Late gadolinium enhancement on an MRI scan of the heart may also carry an increased risk of sudden death. The magnitude of left ventricular hypertrophy on ECG does not help in risk stratification.

6. (A) Amiodarone increases warfarin effect, digoxin and phenytoin levels, and class I antiarrhythmic toxicity. Digoxin is excreted primarily by the kidneys. Digoxin dose should be reduced when given in conjunction with amiodarone. There is no significant interaction between ACE inhibitors or furosemide with amiodarone.

7. (C) This patient is at risk for having episodes of supraventricular tachycardia. The ECG tracing shows intermittent preexcitation (short PR interval and delta wave). In patients with Wolff–Parkinson–White (WPW) syndrome, the preexcitation can often be intermittent and picked up when monitoring for longer periods such as on a Holter monitor. Patients with WPW are at risk for having episodes of supraventricular tachycardia. Although it is possible that these are premature ventricular contractions, the PR interval is exactly the same on all of the beats with the wider QRS complex, making preexcitation much more likely. There is no evidence of an atrial arrhythmia.

8. (B) The ECG shows complete AV block. In combination with the classic rash with central clearing (erythema migrans with a bull's eye rash), this patient likely has Lyme disease caused by the spirochete *Borrelia burgdorferi*. The infection is transmitted to humans by tick bites. In patients with Lyme disease, the incidence of cardiac involvement has been estimated to be 8% and usually occurs within a few weeks of the onset of the illness. The most common feature of Lyme carditis is atrioventricular (AV) block. The AV block usually resolves gradually with normalization of the PR interval in 1 to 2 weeks. Persistence of AV block requiring a pacemaker is unusual. Prompt treatment with antibiotics is the treatment of choice, but temporary pacing may be necessary if the heart rate is very slow. Treatment is usually with doxycycline, but cephalosporins and amoxicillin can also be used. Gentamicin and vancomycin are not typically used. IVIG is used for Kawasaki disease, which typically does not present with AV block. Myocarditis can also present with AV block, but the clinical picture is more consistent with Lyme disease.

9. (C) Neurocardiogenic syncope is very common in the teenage years. These patients may have a myoclonic jerk resembling a seizure or may actually have a seizure when syncopal. In the presence of a single episode and clear

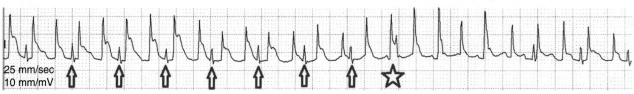

25 mm/sec
10 mm/mV

FIGURE 6.49

history suggesting neurocardiogenic syncope, no further workup may be necessary. Recommending liberalization of fluid intake may be adequate. A neurology referral is not necessary if history is strongly suggestive of neurocardiogenic syncope. Myoclonic jerks are occasionally seen with syncope and may be mistaken for seizures. The lack of a postictal phase goes against (but does not exclude) seizures. A 24-hour ambulatory monitor is unlikely to capture sporadic episodes. An implantable loop recorder is effective at ruling out arrhythmias in patients with syncope, but is typically used in patients with multiple episodes of syncope with no discernable cause and is not indicated for a single episode of syncope classic for neurocardiogenic syncope.

10. (D) The ECG shows left ventricular hypertrophy and T-wave inversion. T-wave inversion on an ECG may be a marker for abnormal ventricular myocardium. The ECG is most consistent with hypertrophic cardiomyopathy. T-wave inversion in the left precordial leads (V5 and V6) is almost always an abnormal finding. In addition, the T waves are inverted in leads I and aVL, which is also an abnormal finding. The forces are suggestive of increased left ventricular hypertrophy (notice that the ECG is half standard in the precordial leads). A complete workup including an echocardiogram to evaluate the coronary arteries is necessary before clearing the patient for sports.

11. (A) The Kearns–Sayre syndrome (characterized by its onset before the age of 20 years, chronic ophthalmoplegia, pigmentary retinal degeneration, and at least one of the following symptoms: ataxia, heart block, and high protein content in the cerebrospinal fluid) is a severe variant of chronic progressive external ophthalmoplegia with frequent rearrangements of the mitochondrial DNA (mtDNA). Patients typically present with a bundle branch block and prolonged QT interval that progress to complete heart block. Prophylactic pacemaker therapy is advisable in patients suffering from the Kearns–Sayre syndrome, who have bifascicular block on the precordial ECG as they may rapidly progress to complete AV block. Steroids or an electrophysiology study is of no benefit, and the risk for progression of conduction disease makes watchful waiting less advisable.

12. (B) The ECG demonstrates long QT syndrome (LQTS) with 2:1 AV block (more appropriately termed pseudo 2:1 AV block as the AV node has normal function). Note the prominent P waves in leads V1 and V2 that fall in the middle of the T wave and are not conducted. Because of the bradycardia and severity of the phenotype, long QT syndrome with 2:1 AVB has a poor prognosis with up to 50% mortality rate in infancy. Mutations of cardiac ion channel genes cause LQTS, manifesting as increased risk of ventricular tachycardia and sudden death. The prognosis is generally poor, but recent data has suggested more optimistic outcomes. β-Blocker therapy alone can have side effects including enhancing the AV block. Hence, β-blocker therapy along with pacemaker implantation is recommended, although a β-blocker may be added to decrease the chance of ventricular arrhythmias. There is no indication for isoproterenol in a stable patient with a reasonable underlying rate. Amiodarone may lengthen the QT interval and is relatively contraindicated in LQTS.

13. (B) The course of the AV node and His–Purkinje system in endocardial cushion defects passes through the central fibrous body beneath the crest of the VSD. It is therefore displaced posteriorly and inferiorly. In the frontal plane, the initial QRS vector forces are usually directed inferiorly to the right, and the QRS loop moves counterclockwise, superiorly and to the left resulting in left axis deviation. The mean QRS axis in the frontal plane ranges between −30 degrees and −180 degrees, with most axes directed between −30 degrees and −120 degrees.

14. (A) Negative predictors of long-term survival after tetralogy of Fallot repair include older age at operation, significant residual hemodynamic abnormalities after surgery, use of an outflow tract patch, a QRS duration >180 ms, elevated left ventricular end-diastolic pressure, and poor left ventricular function. The presence of premature ventricular contractions does not increase the risk of sudden death. Atrial tachycardia is found in 20% to 30% of patients in long-term follow-up and may predispose to sudden death. However, there is no correlation between sinus bradycardia and sudden death. Right bundle branch block and left anterior hemiblock (bifascicular block) were initially thought to be risk factors for long-term development of complete AV block, but this has not been proven to be true.

15. (A) The ECG shows a prolonged PR interval of around 400 ms. ECG evidence of PR interval prolongation is a minor Jones criteria for acute rheumatic fever. To make a diagnosis of acute rheumatic fever, you need two major or one major and two minor criteria. The clinical manifestations of acute rheumatic fever follow the inciting group A streptococcal infection after a period of latency of about 3 weeks. Rheumatic fever is a multisystem disease affecting primarily the heart, the joints, the brain, and the cutaneous and subcutaneous tissues. Carditis associated with acute rheumatic fever is seen in about 50% of the patients. Tachycardia is one of the early signs of myocarditis. Complete heart block is not usually seen in rheumatic carditis. Choreiform movements are rapid jerking movements of the hands, face, and feet and are characteristics of rheumatic fever. Kawasaki disease resulting in coronary artery aneurysms, Marfan syndrome resulting in a dilated ascending aorta, and juvenile rheumatoid arthritis do not typically give a prolonged PR interval. Systemic lupus erythematosus and scleroderma may also be associated with a prolonged PR interval. Glomerulonephritis is not associated with acute rheumatic fever and does not affect the PR interval. A bifid uvula is associated with Loeys–Dietz syndrome, which does not result in PR prolongation.

16. (E) Premature atrial beats are common in the fetus and the neonate and do not warrant any therapy. Blocked premature atrial contractions (PACs) may result in temporary decreases in the heart rate, but these are not concerning in the fetus with good ventricular function and no hydrops. Early delivery is not indicated. The incidence of premature beats detected in utero is approximately 2%, with less than 10% of these arrhythmias persisting in the newborn. In the fetus, PACs account for 80% to 90% of premature beats. In the newborn, premature ventricular contractions are recognized in approximately 30% of infants with extrasystoles.

17. (E) The ECG demonstrates findings consistent with Wolff–Parkinson–White (WPW) syndrome. Propranolol is frequently the first-line therapy for SVT in patients with WPW. Digoxin and verapamil are relatively contraindicated in the presence of WPW as it may increase the risk for ventricular fibrillation. Flecainide is a second-line agent if the patient is not responsive to β-blockers. Mexiletine is a class IB antiarrhythmic not indicated for SVT. Amiodarone has a very long half-life and takes several days to build up a therapeutic level orally. Therefore, a "pill in pocket" strategy of taking medications only after SVT starts will likely not be effective.

18. (C) A change in T-wave polarity from positive to negative in the right precordial leads describes the normal maturation of change in the ECG during the first week of life. The positive T wave in lead V1 in the first days of life most likely results from the early appearance of repolarization in the left ventricle and the late termination of depolarization in the right ventricle. An overall left ventricle to right ventricle sequence results, and this accounts for the upright T wave in lead V1 in the normal term infant. The axis will shift to the left, but not to less than 55 degrees. There are decreased right ventricular forces, so the R wave will typically get smaller in lead V1. The PR interval remains the same, although it will lengthen with age.

19. (A) Permanent junctional reciprocating tachycardia (PJRT) is an accessory pathway-mediated tachycardia due to a slowly conducting accessory pathway typically located in the right posterior septum. The position of the pathway creates P waves with a purely negative polarity in leads II, III, and aVF with a P-wave axis of −90 degrees. Because the accessory pathway conducts slowly, P waves are usually easily visible on the ECG. Because it is an accessory pathway-mediated tachycardia, there is a 1:1 relationship of the ventricles to the atria. PJRT tends to be an incessant form of tachycardia and may cause a cardiomyopathy. PJRT rates tend to be slower (150 to 200 bpm) than other accessory pathway-mediated tachycardias, which makes them more difficult to detect clinically.

20. (C) At K of 5.5 to 6.5 mEq/L, the T waves become tall and peaked. At serum K level above 6.6 mEq/L, QRS widening along with ST-segment elevation is noted. Above 8.5 mEq/L the P waves disappear. At ~9 mEq/L, arrhythmias begin: AV block, ventricular tachycardia, and ventricular fibrillation. Q waves are indicative of infarction and are not typically seen with elevated potassium.

21. (E) Junctional ectopic tachycardia is the most common arrhythmia in the acute postoperative period following congenital heart surgery. It is a focal tachycardia with gradual warm-up and cool-down and rate variability. The P waves may be visible in the terminal portion of or shortly after the QRS complex or be completely dissociated. The rate may be constant or fluctuate with increases and decreases in the catecholamine state. The ECG shown demonstrates VA dissociation with the ventricular rate being faster than the atrial rate. As the ventricular rate is faster than the atrial rate, this excludes atrial flutter and ectopic atrial tachycardia as the cause. In a reentrant SVT using an accessory pathway, there should be a 1:1 relationship between the atria and ventricles. Although VA dissociation can be seen in ventricular tachycardia, the QRS complex is narrow, essentially excluding ventricular tachycardia as a cause.

22. (A) Neonatal thyroid abnormalities (hyper- or hypothyroidism) are the most common sequelae of maternal treatment with amiodarone. There is no significant impact to the neonatal liver, lungs, eyes, or kidneys.

23. (A) The ECG shown demonstrates left axis deviation (axis of −80 degrees). This is seen in patients with a primum atrial septal defect (ASD). The ECG also demonstrates right ventricular hypertrophy (qR in lead V1). Other types of ASDs (secundum, sinus venosus, and unroofed coronary sinus) typically show a normal to rightward axis, and older patients will frequently have an rSR' (or qR) pattern in lead V1. A PFO is seen in 20% to 30% of the normal population and does not result in any changes on the ECG.

24. (D) Erythromycin is associated with prolongation of the QT interval. In patients with baseline-prolonged QT intervals, care should be taken to avoid administration of any medications that have been implicated in drug-induced torsades de pointes, including QT-prolonging antiarrhythmic drugs, tricyclic antidepressants, erythromycin, ondansetron, and chloral hydrate. The other drugs shown do not have a significant effect on the QT interval.

25. (C) Adenosine has a half-life of 2 to 10 seconds and is an excellent drug for acute termination of reentry SVT or diagnosis of atrial arrhythmias such as atrial flutter. DC cardioversion would be indicated in a hemodynamically unstable patient. Verapamil is relatively contraindicated in infants less than 1 year of age. Propranolol is used for long-term prevention of SVT and would not be a first-line IV treatment before adenosine is attempted. Amiodarone may be used when other first-line agents have failed or if the patient is unstable and there is around a 30% chance of significant hypotension with rapid IV administration. IV digoxin may be proarrhythmic and is not generally given as a first-line agent.

26. (B) DC cardioversion is at times used as a first-line therapy for neonatal atrial flutter (rapid atrial pacing using an esophageal catheter is preferred as first-line therapy by many). The recommended energy is 0.5 to 1 J/kg. However, frequently in neonates, a higher dose is required as the energy is not delivered as efficiently through small neonatal pads or patches. If energy delivery of 1 J/kg is unsuccessful, the energy should be increased and cardioversion reattempted. In a stable rhythm with a pulse, synchronized cardioversion is indicated, as unsynchronized cardioversion may result in a shock on a T wave inducing ventricular fibrillation. There is no indication to wait and repeat cardioversion as another 4 J shock is not likely to be successful. IV adenosine will only create temporary AV block and is not helpful in converting atrial flutter. It is important to differentiate failure to convert an arrhythmia and successful cardioversion with immediate reinitiation of the arrhythmia. If cardioversion is successful in restoring sinus rhythm but the tachycardia reinitiates shortly after cardioversion, it may be necessary to begin an antiarrhythmic agent like amiodarone. However, in this instance, where the cardioversion was not successful, the next most appropriate step would be increasing the energy dose.

27. (E) A wide QRS escape rhythm in a patient with complete heart block is a class I indication for a pacemaker. The class I recommendations for permanent pacing in children, adolescents, and patients with congenital heart disease are as follows:

1. Advanced second- or third-degree AV block associated with symptomatic bradycardia, ventricular dysfunction, or low cardiac output.
2. Sinus node dysfunction with correlation of symptoms during age-inappropriate bradycardia. The definition of bradycardia varies with the patient's age and expected heart rate.
3. Postoperative advanced second- or third-degree AV block that is not expected to resolve or persists at least 7 days after cardiac surgery.
4. Congenital third-degree AV block with a wide QRS escape rhythm, complex ventricular ectopy, or ventricular dysfunction.
5. Congenital third-degree AV block in the infant with a ventricular rate less than 55 bpm or with congenital heart disease and a ventricular rate less than 70 bpm.

In this patient, a QRS duration of 130 ms constitutes a wide complex escape, which may be unstable, and therefore requires pacemaker placement. The atrial rate is not important in determining the need for a pacemaker. Although complex ventricular ectopy is an indication for pacemaker placement, rare PVCs would not meet this criterion. In a stable patient and in the absence of congenital heart disease, a heart rate of 60 bpm would not warrant immediate pacemaker placement.

28. (D) Long QT syndrome type 1, the most common form of long QT, presents as syncope or arrhythmias with exercise. The ECG in this patient clearly shows a prolonged QT interval. Genetic testing may reveal a cause in about 75% of patients with a high index of suspicion for long QT syndrome. An echocardiogram may be helpful in identifying hypertrophic cardiomyopathy but the ECG does not suggest hypertrophy. Magnetic resonance imaging may be helpful in identifying arrhythmogenic ventricular cardiomyopathy or myocarditis, but the ECG is consistent with long QT syndrome rather than either of these diagnoses. There are typically no abnormalities of the AH or HV intervals in patients with long QT syndrome and there is no suggestion of conduction disease of the AV node based on the ECG. Procainamide challenge may be helpful in bringing out Brugada syndrome, but there is no indication of Brugada syndrome on the ECG, and procainamide will further prolong the QT, which may precipitate ventricular arrhythmias.

29. (A) For SVT to occur, there need to be two pathways with differences in conduction properties and refractory periods separated by an area of nonconduction. Entrainment is a form of mapping reentry tachycardias, and triggered activity and increased automaticity are properties of focal tachycardias.

30. (D) One of the long-term complications that can manifest in patients who have had surgery for congenital heart disease is the development of heart block. This is more common in patients who had temporary AV block in the immediate postoperative period. Late development of AV block may play a role in sudden cardiac death. The presence of Mobitz type II second-degree heart block implies conduction system disease placing a patient at risk, and pacemaker placement is warranted even with a good underlying heart rate and no symptoms (class IIa). However, in the presence of Mobitz type I second-degree heart block (Wenckebach), pacemaker placement is not warranted unless the patient has a slow underlying rate and/or symptoms. Digoxin and amiodarone may worsen AV conduction. There is no indication for theophylline therapy for the treatment of AV block in the current era.

31. (C) Atrial flutter has traditionally been characterized as a macro reentrant arrhythmia with atrial rates between 240 and 400 bpm. The ECG usually demonstrates a regular rhythm, with P waves that can appear saw-toothed, also called flutter waves. Since the atrioventricular (AV) node cannot conduct at the same rate as the atrial activity, one commonly sees some form of conduction block, typically 2:1 or 4:1. This block may also be variable and cause atrial flutter to appear as an irregular rhythm. Atrial flutter is a common manifestation in patients who have undergone atrial surgery. DC cardioversion is the most effective way to terminate atrial flutter and would be indicated in a patient with hemodynamic instability. An alternative is atrial overdrive pacing that may be performed through atrial pacing wires in the postoperative setting. Temporary overdrive pacing can be an effective means of terminating reentry tachycardias such as atrial flutter and paroxysmal supraventricular tachycardia. Typically, the pacing rate is set at 10 to 20 bpm faster than the tachycardia rate. Progressively faster rates can be tried with multiple attempts although there is a risk of inducing atrial fibrillation. Adenosine and digoxin will block the ventricular response, but not typically terminate the arrhythmia. Correction of hypokalemia is unlikely to terminate the arrhythmia.

32. (B) Atrial fibrillation occurs in 10% to 15% of patients with hyperthyroidism. Thyroid hormone contributes to arrhythmogenic activity by altering the electrophysiologic characteristics of atrial myocytes by shortening the action potential duration and enhancing automaticity and triggered activity in the pulmonary vein cardiac tissue. Decreased voltages on an ECG can result from hypothyroidism, but not usually in hyperthyroidism. Hyperthyroidism may also be associated with a hyperdynamic state with an increased pulse pressure and hypercontractile function, although ejection fraction may decrease in the face of long-standing hyperthyroidism. Hyperthyroidism typically does not affect conduction and does not cause heart block.

33. (A) Surgery within the atrium can result in damage to the sinus node. The risk for sinus node dysfunction is directly related to the extent of surgery within the atrium. Patients after an atrial switch or Fontan procedure are at greatest risk for sinus node dysfunction. Lyme disease, maternal SLE, and myocarditis are more commonly associated with AV block. Patients with cardiomyopathy may present with atrial and ventricular arrhythmias.

34. (B) Sinus node dysfunction is the most common arrhythmia after sinus venosus ASD repair. SVASD differs from secundum atrial septal defect by its atrial septal location and its association with anomalous pulmonary venous connection. The SVASDs tend to have a higher incidence of sinus node dysfunction likely due to their proximity to the sinus node with the potential for direct damage or injury to the sinus node artery during repair. In one study, at follow-up after SVASD repair, 6% of patients had sinus node dysfunction, a permanent pacemaker, or both, and 14% of patients had atrial fibrillation.

35. (D) The Heart Rhythm Society and the British Pacing and Electrophysiology Group have developed a code to describe various pacing modes (NBG code). This is a series of letters used to describe how the pacemaker is programmed. The first position denotes the chamber(s) paced, and the second position denotes the chamber(s) sensed (A for atria, V for ventricles, and D for dual—both atria and ventricles). The third position indicates the response of the pacemaker to a sensed event (I for inhibit, T for track, and D for dual—both inhibit and track). In the inhibit mode, when the pacemaker senses an intrinsic cardiac event, it inhibits pacing. In this manner, it allows intrinsic cardiac events to happen without pacing. In the triggered or tracking mode, the pacemaker actively paces in response to a sensed event (e.g., senses an intrinsic atrial contraction, then paces the ventricle in response). A DDD pacemaker paces both atrium and ventricle, senses both atrium and ventricle, and both inhibits and tracks in response to a sensed event. As the heart rate of the patient is higher than the set rate limit of the pacemaker, the device is sensing the native atrial rate at a rate of 85 bpm and triggering the ventricle to pace at the same rate. If the patient were set AAI or VVI, it would pace only the atria or ventricles at the lower set rate. If a DDI setting was selected, the patient would sense and pace in both the atria and ventricles, but would not have the capability of tracking an atrial rate above the lower rate limit of the pacemaker as it is only set in the inhibit mode. The DDI mode is helpful in patients with atrial arrhythmias to avoid the pacemaker tracking rapid atrial rates with subsequent rapid pacing in the ventricles. In the DOO mode, the pacemaker would pace the atria and ventricle at the lower rate limit with no sensing (i.e., would pace both the atria and ventricles without regard to the intrinsic cardiac activity).

36. (B) Behavioral changes, depression, and mood swings are the most common side effects of β-blockers in children. Other less common side effects include lightheadedness, tiredness, headaches, nightmares, difficulty sleeping, heartburn, diarrhea, and constipation. Rarely, β-blockers can cause a rash. Hypoglycemia has been reported but is also rare. β-Blockers can exacerbate asthma. They should also be used with caution in patients with diabetes as they can block hypoglycemic symptoms in these patients. Amiodarone, rather than β-blockers, causes hypothyroidism.

37. (C) The ECG shows marked ventricular hypertrophy with QRS complexes going off the page as well as a short PR interval. There is also evidence of strain with ST-segment changes and T-wave inversion in the limb leads. Pompe disease is a glycogen storage disease (type II). The disease is linked to an inherited deficiency of the lysosomal enzyme acid α-glucosidase, which is responsible for the breakdown of glycogen to glucose. The result is intralysosomal accumulation of glycogen, primarily in muscle cells, that leads to a progressive loss of muscle function. It is one of the most severe and lethal form of hypertrophic cardiomyopathy, typically causing death within the first 2 years of life. Babies appear clinically well at birth, but within 6 months start developing hypotonia, severe cardiomegaly, hepatomegaly, poor weight gain, difficulty sucking, and an enlarged protruding tongue. The ECG classically shows a short PR interval and extremely large QRS voltages suggestive of left ventricular hypertrophy.

38. (B) Patients with congenitally corrected transposition of the great arteries (ccTGA) are at risk for development of complete AV block. Because of the displacement of the AV node and the abnormal course of conduction tissue that runs very superficially, there is an increased risk for development of complete AV block. Approximately 10% of the patients may present with heart block. Spontaneous complete heart block occurs at a rate of up to 2% per year in this population. These patients also have an increased risk for Wolff–Parkinson–White. The atria are not generally dilated in the absence of AV valve regurgitation and patients are not at a high risk of atrial flutter or sinus node dysfunction. Junctional tachycardia and TdP are also rare in ccTGA.

39. (B) By delivering premature atrial stimuli (S_2 at 320, 310, and 300 ms) after a pacing train (S_1 at 600 ms), there should be a small decremental change in the AH interval. However, if there is a large change (>50 ms) in the AH interval with a 10 ms change in the premature atrial stimulus (S_2), this increase in the AH interval is called an "AH jump" and suggests dual AV node pathways (i.e., both a fast pathway and a slow pathway) that may be a substrate for AV nodal reentry tachycardia. If the S_2 captures the atrium but does not conduct to the ventricles, then the AV node effective refractory period has been reached. If the S_2 fails to capture the atrium, the atrial muscle effective refractory period has been reached. Wenckebach is seen during atrial pacing and not during an extrastimulus protocol. The lengthening of the AV conduction time represented by the AH interval is a normal finding (decremental property of the AV node) and does not indicate AV node conduction system disease.

40. (D) The intracardiac ECG shows a drive train of pacing (S_1) followed by a prematurely paced ventricular stimulus (S_2). The paced beat is delivered creating a pacing spike (excluding failure of output). However, this beat does not capture the ventricle (there is a pacing spike but no resulting QRS on the surface ECG) and therefore represents the ventricular muscle ERP. If the premature stimulus captured the ventricle beat but then blocked going to the atrium (ventricular signal on the ventricular catheter and a QRS on the surface ECG) but did not conduct to the atrium, this would represent the AV node retrograde ERP. There is normal atrial activation and no evidence of an accessory pathway. VA Wenckebach occurs during ventricular pacing and not during a ventricular extrastimulus protocol.

41. (C) The ECG demonstrates pacing in the VVI mode. The rate is 75 bpm. The P waves have no relationship to the QRS complex (are dissociated), indicating that there is no sensing of the atrium, eliminating the possibility of DDD or VDD pacing. There are no atrial pacing spikes eliminating the possibility of DOO (asynchronous dual chamber) pacing. There is pacing in the ventricle, so AAI is not a possibility. The pacemaker could be pacing VOO or VVI (since no intrinsic beats are seen on the tracing), but VOO was not a choice and therefore VVI is the correct answer.

42. (A) The surface tracings show a wide complex tachycardia. The atrial electrical signals (shown in the coronary sinus tracings) have no relationship to (are dissociated from) the ventricular electrical signals (shown on the bottom two ventricular electrogram tracings). As the atrial rate is slower than the ventricular rate, the tachycardia is originating distal to the AV node and is therefore a ventricular tachycardia. As the atrial rate is slower than the ventricular rate, this cannot be an atrial tachycardia. In an accessory pathway-mediated tachycardia, there is a 1:1 relationship between the atria and ventricles as the atria, AV node, ventricles, and accessory pathway are all obligatory parts of the circuit. In AV node reentry tachycardia, the AV relationship is also typically 1:1. As the patient is in a wide complex rhythm with a rapid ventricular rate, although there is VA dissociation, there is no evidence of antegrade complete AV block (to make this diagnosis, the atrial rate must be typically faster than the ventricular rate).

43. (B) This patient has evidence of right ventricular hypertrophy (qR in lead V1) and ST-segment elevation consistent with ischemia in V1 and V2. This is consistent with right ventricular ischemia. This can be seen in patients with pulmonary atresia with intact ventricular septum and right ventricle–dependent coronary circulation. The high pressure in the right ventricle creates sinusoidal connections between the right ventricle and coronary artery circulation that may predispose the patient to ischemia. Tetralogy of Fallot and truncus arteriosus can result in RVH, but not typically ischemia. Total anomalous pulmonary venous return may result in RVH and right atrial enlargement, but also does not give signs of ischemia.

44. (A) The ECG demonstrates atrial sensing followed by ventricular tracking and resultant ventricular pacing. This is a dual-chamber pacemaker and the pacing mode is either DDD or VDD. The VDD mode is capable of atrial sensing but not pacing in the atrium. Most patients have both an atrial and a ventricular lead placed with a dual-chamber pacemaker. However, there are leads that have the capability in a single lead to sense both the atrium and the ventricle as

well as pace the ventricle achieving AV synchrony using a single lead set VDD. If the pacemaker was set VVI or VOO, it would pace at the lower rate limit of 60, not the rate of 80 seen in the tracing. If the pacemaker were set DOO (pacing in the atria and ventricles without sensing), both atrial and ventricular pacing spikes would be present in the tracing and would pace through the tracing without any regard to exiting P waves or QRS complexes.

45. (D) The ECG shows complete AV block. AV conduction block is a complication in 1% to 3% of surgical operations for congenital heart disease. Unless treated with an implanted pacemaker, postoperative complete heart block is associated with 28% to 50% mortality, and permanent pacemaker implantation is a class I indication for surgically induced complete AV block regardless of the ventricular escape rate and condition of the patient. Postoperative heart block often proves to be transient, typically resolving within 7 to 10 days of onset, and it is prudent to wait at least 7 days to determine whether AV nodal conduction will return. In a stable patient with a reasonable escape rate, there is no indication for epinephrine or isoproterenol.

46. (C) Mobitz type I second-degree AV block, also referred to as Wenckebach periodicity, is characterized by progressive PR prolongation, usually owing to changes in the AH interval (reflecting AV node delay), with eventual failure of conduction to the ventricle. In contrast, type II AV block refers to abrupt failure of AV conduction of one or more atrial impulses without prior PR prolongation. Type II block usually occurs below the AV node. In addition to the absence of progressive PR prolongation before block, type II block may abruptly progress to third-degree block with an inadequate escape rhythm and is therefore an indication for a pacemaker, even in the absence of symptoms. Sinus bradycardia, Wenckebach, and a prolonged PR interval are not indications for a pacemaker in an asymptomatic patient, but would be an indication if symptoms correlate with the rhythm. Left bundle branch block by itself is not an indication for pacemaker placement, regardless of QRS duration.

47. (B) The ECG shows bidirectional ventricular tachycardia with the QRS changing in every other beat during the VT. This tachycardia is most consistent with CPVT. Features of CPVT are a catecholamine-driven (typically exercise or emotion) ventricular tachyarrhythmias, a typical pattern of bidirectional ventricular tachycardia during exercise or emotion with a normal resting ECG and a structurally normal heart. CPVT is a genetic disease related most commonly to mutations in the cardiac ryanodine receptor gene (*RYR2*) or calsequestrin 2 gene (*CASQ2*). Long QT syndrome and Brugada syndrome arrhythmias are typically triggered by an early afterdepolarization with a PVC appearing at the end of the T wave and the classic arrhythmia is torsades. Arrhythmogenic right ventricular cardiomyopathy typically produces VT from the right ventricle and hypertrophic cardiomyopathy patients are at an increased risk of VT, but bidirectional VT is the hallmark feature of CPVT.

48. (E) The findings on this ECG are consistent with intermittent capture of ventricular lead. There are pacing spikes with no capture, ventricular escape beats at a slow rate, and intermittent capture of the ventricle by the pacemaker. This is most consistent with a partial fracture of the ventricular lead. The lead impedance will often be out of the normal range when interrogated. This patient will need to be admitted and have the output of the pacemaker adjusted. If this is not successful or there are other indicators of lead malfunction, the pacing lead will need to be replaced. Undersensing is the inability of the pacemaker to sense spontaneous myocardial depolarization and results in paced complexes in the presence of the heart's intrinsic rhythm. This leads to inappropriate pacing complexes after native QRS beats. Oversensing refers to the pacemaker sensing artifacts and hence not pacing when indicated. The pacemaker is continually pacing in the tracing without inhibiting (withholding pacing), so oversensing is not present. ERI is the point in the pacemaker battery life where replacement is needed, but the pacemaker will continue to operate and will still result in ventricular capture. At the end of life when the battery voltage is extremely low, the pacemaker may not be able to generate enough energy to capture the heart which could result in a similar picture to the ECG shown. Placing a magnet over a pacemaker typically causes it to pace asynchronously, but not lose capture. Typically when a pacemaker performs a testing feature, it will not allow loss of capture for even a single beat.

49. (E) Adverse effects of amiodarone include photosensitivity, thyroid dysfunction, weakness, peripheral neuropathy, corneal microdeposits, and elevation of hepatic enzymes. Periodic evaluation of thyroid function and liver function should be performed in patients taking amiodarone chronically. Nausea is common at the initiation of therapy, but generally resolves over time. Photosensitivity is quite common, and patients should be instructed to cover their skin and use skin-blocking agents. Less common but serious side effects include proarrhythmia and pulmonary fibrosis. Corneal microdeposits can also be seen, and a yearly ophthalmology visit is warranted for patients on chronic amiodarone. Renal dysfunction is not a side effect of amiodarone.

50. (B) The ECG shows right atrial enlargement with a right bundle branch block as well as suggestion of preexcitation in leads V2 and V3. These findings are most consistent with Ebstein anomaly of the tricuspid valve. WPW is associated with Ebstein anomaly, hypertrophic cardiomyopathy, and congenitally corrected transposition of the great arteries. Around 30% of patients with Ebstein have preexcitation and 50% of those with an accessory pathway will have more than one accessory pathway. Patients with Ebstein are at risk for reentrant SVT using an accessory pathway, atrial tachycardia and atrial flutter due to the dilated atrium, and atrial fibrillation. A complete AV canal, total anomalous pulmonary venous return, and dilated cardiomyopathy may result in a dilated right atrium, but do not typically have the enormous P waves seen in this ECG and do not usually have a right bundle branch block and preexcitation. Pulmonary stenosis as an isolated finding does not typically result in right atrial enlargement.

51. (C) The patient's presentation is consistent with neurocardiogenic (or vasovagal) syncope. All the therapeutic options can be used for treatment of neurocardiogenic syncope. However, fluid liberalization and behavior modification should be the first steps in the treatment of symptoms. A majority of the patients will improve with this alone and need no further intervention. A tilt table test is useful only when the diagnosis cannot be made by history alone. Although there is a pause of 3.5 seconds, without true episodes of syncope, a pacemaker is not indicated until other therapeutic options have been attempted. In addition, in many patients with neurocardiogenic syncope, there is a combined problem of hypotension and bradycardia, and placing a pacemaker may not alleviate symptoms. An ICD is not indicated in neurocardiogenic syncope. There is no value to an invasive electrophysiology study as this phenomenon is mediated by bradycardia induced by the vagus nerve rather than an arrhythmia.

52. (E) Digoxin toxicity is a relatively rare occurrence and typically occurs in the presence of acute or chronic renal failure. Hypokalemia increases digoxin cardiac sensitivity and should be corrected. Patients with hypomagnesemia, hypokalemia, or both may become cardiotoxic even with therapeutic digitalis levels. Patients with digoxin toxicity should receive IV hydration and oxygen and be admitted to an intensive care unit for monitoring. Arrhythmias play a prominent role in digoxin toxicity. β-Blockers may be helpful for the treatment of supraventricular tachyarrhythmias with rapid ventricular rates. In the presence of sinus node suppression or AV node block, however, they may cause further bradycardia and should be used with caution, and a short-acting β-blocker such as esmolol should be the first line of therapy. Lidocaine can suppress ventricular arrhythmias. Phenytoin (which is a class IB antiarrhythmic in addition to being an antiepileptic medication) is also very effective in treating ventricular arrhythmias. The ventricular arrhythmias from digoxin result from early afterdepolarizations (depolarization of the ventricular myocardium during early repolarization). These early afterdepolarizations are also the mechanism of induction of arrhythmias in long QT syndrome. Temporary pacing is an alternative for patients with severe bradycardia. Digoxin immune Fab is made from immunoglobulin fragments from sheep that have been exposed to a digoxin derivative. It irreversibly binds to digoxin, making it unable to act on its target cells, including those in the heart. Just as with any other antibody product, patients must be monitored for anaphylactic shock, but the product is extremely effective. The onset of action ranges from 20 to 90 minutes with a complete response generally occurring within 4 hours.

53. (C) This rhythm strip shows torsades de pointes (TdP), which is a ventricular tachycardia with a varying QRS morphology. Magnesium sulfate (MgSO$_4$) can be a helpful adjunct in the treatment for TdP. Its use is therefore recommended for therapy of TdP. Magnesium can be given at 5 to 10 mg/kg IV or 1 to 2 g IV in adults initially in a rapid bolus over 30 to 60 seconds. The dose can be repeated in 5 to 15 minutes and a drip can be started at 0.3 to 1 mg/kg/hr. Magnesium can be effective even in patients with normal magnesium levels. Defibrillation should be performed in patients with sustained torsades especially if magnesium is not readily available, but magnesium may prevent further recurrences. There is no significant effect of digoxin, atropine, potassium, or adenosine in torsades.

54. (B) Adenosine is used in the diagnosis and treatment of supraventricular arrhythmias. Adenosine works via a specific adenosine receptor linked to the potassium channel. This results in shortening of the action potential duration and sinus bradycardia as well as AV block. It has a very short half-life of 1 to 5 seconds and is metabolized by erythrocytes and endothelial tissue. It must be given by a rapid push in a large vein as close to the heart as possible. The most likely reason that adenosine is not effective is that it was not given by a rapid push in a large vein. In this case, the 24-gauge IV was likely too small to administer the dose rapidly. Adenosine should be effective in converting AV node reentry tachycardia. The dose is usually 0.1 to 0.3 mg/kg, so an effect should have been seen at the dose given. Adenosine should be effective regardless of the duration and rate of the tachycardia episode.

55. (D) The fourth letter of the NBG pacing code can be used to represent rate response pacing. The pacemaker uses some type of sensor to detect activity and increases the lower rate limit of pacing in conjunction with the level of activity. When the activity ceases, the pacing returns to the set basal rate. Rate response enables a patient's pacemaker to vary heart rate when the sinus node cannot provide the appropriate rate to meet the body's demands. Rate-responsive pacing is indicated for patients who have chronotropic incompetence (heart rate cannot reach appropriate levels during exercise or to meet other metabolic demands).

56. (C) When the pacemaker is programmed AAIR, it is capable of pacing and sensing only in the atrium. This mode of pacing is indicated only when there is a problem with the sinus node. To correct any degree of heart block, a lead in the ventricle is necessary.

57. (C) The patient will receive a defibrillation shock if the ventricular rate goes at or above the programmed shock rate of 180 bpm. In the ventricular fibrillation zone, the patient will receive a shock if the ventricular rate is above the set rate, even if the rhythm is sinus. A separate ventricular tachycardia zone can be set with discriminators to try to determine if the arrhythmia is a sinus tachycardia or atrial tachycardia and can be programmed to withhold shock therapy if the device determines that the patient is not in ventricular tachycardia. In the ventricular fibrillation zone, these discriminators are not available and the device will deliver therapy purely based on the ventricular rate. In addition, the patient will not receive a shock if a ventricular tachycardia occurs at a rate slower than the set shocking rate (in this case, 180 bpm). Sinus tachycardia falling in the VT zone can lead to inappropriate shocks and is one of the most common reasons for inappropriate shocks in patients with an ICD.

58. (B) Electrocautery can create inappropriate noise and sensing within the pacemaker thus causing it to oversense and prevent necessary pacing. Placement of a magnet over a pacemaker causes an asynchronous pacing (no sensing, just pacing at the pacemaker's magnet rate). This avoids inappropriate pacemaker inhibition due to oversensing from electrocautery during surgery.

59. (B) When a magnet is placed over most ICDs, it disables shock therapy but pacing is not affected. This is different from when a magnet is placed over a pacemaker, which enables an asynchronous pacing. By disabling shock therapy, it avoids inappropriate shocks due to oversensing from electrocautery during surgery. However, it also avoids appropriate shocks due to ventricular tachycardias. The effects are temporary and remain there only as long as the magnet is placed over the ICD.

60. (E) The etiology of a cardiac arrest is not always clear despite extensive testing. In the absence of a known reversible or treatable cause of sudden cardiac arrest, ICD is the treatment of choice and a class I indication for ICD placement according to the 2012 Pacemaker/ICD guidelines as this patient is at risk of having another cardiac arrest. β-Blockers and amiodarone are not as effective as an ICD in preventing sudden cardiac death and are not a substitute for ICD placement. An implantable loop recorder is only capable of recording rhythms and not delivering therapy. There is no indication for hemodynamic catheterization in the face of a normal echo and cardiac MRI.

61. (B) The ECG shown demonstrates left axis deviation (axis of 0 degrees), left ventricular hypertrophy, and right atrial enlargement (P wave taller than three boxes) with a marked decrease in right-sided forces. This is most consistent with a diagnosis of tricuspid atresia. Patients with tricuspid atresia may also have a short PR interval without evidence of preexcitation. The major causes of left axis deviation in the pediatric population are complete AV canal, primum ASD, tricuspid atresia, and Wolff–Parkinson–White. Left ventricular hypertrophy only rarely causes left axis deviation in pediatric patients. Hypoplastic left heart syndrome, truncus arteriosus, and tetralogy of Fallot frequently show right axis deviation and right ventricular hypertrophy, which may also be normal in the immediate newborn period. In truncus arteriosus, the axis is typically normal but combined ventricular hypertrophy is commonly seen.

62. (E) Complete heart block (CHB) detected in utero is strongly associated with maternal antibodies to SSA (Ro) and SSB (La). Their pathogenic role in the development of CHB has been established in several studies. The mothers of affected infants often have autoimmune disease (systemic lupus erythematosus, Sjögren syndrome) but are frequently asymptomatic. Although the association of anti-SSA/SSB with CHB is widely accepted, the precise mechanism by which these antibodies cause cardiac conduction abnormalities remains to be defined. Fetal and neonatal diseases are presumed to be due to the transplacental passage of these immunoglobulin G (IgG) autoantibodies from the mother into the fetal circulation. Since these antibodies may have a pathogenic role in CHB, screening of infants with isolated CHB or neonatal lupus and their mothers for the presence of anti-SSA and anti-SSB is strongly recommended. Elevated serum potassium does not cause complete AV block without causing QRS widening. Maternal congenital heart disease does not cause isolated CHB. 22q11 deletions have been reported in patients with CHB, but are a rare cause, and Ro and La antibodies are a much more common finding.

63. (B) The ECG shows a wide complex rhythm at a rate of ~150 bpm. There is a characteristic failure of differentiation between the QRS and the T wave that blend together. This is seen in patients with hypoxia, acidosis, or hyperkalemia. Initial findings of hyperkalemia are tall-peaked T waves. As the potassium level increases, the T waves become more peaked and an intraventricular conduction delay results in a widened QRS along with PR prolongation. The resultant ECG may resemble a "sine wave" ECG pattern or wide ventricular tachycardia. At concentrations >9 mEq/L, atrial standstill, AV block, and ventricular fibrillation can occur. Increased calcium causes a shortened QT interval. The other electrolytes have minimal effect on the ECG.

64. (D) In Wolff–Parkinson–White, there is an accessory connection between the atria and the ventricles bypassing the AV node. These accessory pathways conduct quickly to the ventricles. It normally takes 35 to 70 ms to get through the AV node and bundle of His. This time is represented by the HV (His to ventricle) interval that can be measured in the EP lab. The HV interval is calculated by measuring the distance from the His deflection to the earliest QRS deflection on any lead on the surface ECG. A short HV interval (<25 to 35 ms) indicates an alternative method of conduction other than the AV node, which is only possible in the presence of an accessory pathway. In some cases, the HV interval may actually be negative, with the ventricular myocardium in close proximity to the site of the accessory pathway being activated prior to the bundle of His. Bundle branch block and infra-Hisian conduction delay result in a prolonged HV interval. First-degree AV block typically has a prolonged AH (atrium to His) interval. Dual AV node physiology is seen during an atrial extrastimulus protocol and results in prolongation of the AH interval.

65. (D) The newborn myocardium has unique properties that allow it to conduct impulses very rapidly, and atrial flutter at very fast rates (up to over 400 bpm) can be maintained. Although it is important to perform an echocardiogram on all patients who present atrial flutter, the majority of these patients have no underlying structural heart disease and a low incidence of recurrence of atrial flutter.

66. (A) This ECG shows atrial fibrillation with an irregularly irregular rhythm. This rhythm results in no organized atrial contractions and stasis in the atria. This stasis predisposes patients to thrombi and potential strokes. This risk may persist for some period of time, even after sinus rhythm is restored.

67. (C) This tracing shows Mobitz type I second-degree AV block (Wenckebach) with progressive prolongation of the PR interval followed by a dropped beat. This finding is not uncommon in teenagers and older adults while sleeping but is rare while awake. If it occurs in an otherwise asymptomatic person while sleeping, it likely has no clinical significance and, as an isolated finding, does not require any therapy or further evaluation.

68. (A) This tracing shows loss of preexcitation *in a single beat* (shown in the middle of the tracing with a change from a wide, preexcited QRS to a narrow QRS). The loss in a single beat on an exercise treadmill test indicates an accessory pathway is less likely to rapidly conduct to the ventricle in atrial fibrillation and is therefore at a lower risk for sudden death. The antegrade conduction seen on a resting ECG has no definitive relationship with the retrograde conduction that causes supraventricular tachycardia, and therefore, the risk of SVT cannot be estimated. There is no evidence of ventricular tachycardia.

69. (B) The tracing shows intermittent atrial undersensing as well as atrial pacing with no evidence of capture. This is indicative of atrial lead dysfunction. The ventricular lead shows capture of all beats and there is no evidence of dysfunction. The variability of the rate is due to atrial lead dysfunction and there is no evidence of oversensing or undersensing of the ventricular lead.

70. (E) This ECG shows severe bradycardia, relatively low-voltage QRS complexes, and low-amplitude T waves with no other significant abnormalities. The body's response to nutritional deprivation is to decrease the heart rate. There is no evidence of Wolff–Parkinson–White. Renal failure typically causes electrolyte disturbances that change the QRS or QT intervals. An atrial septal defect usually does not result in severe bradycardia. Thyroid storm involves hyperthyroidism and an elevated heart rate. This ECG could be consistent with hypothyroidism.

71. (D) The intracardiac tracing shows a pattern of activation through the bundle of His, to the atrium followed by the ventricle. This pattern of activation is the classic pattern seen with typical AV node reentry tachycardia. There is 1:1 AV conduction (one atrial impulse for every ventricular impulse), so this is not atrial flutter with 2:1 conduction. The atrial activation is earlier on the His catheter rather than the high right atrial catheter making sinus rhythm unlikely. An accessory pathway-mediated tachycardia has to go down the AV node through the ventricle up the accessory pathway to the atrium and then back down the AV node. This creates a pattern of His deflection, then a ventricular signal *followed* by an atrial activation at least 20 to 40 ms following the QRS. Atypical AV node reentry tachycardia is a long RP tachycardia, and this is a short RP tachycardia.

72. (A) This ECG shows massive right and left atrial enlargement consistent with restrictive cardiomyopathy. It is very unusual to see this degree of biatrial enlargement in any condition other than restrictive cardiomyopathy. Patients with restrictive cardiomyopathy are at risk for pulmonary hypertension. None of the other conditions listed as answers are associated with restrictive cardiomyopathy.

73. (B) This ECG, which is performed at half-standard (any measured voltage should be doubled to determine the true height), shows massive ventricular hypertrophy. There is also a somewhat shortened PR interval. These findings are consistent with a glycogen storage disorder, particularly glycogen storage disease type II (Pompe disease). These patients present with hepatomegaly.

74. (C) This ECG shows the classic pattern for Brugada syndrome with a right bundle branch block pattern and ST-segment elevation in leads V1 and V2. This is a channelopathy affecting ion transport (typically sodium) during cardiac conduction. The clinical manifestations of Brugada syndrome are highly variable. Symptomatic patients experience ventricular tachyarrhythmias that may lead to recurrent syncope and/or sudden cardiac death. In symptomatic patients with Brugada syndrome who have either syncope or ventricular arrhythmias, an ICD is the best option. β-Blockers are not effective at preventing sudden cardiac death, and amiodarone may exacerbate ventricular arrhythmias. Patients with a spontaneous ECG for Brugada syndrome are thought to be at higher risk for arrhythmias. Although ST-segment elevation is present, patients have normal coronary arteries.

75. (E) The genetic defect associated with Brugada syndrome results from a mutation in the SCN5A channel that is a sodium channel. HERG and KCNQ1 mutations cause LQTS. 22q11.2 deletion is associated with DiGeorge syndrome. Trisomy 21 has no relationship to Brugada syndrome.

76. (E) In patients with Brugada syndrome, Vaughan Williams class I drugs such as procainamide that block the sodium channel may bring out a Brugada-type pattern on ECG. Epinephrine may be useful in identifying patients with LQTS, but not Brugada syndrome.

77. (A) This tracing shows progressive prolongation of the atrium to His (AH interval) and consequentially PR intervals followed by a nonconducted beat. This finding can be created by pacing the atria faster and faster during an atrial pacing protocol. There is no evidence on this tracing of supraventricular tachycardia, atrial fibrillation, an abrupt increase in the AH interval, or preexcitation.

78. (D) This tracing shows diffuse ST-segment elevation and PR-segment depression consistent with pericarditis. Coxsackievirus is the most common cause of viral pericarditis. Cocaine can result in coronary vasospasm and ischemia, but the ECG changes are usually localized to one segment (not diffuse ST-segment elevation) and the ECG in cocaine use may appear abnormal without evidence of true acute infarction. A myosin heavy chain mutation may result in hypertrophic cardiomyopathy with subsequent left ventricular hypertrophy with strain, but not the diffuse ST-segment elevation and PR depression seen on this ECG. Patients with hypertrophic cardiomyopathy often have a short PR interval due to true preexcitation or pseudo-preexcitation (rapid AV nodal conduction seen in HCM). Increased intracranial pressure can cause T-wave changes and QT prolongation, but not diffuse ST-segment elevation. Erythromycin prolongs the QT interval, but does not affect ST or PR segments.

79. (A) This tracing shows an irregular wide complex tachycardia. This is atrial fibrillation in the presence of either a preexisting bundle branch block or preexcitation (Wolff–Parkinson–White). The most likely scenario in a previously asymptomatic patient is atrial fibrillation with WPW. The patient has rapid conduction through the accessory pathway and is at risk for ventricular fibrillation. With the rapid ventricular conduction, the patient should be cardioverted as quickly as possible. As the accessory pathway conducts very rapidly, the patient should undergo an ablation to eliminate conduction in the accessory pathway and, if this is not possible, should be treated with an antiarrhythmic medication such as flecainide or amiodarone that can potentially slow conduction in the accessory pathway. Patients with Ebstein anomaly have an increased incidence of WPW and are at risk for atrial fibrillation because of their dilated atria. WPW is classically associated with Ebstein, congenitally corrected transposition of the great arteries, and hypertrophic cardiomyopathy, not the other conditions listed.

80. (B) In the presence of atrial fibrillation and WPW, any drug that can block the AV node, such as adenosine, digoxin, or a calcium channel blocker, is relatively contraindicated. This may cause preferential conduction down the accessory pathway resulting in rapid conduction to the ventricle and subsequently ventricular fibrillation.

81. (A) This ECG shows complete AV block. There is no relationship between the P waves and the QRS complexes, the atrial rate is faster than the ventricular rate, and there are P waves that should conduct, but do not. There is no significant enough increase in ventricular arrhythmias to warrant implantation of an ICD in the absence of other risk factors. β-Blockers will have little effect and may slow the underlying junctional rate. Left stellate ganglionectomy may have some utility in LQTS, but not complete AV block. Cardiac transplantation is not indicated. A pacemaker is indicated in the presence of symptoms, a wide complex escape rhythm, complex ventricular ectopy. In infants, a pacemaker is indicated with symptoms and a heart rate <50 bpm in the absence of congenital heart disease and 70 bpm in the presence of congenital heart disease, while a heart rate of <50 bpm is the threshold for pacemaker placement over 1 year of age, although this is a class IIa indication.

82. (D) Hypertrophic cardiomyopathy is not classically associated with AV block. All the other conditions may result in alterations of AV nodal conduction.

83. (B) This ECG shows a long RP tachycardia (the P wave occurs greater than half the distance between two successive QRS complexes). The P waves are deeply negative in leads II, III, and aVF. This is consistent with either the permanent form of junctional reciprocating tachycardia (PJRT) or atypical AV node reentry tachycardia. PJRT is an accessory pathway-mediated tachycardia due to a slowly conducting accessory pathway typically located in the right posterior septum. Because the accessory pathway conducts slowly, the atrial activation is seen a significant time following the QRS. Both PJRT and atypical AV node reentry tachycardia are dependent on the AV node and will break with adenosine. However, both also tend to be incessant and may reinitiate quickly after termination with adenosine (see tracing below; **Figure 6.50**). Atrial flutter will continue with only P waves in a saw-tooth pattern after adenosine. Sinus tachycardia will slow transiently, then speed back up. A sinus tachycardia or atrial tachycardia in the presence of preexcitation may widen transiently as the AV node blocks and there is preferential conduction down the AV node.

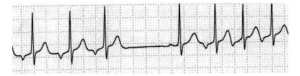

FIGURE 6.50

84. (C) The differential diagnosis for a long RP tachycardia with a narrow-complex QRS includes an atrial tachycardia, PJRT, and atypical AV node reentry tachycardia. A Mahaim fiber is an accessory pathway fiber that conducts antegrade only. Mahaim fiber tachycardias present with a wide complex tachycardia. Atrial flutter can also present as a long RP tachycardia when P waves are hidden in the T wave or QRS.

85. (B) This tracing shows a supraventricular tachycardia. The atrial activation is earliest in the mid-CS, which runs along the AV groove between the left atrium and left ventricle. There are no normal structures that connect the atria and the ventricles present in this location. Therefore, this tracing shows supraventricular tachycardia due to a left-sided accessory pathway.

86. (D) This ECG shows prolonged QT syndrome with QRS alternans. This is an alternating pattern of appearance of the T waves. This is a poor prognostic sign, and these patients are at risk for both 2:1 AV block (which this patient has on other tracings) and sudden death. Methadone prolongs the QT interval and should be avoided. Most cases of LQTS are familial; hence, other family members should be screened. The underlying mutation is typically due to a sodium or potassium channel mutation and only very rarely due to a calcium channel mutation. Calcium channel mutations are a common cause of catecholaminergic polymorphic ventricular tachycardia (CPVT).

87. (A) Pacemakers have a feature that allows the pacemaker to increase the pacing rate in response to patient activity. This is called rate responsiveness and is denoted by the R in the fourth letter of the NBG pacing code (AAIR). The most common mechanism for this to occur is through an accelerometer. An accelerometer senses motion and then increases the patient's pacing rate in response. In this particular instance, the bumpy road creates motion that the pacemaker senses and subsequently increases the pacing rate as a response. The pacemaker cannot determine if the motion is due to exercise, physical activity, or other sources of motion. An atrial arrhythmia would be unlikely to happen at the same time each day. Electromagnetic interference may inhibit the function of the pacemaker or make it pace asynchronously, but would

not give a gradual increase in heart rate. Oversensing would result in a decrease in the rate from inhibition of pacing. When a magnet is placed over the pacemaker, it asynchronously paces at a set rate determined by the pacemaker manufacturer (the magnet rate). While this may cause an increase in the rate, it would pace at a constant rate and not steadily increase.

88. (B) The classic ECG findings of Brugada are ST-segment elevation and a right bundle branch block pattern in leads V1 and V2. A spontaneous Brugada ECG pattern carries the highest risk for arrhythmias. However, some patients may have a normal ECG at rest. Fever can be a trigger for the ECG findings in Brugada syndrome and patients may exhibit an increased incidence of arrhythmias during febrile illnesses. In addition to fever, the ECG findings in Brugada syndrome may be brought out by repeating an ECG with "high-lead" placement of leads V1 and V2 as indicated. This involves moving the two leads up one and/or two intercostal space in an attempt to bring out characteristic changes in the J-point and ST segments of leads V1 and V2. Procainamide may also be infused to bring out the typical ECG findings in Brugada syndrome. Emotional stress is a typical trigger for long QT syndrome type 2. Dehydration may bring out symptoms in patients with hypertrophic cardiomyopathy. Hypertension may result in left ventricular hypertrophy with strain on an ECG, but typically does not affect the right-sided leads (V1 and V2). The majority of events in long QT syndrome type 3 happen during sleep, but sleep does not classically bring out the ECG pattern seen in Brugada syndrome.

89. (C) Chronic resynchronization therapy (CRT) also known as biventricular pacing is used to try to promote ventricular synchrony in patients with heart failure and a wide QRS. The 2012 guidelines state that CRT is indicated for patients who have LVEF less than or equal to 35%, sinus rhythm, LBBB with a QRS duration greater than or equal to 150 ms, and NYHA class II, III, or ambulatory IV symptoms on guideline-directed medical therapy (the only class I indication). It is generally only beneficial when the ejection fraction is less than 35% and is only indicated after medical therapy is optimized. There is some evidence that CRT may be beneficial with more narrow QRS durations and in patients with a right bundle branch block pattern, but it tends to have a lower success rate in these patients and is therefore not a class I indication. CRT is NOT recommended for patients with NYHA class I or II symptoms and non-LBBB pattern with QRS duration less than 150 ms.

90. (D) The ECG shows complete AV block. Mutations in NKX2.5 can be associated with heart block and various forms of congenital heart disease but most commonly a secundum ASD. KCNH2 mutations can cause long QT syndrome type 2. PKP2 mutations can be associated with arrhythmogenic right ventricular cardiomyopathy. PTPN11 mutations are associated with Noonan syndrome which can be associated with dysplastic pulmonary valve and pulmonary stenosis and/or hypertrophic cardiomyopathy. NOTCH1 mutations can be associated with left-sided heart disease including aortic valve stenosis, bicuspid aortic valve, coarctation of the aorta, and/or hypoplastic left heart disease.

91. (A) Kearns–Sayre is a mitochondrial disorder that presents prior to age 20 with ptosis and pigmentary retinopathy. Multiple organ systems can be affected but patient must also have either cerebellar ataxia, a cardiac conduction abnormality, or increased cerebral spinal fluid protein in order to make the diagnosis. Cardiac conduction abnormalities can vary from intraventricular conduction delay or various forms of bundle branch block to various degrees of AV block. Conduction abnormalities may unpredictably and rapidly progress to complete AV block potentially resulting in sudden death. Pacemaker implantation is indicated in patients with Kearns–Sayre and any degree of AV block or conduction abnormality. Prolonged QT is not associated with Kearns–Sayre. Epsilon waves can be associated with arrhythmogenic right ventricular cardiomyopathy (ARVC). ST depression and T-wave inversion would not be expected with a normal echo. Wolff–Parkinson–White is not associated with Kearns–Sayre, so a delta wave would not be expected.

92. (E) The electrograms in the figure demonstrate Wolff–Parkinson–White in the first beat with loss of ventricular preexcitation in the second beat. This is evident from the delta wave and wide QRS seen on the first beat compared to the narrow QRS with no delta wave on the second beat. In addition, on the second beat, the His bundle electrogram becomes evident on the His catheter with loss of ventricular preexcitation. There is also separation of the atrial and ventricular electrogram on the ablation catheter once ventricular preexcitation is lost. Because there is an accessory pathway present, AV reentrant tachycardia is the most likely cause of the palpitations. There is no evidence from the electrograms to suggest any of the other answers presented are present.

93. (D) This patient has type 1 long QT syndrome (due to a mutation in KCNQ1). With type 1 long QT syndrome, episodes of ventricular arrhythmias (torsades de pointes) are more likely with exertion, and β-blockade is considered very effective in preventing episodes (more so than in other long QT subtypes and likely with a greater than 95% efficacy). Nadolol is considered superior for episode prevention compared to other forms of β-blockers. In light of the efficacy of β-blockade (and assuming compliance), a trial of β-blockade is appropriate prior to ICD implantation. A future episode of syncope while on β-blockade would be considered an indication for an ICD. Discussions about avoiding QT-prolonging drugs as well as the potential exercise limitations are appropriate for any subtype of long QT syndrome (with exercise limitations particularly relevant for type 1).

94. (D) In a patient over 1 year of age, a heart rate of <50 bpm is considered an indication for permanent pacing (especially with complex congenital heart disease). A transvenous pacemaker is considered contraindicated with Fontan physiology due to endocardial leads (especially ventricular) mandatorily having to be in the systemic circulation (the risk of thrombus formation on the lead and subsequent embolism is the primary concern). An epicardial pacing system is therefore required in this patient. A Fontan patient is expected to need AV synchrony, so placement of only a ventricular lead (and VVI pacing) is not considered optimal.

95. (C) An ICD is implanted when a patient is considered at high risk for a dangerous ventricular arrhythmia and that arrhythmia is amenable to shock therapy. In a patient with incessant VT, a shock will at most only transiently terminate the rhythm, but a recurrence is expected immediately after (resection of the tumor would be the recommended therapy). The other patients are considered at high risk for ventricular arrhythmias that respond to defibrillation. While a patient with CPVT may be trialed on a β-blocker prior to ICD therapy, an ICD would be indicated if they were to have an episode of syncope while already on a β-blocker.

96. (C) P waves without QRSs are seen marching out for the majority of this rhythm strip despite being in DDD mode (with ventricular pacing expected after each atrial event). The lack of ventricular pacing spikes (or QRS) suggests that ventricular pacing was inhibited (due to pacemaker perceiving ventricular events when they are not there—this is usually seen due to electrical noise). Loss of ventricular capture is manifested by pacing spikes without resulting QRSs. Loss of ventricular sensing results in failure of the pacemaker to inhibit itself when ventricular events are occurring (this manifests as extra pacing spikes resulting in QRSs that were not necessary). Loss of atrial sensing can explain why some atrial beats do not have a paced QRS complex immediately after them (but would not explain that prolonged absence of pacing spikes when a lower rate of 60 bpm is set on the pacemaker).

97. (E) Hypertrophic cardiomyopathy (HCM) is the most common cause of sudden cardiac death among young athletes. Maron et al. from the Minneapolis Heart Institute Foundation Registry (*Circulation* 2007) reported on 1,435 cases of sudden cardiac death and found HCM to be the most common cause, accounting for at least 36% of deaths, and this data has been replicated in other studies of hypertrophic cardiomyopathy. The second most common cause was coronary artery anomalies, accounting for 17% of deaths.

98. (B) According to the 2017 ACC/AHA/HRS guidelines for the evaluation and management of patients with syncope, initial workup should include a thorough history (including the history of the event, past medical history, and family history), a physical examination, and an electrocardiogram. An echocardiogram should not be routinely obtained in the workup of syncope unless there are abnormalities discovered in the aforementioned history or testing.

ACKNOWLEDGMENT

The authors would like to acknowledge Anjan Batra, MD, for his contributions to the first edition of the textbook. Some of the questions included in this edition are modifications of his original questions.

SUGGESTED READINGS

Ackerman MJ, Priori SG, Willems S, et al. HRS/EHRA expert consensus statement on the state of genetic testing for the channelopathies and cardiomyopathies: This document was developed as a partnership between the Heart Rhythm Society (HRS) and the European Heart Rhythm Association (EHRA). *Heart Rhythm.* 2011;8(8):1308–1339.

Antzelevitch C, Brugada P, Borggrefe M, et al. Brugada syndrome: Report of the second consensus conference: Endorsed by the Heart Rhythm Society and the European Heart Rhythm Association. *Circulation.* 2005;111(5):659–670.

Aziz PF, Tanel RE, Zelster IJ, et al. Congenital long QT syndrome and 2:1 atrioventricular block: An optimistic outcome in the current era. *Heart Rhythm.* 2010;7:781–785.

Balli S, Oflaz MB, Kibar AE, et al. Rhythm and conduction analysis of patients with acute rheumatic fever. *Pediatr Cardiol.* 2013;34(2):383–389.

Bartalena L, Bogazzi F, Braverman LE, et al. Effects of amiodarone administration during pregnancy on neonatal thyroid function and subsequent neurodevelopment. *J Endocrinol Invest.* 2001; 24(2):116–130.

Benson DW. The normal electrocardiogram. In: Allen HD, Driscoll DJ, Shaddy RE, et al., eds. *Moss and Adams' Heart Disease in Infants, Children, and Adolescents: Including the Fetus and Young Adult.* 7th ed. Lippincott Williams & Wilkins; 2007:152–165.

Boineau JP, Moore EN, Patterson DF. Relationship between the ECG, ventricular activation, and the ventricular conduction system in ostium primum ASD. *Circulation.* 1973;48:556–564.

Bricker JT, Porter CJ, Garson A Jr, et al. Exercise testing in children with Wolff–Parkinson–White syndrome. *Am J Cardiol.* 1985; 55:1001–1004.

Brito-Zerón P, Izmirly PM, Ramos-Casals M, et al. The clinical spectrum of autoimmune congenital heart block. *Nat Rev Rheumatol.* 2015;11(5):301–312.

Cannon BC, Snyder CS. Disorders of cardiac rhythm and conduction. In: Allen HD, Driscoll DJ, Shaddy RE, et al., eds. *Moss and Adams' Heart Disease in Infants, Children, and Adolescents: Including the Fetus and Young Adult.* 8th ed. Lippincott Williams & Wilkins; 2012:1573.

Carvalho JS. Fetal dysrhythmias. *Best Pract Res Clin Obstet Gynaecol.* 2019;58:28–41.

Casiero D, Frishman WH. Cardiovascular complications of eating disorders. *Cardiol Rev.* 2006;14(5):227–231.

Collins KK, Van Hare GF, Kertesz NJ, et al. Pediatric nonpost-operative junctional ectopic tachycardia medical management and interventional therapies. *J Am Coll Cardiol.* 2009;53(8):690–697.

Costello JM, Alexander ME, Greco KM, et al. Lyme carditis in children: Presentation, predictive factors, and clinical course. *Pediatrics.* 2009;123:e835–e841.

Decker JA, Rossano JW, Smith EO, et al. Risk factors and mode of death in isolated hypertrophic cardiomyopathy in children. *J Am Coll Cardiol.* 2009;54(3):250–254.

Denfield SW, Rosenthal G, Gajarski RJ, et al. Restrictive cardiomyopathies in childhood. Etiologies and natural history. *Tex Heart Inst J.* 1997;24(1):38–44.

Donofrio MT, Moon-Grady AJ, Hornberger LK, et al. Diagnosis and treatment of fetal cardiac disease: A scientific statement from the American Heart Association. *Circulation.* 2014;129(21):2183–2242.

Ellenbogen KA, Wood MA. *Cardiac Pacing and ICDs.* 5th ed. Wiley-Blackwell; 2008.

Fogoros R. *Electrophysiologic Testing.* 4th ed. Wiley-Blackwell Publishers; 2012.

Haverkamp W, Rolf S, Eckardt L, et al. Long QT syndrome and Brugada syndrome: Drugs, ablation or ICD? *Herz.* 2005;30(2):111–118.

Hirschhorn R, Arnold JJR. Glycogen storage disease type II: Acid alpha-glucosidase (acid maltase) deficiency. In: Scriver C, Beaudet A, Sly W, et al., eds. *The Metabolic and Molecular Bases of Inherited Disease.* 8th ed. McGraw-Hill; 2001:3389–3420.

Jayaprasad N, Francis J. Atrial fibrillation and hyperthyroidism. *Indian Pacing Electrophysiol J.* 2005;5:305–311.

Jost CHA, Connolly HM, Danielson GK, et al. Sinus venosus atrial septal defect long-term postoperative outcome for 115 patients. *Circulation.* 2005;112:1953–1958.

Khairy P, Harris L, Landzberg MJ, et al. Implantable cardioverter-defibrillators in tetralogy of Fallot. *Circulation.* 2008;117:363–370.

Kishnani PS, Hwu W-L, Mandel H, et al. A retrospective, multinational, multicenter study on the natural history of infantile-onset Pompe disease. *J Pediatr.* 2006;148:671–676.

Kleinman CS. Prenatal diagnosis and management of intrauterine arrhythmias. *Fetal Ther.* 1986;1:92–95.

Kugler JD, Danford DA, Gumbiner CH. Ventricular fibrillation during transesophageal atrial pacing in an infant with Wolff–Parkinson–White syndrome. *Pediatr Cardiol.* 1991;12(1):36–38.

Laitinen PJ, Brown KM, Piippo K, et al. Mutations of the cardiac ryanodine receptor (RyR2) gene in familial polymorphic ventricular tachycardia. *Circulation.* 2001;103:485–490.

Lehnart SE, Ackerman MJ, Benson DW Jr, et al. Inherited arrhythmias: A National Heart, Lung, and Blood Institute and Office of Rare Diseases workshop consensus report about the diagnosis, phenotyping, molecular mechanisms, and therapeutic approaches for primary cardiomyopathies of gene mutations affecting ion channel function. *Circulation.* 2007;116(20):2325–2345.

Murphy JG, Gersh BJ, Mair DD, et al. Long-term outcome in patients undergoing surgical repair of tetralogy of Fallot. *N Engl J Med.* 1993;329(9):593–599.

Olsson SB, Halperin JL. Prevention of stroke in patients with atrial fibrillation. *Semin Vasc Med.* 2005;5(3):285–292.

Ommen SR, Mital S, Burke MA, et al. 2020 AHA/ACC guideline for the diagnosis and treatment of patients with hypertrophic cardiomyopathy: Executive summary: A report of the American College of Cardiology/American Heart Association Joint Committee on Clinical Practice Guidelines. *Circulation.* 2020;142(25):e533–e557.

Paul T, Guccione P, Garson A Jr. Relation of syncope in young patients with Wolff–Parkinson–White syndrome to rapid ventricular response during atrial fibrillation. *Am J Cardiol.* 1990; 65:318–321.

Pediatric and Congenital Electrophysiology Society (PACES); Heart Rhythm Society (HRS); American College of Cardiology Foundation (ACCF); American Heart Association (AHA); American Academy of Pediatrics (AAP); Canadian Heart Rhythm Society (CHRS); Cohen MI, Triedman JK, Cannon BC, et al. PACES/HRS expert consensus statement on the management of the asymptomatic young patient with a Wolff-Parkinson-White (WPW, ventricular preexcitation) electrocardiographic pattern: Developed in partnership between the Pediatric and Congenital Electrophysiology Society (PACES) and the Heart Rhythm Society (HRS). Endorsed by the governing bodies of PACES, HRS, the American College of Cardiology Foundation (ACCF), the American Heart Association (AHA), the American Academy of Pediatrics (AAP), and the Canadian Heart Rhythm Society (CHRS). *Heart Rhythm.* 2012;9(6):1006–1024.

Petrov D, Petrov M. Widening of the QRS complex due to severe hyperkalemia as an acute complication of diabetic ketoacidosis. *J Emerg Med.* 2008;34:459–461.

Polak PE, Zulstra F, Roelandt JR. Indications for pacemaker implantation in the Kearns–Sayre syndrome. *Eur Heart J.* 1989;10:281–282.

Postema PG, Wolpert C, Amin AS, et al. Drugs and Brugada syndrome patients: Review of the literature, recommendations, and an up-to-date website (www.brugadadrugs.org). *Heart Rhythm.* 2009;6(9):1335–1341.

Shah MJ, Silka MJ, Silva JA, et al. 2021 PACES expert consensus statement on the indications and management of cardiovascular implantable electronic devices in pediatric patients. *Cardiol Young.* 2021;31(11):1738–1769.

Shaw DB, Kekwick CA, Veale D, et al. Survival in second degree atrioventricular block. *Br Heart J.* 1985;53(6):587–593.

Sheldon RS, Grubb BP 2nd, Olshansky B, et al. 2015 Heart Rhythm Society expert consensus statement on the diagnosis and treatment of postural tachycardia syndrome, inappropriate sinus tachycardia, and vasovagal syncope. *Heart Rhythm.* 2015; 12(6):e41–e63.

Shen WK, Sheldon RS, Benditt DG, et al. 2017 ACC/AHA/HRS guideline for the evaluation and management of patients with syncope: A report of the American College of Cardiology/American Heart Association Task Force on Clinical Practice Guidelines and the Heart Rhythm Society. *Circulation.* 2017;136(5):e60–e122.

Tzivoni D, Banai S, Schuger C, et al. Treatment of torsade de pointes with magnesium sulfate. *Circulation.* 1988;77:392–397.

Viera AJ, Wouk N. Potassium disorders: Hypokalemia and hyperkalemia. *Am Fam Physician.* 2015;92(6):487–495.

Vrobel TR, Miller PE, Mostow ND, et al. A general overview of amiodarone toxicity: Its prevention, detection, and management. *Prog Cardiovasc Dis.* 1989;31(6):393–426.

Wren C. Cardiac arrhythmias in the fetus and newborn. *Semin Fetal Neonatal Med.* 2006;11(3):182–190.

Woosley RL, Heise CW, Gallo T, et al. QTdrugs List. *AZCERT, Inc.* 2021. http://www.crediblemeds.org

Exercise Physiology and Testing

Justin M. Horner, Sophia Pillai, and Thomas G. Allison

Questions

1. What is the most commonly accepted method of indexing maximum oxygen uptake (O_{2max}) in clinical pediatric exercise testing?

   A. Age
   B. Sex
   C. Lean body mass
   D. Body weight (kilograms)
   E. Exponent of body length (height)

2. Which method of exercise would achieve a higher maximum oxygen uptake (O_{2max})?

   A. Stationary electronically braked cycle ergometer
   B. Arm crank ergometer
   C. Hand grip ergometer
   D. Treadmill
   E. Stationary mechanically braked cycle ergometer

3. Which physiologic measure has the smallest increase with exercise?

   A. Heart rate (HR)
   B. Minute ventilation
   C. Stroke volume
   D. Respiratory rate
   E. Oxygen uptake

4. What cardiovascular changes would be expected during exercise?

	Cardiac output	HR	EF	Total peripheral resistance	Central venous pressure
A.	↑	↑	↑	↑	↑
B.	↑	↑	↑	↓	↑
C.	↑	↑	↑	↑	↓
D.	↑	↑	↑	↓	NC
E.	↑	↑	↑	↑	NC

5. Which blood pressure change would be expected in a normal 15-year-old male patient (resting blood pressure = 110/61 mm Hg) with isometric hand grip exercise?

   A. 150/60 mm Hg
   B. 155/55 mm Hg
   C. 120/40 mm Hg
   D. 170/65 mm Hg
   E. 140/110 mm Hg

6. Which peak exercise blood pressure would be expected in a normal 15-year-old male patient (resting blood pressure = 110/72 mm Hg) with maximal isotonic (cycle ergometer or treadmill) exercise?

   A. 200/100 mm Hg
   B. 130/60 mm Hg
   C. 120/68 mm Hg
   D. 124/76 mm Hg
   E. 170/50 mm Hg

7. What maximum HR and oxygen consumption would best represent a normal (untrained) 15-year-old female patient during maximal isotonic (cycle ergometer or treadmill) exercise?

	HR (bpm)	$\dot{V}O_{2max}$ (mL/kg/min)
A.	200	35
B.	140	25
C.	200	65
D.	200	25
E.	140	55

BONUS REVIEW

7.1. Based on the answer choices in Question 7, what maximum HR and oxygen consumption would best represent a 15-year-old female who was a cross-country champion and a patient with an unrepaired Ebstein anomaly?

8. A healthy 21-year-old woman without known heart disease who is not on medications just finished a treadmill exercise test. She exercised for a total of 6 minutes. The exercise physiologist questioned her effort. However, the patient claimed she "gave it her all." What is her expected maximal HR if she gave an intense effort?

   A. 123 bpm
   B. 158 bpm
   C. 183 bpm
   D. 196 bpm
   E. 229 bpm

9. As a normal child ages, what ventilatory changes at peak exercise would be expected?

	Maximum RR	Tidal volume	Minute ventilation ($\dot{V}_E$)
A.	↑	↔	↑
B.	↔	↑	↑
C.	↑	↑	↑
D.	↓	↑	↔
E.	↔	↔	↔

10. What cardiovascular changes would be expected with improved fitness?

	Stroke volume	HR (resting)	HR (max)	Cardiac output
A.	↑	↓	↑	↑
B.	↑	↑	↑	↑
C.	↑	↑	↔	↑
D.	↔	↓	↑	↔
E.	↑	↓	↔	↑

11. Choose the correct statement about units of work, power, and $\dot{V}_{O_2}$:

   A. 1 MET = 5.0 mL/kg/min
   B. Watts and MET hours are both measures of work performed
   C. Multiply watts by 6.12 to convert to kilopond meters (kpm)/min
   D. Body weight of the patient affects the MET level associated with a particular speed and grade on a treadmill test
   E. The same formula is used to predict $\dot{V}_{O_2}$ from work rate for both arm and leg cycle ergometry

12. Which condition would be considered "higher risk" for exercise testing?

   A. Atrial septal defect (ASD)
   B. Ventricular septal defect (VSD) with left-to-right shunt
   C. Primary pulmonary hypertension
   D. Severe aortic regurgitation
   E. Prior repair of tetralogy of Fallot

13. Which condition would be considered "lower risk" for exercise testing?

   A. Greater than moderate airway obstruction with baseline FEV_1 less than 60%
   B. Unexplained exertional syncope
   C. Hypertrophic obstructive cardiomyopathy with severe LVOT obstruction
   D. Documented long-QT syndrome
   E. Ebstein anomaly with severe tricuspid regurgitation

14. Which diagram is correct (**Figure 7.1**)? Four conditions are depicted.

   A. Figure 7.1A
   B. Figure 7.1B
   C. Figure 7.1C
   D. Figure 7.1D
   E. None of the above

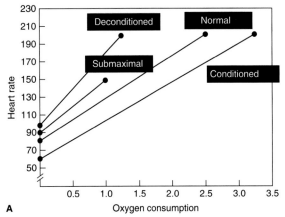

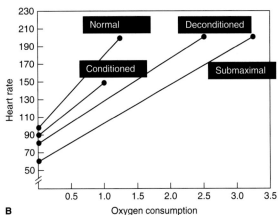

FIGURE 7.1 Oxygen consumption versus heart rate. (Derived from Pianosi PT, Driscoll DJ. Exercise testing. In: Allen HD, Driscoll DJ, Shaddy RE, et al., eds. *Moss & Adams' Heart Disease in Infants, Children, and Adolescents: Including the Fetus and Young Adult.* 8th ed. Wolters Kluwer; 2013. Figure 7.6.)

continued

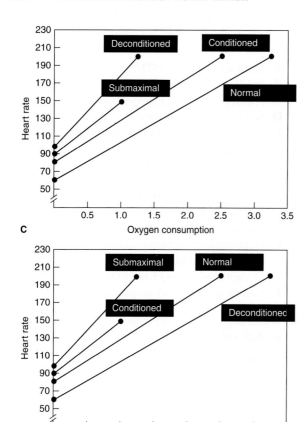

FIGURE 7.1 (continued)

15. Identify the correct statement regarding ventilatory anaerobic threshold (VAT).

  A. The VAT is the O_2 uptake at which there is a disproportionate decrease in CO_2 production and minute ventilation relative to oxygen uptake

  B. VAT is synonymous with the threshold for decompensated metabolic acidosis

  C. There is commonly a relative drop in lactate production when VAT is reached

  D. When VAT is reached, there is a decrease in mixed expired O_2 concentration

  E. During incremental exercise, VAT reflects the onset of anaerobic metabolism

16. As compared to a normal patient, an unrepaired, cyanotic patient at peak exercise will exhibit higher:

  A. Heart rate

  B. Ventilatory equivalent for O_2

  C. Blood oxygen saturation

  D. Maximum oxygen uptake

  E. Systolic blood pressure

17. Which statement is correct regarding an exercise protocol?

  A. Target duration of an exercise test should be between 15 and 20 minutes

  B. The Bruce and Balke protocols were developed specifically for exercise testing of children

  C. Ramp protocols feature small increments in workload updated frequently

  D. Exercise-testing protocols in which HR response to the first workload determines when to change stages and by how much are best for testing children.

  E. A ramp protocol is appropriate for assessing steady-state exercise

18. Which statement is correct regarding the ventilatory response to exercise?

  A. Total ventilation increases because of increased respiratory rate, while tidal volume remains constant during exercise

  B. Tidal volume increases predominately by tapping into the expiratory reserve volume

  C. $\dot{V}_E/\dot{V}CO_2$ declines early in exercise due to a reduction in respiratory dead space as a fraction of tidal volume

  D. Normal subjects terminate exercise because ventilation cannot increase further while cardiac output can continue to increase

  E. Diffusion limitation is a common problem during routine clinical exercise testing

19. Which of the following statements about exercise-testing techniques for noninvasive assessment of cardiac output is correct?

  A. Indirect Fick techniques to measure cardiac output during exercise require placement of a catheter in the right atrium via the jugular vein as in the direct Fick procedure

  B. Measurement of cardiac output is easier during treadmill exercise than during cycle ergometry

  C. The assumption that acetylene–helium technique approximates cardiac output would be valid despite a large atrial septal defect and left-to-right shunt

  D. The acetylene–helium technique is dependent on even distribution of inspired gas in the lungs

  E. The acetylene–helium technique to measure cardiac output is less well tolerated in children than the CO_2 rebreathing technique

20. Which of the following exercise-testing technique statements about blood pressure measurement is correct?

    A. Circling 60% of the patient's arm with the sphygmomanometer cuff is appropriate

    B. Sphygmomanometer cuff width equals 30% of the upper arm length

    C. A peak systolic blood pressure >200 mm Hg in a high school male cross-country runner performing a $\dot{V}O_2$ max exercise test is highly unusual and should be an indication to stop exercise

    D. Exercise blood pressure is higher in prepubertal versus postpubertal children

    E. A drop in systolic blood pressure in early active recovery is a normal finding during treadmill testing

21. A 20-year-old male, well-trained American football player (linebacker) underwent a treadmill exercise study midseason. Shortly thereafter, he sustained a lower limb injury and was unable to train for 3 months during recovery. He completed a second treadmill exercise test at the start of retraining after the injury was fully healed. Both exercise studies were maximum effort with peak respiratory exchange ratio (RER) >1.15 and rating of perceived exertion 19/20 on the Borg scale. Which data would best describe his situation?

		Test 1	Test 2
A.	HR (bpm) maximum	200	150
B.	Maximum $\dot{V}O_2$ (mL/kg/min)	55	45
C.	Maximum $\dot{V}E$ (L/min)	80	70
D.	Maximum O_2 saturation (%)	98	92
E.	Maximum $\dot{V}O_2$ (mL/kg/min)	75	65

22. In a healthy 15-year-old female without lung disease who gave maximum effort on spirometry before exercise testing, which statement about maximal voluntary ventilation (MVV) is correct?

    A. MVV is reliably measured as it is independent of subject effort

    B. Maximal $\dot{V}E$ <70% of resting MVV suggests pulmonary limitation to exercise

    C. MVV is ~35 to 40 times FEV_1

    D. MVV is typically measured during early exercise

    E. MVV can also detect vocal cord dysfunction as a cause for exertional dyspnea

23. In healthy patients, which of the following is a normal physiologic response during treadmill or cycle ergometer exercise?

    A. Increased end-systolic volume

    B. Increased diastolic pressure

    C. Among similar-sized children, girls have a higher peak systolic blood pressure than boys

    D. African-American children have a higher blood pressure response to exercise when compared to Caucasian children

    E. Blood pressure increases during exercise are due to increased systemic resistance

24. Which patient would be a good candidate for the use of acetylene–helium rebreathing technique during exercise testing for the measurement of cardiac output?

    A. A 15-year-old boy with Ebstein anomaly and a large secundum ASD with right-to-left shunt

    B. A 12-year-old girl s/p Fontan operation with arteriovenous pulmonary fistulas

    C. A 14-year-old boy with a patent foramen ovale with trivial left-to-right shunt

    D. An 8-year-old boy with a moderate membranous ventricular septal defect with left-to-right shunt

    E. A 10-year-old girl with a persistent left superior vena cava and unroofed coronary sinus

25. During exercise stress testing, what direct measurement can be performed by using acetylene–helium rebreathing technique?

    A. Systemic blood flow

    B. Pulmonary oxygen exchange

    C. Cardiac output

    D. Shunt volume

    E. Effective pulmonary blood flow

26. In a healthy, normal child, what organ system is most commonly responsible for limiting maximal achievable workload?

    A. Pulmonary

    B. Cardiovascular

    C. Musculoskeletal

    D. Neurologic

    E. Gastrointestinal

27. The calculation of work can be completed with which equation?

    A. Work = force × distance

    B. Work = force/distance

    C. Work = distance/force

    D. Work = mass × acceleration

    E. Work = mass/acceleration

28. Which statement about exercise-testing physiology is correct?

    A. An increase in stroke volume is the major determinant of an increased cardiac output during exercise in a normal patient

    B. Girls, particularly after puberty, have a slightly lower HR when compared to boys at any given workload

    C. For patients >20 years of age, maximum HR decreases progressively with age

    D. For patients >20 years of age, maximum HR increases with level of conditioning

    E. Total systemic vascular resistance increases with increased workload

29. Assuming a maximal effort achieved and structurally normal hearts, which of the following patients would likely result in a higher maximal $\dot{V}o_2$ (as measured in mL/kg/min)?

    A. A 17-year-old female performing leg cycle ergometer test
    B. A 17-year-old male performing leg cycle ergometer test
    C. A 19-year-old anemic male (hemoglobin 10 g/dL) performing leg cycle ergometer test
    D. An 11-year-old male performing leg cycle ergometer test
    E. A 19-year-old male performing arm ergometer test

30. Which of the following echocardiographic findings would be most consistent with the heart of a well-trained, normal athlete?

    A. Decreased left ventricular end-diastolic dimension
    B. Decreased left ventricular wall thickness
    C. Decreased stroke volume
    D. Increased left ventricular end-diastolic volume
    E. Increased left ventricular end-systolic dimension

31. Which of the following patients with congenital heart disease would likely have a normal maximal $\dot{V}o_2$ (as measured in mL/kg/min) for age and sex (assume all are at normal weight)?

    A. Long-QT syndrome type 1 treated with nadolol 80 mg daily
    B. Congenitally corrected TGA (ccTGA)
    C. Bicuspid aortic valve with mild regurgitation
    D. Unrepaired Ebstein anomaly
    E. Unrepaired Scimitar syndrome with two anomalous pulmonary veins

32. Which of the following conditions is not considered a higher risk to exercise testing in a pediatric patient?

    A. Second-degree AV block
    B. Asymptomatic severe aortic stenosis
    C. Catecholaminergic polymorphic ventricular tachycardia (CPVT)
    D. Long QT syndrome
    E. Anomalous origin of a coronary artery

33. Which of the following statements comparing treadmill exercise testing to cycle ergometry is correct?

    A. Cycle ergometry–derived maximum oxygen uptake ($\dot{V}o_{2max}$) is higher than treadmill testing
    B. Noise and artifact are less during treadmill exercise testing
    C. Treadmill allows for a better work measurement to perform measures like cardiac output assessment or exercise flow-volume loops than cycle ergometer
    D. Cycle ergometry is potentially more dangerous than treadmill ergometry
    E. Younger children (4 to 6 years of age) often require a special pediatric cycle ergometer

34. Which statement is most accurate regarding aortic stenosis (AS) and exercise stress testing?

    A. Exercise capacity has a positive linear relationship with transaortic pressure gradient in AS
    B. There is a greater increase in systolic blood pressure with exercise in AS when compared to normal patients
    C. The higher the transaortic pressure gradient, the lower the expected ST segment change during exercise
    D. The higher the transaortic gradient, the higher the maximum oxygen uptake ($\dot{V}o_{2max}$) achievable
    E. Exercise capacity has an inverse relationship with transaortic pressure gradient

35. Which exercise-testing statement would be most correct in an 8-year-old boy with pulmonary atresia, ventricular septal defect, and a systemic arterial-to-pulmonary arterial anastomosis?

    A. Achievement of normally expected maximum aerobic power
    B. Normal ventilation relative to oxygen uptake ($\dot{V}o_2$) and $\dot{V}co_2$
    C. Blood oxygen saturation is low at rest but improves with exercise
    D. Complete repair would improve the blood oxygen saturation at rest and with exercise
    E. Complete repair would allow patients to achieve $\dot{V}o_{2max}$ equal or even superior to normal patients

36. Which statement is consistent with an appropriate exercise technique for evaluating pediatric patients with clinically significant or suspected heart disease?

    A. Only two surface electrocardiographic (ECG) leads need to be recorded during the exercise study
    B. A complete 12-lead ECG, along with a rhythm strip in one or two leads, should be obtained at rest, at the end of each workload, and several times in active and passive recovery
    C. Avoid placing electrodes above bone, as that will distort the signal
    D. Diastolic blood pressure measurement is typically made with ease during treadmill ergometry
    E. Direct blood pressure measurement in the radial artery underestimates the central aortic blood pressure

37. As compared to an acyanotic patient, a cyanotic patient at peak exercise will exhibit a higher:

    A. Heart rate
    B. Ventilatory equivalent for oxygen
    C. Arterial blood oxygen saturation
    D. Arterial pCO_2
    E. Diastolic blood pressure

38. Using the CO_2 rebreathing technique during an exercise study, which statement is most correct?

A. The CO_2 rebreathing technique is well tolerated by all patients and is noninvasive

B. The CO_2 concentration in the rebreathing technique does not need to be adjusted for the patient's size and exercise intensity

C. The CO_2 rebreathing technique does not obtain enough information to use the Fick principle for determining the cardiac output

D. The instrument dead space in the tubing does not need to be accounted for

E. The CO_2 rebreathing technique can be completed noninvasively by using the Bohr equation

39. A 20-year-old female with congenital complete heart block is now A-sensed, V-paced. She also has a known coronary anomaly with RCA coming off the left coronary cusp. She performs an exercise test. As her ventricular rate reaches 180 bpm, she begins to drop beats, and the HR ultimately slows down to about 120 bpm, limiting exercise, and returns to 180 during minute 2 of active recovery. What is your diagnosis of the problem?

A. The ventricular lead is not sensing properly

B. The patient is having frequent sinus pauses

C. Pacemaker Wenckebach

D. SA node ischemia due to RCA compression between aorta and pulmonary artery

E. Pacemaker battery problem—schedule replacement

*For the following five questions, correctly match the patient with the graphic exercise data in Tests A–F (**Figure 7.2**). All patients are of normal weight, young adults aged 18 to 26. The exercise data include HR (red) in bpm, $\dot{V}o_2$ (green), and $\dot{V}co_2$ (blue)—both in mL/min. The predicted $\dot{V}o_2$ is given as a green dashed horizontal line.*

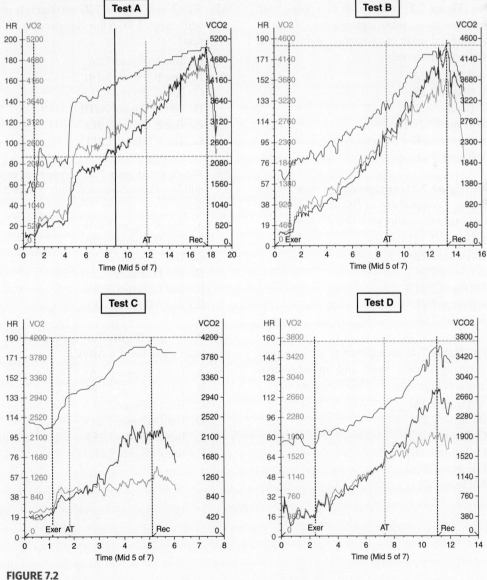

FIGURE 7.2

continued

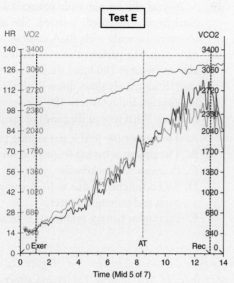
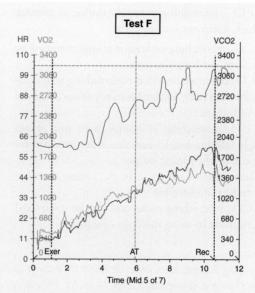

FIGURE 7.2 (continued)

40. Which test (**Figure 7.2**) corresponds to a young man with severe neo-aortic valve regurgitation, s/p prior Ross procedure and repair of coarctation of the aorta in setting of Shone syndrome?

A. Test A (Figure 7.2A)
B. Test B (Figure 7.2B)
C. Test C (Figure 7.2C)
D. Test D (Figure 7.2D)
E. Test E (Figure 7.2E)
F. Test F (Figure 7.2F)

41. Which test (**Figure 7.2**) corresponds to a male college basketball player complaining of fatigue and found to have dilated cardiomyopathy with LVEF = 46%?

A. Test A (Figure 7.2A)
B. Test B (Figure 7.2B)
C. Test C (Figure 7.2C)
D. Test D (Figure 7.2D)
E. Test E (Figure 7.2E)
F. Test F (Figure 7.2F)

42. Which test (**Figure 7.2**) corresponds to a young man with structurally normal heart and mitochondrial myopathy due to heterozygous YARS-2 mutation?

A. Test A (Figure 7.2A)
B. Test B (Figure 7.2B)
C. Test C (Figure 7.2C)
D. Test D (Figure 7.2D)
E. Test E (Figure 7.2E)
F. Test F (Figure 7.2F)

43. Which test (**Figure 7.2**) corresponds to a young man with repaired TGA but experiencing SA node dysfunction?

A. Test A (Figure 7.2A)
B. Test B (Figure 7.2B)
C. Test C (Figure 7.2C)
D. Test D (Figure 7.2D)
E. Test E (Figure 7.2E)
F. Test F (Figure 7.2F)

44. Which test (**Figure 7.2**) corresponds to an elite female middle distance runner with a structurally normal heart?

A. Test A (Figure 7.2A)
B. Test B (Figure 7.2B)
C. Test C (Figure 7.2C)
D. Test D (Figure 7.2D)
E. Test E (Figure 7.2E)
F. Test F (Figure 7.2F)

45. Which test (**Figure 7.2**) corresponds to a recent male heart transplant for ARVC?

A. Test A (Figure 7.2A)
B. Test B (Figure 7.2B)
C. Test C (Figure 7.2C)
D. Test D (Figure 7.2D)
E. Test E (Figure 7.2E)
F. Test F (Figure 7.2F)

46. Which of the following is not a recommended indication for exercise testing in pediatric patients?

  A. Evaluate specific signs or symptoms that are induced or aggravated by exercise

  B. Assess or identify abnormal responses to exercise in children with cardiac, pulmonary, or other organ disorders, including the presence of myocardial ischemia and arrhythmias

  C. Assess efficacy of specific medical or surgical treatments

  D. Assess functional capacity for recreational, athletic, and vocational activities

  E. Required part of the pre-participation screening for all athletes <18 years of age

47. Exercise-induced cardiac remodeling can produce a series of characteristic ECG findings considered "normal." Which of these findings on the resting ECG would be considered a normal response to exercise training in a 15-year-old black male 800-m runner?

  A. Mobitz type II second-degree block

  B. Left bundle branch block (LBBB)

  C. Resting heart rate of 40 bpm with junctional rhythm

  D. T-wave inversions in leads V1–V6

  E. Ventricular bigeminy

48. Which of the following statements about cardiac channelopathies is correct?

  A. Brugada pattern frequently disappears during exercise

  B. In long-QT syndrome type 2, the QT interval may appear normal but is highly subject to drug-induced prolongation

  C. In catecholaminergic polymorphic ventricular tachycardia (CPVT), PVCs may appear throughout exercise and active recovery

  D. As many as 50% of deaths in long-QT 3 occur during heavy exercise

  E. Amiodarone is the first line of treatment for long-QT 1

*For the next five questions, please select the correct resting ECG (**Figure 7.3A–E**) to the patient.*

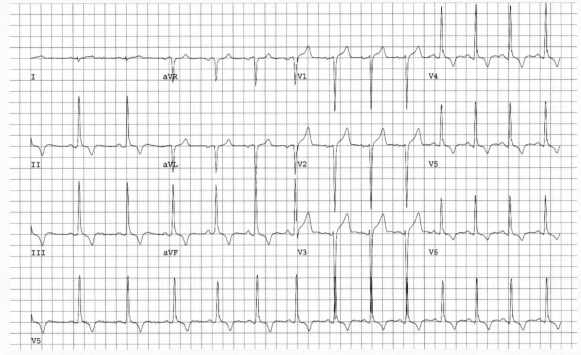

A

FIGURE 7.3A

continued

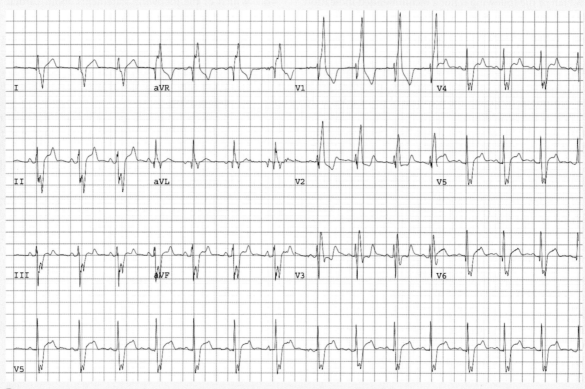

B

FIGURE 7.3B

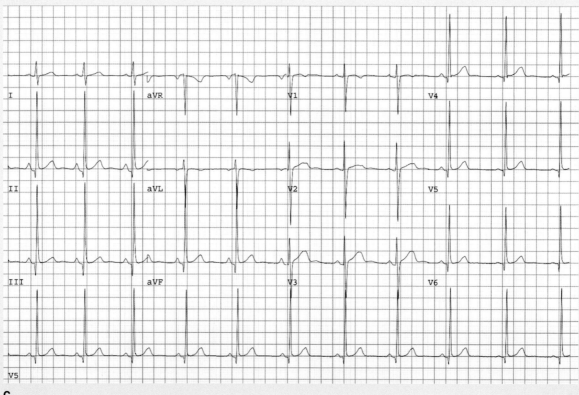

C

FIGURE 7.3C

continued

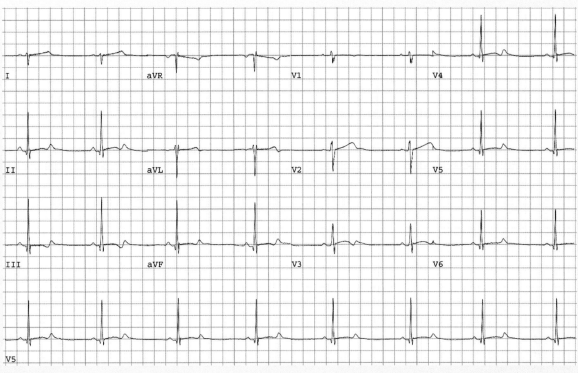

D

FIGURE 7.3D

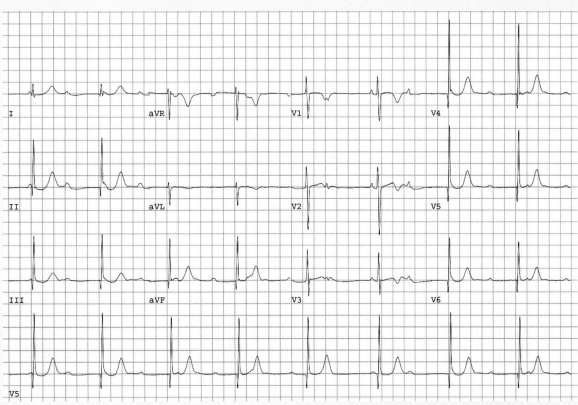

E

FIGURE 7.3E

continued

49. Which ECG corresponds to a normal pediatric ECG in a 15 year old male soccer player?

  A. Figure 7.3A
  B. Figure 7.3B
  C. Figure 7.3C
  D. Figure 7.3D
  E. Figure 7.3E

50. What ECG corresponds to a 19-year-old African-American male basketball player with hypertrophic obstructive cardiomyopathy (HOCM)?

  A. Figure 7.3A
  B. Figure 7.3B
  C. Figure 7.3C
  D. Figure 7.3D
  E. Figure 7.3E

51. Which ECG corresponds to a 10-year-old male baseball player with congenital complete heart block?

  A. Figure 7.3A
  B. Figure 7.3B
  C. Figure 7.3C
  D. Figure 7.3D
  E. Figure 7.3E

52. Which ECG corresponds to a 20-year-old female cross-country runner with long-QT 3?

  A. Figure 7.3A
  B. Figure 7.3B
  C. Figure 7.3C
  D. Figure 7.3D
  E. Figure 7.3E

53. Which ECG shows an Ebstein anomaly in a 19-year-old male with severe tricuspid regurgitation massive right atrial enlargement?

  A. Figure 7.3A
  B. Figure 7.3B
  C. Figure 7.3C
  D. Figure 7.3D
  E. Figure 7.3E

54. **Figure 7.4** shows peak exercise ECG in an 18-year-old woman referred for evaluation of exercise intolerance.

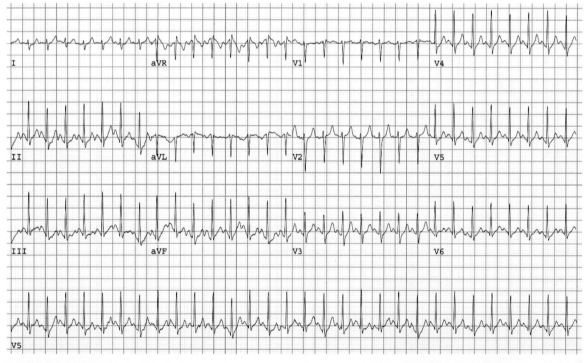

FIGURE 7.4

Which of the following is her likely diagnosis?

A. Postural orthostatic tachycardia syndrome (POTS)
B. Catecholaminergic polymorphic ventricular tachycardia (CPVT)
C. Hypertrophic obstructive cardiomyopathy (HOCM)
D. Mobitz II AV block
E. Wolff–Parkinson–White (WPW) syndrome

*For the next five questions, please select the exercise-induced arrhythmia (shown in **Figure 7.5A–E**) to the diagnosis.*

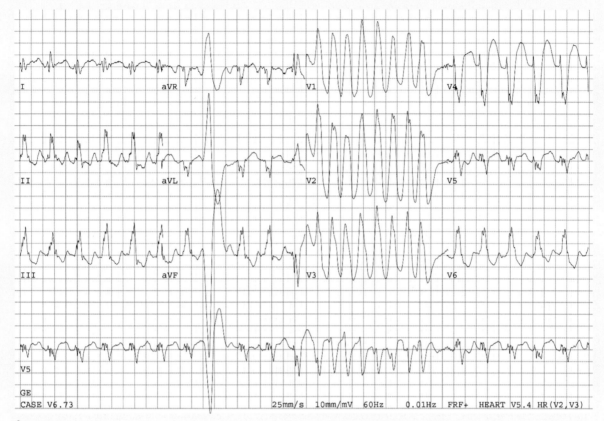

A

FIGURE 7.5A

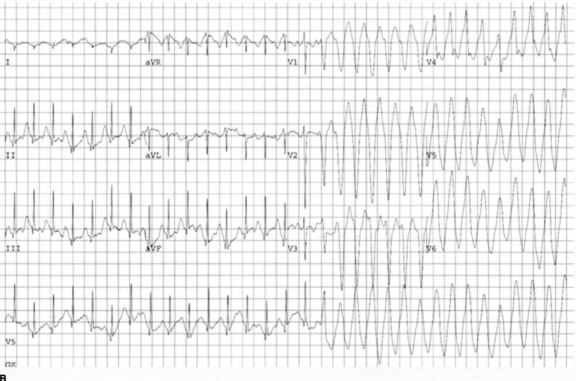

B

FIGURE 7.5B

continued

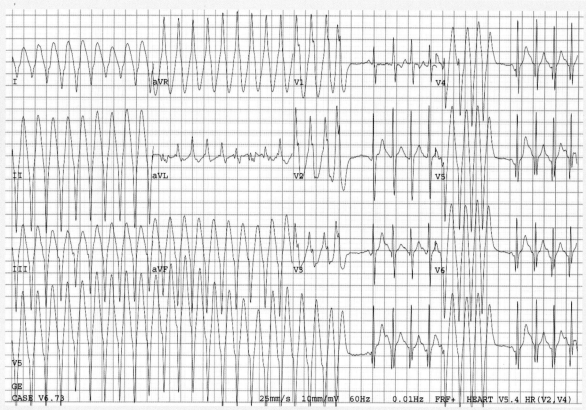

C

FIGURE 7.5C

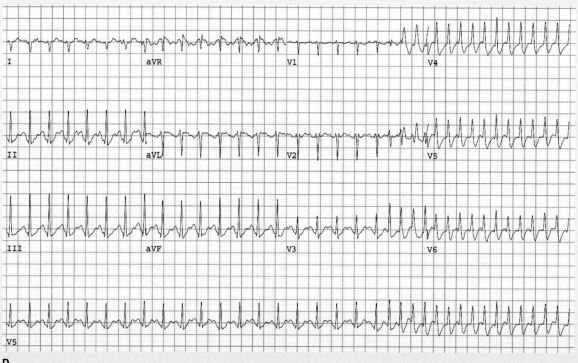

D

FIGURE 7.5D

continued

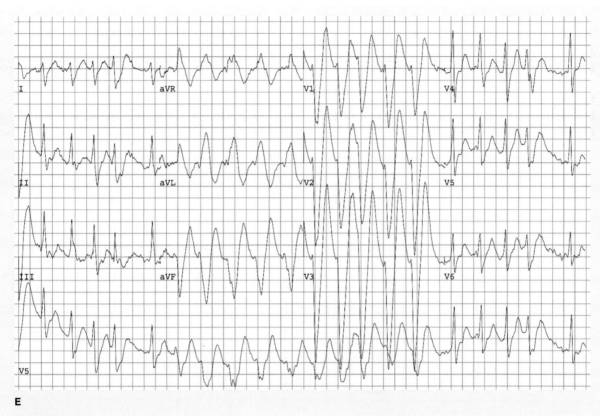

E

FIGURE 7.5E

55. A 21-year-old male with hypertrophic obstructive cardiomyopathy (HOCM) post myectomy.

A. Figure 7.5A
B. Figure 7.5B
C. Figure 7.5C
D. Figure 7.5D
E. Figure 7.5E

56. A 19-year-old male basketball player with dilated cardiomyopathy.

A. Figure 7.5A
B. Figure 7.5B
C. Figure 7.5C
D. Figure 7.5D
E. Figure 7.5E

57. A 20-year-old female swing dancer with WPW with orthodromic reciprocating tachycardia.

A. Figure 7.5A
B. Figure 7.5B
C. Figure 7.5C
D. Figure 7.5D
E. Figure 7.5E

58. A 17-year-old male soccer player with CPVT and flecainide-induced wide-complex SVT.

A. Figure 7.5A
B. Figure 7.5B
C. Figure 7.5C
D. Figure 7.5D
E. Figure 7.5E

59. An 18-year-old female volleyball player with fascicular VT with structurally normal heart.

A. Figure 7.5A
B. Figure 7.5B
C. Figure 7.5C
D. Figure 7.5D
E. Figure 7.5E

60. All but which one of the following conditions might likely result in a high $\dot{V}_E/\dot{V}CO_2$ during exercise?

  A. Volitional hyperventilation
  B. Hypertrophic cardiomyopathy with an instantaneous peak gradient of 80 mm Hg and LVEF of 75%
  C. Chronic thromboembolic pulmonary hypertension
  D. Interstitial lung disease with resting SpO_2 of 88%
  E. ASD with right-to-left shunt

61. After reviewing the rest and exercise ECG (**Figure 7.6**) on this 19-year-old white male, what is your diagnosis?

  A. Long-QT syndrome type 1
  B. Arrhythmogenic right ventricular cardiomyopathy (ARVC)
  C. SVT with LBBB aberrancy
  D. Ischemic VT from an anomalous left coronary artery
  E. Catecholaminergic polymorphic ventricular tachycardia (CPVT)

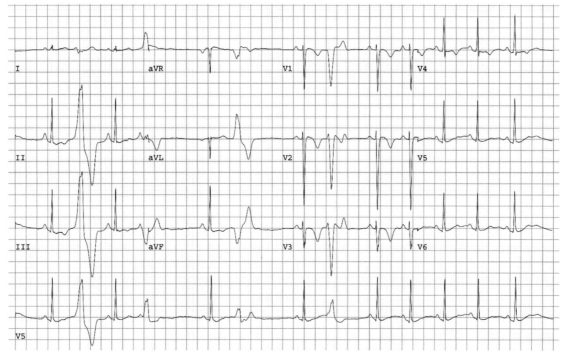

A

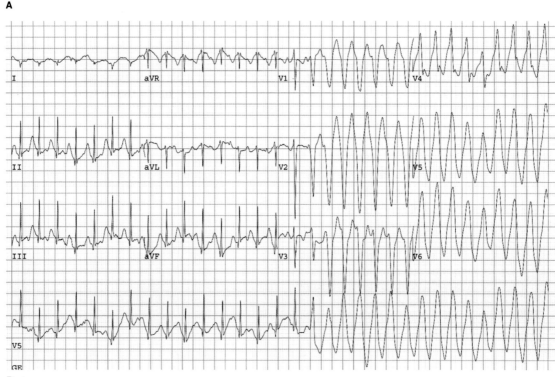

B

FIGURE 7.6

62. How would you interpret this ECG (**Figure 7.7**) at peak exercise on an 8-year-old boy?

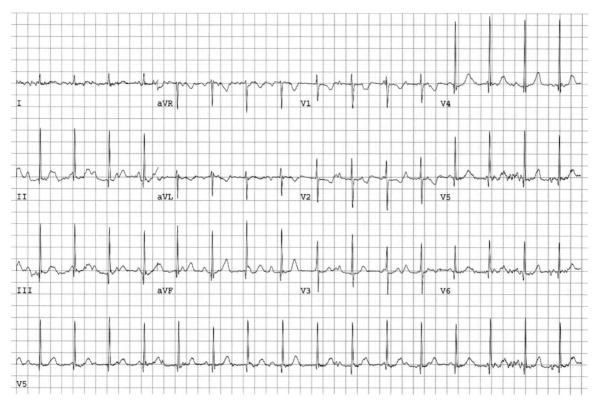

FIGURE 7.7

A. Second-degree AV block Mobitz type I
B. Normal exercise ECG; low peak HR due to poor effort or excessive beta blockade
C. Third-degree AV block
D. Second-degree AV block Mobitz type II
E. Atrial tachycardia with second-degree AV block

63. Nuclear stress testing to determine myocardial perfusion is being increasingly employed in pediatric patients, especially as more and more children undergo surgical procedures which report some late consequences producing ischemia. All but which one of these conditions might be an indication for myocardial perfusion imaging?

A. An 18-year-old girl reports chest pain during 400-m races in track. CTA shows an anomalous RCA coming off the left coronary cusp with a slit-like orifice and long intramural segment.
B. An 11-year-old girl reports chest pain and reduced performance during age group swimming meets. She was born with anomalous left coronary artery from the pulmonary artery (ALCAPA) which was repaired using a Gortex graft at age 3 months.
C. A 17-year old boy with Ebstein anomaly continues to experience exercise intolerance after tricuspid valve repair.
D. A 15-year-old female equestrian complains of chest pain during gym class and has ST abnormalities on an exercise test. Six-weeks prior she suffered a mid-chest contusion with a large bruise as a result of being kicked by her horse
E. A 7-year-old boy reports reduced exercise capacity and experiences syncope while playing soccer. He was born with D-transposition of the great arteries and underwent an arterial switch operation during infancy.

64. A 19-year-old man from rural Wisconsin performs an exercise test as part of a workup for syncope while performing farm work. The ECG at peak exercise is shown in **Figure 7.8A**, along with a repeat test done 3 months later (**Figure 7.8B**).

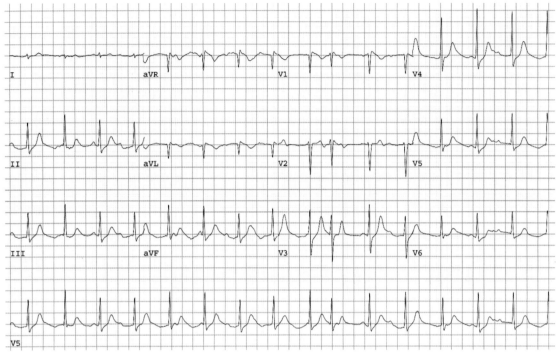

A

FIGURE 7.8A

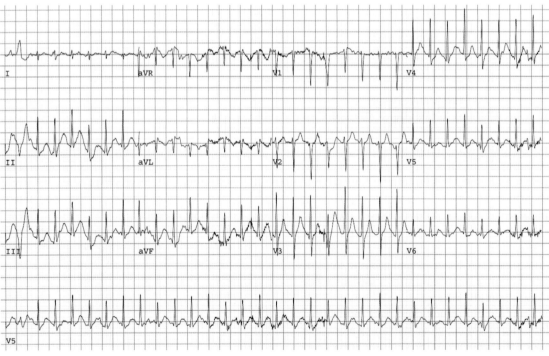

B

FIGURE 7.8B

What is the most likely scenario explaining these findings?

A. His beta blocker was stopped

B. He underwent radiofrequency (RF) ablation

C. A permanent pacemaker was implanted

D. Myocardial bridge of the mid-LAD was surgically unroofed

E. Lyme disease resolved with ceftriaxone therapy

65. A 13-year-old boy performs an exercise test, which he tolerated well without symptoms other than fatigue. How would you interpret the peak exercise ECG shown in **Figure 7.9**?

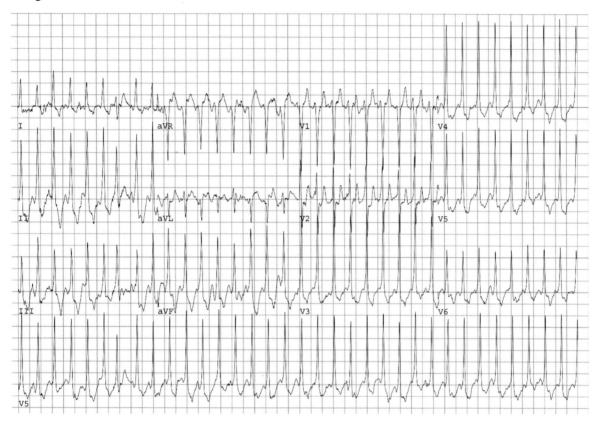

FIGURE 7.9

A. Normal peak HR for age with pre-excitation indicating Wolff–Parkinson–White (WPW) syndrome
B. Hypertrophic obstructive cardiomyopathy (HOCM)
C. Myocardial ischemia
D. Atrial fibrillation
E. Right ventricular outflow tract (RVOT) VT

66. Review the graphic data from the cardiopulmonary exercise test (**Figure 7.10**) on a 20-year-old woman and decide on the most likely diagnosis. Dashed horizontal lines represent (going clockwise from top left): maximal voluntary ventilation; predicted $\dot{V}o_{2max}$; the upper limit of the $\dot{V}_E/\dot{V}co_2$ nadir; and predicted oxygen pulse.

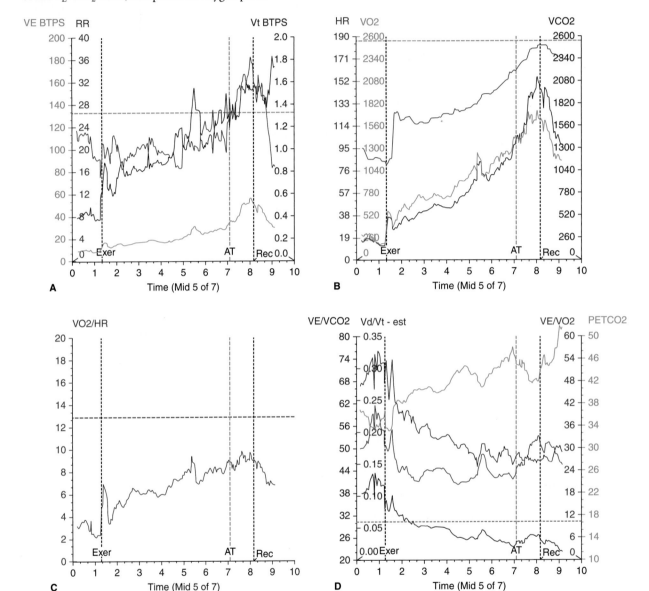

FIGURE 7.10

A nine-panel plot (**Figure 7.11**) is also supplied for review.

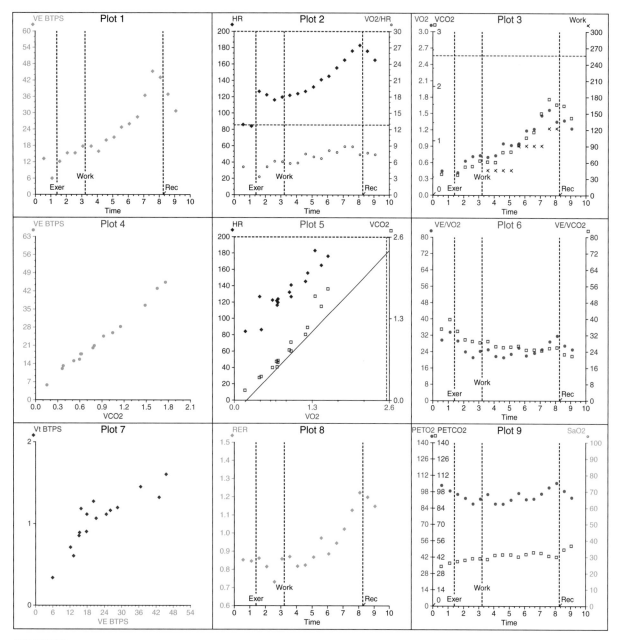

FIGURE 7.11

A. Normal test on healthy young woman with average cardiorespiratory fitness
B. Reduced peak Vo_2 due to limited breathing reserve secondary to uncontrolled asthma
C. Thromboembolic pulmonary hypertension
D. Poor effort
E. Pulmonary regurgitation

67. Review the graphic data from the cardiopulmonary exercise test (**Figure 7.12**) on a 12-year-old boy who is 149.5 cm tall—50th percentile for age, and a weight of 36.5 kg—only at the 25th percentile for weight. Decide on the most likely diagnosis. Dashed horizontal lines represent (going clockwise from top left): maximal voluntary ventilation; predicted $\dot{V}o_{2max}$; the upper limit of the $\dot{V}_E/\dot{V}co_2$ nadir; and predicted oxygen pulse.

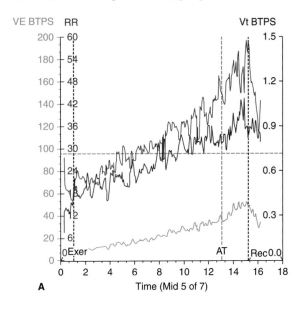

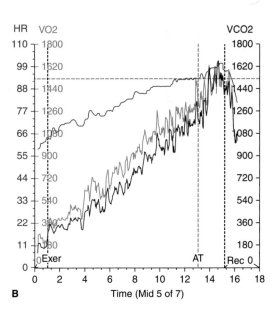

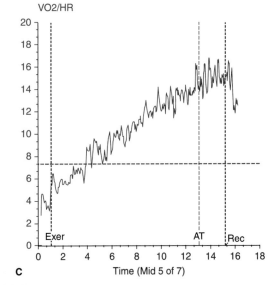

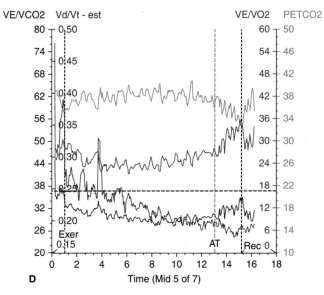

FIGURE 7.12

A nine-panel plot (**Figure 7.13**) is also supplied for review.

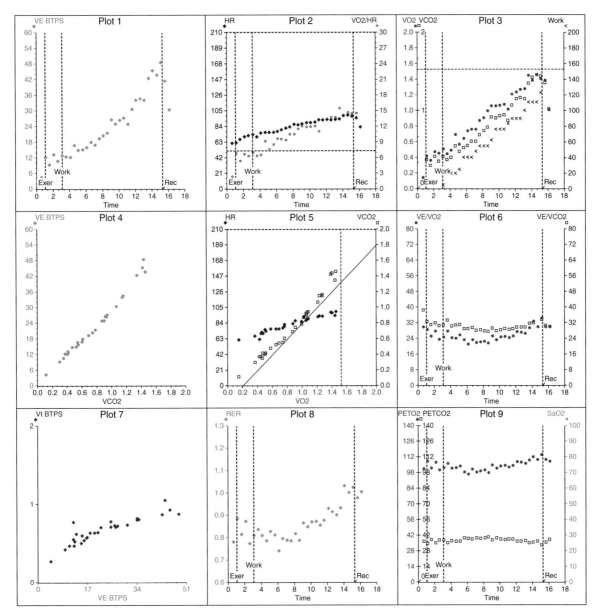

FIGURE 7.13

A. Congenitally corrected TGA (ccTGA)
B. Soccer player with no cardiac or pulmonary disease
C. Long-QT syndrome type 1
D. Ebstein anomaly
E. Bicuspid aortic valve with moderate regurgitation

68. A 16-year-old high school student undergoes CPET spirometry for evaluation of exertional dyspnea. He has a remote history of viral induced wheezing during early childhood. Chest x-ray and baseline spirometry are normal. He is not taking any medications. Which of the following would be consistent with exercise-induced bronchoconstriction (EIB)?

  A. The symptoms of EIB are fairly typical and specific to exercise triggers and have a good correlation to objective assessments

  B. EIB symptoms are thought to occur within 5 minutes of peak exercise with a rapid resolution of symptoms once the exercise trigger is stopped

  C. Airway response to exercise defines EIB as a fall in FVC of >10% from baseline spirometry assessments.

  D. The pathophysiology of EIB includes airway narrowing thought to be brought on by rapid exchange of air with the bronchial wall mucosa and smooth muscles causing dehydration, rapid cooling of the airway surfaces, and release of mast cell–related inflammatory mediators

  E. Children with EIB are recommended to refrain from any form of physical exertion immediately prior to exercise as this may worsen the subsequent EIB symptoms

69. During a CPET test, which of the following features indicate a pulmonary origin to exercise limitation?

  A. A reduction in the breathing reserve to less than 20% of the predicted maximal ventilation is an indication of pulmonary limitation

  B. The maximal voluntary ventilation (MVV) is a reproducible maneuver and fairly representative of the ventilatory response during incremental exercise

  C. Minute ventilation, the product of tidal volume and respiratory frequency is primarily driven by an increase in tidal volume during the latter part of the exercise

  D. With the minute ventilation increasing manyfold from baseline during incremental exercise, the exercise tidal volumes approach the resting inspiratory capacity

  E. End-tidal CO_2 ($ETCO_2$) values of >35 mm Hg at peak are considered abnormal and is suggestive of ventilatory limitation

70. Which of the following regarding arterial, alveolar, and end-tidal O_2 tensions and arterial oxygen saturations (SpO_2) is inaccurate?

  A. Arterial oxygen desaturations during exercise are common in disorders of pulmonary origin including pulmonary vascular disorders

  B. Arterial oxygen desaturation is defined as an absolute value of 88% or below or a decrease in oxygen saturation of more than 4% from resting values

  C. A right-to-left shunt may suddenly open causing an acute fall in O_2 saturation during progressive exercise

  D. Individuals with chronic heart failure frequently have oxygen desaturation due to ventilation–perfusion mismatch

  E. A transient fall in both the alveolar (PAO_2) and arterial (PaO_2) O_2 tension at the beginning of exercise is a normal phenomenon

Answers

1. (D) Body weight. Maximum oxygen uptake is closely related both to cardiac output, which in turn is related to heart size and blood volume, and the mass of the working muscles. The more work/exercise a patient does, the more oxygen uptake will be needed, and larger people with more muscle mass can perform more work. Age, sex, lean body mass, body weight, and height will thus to some degree each correlate with $\dot{V}_{O_{2max}}$, though body weight is generally the most common way of predicting $\dot{V}_{O_{2max}}$ in pediatric patients. Lean body mass would be more accurate but requires more extensive measurement issues. Postpubertal males tend to have a higher lean body mass than females, which causes differences in $\dot{V}_{O_{2max}}$ between the sexes, but there is also great variation within each sex, and younger children generally show less male–female difference in $\dot{V}_{O_{2max}}$ than older children. In children, muscle mass (and $\dot{V}_{O_{2max}}$) increases also changes with increasing age (and this is the usual way of referencing $\dot{V}_{O_{2max}}$ in adults, but $\dot{V}_{O_{2max}}$ is decreasing rather than increasing with age), though age can be misleading around the age of puberty. Previous studies have revealed an exponent of body length (1.5 to 3.21) has

also been unreliable, likely because body mass can vary considerably at any given height.

A caveat is that boys and girls diverge at puberty, with boys becoming taller and gaining muscle mass, whereas height in girls levels off and there is an increase in the weight or adipose tissue. Whereas $\dot{V}_{O_{2max}}$ is similar in young boys and girls and increases with weight in both sexes, there is generally a plateau in $\dot{V}_{O_{2max}}$ in girls between ages 12 and 18.

There are a couple of other complexities here. First, $\dot{V}_{O_{2max}}$ can be expressed in absolute (mL/min) or relative (mL/kg/min) terms. Cardiorespiratory fitness (CRF) is generally rated according to $\dot{V}_{O_{2max}}$ in mL/kg/min and will correlate well with treadmill performance (where excess weight is not a hindrance), whereas $\dot{V}_{O_{2max}}$ in mL/min correlates better with cycle performance (where excess weight is not a hindrance since the frame of the cycle bears with height and work is related only to the resistance of turning the pedals). A lean patient will thus outperform a heavier patient on the treadmill, whereas the opposite will occur on the cycle ergometer. To achieve a constancy of $\dot{V}_{O_2}$ in mL/kg/min versus time on a cycle protocol, workloads will need to be adjusted for weight, whereas this is not necessary for treadmill exercise.

Second, level of physical activity, particularly aerobic training, can markedly affect $\dot{V}o_{2max}$, perhaps by as much as 35% to 40%. This means that any indexing of $\dot{V}o_{2max}$ according to body weight, age, or any other variable will yield only modest correlations since varying levels of activity are so contributory.

2. (D) Cardiorespiratory or aerobic fitness is defined as the highest rate of oxygen consumption, $\dot{V}o_{2max}$, achieved during exercise. The highest $\dot{V}o_{2max}$ that can be achieved depends on the type of work performed and the muscle mass utilized during exercise. One uses more muscle groups when exercising on a treadmill—which requires energy expenditure to bear the patient's weight—than when using the ergometers listed in the question. On average, values for $\dot{V}o_{2max}$ in children, like adults are 5% to 15% higher on the treadmill than the cycle ergometer. Aerobic fitness data on children aged 8 years and above show that the absolute values ($\dot{V}o_2$ in L/min) or peak $\dot{V}o_2$ increases during childhood and mostly attributable to the increase in muscle mass and strength in both sexes.

3. (C) Stroke volume is dependent on the left ventricular end-diastolic volume and ejection fraction. Stroke volume increases 50% to 100% above baseline during exercise. Stroke volume primarily increases early in exercise (up to an HR of about 130 bpm) due to enhanced venous return and to a less extent, cardiac contractility, but will increase little thereafter as it becomes limited by progressively shorter diastolic filling time.

In comparison, HR increases two- to threefold—even higher for trained athletes who may have resting rates of <50 bpm with peak rates of 200 bpm or higher. Minute ventilation may increase more than 10-fold with exercise—due to a two- to threefold increase in respiratory rate and even larger increases in tidal volume. Oxygen consumption will have the greatest increase of all these physiologic variables, being the product of HR × stroke volume × arteriovenous oxygen difference, producing an overall increase of 10- to 20-fold from rest to peak exercise.

4. (D) In the normal patient, exercise is associated with an increase in cardiac output, HR, and ejection fraction. A decrease in the total peripheral resistance will occur, and no change occurs in central venous pressure. These changes primarily are due to the large increase in sympathetic activity during exercise. The decreased total peripheral resistance primarily is due to decreased skeletal muscle vascular resistance allowing more blood flow to the muscles. Sympathetic stimulation of the beta fibers in skeletal muscle, heart, and lungs cause dilatation of the arterioles, which more than compensates for the constriction produced by stimulation of alpha fibers in the skin and splanchnic beds. Finally, central venous pressure remains relatively unchanged due to the compensatory mechanisms of the skeletal muscle pump and the respiratory pump that both promote increased venous return without significant change in central venous pressure.

5. (E) Isometric exercise consists of constant muscle length (no change) against a force/tension. Examples include holding a weight in a fixed position, pushing against a door frame, or hand grip exercise. During isometric exercise, systolic and diastolic blood pressure both increase significantly. In isotonic exercise, like cycling or walking/running, however, cardiac output increases while peripheral resistance decreases.

6. (E) During isotonic exercise, systolic blood pressure increases due to increased cardiac output (with more forceful ejection of larger boluses of blood into the aorta). The systolic blood pressure increase during exercise is attenuated, however, by a reduction in total systemic resistance. Diastolic blood pressure normally decreases by at least 10 mm Hg with exercise. (Note: Measurement of diastolic blood pressure during exercise can be challenging, and the laboratory must decide on recording the 4th or 5th Korotkoff phase or both.) Blood pressure changes depend on the patient's size as well as gender. Larger patients and/or males will have a higher blood pressure at rest and during exercise compared to smaller patients and/or females. Because of greater arterial compliance, exercise blood pressures are generally lower in children than adults. Higher exercise blood pressures are typically seen during cycle ergometry (due to contribution isometric grip on the handlebars) versus the treadmill.

7. (A) There is a linear relationship between HR and $\dot{V}o_{2max}$ until maximum workload is reached. Every individual has a maximum HR that is achievable, usually ranging between 195 and 215 bpm in adolescents. Normal oxygen consumption ($\dot{V}o_{2max}$) is roughly 35 (females) to 45 mL/kg/min (males), though higher $\dot{V}o_{2max}$ would be seen in athletes. Therefore, an HR of 200 bpm and oxygen consumption of 45 mL/kg/min would be normal for a 15 year old. HR of 145 bpm and oxygen consumption of 1.0 L/min would represent a submaximal exercise test/effort or chronotropic insufficiency.

BONUS REVIEW ——————————————

7.1. The answers to the bonus review questions are **(C)** for the cross-country champion, and **(D)** for the unrepaired Ebstein patient. Neither of these conditions—endurance training nor atrialization of the right ventricle—should significantly affect exercise HR (unless the Ebstein patient has accessory-pathway–mediated tachycardia), whereas $\dot{V}o_{2max}$ will improve with endurance training, while severe tricuspid regurgitation will reduce right ventricular cardiac output, significantly lowering peak $\dot{V}o_2$.

——————————————

8. (D) The accepted maximum HR for patients 5 to 20 years of age is roughly 195 to 215 bpm. However, for patients >20 years of age, various HR prediction equations might give estimates of peak HR for a 21-year-old female of 193 to 199 bpm. Therefore, the best estimate of this patient's maximum HR is 196 bpm. However, there is a large enough standard deviation in peak HR to make **(C)** 183 bpm a possible, though less probable, peak HR for this woman. Inability to keep up with the treadmill, sweating, and loud, labored breathing might be other signs that exercise was really maximal. These signs with a peak HR of only 123 **(A)** or 158 **(B)** might be a cause for further investigation, unless the electrocardiogram showed the abnormality (e.g., AV block). A peak HR of 229 **(E)** would again prompt close examination of the electrocardiogram, as this is suggestive of some form of supraventricular tachycardia (SVT).

We might also consider why the performance was so limited if the HR of 196 bpm (assuming sinus rhythm) was achieved, indicating a maximal effort. Obviously, severe obesity could be the cause or, conversely, an eating disorder if BMI was extremely low. A young woman of this age might also suffer from anemia, and recent, prolonged illness producing severe deconditioning and postural orthostatic tachycardia syndrome (POTS) could also cause a poor performance despite a good heart rate response.

9. (B) During exercise, minute ventilation increases to provide more oxygen and carbon dioxide exchange with the blood. This occurs by an increase in both ventilation frequency (respiratory rate) and tidal volume. Young children have relatively smaller lungs relative to height versus adults, and the lung volume increases with age, allowing for greater tidal volumes. Oxygen consumption also increases with growth and maturation, as there is a greater muscle mass to perform work and consume oxygen. This is what drives higher exercise ventilation. Tidal volume and ventilation during exercise will continue to increase with increasing age, at least until adult height and torso size are attained. However, the maximum respiratory rate that can be achieved at peak exercise is unchanged or may even decrease slightly. This is a consequence of increasing peak expiratory force with age, on one hand, but larger volumes of air to move, on the other hand.

10. (E) Regular, repetitive aerobic exercise will usually result in improved cardiorespiratory fitness and $\dot{V}o_{2max}$ fitness. Physiologic changes that occur with increased exercise include higher mass of mitochondria and aerobic enzymes in the trained muscles. This increases oxygen extraction and utilization at the tissue level. Heart volume and weight also increase, and there is an increased blood volume. These changes enhance stroke volume, and there is a secondary increase in vagal tone with decreased resting HR. With intense, prolonged training, there may also be some remodeling of the sodium and potassium channels in cardiac muscle, contributing further to a lower resting HR. Peak HR is generally unchanged, though there are published studies suggesting a small decrease, but heart rate reserve (peak resting heart rate) is significantly increased. This greater increase in HR reserve along with higher stroke volume translates to higher cardiac output.

11. (C) 1 watt = 6.12 kpm/min. Both are measures of power = rate at which work is being performed. 1 MET = 3.5 mL/kg/min. Watts represents power, as does METs, so MET hours measures power × time = work. Body weight does not affect the MET level on a treadmill. Increased body weight translates to more work being performed per time, but METs represents mL/kg/min, so body weight is canceled out of the equation. Arm cycle exercise requires approximately 1.5 times as much $\dot{V}o_2$ per watt as does leg cycling.

12. (C) Of the answers listed, the only "higher-risk condition" for exercise testing would be primary pulmonary hypertension according to AHA guidelines for pediatric stress testing. An ASD would not be higher risk for exercise testing. A left-to-right shunt would not cause increased hypoxia with exercise. A right-to-left shunt would—though that is not a reason to avoid an exercise test or contribute to significantly increased risk on the test. In some cases, the direction of the shunt changes with exercise—bidirectional shunts become steadily right to left. A VSD will likely decrease $\dot{V}o_{2max}$ but does not affect patient safety. Regurgitant lesions are graded as lower risk regardless of severity. Repaired tetralogy per se is also not a contraindication to exercise testing. However, a history of any of these conditions, including primary pulmonary hypertension may be an indication for exercise testing to assess symptoms, determine exercise capacity, and adjust therapy, including surgical referral.

13. (E) All of these conditions might potentially result in untoward events during maximal exercise testing except Ebstein anomaly. All regurgitant lesions are considered lower risk regardless of severity. However, for evaluating patients in these categories, the potential benefit of the information gained from the exercise test may exceed the risk of testing in experienced exercise labs with good understanding of the underlying anatomy and physiology of patients with cardiac disease and readily available emergency equipment and code teams that can respond promptly.

14. (A) As one becomes better conditioned, rest HR declines and $\dot{V}o_{2max}$ increases but HR_{max} does not change. As one becomes deconditioned, rest HR increases and $\dot{V}o_{2max}$ decreases but HR_{max} remains the same. If one fails to reach predicted HR_{max}, either the effort was submaximal or the patient has chronotropic insufficiency.

15. (E) The VAT refers to a point beyond which both aerobic and anaerobic metabolism contributes to the work done. This is seen as a disproportionate increase in CO_2 production (and minute ventilation) relative to oxygen uptake thought to reflect to the contribution of anaerobic metabolism to energy production. In adults, a disproportionate increase in lactate is also frequently observed. Decompensated acidosis is not synonymous with VAT. Decompensated acidosis occurs later in exercise, after the VAT has occurred. $\dot{V}o_2$ at VAT less than 40% is abnormal and is indicative of reduced cardiac output or abnormal O_2 delivery to the tissues.

16. (B) The ventilatory equivalent for oxygen is minute ventilation divided by oxygen uptake ($\dot{V}_E/\dot{V}o_2$). Patients with cyanotic heart disease typically have more hypoxemia at rest and during exercise. The presence of a large right-to-left shunt is a major determinant of this abnormal exercise response. At peak exercise, cyanotic patients increase their minute ventilation ($\dot{V}_E$) disproportionately to their oxygen uptake ($\dot{V}o_2$), resulting in a higher ventilatory equivalent for oxygen than acyanotic patients. The blood oxygen saturation and maximum oxygen uptake ($\dot{V}o_{2max}$) will be lower, not higher, than for an acyanotic patient. HR and blood pressure should not be systematically affected by the right-to-left shunt.

17. (C) There is no one "best" exercise protocol. The choice of exercise protocol depends on the complaints and exercise symptoms as well as the fitness of the child being tested. For example, in children with reduced exercise capacity due to chronic conditions, an exercise protocol in which the work rate increases slowly is preferred; otherwise, the test will be prematurely terminated due to fatigue without stressing the cardiopulmonary system adequately. The ramp treadmill protocol is becoming more and more popular due to a somewhat constantly increasing workload (small, frequent increments), especially during cycle ergometry testing. The ramp can be adjusted to have the test last 8 to 12 minutes, which is considered optimal. However, this protocol does not allow assessment of steady-state exercise due to the constant changing workload. The Bruce and modified Bruce treadmill protocols were developed for testing adult patients, but they are often used to also test children—and some normative values have been published, particularly for the standard Bruce protocol. Protocols based on HR response are difficult to implement and are not generally used in clinical practice.

18. (C) At rest, tidal volumes are low and respiratory dead space (in which gas exchange does not occur) maybe be as high as 30% of the tidal volume. With increased work, the ventilatory response includes increased minute ventilation due to increases in both respiratory rate and tidal volume. At the onset of exercise, tidal volume increases predominate while respiratory rate increases only modestly. Hence ventilation becomes more efficient with dead space falling to 10% to 15% of the tidal volume, and $\dot{V}_E/\dot{V}co_2$ decreases. At high levels of exercise, above the VAT, tidal volume begins to plateau as expiratory flow limits are reached, so respiratory rate accounts for most of the increase. As a result, $\dot{V}_E/\dot{V}co_2$ may increase, indicating less efficient ventilation. Normal patients terminate exercise because cardiac output can no longer increase, even though there typically is still ventilatory reserve available (20% to 30% in healthy individuals with normal heart and lungs). Diffusion limitation is rarely a problem during routine clinical exercise testing, though it can be observed in patients with restrictive lung disease or heart failure.

19. (D) The acetylene–helium rebreathing is an indirect Fick technique used to measure cardiac output noninvasively. It is dependent upon even distribution of the inspired gas throughout the lungs, so it will not be a reliable method for cardiac output measurement in patients with lung disease that involves mismatching of ventilation and perfusion or in the presence of significant intracardiac shunts. Indirect Fick techniques are used because they avoid the arterial puncture and jugular vein catheterization required in direct Fick techniques. The acetylene–helium rebreathing technique is easier to perform during cycle ergometry versus treadmill exercise. The acetylene–helium rebreathing technique is generally better tolerated than the older, CO_2 rebreathing technique, especially in younger children.

20. (E) The sphygmomanometer cuff should have a bladder length that covers at least 80% of the circumference of the upper arm and at least 40% width of the upper arm. Improper cuff size may cause measurement artifacts. Blood pressure increases with age in children and is generally higher in boys than girls, especially after puberty. While an exercise blood pressure of 200 mm Hg is above the median for healthy boys 15 to 17 years of age, it is common enough to be seen on about 8% to 9% of exercise tests and poses no immediate threat of harm to an otherwise normal patient. Athletes may generate higher exercise blood pressure due to higher cardiac output. Blood pressure usually falls in early active recovery due to venous pooling as the muscle pumping action decreases as the speed of the treadmill decreases. This may cause mild lightheadedness. Symptoms will quickly resolve, and blood pressure will increase as active recovery progresses. Abruptly stopping the treadmill at peak exercise without an active recovery may precipitate presyncope or even syncope. Fall in systolic blood pressure and pulse pressure with increasing workload suggests cardiac dysfunction and is an indication for termination of the test.

21. (B) With improved fitness, a patient can complete more work; thus, a higher maximum $\dot{V}o_2$ is achieved. Choice **(E)** also shows a lower $\dot{V}o_{2max}$, but values this high would be characteristic of athletes in endurance sports, not large, muscular American football players. Maximum minute ventilation is a product of tidal volume and respiratory rate ($\dot{V}_E = Vt \times RR$). Minute ventilation at rest is roughly 9 L/min. The rule of nine states that for every 25 watts increase the minute ventilation increases by 9 L/min. Maximum minute ventilation ($\dot{V}_E$) also increases with improved fitness and might thus decrease with deconditioning, but these values are much too low for a large 20-year-old male. An athlete's ability to reach maximum HR will not be limited by deconditioning, assuming his injury was fully healed such that he was not limited by musculoskeletal factors on the test. The oxygen saturation during an exercise test should not decrease as a result of deconditioning. A value of 98% at peak exercise is normal for a team sport athlete, though extremely well-trained endurance athletes may show mild desaturation because their cardiac outputs become too high for blood to be fully oxygenated in the lungs (which, unlike the heart, do not increase in size with training).

22. (C) MVV is obtained at rest and difficult to perform correctly and does not compare well to the actual breathing during exercise. Owing to the dependence on the patient's effort, MVV must cautiously be used for suggesting pulmonary limitation. The ATS/ACCP statements on CPET testing recommend the use of $FEV_1 \times 35$ or $FEV_1 \times 40$ as the predicted MVV. At the point of exercise termination in a normal patient, minute ventilation ($\dot{V}_E$) is 60% to 80% of MVV. Patients with lung disease and pulmonary limitation will achieve $\dot{V}_E >70\%$ by tapping into the ventilatory reserve. Tidal flow–volume loops are a more accurate method of assessing pulmonary limitation to exercise than MVV. Tidal flow–volume loops also have the advantage of assessing vocal cord dysfunction, which is an increasingly common cause for exertional dyspnea.

23. (D) African-American children have a higher blood pressure response to exercise than Caucasian children. The same holds true for larger-sized children when compared to smaller-sized children. Of similar-sized patients, boys have a greater blood pressure response than girls, especially after puberty. During exercise, contractility improves resulting in lower end-systolic volume. During treadmill or cycle ergometer exercise, the diastolic pressure generally decreases (though diastolic blood pressure increases during isometric exercise). Blood pressure increases during exercise predominately occur by increased cardiac output. The total systemic resistance generally decreases during exercise.

24. (C) Acetylene–helium rebreathing technique, which is dependent on even distribution of the inspired gas throughout the lungs, is used to measure cardiac output indirectly by measuring effective pulmonary blood flow in the absence of significant intracardiac shunts. It will not be a reliable method of cardiac output measurement in patients with lung disease that involves mismatching of ventilation and perfusion or those patients with significant intracardiac or intrapulmonary shunts. Therefore, the only patient with an insignificant intracardiac shunt of those listed would be the 14-year-old boy with a patent foramen ovale with trivial left-to-right shunt.

25. (E) Acetylene–helium rebreathing technique is noninvasive, and it is usually well tolerated by children. This method directly measures the effective pulmonary blood flow in the absence of significant intrapulmonary or intracardiac shunts. This allows for an effective method to estimate cardiac output. Acetylene diffuses from the alveolus into the pulmonary capillary blood, and thus the acetylene concentration declines relative to the volume of effective pulmonary blood flow. This technique depends on an even distribution throughout the lungs.

26. (B) In the normal, healthy child, the cardiovascular system will be the limiting factor to exercise—assuming an appropriate exercise protocol that does not exceed a young child's capacity for work from a muscular standpoint. Maximum cardiac output will be achieved when the maximum HR limits ventricular filling during diastole and in turn stroke volume. The pulmonary system in a normal, healthy child will not limit exercise capacity. Minute ventilation ($\dot{V}_E$) and work have a linear relationship until the ventilatory anaerobic threshold (VAT) is achieved. At this point, there is a disproportionate increase in $\dot{V}_E$ relative to $\dot{V}o_2$. At the point of exhaustion, $\dot{V}_E$ is generally 60% to 80% of the maximum ventilatory volume. This percentage increases with aerobic fitness.

27. (A) A few equations for exercise are needed to calculate the total work accomplished as well as the total power achieved. Work is defined by force multiplied by distance or, in other words, the force needed to move a mass a given distance. The unit for work is the Newton-meter or joule (J). Force is mass × acceleration. Power is the work performed per unit time. The other equations listed are not correct. On exercise testing, power is the quantity usually expressed. For cycle ergometry, it can be kilopond meters/min or watts (1 watt = 6.12 kilopond meters/min). Watts can be converted to METs, which is an expression of power based on rate of oxygen consumption (1 MET = 3.5 mL of O_2 consumed/kg of body weight/min).

28. (C) For patients between the ages of 5 and 20, the HR_{max} reported in several large cohorts ranges from 195 to 215 bpm with little consistent impact of age or sex on HR. For patients >20 years of age, however, the maximum HR will decrease with increasing age. The most commonly used equation to determine a patient's maximum HR is a simple $HR_{max} = 220 - age$, though other formulas with larger datasets have been published, including $HR_{max} = 210 - 0.65 \times age$. Some studies have produced different equations for women ($210 - 0.8 \times age$) versus men, reflecting perhaps different hormonal changes with age. The reason for this decline in HR_{max} is decreased nerve conduction; during aging, a gradual shift toward higher sympathetic versus parasympathetic balance attenuates the decline in HR with age. Stroke volume increases early in exercise with little change thereafter, except in highly trained endurance athletes. The HR increases, then accounts for increasing cardiac output. With exercise, the total systemic vascular resistance declines. Systolic blood pressure will increase with isotonic exercise while the diastolic blood pressure remains relatively unchanged. With isometric exercise, both systolic and diastolic blood pressures rise.

29. (B) Maximal $\dot{V}o_2$ achieved is dependent on age, sex, hemoglobin level, and type of work completed. As age increases in childhood, the maximal $\dot{V}o_2$ achievable also increases. Between the sexes, the maximal $\dot{V}o_2$ achievable is relatively the same before puberty (about 35 mL/kg/min at age 11), but thereafter, males have a higher $\dot{V}o_{2max}$ (45–50 vs. 35–40 mL/kg/min at age 17). Anemic patients have a lower achievable $\dot{V}o_{2max}$ than patients with normal hemoglobin; hemoglobin of 10 g/dL would lower $\dot{V}o_{2max}$ by about 15% to 20%. By age 17, $\dot{V}o_{2max}$ would have largely reached adult levels, so the added 2 years of age in the anemic patient versus the normal 17-year-old boy would not be expected to matter significantly. Finally, achievable $\dot{V}o_{2max}$ depends on the type of work completed; the more muscle groups involved, the higher the $\dot{V}o_2$ achieved. Therefore, a higher $\dot{V}o_{2max}$ is achieved with treadmill ergometry > cycle ergometry > arm crank ergometry > hand grip ergometry. Therefore, the older, nonanemic male would likely achieve the highest $\dot{V}o_{2max}$ during cycle exercise testing. The arm ergometer test might be expected to produce a $\dot{V}o_{2max}$ of 65% to 75% of the leg cycle ergometer test. Caveat: level of physical activity and degree of exercise training can greatly impact $\dot{V}o_{2max}$. A 17-year-old girl on the cross-country team could certainly achieve a higher $\dot{V}o_{2max}$ than her sedentary 17-year-old male classmate; even the 11-year-old boy could have the highest $\dot{V}o_{2max}$ of the group based on level of physical activity—and degree of adiposity (if the 17-year old children were obese), which is another important contributor to $\dot{V}o_{2max}$.

30. (D) In a well-trained athlete higher blood volume and lower resting HR will result in increased end-diastolic volume—producing a higher stroke volume at rest (and during exercise). A decreased left ventricular end-systolic dimension volume during exercise will also occur as a result of greater contractility.

31. (C) Bicuspid aortic valve with mild AR should not affect cardiac output and $\dot{V}o_{2max}$ during exercise. Though the heart has normal macrostructure in LTQS type 1, the beta blocker will reduce peak HR and $\dot{V}o_{2max}$. The patient with ccTGA has a systemic right ventricle with likely a significant reduction in cardiac output. Ebstein anomaly to varying degrees reduces forward RV stroke volume resulting in decreased blood flow to the lung. Anomalous pulmonary veins in Scimitar syndrome recycle oxygenated blood back to the inferior vena cava, reducing LV filling and decreasing A-$\dot{V}o_2$ difference in mixed venous blood.

32. (A) Of the answers listed, the only condition not considered as higher risk to exercise testing in pediatric patients is second-degree AV block. Mostly likely, a type 1 second-degree block will resolve with exercise, whereas a type 2 will not—and ultimately limit exercise, but not constitute a risk of sudden death. Severe aortic stenosis with clear symptoms or an ejection fraction <50% would be an indication for surgery; exercise testing is not required or recommended. Known exercise-induced arrhythmias can be higher-risk conditions; however, exercise testing is a useful provocative test in the diagnosis of CPVT and long QT syndrome—or to determine adequacy of antiarrhythmic therapy and confirm that defibrillator settings are appropriate. Therefore, exercise testing can be carried out in these patients. Finally, anomalous origin of a coronary artery might be a higher-risk condition, especially if it is a left coronary anomaly or a single coronary artery, but exercise testing is needed to help determine the necessity for operative repair.

33. (E) Neither treadmill nor cycle ergometry is superior to the other. Even children as young as 10 years can be tested using the child cycle ergometer or treadmill. However, there are advantages and disadvantages to each type. Small children generally cannot reach the pedals of a cycle ergometer designed for adult testing, but the availability of a child cycle ergometer circumvents this, and they may also need a lower front handrail on the treadmill for safety concerns. Treadmill ergometry will allow a patient to derive a higher $\dot{V}o_{2max}$ and HR due to the use of more muscle groups during exercise. However, the treadmill is potentially more dangerous due to the potential of the patient falling, especially if syncope is a potential concern or the patient has neurologic issues; and there is more noise and artifact while running when compared to stationary cycling. A more accurate and controlled measurement of work can be obtained with cycle ergometry. The patient is not moving as much back and forth and up and down as grade increases. And work/power changes are more closely tied to $\dot{V}o_2$—especially with an electronically braked cycle ergometer when compared to a treadmill—where degree of handrail support and familiarity with treadmill walking may affect $\dot{V}o_2$. Continuous video laryngoscopy, where a flexible laryngoscope is passed trans nasally to determine movements of the laryngeal structures during exercise to evaluate for vocal cord dysfunction/

exercise-induced laryngeal obstruction can be safely done with the child in a seated position on a cycle ergometer.

34. (E) Exercise testing in AS patients can be helpful in the assessment of mild-to-moderate stenosis for significant ST segment changes with exercise as well as distinguishing between chest wall pain and more significant causes of chest pain. However, severe, symptomatic AS or severe AS with LVEF <50% is a contraindication to exercise testing; surgery is indicated for these patients. In AS, there is an inverse relationship between the total cardiac work performed and transaortic pressure gradient. Also, patients with more severe AS (i.e., higher transaortic gradient) have a lower increase in their blood pressure response during exercise than less severe AS patients. The higher the transaortic gradient, the more likely that ST segment changes occur. VT may also occur in the setting of AS. Dyspnea on exertion, poor blood pressure response, ST changes, limited exercise capacity, and VT are all considered to indicate poor prognosis in AS. Not surprisingly, it has been shown that patients with more severe AS achieve a lower $\dot{V}o_{2max}$, though few patients with even moderate AS achieve a normal $\dot{V}o_{2max}$, since many are treated with beta blockers limiting maximal HR. Several papers have demonstrated that survival in AS is impaired when $\dot{V}o_{2max}$ is <80% predicted. An important caveat is that transaortic pressure gradient is not the sole driver of exercise capacity in AS patients. The usual factors—amount of beta blockade, degree of adiposity, level of physical activity, and the presence of other diseases like coronary artery disease or COPD also influence exercise performance and $\dot{V}o_{2max}$. Finally, there is a class of patients with low transaortic gradients despite severe AS according to valve area (<1.0 cm^2) and valve area index (<0.6 cm^2/m^2 of body surface area) who are at very high risk. A second caveat is that these data have been derived by studying outcomes in adults with mostly acquired AS, not pediatric patients with congenital AS. AS in pediatric patients is often part of a larger set of cardiac abnormalities requiring early surgical intervention even when AS is not severe enough to consider surgical intervention by itself.

35. (D) Unrepaired single ventricle patients will have reduced maximum aerobic power and excessive ventilation relative to $\dot{V}o_2$ and $\dot{V}co_2$. Specifically, unrepaired patients with pulmonary atresia with VSD have exercise performance and maximum oxygen uptake when compared to first stage repaired or complete repaired patients as well as normal patients. Blood oxygen saturation levels in unrepaired and first-stage repaired patients are lower at rest than normal patients and decrease significantly with exercise. After complete repair, patients will have a relatively normal resting blood oxygen saturation level but may have a small decrease with exercise. Exercise capacity and peak $\dot{V}o_2$ in repaired single ventricle patients normally does not improve to 100% or greater of normal for age and sex.

36. (B) A complete 12-lead ECG should be obtained at least once at rest, at each workload, and several times after completion. A typical recording includes at rest sitting, supine, and standing; then at each workload and peak exercise, as well as each minute (1 to 5 or 6) of recovery. At least three standard surface ECG leads should be continuously displayed and recorded during the exercise study as well as for 5 to 10 minutes after the study is completed. For fitness tests performed on healthy subjects where the ECG is primarily used to measure heart rate, sometimes only one surface lead is monitored, but this is inappropriate for testing patients with known or suspected cardiac disease, as the ECG provides more information than just HR response. Operators should have the option of switching between various combinations of those leads (i.e., inferior leads, anterior right, anterior left). Appropriate ECG electrode and lead placement should be used in all types of ergometry to limit artifact. Placing the electrode above bone rather than on muscle or adipose tissue usually improves the stability of the tracing and limits random motion artifact. Good skin cleansing with alcohol and abrading a small area with sandpaper to remove dead skin is important. Securing the ECG lead cables with an elastic band or knit shirt may be helpful, especially if the patient is obese or sweats profusely, and if treadmill running is expected. Vigorous exercise itself often produces ECG artifact even with good skin preparation, so obtaining a 12-lead ECG in the first 15 to 30 seconds of active recovery when the HR is still near the peak level attained during exercise is helpful in more accurately interpreting ST-T response. Owing to the typical noise artifact with treadmill exercise testing, the Korotkoff sounds, especially diastolic, can be very difficult to measure accurately. There is some variance as to whether diastolic pressure during exercise should be taken as the 4th or the 5th Korotkoff sound (the 5th phase sound can sometimes be heard down to 0 mm Hg), and some laboratories record both. Published data are mixed as to whether diastolic blood pressure provides any important and independent prognostic information. Direct blood pressure measurement through arterial access in the peripheral arteries will overestimate the central aortic pressure due to peripheral pulse amplification. Aortic puncture for the purpose of blood pressure measurement during exercise is seldom justified.

37. (B) Because of the right-to-left shunt and resultant increase in dead space, cyanotic patients hyperventilate in order to remove additional CO_2. Hence ventilation is disproportionately high relative to $\dot{V}CO_2$ (and $\dot{V}O_2$). Exercise capacity is reduced in cyanotic patients, but peak exercise HR is not likely affected. Because of reduced oxygen uptake relative to cardiac output, submaximal heart rates will likely be higher in the cyanotic patient. There is no clear indication of how diastolic blood pressure would be affected, though peak systolic blood pressure would likely be lower as less work could be performed and reduced pO_2 might be expected to promote lower vascular resistance at the level of autoregulation in the active muscles.

38. (E) The CO_2 rebreathing technique is one of the two most frequently used techniques (other being acetylene–helium rebreathing technique) for measuring cardiac output noninvasively. The CO_2 rebreathing technique is based on the Fick principle for CO_2 {Cardiac output = VEcontent} needs to be directly measured from systemic arterial blood pCO_2 or, noninvasively, by estimating this by using the Bohr equation. This is accomplished by solving for $PaCO_2$ (systemic arterial

pCO_2): $Vd/Vt = (PaCO_2 - PeCO_2)/PaCO_2$. This technique is not well tolerated by all, especially children, because rebreathing CO_2 can cause dyspnea, an unpleasant taste, and a transient headache. This technique involves a few areas of potential error. These include the need to adjust CO_2 concentration used for the patient's size and exercise intensity as well as taking into account dead space (mouthpiece, etc.).

39. (C) These heart rate changes are characteristic of pacemaker Wenckebach. The upper rate was likely set at 180 bpm. An atrial rate above 180 cannot be followed 1-to-1 by the ventricular lead, so it begins to drop beats. If the patient is not an athlete and is not reporting any limitations to physical activity, nothing may need to be done; otherwise the upper rate limit can be increased. Anomalous origin of the RCA may sometimes produce ischemia if there is a slit-like ostium and/or a long intramural course. SA node ischemia would manifest as a gradual slowing of the sinus rate, not dropped beats. An example of pacemaker Wenckebach with corresponding drop in $\dot{V}O_2$ in a patient with repaired Shone complex is shown in **Figure 7.14**.

Figure 7.15 shows the low HR point at peak exercise and the return to 1:1 pacing in active recovery 2 minutes later.

40. (D) Young man with severe neo-aortic valve regurgitation, s/p prior Ross procedure and repair of coarctation of the aorta in setting of Shone syndrome performed **Test D**. Quite low $\dot{V}O_{2max}$ (20.1 mL/kg/min) despite a reasonable HR response and good effort (noted by high $\dot{V}CO_2$ relative to $\dot{V}O_2$ at peak exercise).

41. (B) Male college basketball player complaining of fatigue and found to have dilated cardiomyopathy with LVEF = 46% performed **Test B**. Slightly reduced $\dot{V}O_{2max}$ (39.1 mL/kg/min) with normal HR response and good effort.

42. (C) Young man with structurally normal heart and mitochondrial myopathy due to heterozygous YARS-2 mutation performed **Test C**. Extremely low $\dot{V}O_{2max}$ (13.7 mL/kg/min) with normal HR response. Note very high $\dot{V}CO_2$ relative to $\dot{V}O_2$; peak respiratory exchange ratio (RER) was 1.86. While aerobic metabolism is markedly impaired, anaerobic metabolism is normal and provides most of the energy for exercise once the work level exceeds 100 mL/min—in this case about 3 METs.

43. (F) Young man with repaired TGA but experiencing SA node dysfunction performed **Test F**. We can see the inadequate HR response with considerable variation. The limited HR reserve and systemic right ventricle (he had a Senning operation) with EF of 30% to 35% combine to produce a low $\dot{V}O_{2max}$ of 18.9 mL/kg/min.

44. (A) An elite female middle distance runner with a structurally normal heart performed **Test A** in which a very high $\dot{V}O_{2max}$ (66.4 mL/kg/min) was attained.

45. (E) Recent male heart transplant performed **Test E**. $\dot{V}O_{2max}$ is mild to moderately low (34 mL/kg/min) with adequate effort. What identifies this as a recent heart transplant is the HR response with high resting HR, limited HR reserve,

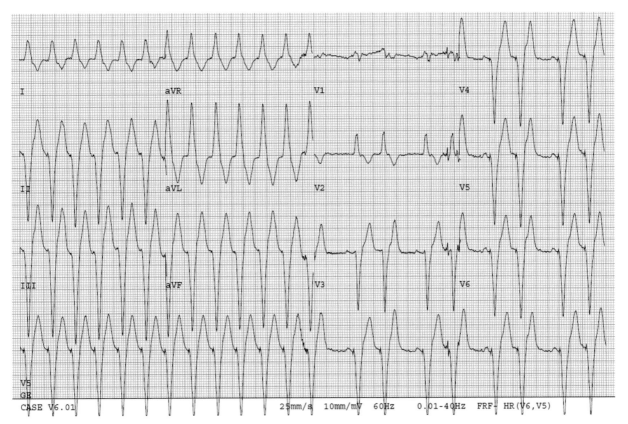

A

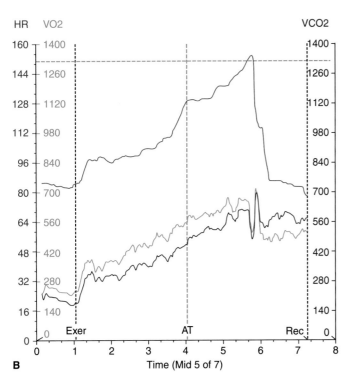

B

FIGURE 7.14

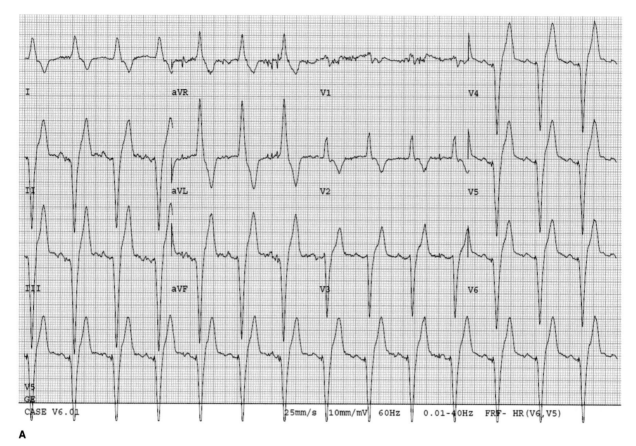

A

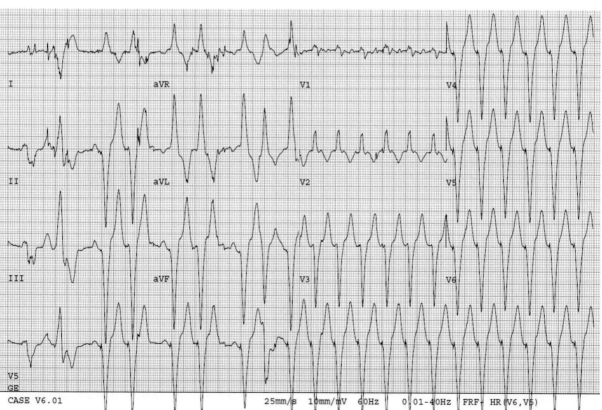

B

FIGURE 7.15

and HR recovery of 0 bpm due to the denervated heart. Sympathetic fibers will often at least partially re-enervate the heart during the first 1 to 2 years, but parasympathetic tone will remain absent.

46. (E) While testing of athletes to determine performance potential or to evaluate problems with performance is a listed indication for exercise testing in the pediatric population, a stress test is not required for participation in sports for healthy asymptomatic children with a normal physical examination and no concerning family history of cardiovascular disease or early sudden death.

47. (C) A resting heart rate as low as 30 bpm can be considered a normal finding in a young athlete. Junctional rhythms and Mobitz type I—but not type II—are normal consequences of high vagal tone. There would be concern if the heart rate did not increase with conversion to sinus rhythm with physical activity. T-wave inversion in a young black athlete would be considered normal out to V4, but not in V5 and V6. LBBB and PVCs ≥3 in a 10-second strip are considered abnormal findings requiring further evaluation.

48. (B) Long-QT 2 is most highly subject to drug-induced prolongation. Only 10% of deaths in long-QT 3 occur during exercise. Brugada patterns may commonly be intermittent; exercise is one technique to bring out Brugada pattern. Fever, drug challenge, and moving electrode for V1, V2, and V3 up or down may bring out the characteristic pattern. CPVT usually occurs only at or near peak exercise. Beta blocker is also first-line therapy in this channelopathy. Fewer than 10% of deaths in long-QT 3 occur during exercise. Exercise-related sudden death is most common in long-QT 1; hence, beta blockade is the first choice of therapy for long-QT 1. Since this disorder is often discovered at a young age and lifetime therapy is indicated, potential pulmonary side effect of long-term amiodarone therapy makes it a poor choice for treatment of this channelopathy.

49. (C) Normal pediatric ECG soccer player aged 15. Sinus arrhythmia, short PR interval, early repolarization, somewhat prominent voltages, and narrow Q-waves anterolaterally are normal pediatric ECG findings. Interestingly, this patient has CPVT, but the heart is structurally normal, so the resting ECG is normal.

50. (A) African-American basketball player aged 19 with HOCM. ST-T abnormalities with asymmetric T-wave inversion indicating LV strain.

51. (E) Baseball player aged 10 with congenital complete heart block. P-waves and QRS complexes march out independently. Patient has chronotropic incompetence with exercise but manages to keep up adequately with peers in baseball. If playing other sports, like swimming or cross-country running, a rate-responsive pacemaker would likely be indicated.

52. (D) Cross-country runner aged 20 with long-QT 3. The T-waves in long-QT 3 are often small and somewhat peaked with a long, flat ST segment. Risk of sudden death during exercise is low in this type of long QT syndrome compared with the more common type 1, but overall mortality is high in long-QT 3. The same SCN5A gene may produce atrial fibrillation, dilated cardiomyopathy, or Brugada syndrome.

53. (B) Ebstein anomaly with severe tricuspid regurgitation aged 19. Right bundle branch block with prominent voltages in V1 and V2 are consistent with RV enlargement.

54. (A) POTS. She has a normal exercise ECG with normal peak HR. There are no ventricular ectopics, which likely rules out CPVT. No ST-T abnormalities or prominent voltages to suggest HOCM. A Mobitz II AV block would not likely resolve with exercise. There is no evidence of pre-excitation, and the peak heart rate is normal for age.

55. (A) A 21-year-old male with HOCM post myectomy. ECG shows an LBBB pattern typical after myectomy. VT is very concerning in HOCM. This patient died from an arrhythmia despite presence of an ICD approximately 4 years after this exercise test.

56. (C) A 19-year-old male basketball player with dilated cardiomyopathy. VT is fast. The axis is very different that his baseline ECG, making SVT unlikely—and it is not initiated with a long–short pattern typical for SVT with aberrancy. Exercise capacity and $\dot{V}o_{2max}$ (36.4 mL/kg/min = 73% predicted) were reduced. Subsequent evaluation showed LVEF of 50%. There was a family history of tachyarrhythmia (father). It was recommended that he discontinue competitive sports, as per 2018 AHA/ACC guidelines.

57. (D) A 20-year-old female swing dancer with WPW with orthodromic reciprocating tachycardia. There is no delta wave or pre-excitation, so this is an orthodromic tachycardia with forward conduction through the AV node/His bundle and retrograde conduction back to the atrium via the accessory pathway. The rate of 285 bpm is too rapid for AVNRT. Subsequent ablation was successful.

58. (E) A 17-year-old male soccer player with CPVT and flecainide-induced wide-complex SVT. The tachycardia is relatively slow (<150 bpm) with wide QRS complexes. The patient is also taking a beta blocker (nadolol). He reported no palpitations or presyncope. Repeat testing 1 year later on reduced dose of flecainide did not show this wide complex SVT, only single PVCs near peak exercise, consistent with known CPVT.

59. (B) An 18-year-old female volleyball player with fascicular VT with structurally normal heart. This tachycardiac was well tolerated, resolved spontaneously after 23 minutes without syncope or hemodynamic compromise. The negative deflections indicate that this focus was lower than usual for LV fascicular tachycardia, and this was confirmed during the EP study as being just below the papillary muscle. Ablation was not performed due to proximity to the papillary muscle, and both verapamil and nadolol were unfortunately not tolerated. Since extreme exercise regularly precipitated the arrhythmia, the patient was ultimately forced to give up sports competition.

60. (B) HOCM produces a high $\dot{V}_E/\dot{V}CO_2$ only in the case of "burnt out" HOCM where the LVEF has dropped significantly and the patient is in left heart failure. In that scenario, there can be a significant increase in pulmonary wedge pressure with exercise causing impaired diffusing capacity in the lungs. $\dot{V}_E/\dot{V}CO_2$ will be high with volitional hyperventilation due to high dead space ventilation (where there is no gas exchange). Interstitial lung disease impairs diffusing capacity, causing an elevation of $\dot{V}_E/\dot{V}CO_2$. Pulmonary emboli impair lung blood flow creating a ventilation:perfusion mismatch that typically worsens with exercise, sometimes leading to extremely high $\dot{V}_E/\dot{V}CO_2$ levels >80 or even >100 at peak exercise. An ASD with L-R shunt will reduce CO_2 delivery to the lungs, shunting it directly into the left atrium, thus raising the ratio of $\dot{V}_E$ to $\dot{V}CO_2$. From another point of view, mixing arterial and venous blood will reduce the A-V CO_2 difference and reduce CO_2 exchange in the lungs.

61. (B) This is ARVC. Note T-wave inversion in V1–V4 and PVCs at rest (inconsistent with CPVT). The QT interval appears to be very normal. The tachyarrhythmia starts with a fusion beat, ruling out SVT. ST segments are normal, indicating this was not of ischemic origin. The patient had a family history or ARVC, and the cardiac HR showed dilated RV with EF of 30%.

62. (C) This is a third-degree AV block. There are separate atrial and ventricular rates with no variation in the ventricular rate to suggest any AV conduction. All other answers can be easily ruled out—no dropped beats, no consistent PR intervals.

63. (C) It is unlikely that tricuspid valve repair would cause coronary insufficiency. All the other conditions might represent ischemia due either to congenital (in the case of anomalous RCA) or acquired coronary artery disease. The Gortex graph may have become occluded in the ALCAPA patient. Chest trauma may have damaged the left anterior descending coronary artery. Coronary occlusion after arterial switch is rare but has been reported.

64. (E) The first exercise ECG (**Figure 7.8A**) shows complete heart block. Lyme disease is known to cause complete heart block, which will resolve with appropriate therapy. Beta blockers are used in young people for a variety of reasons, but they should not cause complete heart block or this degree of chronotropic incompetence. While a pacemaker is often indicated for complete heart block, the second exercise ECG (**Figure 7.8B**) shows no signs of either atrial or ventricular pacing. RF ablation is not a treatment for complete heart block, but it rather is used to treat tachycardias, not bradycardia or chronotropic incompetence. In some circumstances, a myocardial bridge of the LAD may cause exercise-induced ischemia. Though a bridge in the mid-LAD should not cause SA node ischemia and certainly not complete heart block. In this ECG, the ST segments are normal. This patient had a tick bite with characteristic rash and had a positive ELISA for Lyme. Second- or third-degree heart blocks are seen in about 1% of cases of Lyme disease. Wisconsin has a high incidence of Lyme disease, and Lyme is more common in rural areas that are deer tick habitat.

65. (A) Normal peak HR for age (196 bpm) with pre-excitation (short PR with delta wave) indicating WPW. The ST-T abnormalities may be explained by WPW (though in other scenarios HOCM or myocardial ischemia could produce similar ST-T patterns). The rate is regular, ruling out atrial fibrillation, and the QRS is narrow, excluding RVOT VT, which can also be well tolerated.

66. (E) Reviewing the data on this cardiopulmonary exercise test, we see that $\dot{V}O_{2max}$ (**Figure 7.10B**) is reduced (63% predicted), ruling out a normal test with average cardio-respiratory fitness, and there is also a low oxygen pulse (**Figure 7.10C**) suggesting some impairment of cardiac output. Neither $\dot{V}O_2$ nor oxygen pulse are indexed here for body weight, so being overweight (her BMI is 27 kg/m^2 indicating a mild degree of excess weight) would not explain the low values. In **Figure 7.10B**, we can also see that HR reaches 184 bpm (95% predicted) with a peak RER of 1.22 (which we can confirm by comparing $\dot{V}CO_2$ with $\dot{V}O_2$ at peak exercise). This rules out poor effort on the test. Clearly there is a large breathing reserve (**Figure 7.10A**), and gas exchange data in **Figure 7.10D** appear to be normal, ruling out both a ventilation limitation due to uncontrolled asthma and thromboembolic pulmonary hypertension. While the SpO_2 response is not shown, we can assume from our other data ($\dot{V}_E/\dot{V}CO_2$ and $\dot{V}_E/\dot{V}O_2$) that it was likely normal (it was 98% at peak exercise by forehead oximetry). This leaves pulmonary regurgitation as the only diagnosis that would explain a low peak $\dot{V}O_2$ with large breathing reserve despite good effort, normal HR response, and normal gas exchange in the lungs. Of course, other abnormalities could explain similar findings (aortic regurgitation, Ebstein anomaly, and dilated cardiomyopathy without heart failure are three examples).

67. (C) Reviewing the data on this cardiopulmonary exercise test (**Figure 7.12**), we see that peak $\dot{V}O_2$ (Figure 7.12B) is normal (100% predicted) despite a low peak HR of 98 bpm and an RER just over 1.0 (1.04 to be exact). Young children generally have a somewhat lower peak RER during an exercise test than adults—due to lower muscle mass and anaerobic power, and at age 12 the stage of sexual maturity—and hence the RER—can be somewhat variable. Our patient was 149.5 cm tall—50th percentile for age, but weight of 36.5 kg was only at the 25th percentile for weight (see also: (https://www.cdc.gov/growthcharts/clinical_charts.htm). Thus, his RER of 1.04 probably represents near-maximal effort. The oxygen pulse (**Figure 7.12C**) is quite high, indicating a structurally normal heart that has good diastolic and systolic reserve. The normal peak $\dot{V}O_2$ in the setting of a low HR suggests athletic training, though the option of soccer player with normal heart and lungs is unlikely in the setting of such a low peak HR. Gas exchange in the lungs appears to be normal from data in **Figure 7.12D**. Notice how $PETCO_2$ and $\dot{V}_E/\dot{V}CO_2$ are exact mirror images of each other, as would be expected from the mathematics of how they are calculated. Some investigators have proposed that these should be considered separately as independent predictors of outcome in heart failure, but here we can see that they are tightly correlated. There is a normal-to-high breathing reserve (**Figure 7.12A**), somewhat high because cardiac output is reduced by beta blockade. The normal peak $\dot{V}O_2$

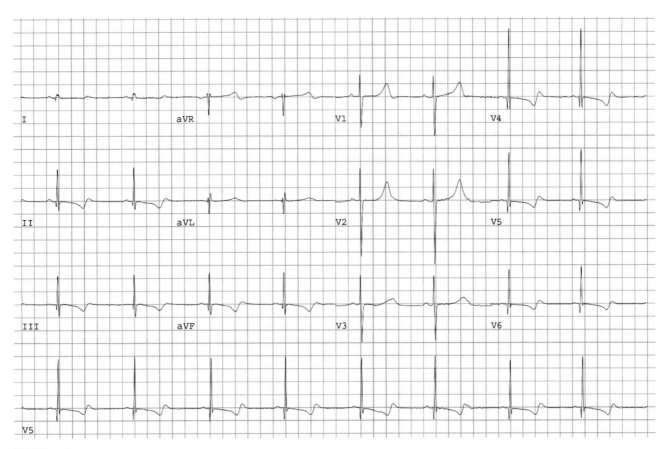

FIGURE 7.16

rules out ccTGA—which has a systemic right ventricle—and Ebstein anomaly—which reduces RV cardiac output. Average peak $\dot{V}o_2$ might be achieved in either Ebstein or moderate aortic regurgitation, but one would not expect such a dramatic response of the oxygen pulse in the presence of structural heart disease—and beta blocker is not generally used in regurgitant lesions. Our patient has both genetically confirmed paternal and maternal long-QT 1. He has a history of cardiac arrest and is being treated with nadolol. He is also post-sympathetic denervation (to keep nadolol dose low and tolerable) and has a CD. He participates in sports, soccer and snowboarding, hence has at least moderately well-trained status. The 2018 AHA/ACC guidelines do allow competitive sport for patients with cardiac channelopathies who are asymptomatic on therapy and have no evidence of significant arrhythmia on a maximal exercise test. Resting ECG is shown in **Figure 7.16**.

68. (E) Exercise is a common trigger for airway bronchospasm both in children with and without asthma. The EIB symptoms are variable and nonspecific and cannot be diagnosed on the basis of symptoms alone as there is a poor correlation to objectively confirmed EIB. EIB is reported in a substantial proportion of children with asthma (80% to 90%) and among elite athletes (20% to 70%). Bronchial provocation tests elicit airway bronchoconstriction either through a direct stimulus like methacholine challenge or an indirect stimulus like exercise challenge, which is more specific for a diagnosis of asthma in the right clinical context. Progressive exercise causes minute ventilation to increase manyfold from baseline. The bronchoconstrictive effects of exercise are thought to be due to airway smooth muscle contraction brought on by the rapid exchange of air with the bronchial mucosal surfaces causing dehydration, cooling of the airway surfaces and release of mast cell–mediated inflammatory markers. The assessment of EIB includes spirometry assessment of airway response to exercise, expressed as a percent fall in FEV_1 from the baseline value with measurements of FEV_1 taken at intervals of 5, 10, 15, and 30 minutes after exercise. Airway narrowing is characteristically maximal at 5 to 15 minutes of exercise. Rapid onset of exertional symptoms with peak exercise and rapid resolution with rest is suggestive of dynamic upper airway obstruction during exercise. A fall in FEV_1 of 10% or more compared to baseline value is diagnostic for EIB. Many healthy individuals show a bronchodilator effect with exercise with FEV1 improving by 3% to 5% from baseline. Engaging in a short burst of physical activity as part of warmup session is known to induce a state of refractoriness for the next 2 hours and minimizes EIB. Pretest administration of bronchoprotective medications can alter the airway response to exercise and ideally should be withheld prior to testing; 4 hours for short-acting beta-2 agonists (SABA) and 24 hours for long-acting beta agonists (LABA).

69. (E) The gold standard for determining a ventilatory limitation is when the maximal minute ventilation exceeds 85% of the predicted maximal minute ventilation or breathing reserve <15% to 20%. Breathing reserve is calculated by the following equation: $100 - (\dot{V}_E \text{ peak}/MVV) \times 100\%$. Maximal voluntary ventilation is obtained at rest, difficult to perform correctly, and it does not compare well to actual breathing during exercise. Owing to the dependence on the patient's effort, MVV must cautiously be used for suggesting pulmonary limitation. The predicted MVV is calculated from the FEV_1 obtained from baseline spirometry ($MVV = 40$ (or 35) $\times$ FEV_1. Ventilation limitation is more certain when the limiting symptom is dyspnea and the RER is submaximal. The lower the breathing reserve (even be negative on some tests), the more likely that the patient is ventilation limited. A low breathing reserve with high RER may represent simultaneous cardiac and pulmonary limitation.

Resting tidal volumes are usually in the range of 0.5 to 1.0 L. Normal tidal volume augmentation from rest to peak is at least two to three times the baseline value. With progressive exercise, tidal volume initially increases until 50% to 60% of the resting inspiratory capacity is reached. Further increase in minute ventilation is achieved through increase in respiratory frequency. Breathing frequency usually does not exceed 50 breaths/min. In lung disease due to a restrictive physiology (limited tidal volume augmentation), an abnormal ventilatory response includes a respiratory frequency of more than 55/min. $PETCO_2$ values typically increase several mm Hg from resting levels up to VAT and decrease toward peak as the ventilation increases in response to accumulation of lactic acidosis. $PETCO_2$ levels of 35 mm Hg and above are normal at peak exercise. Unchanging or low $PETCO_2$ levels with progressive exercise are an indication of poor perfusion as seen in PAH.

70. (B) The oxygen saturation at rest is normally 95% and above and it does not change more than 2% from rest to maximal exercise. The PaO_2 at rest in healthy individuals at sea level is around 80 mm Hg and the alveolar–arterial O_2 difference (A-a DO_2) is 5 to 15 mm Hg and increases to 20 to 30 mm Hg with maximal exercise. A transient fall in both the alveolar (PAO_2) and arterial (PaO_2) O_2 tension at the beginning of exercise is a normal phenomenon due to a lag in the increase in minute ventilation compared to the rise in $\dot{V}O_2$. Exercise-induced arterial hypoxemia (EIAH) is defined as an absolute reduction in the oxygen saturation below 88% or a fall in oxygen saturations of 4% or more from resting/baseline values. EIAH is most commonly seen in airway diseases with worsening of ventilation–perfusion mismatch during exercise with increasing pulmonary blood flow. The poorly ventilated alveoli act like an intrapulmonary shunt causing fall in arterial oxygen saturation and increase in A-aDO_2. In patients with pulmonary vascular disorders (reduction in size of the available capillary bed at baseline), the increase in pulmonary blood flow with exercise causes arterial oxygen desaturation as no additional recruitable pulmonary capillary beds are available. In some individuals with lung disease, a right-to-left shunt develops through atrial septal defect during exercise as the right atrial pressure exceeds the left atrial pressure. In patients with chronic heart failure, a slow pulmonary blood flow allows adequate time for the RBC in the alveolar capillary bed to be oxygenated fully through diffusion equilibration. Furthermore, during strenuous exercise, the greatly reduced transit time for the RBC in the alveolar capillary bed impacts the O_2 diffusion equilibration causing exercise hypoxemia. Finally, artifactual O_2 desaturation could occur due to finger probes used for pulse oximetry. Alternatively, the use of forehead probes can provide reliable oxygen saturations during the test.

Fetal and Neonatal Cardiology

Benjamin W. Eidem, M. Yasir Qureshi, and Jay D. Pruetz

Questions

1. Which of the following is the most common indication to refer for formal fetal echocardiography?

   A. Maternal TORCH infection
   B. First-degree relative with congenital heart disease
   C. Fetal arrhythmia
   D. Suspected cardiac anomaly on obstetrical screening ultrasound
   E. Maternal phenylketonuria (PKU) with phenylalanine level >10 mg/dL

2. Doppler flow studies in the human fetus have shown that the ratio of right-to-left ventricular combined output is approximately which of the following?

   A. 10%/90%
   B. 25%/75%
   C. 55%/45%
   D. 25%/75%
   E. 90%/10%

3. While fetal teratogen exposure is rare, it is still a known risk factor for the development of congenital heart disease. Which of the following fetal teratogen and CHD pairs is correct?

   A. Alcohol and Ebstein anomaly
   B. Salicylates and ventricular septal defects (VSDs)
   C. SSRIs and premature ductus arteriosus closure
   D. Lithium and persistent pulmonary hypertension in the newborn
   E. Retinoic acid and conotruncal anomalies

4. Fetal echocardiography often employs many different views to confirm normal cardiac anatomy in the fetus and rule out congenital heart defects. Which of the following congenital heart lesions is most likely to be detected on a standard four-chamber view of the fetal heart?

   A. Vascular ring
   B. Large muscular ventricular septal defect (VSD)
   C. d-Transposition of the great arteries (d-TGA) with intact ventricular septum
   D. Right aortic arch
   E. Coarctation

5. A fetal echocardiogram uses various imaging modalities in addition to standard 2D views (grayscale) including the use of spectral Doppler (pulsed-wave) and color Doppler. The use of spectral Doppler (pulsed-wave) is often essential to making which one of the following diagnoses?

   A. Vascular ring
   B. d-Transposition of the great arteries (d-TGA)
   C. Premature atrial contractions (PACs)
   D. Hypoplastic left heart syndrome (HLHS)
   E. Anomalies of the branch pulmonary arteries

6. Which is the most common fetal arrhythmia?

   A. Premature atrial contractions (PACs)
   B. Premature ventricular contractions (PVCs)
   C. Supraventricular tachycardia (SVT)
   D. Atrial flutter
   E. Complete heart block

7. What is the normal range for fetal cardiothoracic area ratio?

   A. <20%
   B. 25% to 35%
   C. 40% to 50%
   D. 55% to 70%
   E. >70%

8. Which form of critical CHD listed below is most likely to require an emergent postnatal cardiac intervention (surgery or catheterization) within hours of birth?

   A. Coarctation of the aorta
   B. Obstructed total anomalous pulmonary venous return (TAPVR)
   C. Complete atrioventricular canal (CAVC) defect with pulmonary atresia
   D. Tetralogy of Fallot (TOF) with pulmonary stenosis
   E. Truncus arteriosus

9. From the fetal Doppler interrogation in **Figure 8.1**, what interval is being measured between the parallel lines?

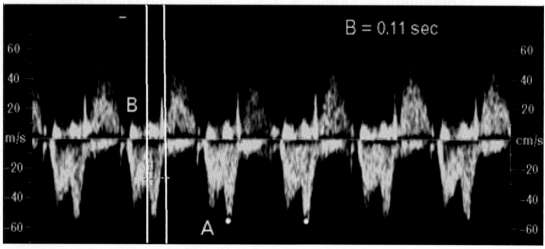

FIGURE 8.1

   A. PP interval
   B. RR interval
   C. QT interval
   D. PR interval
   E. VA interval

10. While performing a fetal echocardiogram, you notice flow reversal across the ductus arteriosus. Which of the following defects is most likely to explain this finding?

    A. d-TGA
    B. AVSD
    C. Critical aortic stenosis
    D. Total anomalous pulmonary venous connection
    E. Pulmonary atresia with intact ventricular septum

11. The normal fetal heart rate ranges from which of the following?

    A. 80 to 120 bpm
    B. 60 to 100 bpm
    C. 100 to 180 bpm
    D. 140 to 220 bpm
    E. 100 to 140 bpm

12. What percentage of fetal cardiac output at term perfuses the lungs?

    A. 10%
    B. 30%
    C. 50%
    D. 75%
    E. 100%

13. The normal fetal cardiac axis is between which of the following?

    A. 30 degrees and 60 degrees
    B. 60 degrees and 90 degrees
    C. 90 degrees and 150 degrees
    D. 60 degrees and 180 degrees
    E. 0 degrees and 90 degrees

14. While performing a fetal echocardiogram, you notice retrograde flow into the aortic arch. Which of the following defects is most likely to explain this finding?

    A. d-TGA
    B. AVSD
    C. Critical aortic valve stenosis
    D. Total anomalous pulmonary venous connection
    E. Pulmonary atresia with intact ventricular septum

15. Match the fetal teratogen and its most commonly associated fetal congenital heart lesion:

    A. Ductal constriction
    B. VSD
    C. Coarctation of the aorta
    D. Ebstein anomaly
    E. d-TGA
    1. Lithium
    2. Fetal alcohol syndrome
    3. Indomethacin
    4. Fetal hydantoin syndrome
    5. Isotretinoin

16. Which of the following congenital heart lesions should be excluded in the fetus with SVT?

    A. Ebstein anomaly
    B. Ventricular septal defect
    C. Coarctation of the aorta
    D. d-TGA
    E. Complete AVSD

17. Which of the following forms of congenital heart disease is at greatest risk for needing emergent neonatal cardiac intervention and often requires a highly coordinated delivery at a tertiary care hospital to ensure immediate access to cardiac treatment?

    A. Tetralogy of Fallot with pulmonary stenosis
    B. Hypoplastic left heart syndrome (HLHS) with restrictive atrial septum
    C. Complete atrioventricular canal defect
    D. Coarctation of the aorta
    E. Double-outlet right ventricle

18. A mother has a fetal echo at 24-week gestation that reveals the diagnosis shown below (**Figure 8.2**). After counseling the family on the diagnosis, you explain that postnatal management of their newborn will include which of the following immediately after birth:

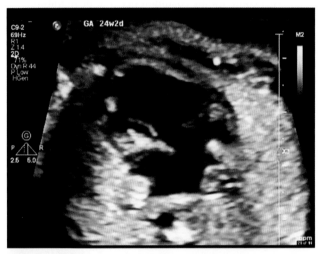

FIGURE 8.2

    A. Balloon atrial septostomy
    B. PGE infusion
    C. Surgery
    D. Intubation
    E. Central venous line placement

19. In specific cases of CHD, there can be additional concerns during the pregnancy. Progression of heart disease or associated comorbidities are often of great concern and need to be monitored closely during the second and third trimesters. For the fetal diagnosis pictured below (**Figure 8.3**), what is of greatest concern for the fetus during the remainder of the pregnancy:

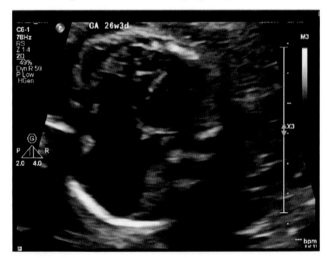

FIGURE 8.3

    A. Hydrops
    B. Supraventricular tachycardia
    C. Growth restriction
    D. Polyhydramnios
    E. Prematurity

20. A fetal echocardiogram performed at 24 weeks EGA confirmed the diagnosis of congenital heart disease with no evidence of heart failure. There was normal fetal heart size, heart function, valve function, and heart rate and rhythm. For the diagnosis pictured below (**Figure 8.4**), what complicating condition needs to be monitored for during the remainder of gestation:

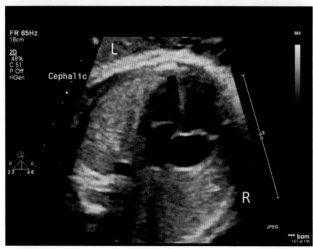

FIGURE 8.4

A. Supraventricular tachycardia
B. Growth restriction
C. Hydrops
D. Heart block
E. Polyhydramnios

21. The following fetal echocardiogram image (**Figure 8.5**) shows an abnormal three-vessel view in a fetus at 27 weeks gestation. Based on these findings, what other organ system is most likely to be significantly affected in the fetus and may even lead to critical presentation at birth requiring neonatal intervention?

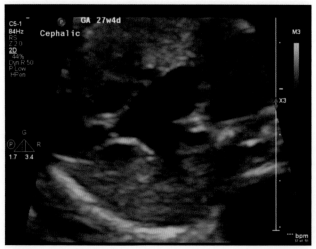

FIGURE 8.5

A. Kidneys
B. Liver/Spleen
C. Brain/Nervous system
D. Lungs/Airways
E. Musculoskeletal

22. A fetal M-mode tracing (**Figure 8.6**) is shown below to assess fetal heart rate and rhythm. What is the most likely cause of this condition in the fetus?

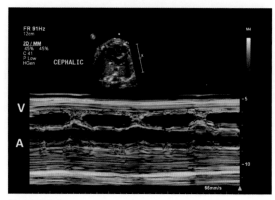

FIGURE 8.6

A. Congenitally corrected transposition of the great arteries (ccTGA)
B. Heterotaxy syndrome
C. Nothing, this fetus has a normal heart rate and rhythm
D. Long QT syndrome
E. Maternal SSA/SSB antibodies

23. Indications for a fetal echocardiogram usually fall into three categories: maternal risks, fetal risks, and familial (inheritable) risks. All the following are indications for formal fetal echocardiography EXCEPT:

A. Maternal pregestational diabetes
B. First-degree relative with congenital heart disease
C. Placenta previa
D. Extracardiac anomaly in the fetus
E. Suspected chromosomal anomaly

24. Which one of the following congenital heart lesions is not considered in the differential diagnosis when a ventricular septal defect (VSD) with overriding great artery is seen on fetal echocardiography (**Figure 8.7**):

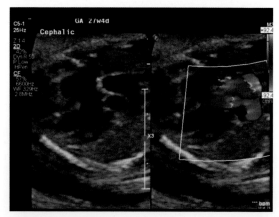

FIGURE 8.7

A. Tricuspid atresia
B. Tetralogy of Fallot
C. Truncus arteriosus
D. Pulmonary atresia with VSD
E. Double-outlet right ventricle (DORV)

25. Fetal echocardiography demonstrates tachycardia. You and your colleagues agree that the fetus has sustained ventricular tachycardia (VT) and evidence of hydrops fetalis. The mother desires that "everything be done" for the fetus. The fetus is at 22 weeks gestation. What is your recommendation?

    A. Give betamethasone immediately
    B. Order anti-SSA/Ro and anti-SSA/La antibody panels and treat with prednisolone if positive
    C. Start sotalol 80 mg PO BID
    D. Load with digoxin 10 mcg IV
    E. Observe only

26. Insulin-dependent maternal diabetes is a maternal risk factor for congenital heart disease. Which of the following statements regarding this referral for fetal echocardiography is *false*?

    A. The incidence of congenital heart disease is lower than referrals with a family history of congenital heart disease
    B. The most common cardiac lesions include d-TGA
    C. A hemoglobin A1C above 8% predicts a high risk of congenital heart disease
    D. The incidence of congenital heart disease is 3% to 7%
    E. The cardiomyopathy is usually reversible

27. Which of the following forms of complex congenital heart disease requires an adequate-size atrial communication (ASD) at birth to maintain adequate systemic oxygenation?

    A. Tetralogy of Fallot with pulmonary atresia
    B. Complete atrioventricular canal defect
    C. d-Transposition of the great arteries
    D. Truncus arteriosus
    E. Coarctation of the aorta

28. Prostaglandin E1 (PGE1) infusion is needed to maintain the patency of the ductus arteriosus (ductal dependent) in certain forms of congenital heart disease. All the following forms of CHD likely require initiation of PGE at birth EXCEPT:

    A. Critical coarctation of the aorta
    B. Hypoplastic left heart syndrome
    C. Truncus arteriosus
    D. Tetralogy of Fallot with severe pulmonary stenosis
    E. Pulmonary atresia with intact ventricular septum

29. A full-term neonate is born via C-section with a birth weight of 3.5 kg to an insulin-dependent diabetic mother. The fetal echocardiogram performed at 20 weeks of gestation was normal with good image quality. The newborn was noted to be mildly tachypneic with mild retractions. Pulse oximetry showed oxygen saturation of 97% on the right arm, and 85% on the left leg. Which of the following congenital heart disease are likely in this neonate?

    A. Complete transposition with patent ductus arteriosus
    B. Congenitally corrected transposition with pulmonary hypertension
    C. Coarctation of the aorta with patent ductus arteriosus
    D. Total anomalous pulmonary venous return with pulmonary hypertension
    E. Tricuspid atresia with normally related great arteries and restrictive VSD

30. A 36-hour-old newborn was noted to have a 1 to 2/6 ejection systolic murmur at the left and right upper sternal border. The rest of the physical examination is unremarkable and the newborn is breathing comfortably in room air. The 25-year-old mother has a history of bicuspid aortic valve without significant stenosis or regurgitation. A transthoracic echocardiogram is ordered for the newborn. All of the following have increased incidence in first-degree family members of patients with bicuspid aortic valve EXCEPT:

    A. Bicuspid aortic valve
    B. Transposition of the great arteries
    C. Hypoplastic left heart syndrome
    D. Dilated ascending aorta
    E. Shone complex

31. A 30-hour-old newborn was noted to have a 2/6 systolic murmur at the left upper sternal border. The rest of the physical examination is unremarkable. Pulse oximetry showed SaO_2 of 98% in the right arm and right leg. A transthoracic echocardiogram showed a pulmonary valve systolic mean Doppler gradient of 22 mm Hg. Which of the following is the next best management step?

    A. Immediate initiation of prostaglandin infusion
    B. Pulmonary balloon valvuloplasty in the next 2 to 3 days
    C. Cardiac magnetic resonance imaging in 1 week
    D. Outpatient follow-up in 6 to 8 weeks with a repeat echocardiogram
    E. None (no further cardiology follow-up needed)

CHAPTER 8

32. A 2 month old was noted to have a grade 3/6 systolic murmur by the pediatrician, radiating to both lung fields. A transthoracic echocardiogram was ordered (**Figure 8.8**).

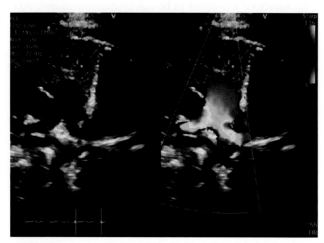

FIGURE 8.8

Which of the following is the best management strategy for this infant?

A. No cardiology follow-up is needed
B. Follow-up with pediatric cardiology in 6 to 8 weeks
C. Cardiac magnetic resonance imaging
D. Start prostaglandin infusion
E. Cardiac cathetcrization and balloon angioplasty of the pulmonary arteries

33. A 4-week-old infant was noted to have increased respiratory distress. On examination, he has a grade 4/6 holosystolic murmur at the cardiac apex, radiating to the left axilla. Pulse oximetry showed a pre- and postductal oxygen saturation of 97%. A chest radiograph showed pulmonary edema with increased pulmonary vascular markings. An ECG showed left superior axis and left atrial enlargement. An echocardiogram is being performed. Which of the following is the most likely cardiac diagnosis in this infant?

A. d-Transposition of the great arteries
B. Partial atrioventricular septal defect
C. Ebstein anomaly
D. Large ventricular septal defect
E. Unobstructed total anomalous pulmonary venous connection

34. An asymptomatic 1-day-old newborn was noted to have a murmur. The mother has insulin-dependent diabetes mellitus that was poorly controlled throughout the pregnancy. An echocardiogram was performed that showed moderate right ventricular hypertrophy. The left ventricular wall thickness was normal. The rest of the cardiac anatomy was normal. What is the next best step in the management of this newborn?

A. Genetic testing for hypertrophic cardiomyopathy
B. β-Blocker therapy
C. Cardiac MRI to look for delayed enhancement
D. Outpatient follow-up in 2 months
E. Surgical consultation for myectomy +/− ICD implantation

35. Atrial flutter was noted on the electrocardiogram of a newborn. A 2:1 atrioventricular conduction was noted with a ventricular rate of 230 beats per minute. A successful DC cardioversion was performed and sinus rhythm was sustained. An echocardiogram was performed that revealed normal cardiac anatomy and function. The newborn was monitored on telemetry for 2 days without any recurrence or any other arrhythmia. What is the next best step for the management of this newborn?

A. Start propranolol
B. Start amiodarone
C. Start digoxin
D. No medical therapy, follow-up in the outpatient clinic
E. Schedule for electrophysiology study

36. A 4-week-old infant carries a prenatal diagnosis of d-transposition of the great arteries, a large posterior malalignment ventricular septal defect and left ventricular outflow tract obstruction, and is being seen in the outpatient clinic. A successful balloon atrial septostomy was performed on the day of birth. The infant was noted to have increased work of breathing. A follow-up echocardiogram showed a widely patent atrial communication, large VSD, LVOT mean Doppler gradient of 20 mm Hg, and a tiny PDA with left-to-right shunt. A chest radiograph has been ordered. What is the best management plan for this patient?

A. Start oxygen by nasal cannula
B. Repeat balloon atrial septostomy
C. Device closure of the PDA
D. Ductal stent implantation
E. Oral furosemide

37. A 5-week-old infant is seen in the outpatient clinic. She carries a diagnosis of double-outlet right ventricle with pulmonary valve atresia. A ductal stent was implanted on day 3 of life. The parents report that her oxygen saturation has been stable between 75% and 85% at home. The PDA murmur is audible on examination. There is no increased work of breathing. Her hemoglobin is normal at 12.5 g/dL. What is the next best management step for this patient?

   A. Start heparin infusion
   B. Give blood transfusion
   C. Start furosemide
   D. Start iron
   E. Emergent cardiac catheterization for ductal stent dilation

38. A 5-day-old infant is brought to the emergency room with excessive lethargy and poor oral intake. The oxygen saturation on the right arm is 98% but the one on the foot is not reading. On examination, he has cold lower extremities with barely palpable pulses. A ductal-dependent lesion was assumed and prostaglandin infusion was started at a high dose. An echocardiogram was performed that confirmed the diagnosis of severe, discrete juxtaductal coarctation of the aorta with a mean Doppler gradient of 38 mm Hg. No patent ductus arteriosus was seen despite the child being on prostaglandin for over an hour. The left ventricular function was mildly decreased with a calculated ejection fraction of 50%. A bicuspid aortic valve with no stenosis or regurgitation was noted. A cardiac surgeon will not be available for several hours. What is the next best management step for this patient?

   A. Call for ECMO support
   B. Transcatheter ductal stent placement
   C. Start furosemide infusion
   D. Start epinephrine infusion
   E. Give oral digoxin

Answers

1. (D) Abnormal findings suggestive of a fetal cardiac anomaly on obstetrical screening ultrasound is the most common reason to refer for formal fetal echocardiography, and in ~40% to 50% of these pregnancies, CHD is confirmed. However, all of these are appropriate indications for performing a fetal echocardiogram. Of note, rubella is an extremely rare maternal infection, but does carry increased risk for CHD, especially pulmonary stenosis. Fetal rhythm abnormalities affect ~1% to 2% of pregnancies and account for <10% of referrals for formal fetal echocardiography. PKU is a rare metabolic disorder that in pregnant women is associated with CHD, particularly when the mother's diet is not well controlled. There is a 10- to 15-fold increased risk of CHD in the fetus when the mother has elevated maternal serum levels of phenylalanine >15 mg/dL. However, if the mother has good preconception control and maintains levels <10 mg/dL during the first trimester, the risk is greatly reduced and a fetal echocardiogram may not be necessary.

2. (C) The right ventricle ejects 55% to 60% of combined fetal cardiac output while the left ventricle ejects 40% to 45%. Cardiac output increases significantly during gestation, but the relative amounts of output from these two parallel circulations remain relatively the same.

3. (E) Retinoic acid is a vitamin A derivative used to treat severe acne and has been associated with increased risk of fetal anomalies in multiple organ systems (CNS, craniofacial, branchial arches, and cardiac). Cardiac anomalies most often seen in retinoic acid exposure included conotruncal defects and aortic arch anomalies. The other answers are

paired incorrectly. Alcohol exposure has an increased risk of septal defects such as VSD in association with fetal alcohol syndrome. Salicylates such as NSAIDs (indomethacin) are associated with premature ductus arteriosus closure usually due to exposure with the highest risk in the third trimester. Fortunately, the constriction is usually mild and can be reversed with discontinuation of the drug if recognized early. Lithium is associated with Ebstein anomaly, but more recent studies have suggested lower risk level than previously thought.

4. (B) The standard four-chamber view of the heart is good for visualizing the atria, ventricles, atrioventricular valves, pulmonary veins, and ventricular septum. In addition, it is good for assessing cardiac size and position within the fetal thorax. The three-vessel view and three-vessel tracheal views are used to assess for arch anomalies such as vascular ring and right aortic arch. The outflow tract views are used to assess for conotruncal defects such as tetralogy of Fallot and d-TGA. The sagittal arch views are best for assessing the ductal and aortic arch for conditions such as coarctation, but the three-vessel tracheal view can also be used to assess these structures.

5. (C) Pulsed-wave Doppler of mitral valve inflow and aortic outflow can be used to assess irregular fetal rhythm (**Figure 8.9**). In addition, M-mode and TDI modalities can also be used to assess irregular fetal rhythm. PACs are the most common cause of fetal arrhythmia. Vascular ring, HLHS, d-TGA, and anomalies of the branch pulmonary arteries are best assessed using sweeps with 2D (grayscale) and color Doppler.

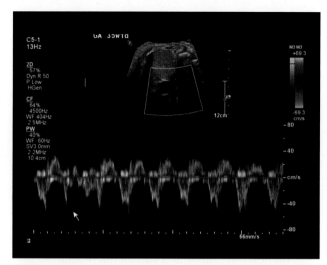

FIGURE 8.9 Pulsed-wave Doppler of AV valve inflow. Doppler demonstrates early premature atrial contraction (*arrow*).

6. (A) Fetal arrhythmias occur in 1% to 3% of all pregnancies. PACs comprise the largest percentage of these rhythm abnormalities followed by PVCs. Fetal SVT, atrial flutter, and complete heart block account for <10% of all reported fetal arrhythmias.

7. (B) The normal fetal heart comprises about one-third of the fetal thorax, ranging from 25% to 35%.

8. (B) Obstructed TAPVR is still a surgical emergency because these patients cannot be fully stabilized with medical intervention alone. Due to the inability of blood to exit the lungs effectively and provide proper oxygen delivery to the body, these neonates are at risk for progressive hypoxia (cyanosis) and acidosis.

9. (D) This is the mechanical PR interval, measured from the beginning of atrial inflow (mitral A wave) to the beginning of ventricular ejection.

10. (E) With lack of antegrade flow across the atretic pulmonary valve, fetuses with pulmonary atresia with intact ventricular septum often have reversal of flow across the ductus arteriosus into the hypoplastic main pulmonary artery and branch pulmonary arteries. The other listed congenital heart lesions all typically have a normally functioning pulmonary valve with antegrade flow into the main pulmonary artery and ductus arteriosus.

11. (C) The normal fetal heart rate ranges from 100 to 180 bpm throughout gestation. Fetal bradycardia is defined as a sustained heart rate less than 100 bpm while fetal tachycardia as a sustained rate greater than 180 bpm.

12. (A) At term, 10% of fetal cardiac output perfuses the lungs. The remainder of this deoxygenated blood is directed through the ductus arteriosus to the descending aorta and placenta for oxygenation.

13. (A) The normal leftward axis of the fetal heart (relative to the midline) ranges from 30 degrees to 60 degrees.

14. (C) Because of limited antegrade blood flow across the critically stenotic aortic valve, flow within the aortic arch is supplied retrograde from the ductus arteriosus. The other listed congenital heart lesions all typically have a normally functioning aortic valve with antegrade flow into the ascending aorta and transverse aortic arch and antegrade flow from the ductus arteriosus to the descending aorta.

15. (1-D, 2-B, 3-A, 4-C, 5-E) Lithium has been shown in studies to be associated with fetal Ebstein anomaly as well as atrial septal defects and atrioventricular valve atresia. Fetal alcohol syndrome has been commonly associated with septal defects including atrial and ventricular septal defects and is less commonly associated with coarctation and conotruncal defects. Indomethacin is a potent ductal constrictor. Coarctation of the aorta and LVOT obstruction have been described in fetal hydantoin syndrome. Exposure to isotretinoin during gestation has been associated with fetal d-TGA as well as septal defects and conotruncal anomalies.

16. (A) Ebstein anomaly is associated with a 15% to 20% incidence of rhythm abnormalities, most notably Wolff–Parkinson–White syndrome and SVT.

17. (B) HLHS with restrictive atrial septum. In HLHS, there is often mitral and/or aortic atresia such that blood cannot exit the left heart. Therefore, HLHS requires an adequate atrial communication to allow the blood to exit the left atrium and join the rest of the circulation to the body. If there is not an adequate atrial communication, these patients can present like obstructed TAPVR due to back up of blood into the lungs resulting in severe pulmonary congestion, worsening hypoxia, and acidosis. These infants are often critically ill at birth and require either emergent opening of the atrial septum via catheterization or surgical septectomy.

18. (B) PGE infusion. This image shows a fetus with HLHS of the mitral atresia and aortic atresia variety. There is a single RV that has enlarged to take over the apex of the heart. The RA and LA are also seen with a wide-open atrial communication between them such that this child does not appear to be at risk for restrictive atrial septum, so a balloon atrial septostomy or immediate surgery should not be warranted. PGE infusion is indicated to maintain ductal patency for systemic blood flow and can be given through a peripheral IV, so placement of a central venous line is not always necessary. PGE causes the side effect of apnea in ~50% of babies so intubation may be necessary, but not in all patients. Therefore, PGE1 is the only therapy that needs to be started in this patient with 100% certainty, shortly after birth.

19. (A) Hydrops. This image depicts a fetus with Ebstein anomaly (EA) as noted by the inferiorly displaced tricuspid valve leaflets, severe RA, and RV dilation with massive cardiomegaly (wall-to-wall heart). EA fetuses can develop all the problems listed above, but the highest risk and one of the greatest concerns is hydrops because it can lead to fetal demise. Development of hydrops and/or fetal demise has been reported in up to 45% of fetal EA cases. Rhythm disturbances have been reported in up to 17% of EA fetuses, with the most common being SVT. Growth restriction and prematurity also occur more frequently in EA and must be monitored closely. Polyhydramnios can be part of the constellation of hydrops and can also increase the risk for prematurity.

20. (D) Heart block. The diagnosis pictured is congenitally corrected transposition of the great arteries (ccTGA). Note that the left-sided ventricle has a lower attachment of the AV valve which is the tricuspid valve, has a moderator band across the apex, and is more trabeculated because it is the morphologic RV. By comparison, the more anterior and rightward ventricle has a higher-inserted AV valve which is the mitral valve, smooth-walled septum with no AV valve attachments, and bullet chamber with no moderator band. Not pictured here are the outflow tracts which are usually oriented in an L-TGA configuration with the aorta arising anterior and leftward from the left-sided RV and the pulmonary artery arising posterior and rightward to the aorta from the right-sided LV. There are often associated heart defects in ccTGA, such as VSD, pulmonary stenosis, and tricuspid valve abnormalities which can be seen in up to 80% of cases. Growth restriction, hydrops, and polyhydramnios are unlikely to occur in cases of ccTGA unless there is associated extracardiac disease, a genetic syndrome, or fetal CHF (in this case it was noted that the heart function and valve function were normal). SVT is rarely noted to occur in ccTGA, but heart block is a well-known risk due to the abnormal position of the AV node and bundle of His which can lead to early fibrosis. Up to 20% of fetuses with ccTGA have been reported to have varying degrees of AV block and associated bradycardia. If complete heart block develops, this can put the fetus at risk of developing hydrops if the ventricular escape rate is very slow. This would also change the delivery management.

21. (D) Lungs/Airways. The image shows a three-vessel view in the setting of TOF with absent pulmonary valve. Both branch pulmonary arteries are severely dilated in this image and there is absence of the ductus arteriosus which is common in this diagnosis. The massive dilation of the branch pulmonary arteries can lead to compression of the proximal and distal airways as well as aberrant branching of the intrapulmonary bronchi and inhibition of alveolar growth. At birth, the result can be severe, extrinsic airway compression from the dilated pulmonary arteries and hypoxemia due to pulmonary hypoplasia. These patients can be difficult to manage with traditional positive pressure ventilation and sometimes will ventilate without mechanical support when placed in the prone position because it "lifts" the dilated pulmonary vessels off the airways. Of note, the diagnosis of TOF/APV is also highly associated 22q11 microdeletion syndrome (DiGeorge), which is seen in approximately 21% to 38% of patients.

22. (E) Maternal SSA/SSB antibodies. The M-mode tracing displays congenital complete heart block with a slow ventricular escape rate of ~60 bpm (top) compared to atrial rate of ~140 bpm (bottom) with complete A to V dissociation. While ccTGA, heterotaxy syndrome (polysplenia type), and long QT syndrome can be associated with heart block, it is maternal SSA/SSB antibody exposure that is the most

common cause of complete heart block in the fetus. This occurs during the second trimester (16 to 24 weeks GA) in ~2% of antibody-positive mothers. Risks are higher for subsequent pregnancies after one affected child (15% to 20%). Fetal mortality rate is ~10% to 20%, but the highest risk is when the fetal heart rate drops to <55 bpm due to the slow ventricular escape rate.

23. (C) Placenta previa is an abnormality of placental implantation that is not associated with congenital heart disease (CHD) and thus not an indication for formal fetal echo. Answer A is a common maternal risk factor for CHD as well as the development of hypertrophic cardiomyopathy in the third trimester which correlates directly with the degree of DM severity (i.e., average blood sugar levels as measured by maternal HgbA1C level). Answer B is a familial risk for CHD which varies depending on the type of CHD and family member affected. In general, recurrence risk ranges from 3% to 7% but can be higher for certain types of CHD such as aortic stenosis and AV septal defects. Answers D and E are both fetal risk factors for CHD. Suspected chromosomal anomaly has a high risk for CHD which varies depending on the specific syndrome. Extracardiac anomalies in the fetus are also frequently associated with CHD as well as chromosomal anomalies. The risk of CHD is dependent on the type of fetal malformation with some organ systems having a very high risk (CNS and renal, >70%) with others being lower risk (pulmonary and craniofacial, 35%).

24. (A) Tricuspid atresia. The long-axis view on fetal echo is often used to demonstrate outflow tract lesions. When there is a large VSD with an overriding great artery, this likely denotes a conotruncal anomaly which includes TOF, truncus arteriosus, DORV, d-TGA with VSD, and pulmonary atresia with VSD. Tricuspid atresia typically involves an underdeveloped (hypoplastic) right ventricle with VSD and sometimes transposition of the great arteries but does not usually have an overriding outflow tract.

25. (C) This fetus has significant hemodynamic compromise by the underlying fetal tachycardia. Starting sotalol is the most effective therapy to treat this hydropic fetus. Digoxin has poor maternal–fetal transfer in the hydropic fetus and is not the first-line drug therapy in this clinical scenario. Maternal lupus is associated with fetal heart block and bradycardia; hence, evaluation of ant-SSA/Ro and anti-SSA/La antibodies is not indicated. At 22 weeks, delivery of a live fetus is not an optimal strategy either, so pretreatment of the mother with betamethasone is not indicated.

26. (A) The incidence of congenital heart disease in maternal diabetes (4% to 10%) is higher than those with a previous family history of congenital heart disease (2% to 4%). The most common cardiac lesions in fetuses of diabetic mothers include d-TGA, truncus arteriosus, and tetralogy of Fallot. Risk of congenital heart disease in the fetus has been directly associated with the maternal hemoglobin A1C level during early gestation. HCM associated with poor maternal glucose control is most often reversible within weeks or months post delivery.

27. (C) d-Transposition of the great arteries (d-TGA) requires an atrial communication for blood to mix between the right and left heart so that there can be effective systemic and pulmonary blood flow. When the atrial septum is restrictive or intact in d-TGA, the circulations are no longer in series but rather in parallel. Thus, the infant has adequate pulmonary blood flow, but this oxygenated blood does not make it back to the systemic circulation and therefore it is not effective pulmonary blood flow. The infant will become progressively more cyanotic as the systemic venous return is recirculated back to the body with lower and lower oxygen content. PGE alone would not help, as the flow in the ductus arteriosus tends to become one directional with time (shunting from aorta to pulmonary artery). This results in a medical emergency that will require either opening of the atrial septum via catheterization with balloon atrial septostomy (BAS) or intraoperative atrial septectomy.

28. (C) Truncus arteriosus does not require PGE infusion because the common arterial trunk provides blood flow to both the aorta and the pulmonary arteries. In fact, truncus arteriosus often is associated with complete absence of the ductus arteriosus. The only type of truncus arteriosus that requires PGE infusion is when there is associated interruption of the aortic arch. In this case, there is a ductus arteriosus, and PGE is indicated to maintain patency of flow to the lower half of the body. Critical coarctation and HLHS both require PGE to maintain ductus arteriosus patency for systemic blood flow after birth. TOF with severe pulmonary stenosis and PA/IVS require PGE to maintain ductus arteriosus patency for pulmonary blood flow after birth.

29. (C) Coarctation of the aorta is the most common missed diagnosis on fetal echocardiography. A right-to-left shunt at the ductal level in coarctation leads to differential cyanosis of the lower extremities. Pulmonary venous anomalies can also be missed (less frequently) on fetal echocardiography but will not result in differential cyanosis. All other diagnoses do not cause differential cyanosis and should be identifiable on a fetal echocardiogram with good-quality images.

30. (B) Transposition of the great arteries is not associated with a family history of bicuspid aortic valve. All others have known increased incidence in the first-degree family members of patients with bicuspid aortic valve and hypoplastic left heart syndrome.

31. (D) A pulmonary valve mean Doppler gradient of 22 mm Hg is not critical and does not require prostaglandin infusion or balloon valvuloplasty at this time. This gradient is likely to increase as the pulmonary vascular resistance drops. Therefore, a follow-up echocardiogram in 6 to 8 weeks is important to reassess the pulmonary valve gradient. Cardiac magnetic resonance imaging is not needed at this time.

32. (A) The infant has physiologic peripheral pulmonary stenosis causing the murmur. The infant does not need any cardiology follow-up as this is an innocent murmur of childhood that is expected to go away by 6 months of age.

33. (B) Partial atrioventricular septal defect with significant left AV valve regurgitation presents early with respiratory distress due to left atrial hypertension and pulmonary venous congestion. Left axis deviation on ECG is notable on any atrioventricular septal defect.

34. (D) Hypertrophic cardiomyopathy is common in infants of a diabetic mother, especially in insulin-dependent diabetes. This hypertrophy does not pose a risk of sudden death and usually resolves postnatally in a few weeks. Therefore, outpatient follow-up in a few months is reasonable. No other testing, therapy, or intervention is needed.

35. (D) Atrial flutter in newborns with normal cardiac anatomy and function usually does not recur. Therefore, antiarrhythmic therapy is not indicated. An electrophysiology study is not needed.

36. (E) An LVOT mean Doppler gradient of 20 mm Hg suggests inadequate pulmonary stenosis to prevent pulmonary overcirculation. Diuretic therapy will help decrease the pulmonary edema from pulmonary overcirculation and improve the respiratory status of the infant.

37. (D) A normal hemoglobin in single ventricle physiology with oxygen saturation of 75% to 85% suggests iron deficiency anemia. These patients are generally polycythemic as they require increased hemoglobin to improve oxygen-carrying capacity.

38. (D) If the ductus arteriosus does not open after prostaglandin infusion in severe coarctation of the aorta, inotropic support should be used to improve left ventricular function and augment flow across the coarctation. Neonatal coarctation should not be managed with ductal stent. Diuretics and digoxin do not help in this situation and the patient should be kept NPO.

SUGGESTED READINGS

Abuhamad A, Chaoui R. *A Practical Guide to Fetal Echocardiography : Normal and Abnormal Hearts.* 3rd ed. Wolters Kluwer Health; 2016.

AIUM practice parameter for the performance of fetal echocardiography. *J Ultrasound Med.* 2020;39(1):E5–E16. doi:10.1002/jum.15188

Donofrio MT, Moon-Grady AJ, Hornberger LK, et al. Diagnosis and treatment of fetal cardiac disease: A scientific statement from the American Heart Association. *Circulation.* 2014;129(21):2183–2242. doi:10.1161/01.cir.0000437597.44550.5d

Simpson JM, Hunter LE. Fetal echocardiography. In: Eidem BW, Johnson J, Lopez L, et al., eds. *Echocardiography in Pediatric and Adult Congenital Heart Disease.* 3rd ed. Wolters Kluwer; 2021:595–613.

Freud LR, Escobar-Diaz MC, Kalish BT, et al. Outcomes and predictors of perinatal mortality in fetuses with Ebstein anomaly or tricuspid valve dysplasia in the current era: A multicenter study. *Circulation*. 2015;132(6):481–489. doi:10.1161/CIRCULATIONAHA.115.015839

Pruetz JD, Miller JC, Loeb GE, et al. Prenatal diagnosis and management of congenital complete heart block. *Birth Defects Res*. 2019;111(8):380–388. doi:10.1002/bdr2.1459

Pruetz JD, Votava-Smith J, Tesoriero L. Neonates with critical congenital heart disease: Delivery room management and stabilization before transfer to the cardiac ICU. In: Polin RA, ed. *Hemodynamics and Cardiology: Neonatology Questions and Controversies*. 3rd ed. Elsevier; 2019.ISBN: 978-323-533 669

Rychik J, Tian Z. *Fetal Cardiovascular Imaging: A Disease-Based Approach*. Saunders; 2012.

Sanapo L, Pruetz JD, Słodki M, et al. Fetal echocardiography for planning perinatal and delivery room care of neonates with congenital heart disease. *Echocardiography*. 2017;34(12): 1804–1821.

Outpatient Cardiology

Frank Cetta, Nibras E. El Sherif, Carolina P. Larmeu, and Adam Cassidy

Questions

1. Three months ago, a 15 year old was found to have a consistently elevated blood pressure to 140/84 and she instituted lifestyle modifications. During this timeframe she lost 5 kg and her most recent blood pressure was 135/85. An ambulatory blood pressure monitor was consistent with these readings. What is the best next step in management?

   A. Continue lifestyle modifications
   B. Start ACE inhibitor
   C. Start β-blocker
   D. Start hydrochlorothiazide
   E. Start amlodipine

2. A healthy 13 year old was referred to cardiology clinic following an episode of syncope. She was walking to class when her friend surprised her with a loud noise. She lost postural tone and was unconscious for 30 seconds. She regained consciousness spontaneously afterward and was quickly back to her usual state of health. What would you recommend?

   A. Increase hydration and salt intake
   B. Reassurance only
   C. Baseline ECG
   D. Start β-blocker therapy
   E. Exercise test

3. A 16-year-old boy was referred to your clinic. You determine that this is most likely a benign murmur, common in his age group. Which of the following best describes the most common benign murmur in a teenager?

   A. Midsystolic click followed by a II/IV late systolic murmur at the apex
   B. II/IV ejection systolic murmur at the second left intercostal space
   C. Soft continuous murmur at the left upper chest
   D. II/IV vibratory murmur at the left lower sternal border
   E. III/IV harsh holosystolic murmur at the left lower sternal border

4. A 10 year old has a bicuspid aortic valve with a mean gradient of 10 mm Hg and a 3/6 blowing decrescendo diastolic murmur. Which of the following physical examination findings would be expected in this patient?

   A. Narrow pulse pressure
   B. Prominent jugular venous V wave
   C. Bounding pulses
   D. Radial-femoral pulse delay
   E. Prominent hepatojugular reflex

5. You are evaluating a 10-year-old girl who was referred for hypertension. On physical examination, she has a 2/6 systolic ejection murmur and diminished lower extremity pulses. She has no physical stigmata suggestive of a syndrome. An echocardiogram confirmed the diagnosis of bicuspid aortic valve and coarctation of the aorta with a mean gradient of 35 mm Hg across the coarctation site. Which of the following is true regarding further workup?

   A. Repeat echocardiogram in 6 months to follow the coarctation gradient
   B. Perform transesophageal echocardiogram
   C. Obtain karyotype and chromosomal microarray
   D. Obtain a fasting lipid profile

6. Which of the following disorders is associated with a short PR interval on ECG?

   A. Duchenne muscular dystrophy
   B. Marfan syndrome
   C. Pompe disease
   D. Turner syndrome
   E. Alagille syndrome

7. A 5 year old was seen in the outpatient clinic. He was discharged from the hospital 2 weeks ago for Kawasaki disease. An echocardiogram performed on the day of hospital discharge showed normal coronary arteries. His parents asked when would be the appropriate time to return to sports participation?

   A. Now, since he does not have any evidence of coronary aneurysms
   B. He cannot play until 4 weeks from the time of hospital dismissal
   C. He should be restricted from sports for 6 months from the date of diagnosis
   D. He should be restricted from sports for 8 weeks from the date of diagnosis
   E. He can participate in low-impact sports only in 6 weeks

8. A 16-year-old high school basketball player is presenting for a follow-up visit. He was discharged 2 weeks ago from the hospital after a 1-week stay for MIS-C. He transiently required vasoactive support due to LV dysfunction. But his EF was 62% at the time of hospital discharge. He reports that he is feeling well and is back to his baseline. He is wondering if he can return to playing basketball?

   A. He can return to sports now because his EF normalized prior to hospital discharge
   B. Repeat echocardiogram in 2 weeks and if it continues to show normal function, clear for sports participation at that time
   C. He will need an echocardiogram, 24-hour Holter monitor, and exercise ECG in 3 to 6 months after the initial illness
   D. Sports restriction is based on the development of coronary artery aneurysms
   E. Sports participation is allowed only if cardiac MRI shows no evidence of inflammation

9. Which of the following is a key difference between MIS-C and Kawasaki disease (KD)?

   A. Coronary artery aneurysms are associated only with KD
   B. Steroids are not first-line agents for MIS-C, but they are for KD
   C. Gastrointestinal symptoms are more common with KD rather than MIS-C
   D. Desquamative rash is exclusively a feature of KD
   E. Systemic hypotension and shock are more common in MIS-C

10. Which of the following is a supplemental laboratory finding used to diagnose Kawasaki disease?

    A. Hyperalbuminemia
    B. Thrombocytopenia
    C. Erythrocytosis
    D. Leukopenia
    E. Sterile pyuria

11. A 3-year-old boy is referred because a new murmur was auscultated during a routine well-child visit. He is adopted. His adoptive mother tells you that his birth mother died suddenly and no records are available. Which of the following is most likely to prompt you to order an echocardiogram?

    A. The second heart sound splits with inspiration
    B. The murmur is loudest in the standing position
    C. The murmur is not heard over the neck
    D. The patient has a normal ECG and chest x-ray
    E. The murmur is heard best at the LUSB

12. A 6-year-old boy is referred to pediatric cardiology secondary to an LDL concentration of 170 mg/dL. Pertinent family history includes a grandfather with coronary vascular disease and first myocardial infarction at age 50. The patient has a BMI that puts him in the 90th percentile. Which of the following is the best management step?

    A. Weight management including nutritional counseling and increased physical activity should be started while initiating a bile acid–binding resin, such as cholestyramine

    B. Single pharmacotherapy with a statin should be initiated

    C. Niacin should be initiated in addition to weight management

    D. Repeat cholesterol screening should be performed at age 8 years

    E. Weight management should be the primary method of control

13. A 17-year-old girl is referred to pediatric cardiology clinic after ascending aortic dilation was found on an echocardiogram performed secondary to chest pain complaints. The remainder of the echocardiogram was normal. On review of the echocardiogram, the sinus of Valsalva is dilated with a Z-score of +3.4. A physical examination reveals the patient has scoliosis, pectus carinatum, and a hindfoot deformity. Family history is positive for a maternal grandfather with ascending aortic dissection. Which of the following genes should be tested for maximum yield?

    A. Transforming growth factor β receptor 1 (*TGFBR1*)
    B. Fibrillin 1 (*FBN1*)
    C. Collagen, type III, α 1 (*COL3A1*)
    D. ADAM metallopeptidase with thrombospondin type 1 motif, 10 (*ADAMTS10*)
    E. Actin, α 2, smooth muscle, aorta (*ACTA2*)

14. Which of the following medications is not indicated for a 16 year old with *FBN1* mutation and sinus of Valsalva dilation measuring 42 mm?

    A. Losartan
    B. Enalapril
    C. Digoxin
    D. Atenolol
    E. Amlodipine

15. A 13-year-old boy is referred to pediatric cardiology clinic secondary to hypertension. His blood pressure was recorded as 128/78 at his last health maintenance visit. On the basis of age and height, he is greater than the 95th percentile for systolic and the 90th percentile for diastolic blood pressure. In pediatric cardiology clinic, his blood pressure is 130/80, using auscultation and an appropriate cuff size. Which is the next best step in evaluation and treatment?

    A. Ambulatory blood pressure monitoring
    B. Recommend dietary modifications as a primary therapy
    C. Echocardiogram to evaluate end-organ damage
    D. Renal ultrasound
    E. Initiation of atenolol

16. An 8-year-old boy has blood pressures in the 92nd to 94th percentile range on multiple readings over the past several visits at his pediatrician's office. Which category does this child fall into and what is the next best step?

    A. Stage 2 hypertension; initiate pharmacotherapy
    B. Stage 1 hypertension; echocardiogram
    C. Prehypertension; echocardiogram
    D. Prehypertension; lifestyle changes and repeat BP check in 6 months
    E. Normal; annual blood pressure monitoring

17. A 16-year-old girl is referred to pediatric cardiology clinic secondary to a murmur heard at a sports physical. On auscultation, there is a I–II/VI systolic ejection murmur best heard over the upper sternal border and a blowing decrescendo diastolic murmur radiating toward the apex. What other finding on physical examination might be expected?

    A. Narrowed pulse pressure
    B. Systolic ejection click at the apex
    C. Displaced right ventricular impulse
    D. Elevated diastolic blood pressure
    E. Decreased femoral pulses

18. A 12-year-old girl presents with a high-pitched, blowing, holosystolic murmur heard best over the apex of the chest. An echocardiogram confirms moderate mitral valve regurgitation with thickening of the mitral valve. Suspecting rheumatic heart disease (RHD), you send streptococcal antibody titers, which are elevated. Which of the following additional findings would most strongly support the diagnosis of acute RHD?

    A. Arthralgia
    B. Fever
    C. Elevated ESR or CRP
    D. Prolonged PR interval
    E. Erythema marginatum

19. In a patient with a syncopal episode, which of the following features would prompt hospitalization or intense outpatient workup?

    A. Syncope with exertion
    B. Syncope after rising from supine to standing position
    C. Family history of bicuspid aortic valve
    D. Previous near-syncopal episode
    E. Loss of bladder control during syncopal episode

20. A 14-year-old girl is referred following two episodes of loss of consciousness, both occurred during soccer practice while she was sprinting down the field. Each episode lasted 1 minute, and the patient returned quickly to baseline. She denies nausea, vomiting, sweating, or blurred vision prior to the episodes but reports that her heart was beating "funny" prior to the episodes. Family history is negative for sudden cardiac death. Physical examination is unremarkable. Which of the following is the next best step in evaluation?

    A. Exercise stress test
    B. Electrocardiogram
    C. 24-Hour Holter monitor
    D. In-hospital monitoring

21. Which of the following is considered the gold standard for diagnosis of myocarditis?

    A. Viral cultures and titers
    B. Electrocardiogram
    C. Endomyocardial biopsy
    D. Magnetic resonance imaging
    E. Echocardiography

22. Which of the following accounts for the findings of cardiomegaly, left ventricular hypertrophy, and a flow murmur observed in patients with sickle cell anemia?

    A. Chronic anemia
    B. Thrombotic crisis
    C. Arrhythmia
    D. Iron overload
    E. Pulmonary hypertension

23. A 16-year-old boy is referred because an elevated BP was detected during a high school sports screen. His examination reveals a normal precordial impulse and a normal S_1 with an S_2 that splits appropriately. His BMI is >99th percentile. There is a 2/6 systolic murmur best heard at the LUSB that is accentuated with lying down. The murmur resolves when he sits upright. His blood pressure is 135/75 mm Hg in the right arm. In this patient, which of the following is the best next step?

    A. BP measurement is likely falsely elevated. BP should be repeated using a cuff with a bladder size that is at least 80% of the upper arm circumference
    B. BP measurement is likely falsely elevated. BP should be repeated using a cuff that is two-thirds the length of the upper arm
    C. BP measurement is likely falsely elevated. BP should be repeated with the same cuff but at a more inferior level on the arm
    D. BP measurement is likely accurate, patient should begin antihypertensive medication
    E. BP measurement is likely accurate, an echocardiogram should be ordered

24. A 3-year-old girl is referred to the pediatric cardiology clinic for a murmur. The child is at the 3rd percentile for weight and 45th percentile for height. She has no cyanosis, dyspnea, or syncope. On examination, there is a 3/6 systolic murmur best heard in the left upper sternal border that has a crescendo–decrescendo quality. There is no diastolic murmur. She has a normal S_1 and a fixed split S_2. Pulses are normal. Which of the following is the most likely source of murmur?

    A. Increased flow across the tricuspid valve
    B. Increased flow across the pulmonary valve
    C. Flow across the atrial septum
    D. Flow across the ventricular septum
    E. Increased flow across the aortic valve

25. A 13-year-old boy with an ASD, diagnosed in infancy, was lost to follow-up. His last echocardiogram was 10 years ago. During your examination, he has a normal S_1, his S_2 splits with expiration, and it is prominent. He has a short systolic murmur heard along the LUSB. There is no diastolic murmur. His liver is palpable 1 cm below the costal margin. Which of the following is the best explanation for his physical examination findings?

    A. The absence of a diastolic murmur indicates a decrease in left-to-right shunting as a result of the decreasing size of the ASD
    B. The prominent S_2 indicates increased left-to-right shunt
    C. The absence of a fixed split S_2 and increased S_2 prominence indicate a decrease in left-to-right shunting as a result of increased pulmonary artery pressures
    D. The systolic murmur is from tricuspid regurgitation as a result of RV enlargement
    E. The splitting of S_2 indicates a decrease in left-to-right shunting as a result of the decreasing size of the ASD

26. You are evaluating a 2-month-old infant who weighs 3.9 kg. He was full term, and his birth weight was 3.6 kg. The infant has a large VSD that was demonstrated on echocardiography obtained soon after birth. Currently, his respiratory rate is 60 breaths per minute. The parents report that he is not cyanotic, but he does take 40 minutes to complete a 2-oz bottle of formula. What is the next most appropriate step for this infant?

    A. Dietician referral to increase caloric intake
    B. Cardiology follow-up in 2 months
    C. Begin treatment with sildenafil
    D. Begin treatment with furosemide 4 mg orally twice daily
    E. Pulmonary consult to evaluate for noncardiac etiologies of tachypnea

27. A 9-year-old girl is referred for evaluation of a murmur. She is an otherwise healthy child. There is no parasternal lift. She has a 2/6 early systolic murmur best heard between the apex and left lower sternal border. It is of low pitch and has a musical quality. It is best heard with the bell of the stethoscope and decreases with standing upright. Pulses are normal. What is the most appropriate next step in evaluating this patient?

    A. Obtain an electrocardiogram
    B. Obtain an echocardiogram
    C. Reassurance only
    D. Obtain a chest x-ray
    E. Obtain a chest x-ray and electrocardiogram

28. A 3-week-old, full-term, infant is referred for evaluation of a murmur. The pregnancy was complicated by gestational diabetes. There is a 2/6 midsystolic murmur heard at the left upper sternal border and radiating to both axillae and the back. The first and second heart sounds are normal. No click is audible. The child has oxygen saturations of 97% in the upper and lower extremities and is growing at the 30th percentile for weight. What is the most likely cause of the murmur in this child?

    A. Increased blood flow velocity across the pulmonary valve due to subvalvar obstruction
    B. Normal transitioning of the pulmonary vasculature as pulmonary pressures drop
    C. Right to left blood flow across the ventricular septum
    D. Right-to-left shunting across a PDA
    E. Flow through a pulmonary AV fistula

29. In which patient is administration of bacterial endocarditis prophylaxis most appropriate based on the 2007 American Heart Association guidelines?

    A. A 12 year old after orthotopic heart transplant 3 years ago, now with moderate–severe tricuspid valve regurgitation undergoing teeth cleaning
    B. An 8 year old after VSD patch closure 5 months ago undergoing a bronchoscopy without biopsy for evaluation of chronic cough
    C. A 15 year old with Ebstein anomaly and moderate tricuspid regurgitation undergoing tooth extraction
    D. A 22 year old after extracardiac Fontan undergoing colonoscopy due to hematochezia
    E. A 20 year old with history of aortic stenosis, status post Ross procedure with an RV-to-PA conduit 10 years ago, undergoing cesarean section for failure to progress

30. An 8-year-old patient with repaired tetralogy of Fallot and placement of a bioprosthetic pulmonary valve is scheduled for a tonsillectomy next week. She is penicillin allergic. In this patient, what is the best strategy for infective endocarditis prophylaxis?

    A. Ceftriaxone IM
    B. Azithromycin PO
    C. Cefepime IV
    D. Amoxicillin PO
    E. Prophylaxis is not indicated

31. Which of the following is correct regarding risk of cardiotoxicity related to chemotherapy in children?

    A. Acute cardiotoxicity occurs in >25% of children receiving anthracyclines
    B. The greatest risk factor for the development of cardiotoxicity is cumulative anthracycline dose
    C. Clinical heart failure symptoms only occur within 5 years of receiving anthracyclines
    D. Early-onset, chronic progressive cardiomyopathy related to chemotherapy toxicity is usually a transient phenomenon with recovery of cardiac function in the majority of cases

32. A 13-year-old boy with severe pulmonary arterial hypertension (PAH) is seen for follow-up care. He takes sildenafil and bosentan. Which of the following is most accurate regarding the natural history of patients with PAH?

    A. The 5-year survival for an untreated child with idiopathic PAH is 65%
    B. Targeted PAH therapies have improved symptomatology, but have not significantly altered long-term survival
    C. Children with PAH are more likely to present with syncope than with right heart failure
    D. The least common presentation of PAH in children is dyspnea and fatigue
    E. Patients with Eisenmenger syndrome typically have a greater mortality than patients with idiopathic PAH

33. An 11-year-old boy with type 1 diabetes has a persistent serum low-density lipoprotein (LDL) cholesterol concentration of 180 mg/dL. His LDL was 175 mg/dL last year, and at that time diet and exercise modifications were recommended. On the basis of the current guidelines for management of hyperlipidemia in childhood, which of the following would be the most appropriate next step?

   A. Obtain an echocardiogram
   B. Measure the carotid artery intimal thickness
   C. Enroll the patient in a disciplined exercise training program
   D. Begin statin therapy
   E. Tighten diabetic control

34. A 13-year-old girl who recently immigrated to the United States with her parents is evaluated in a pediatric cardiology clinic. She has a reported history of a VSD. Her examination reveals a parasternal lift over the xiphoid area. There is a 3/6 holosystolic murmur coincident with S_1 best heard at the right lower sternal border (RLSB). There is a single, loud, palpable S_2 and no diastolic murmur. Her systemic oxygen saturation is 85% in room air. Regarding this patient's examination, which of the following is correct?

   A. The murmur is likely from left-to-right shunting through a membranous VSD
   B. The murmur is likely from right-to-left shunting through a membranous VSD
   C. The murmur is likely from tricuspid regurgitation
   D. The parasternal lift is from LVH
   E. The systolic murmur is likely from flow across the pulmonary valve

35. Two sisters present for a second opinion regarding sports participation. They are both competitive swimmers. During routine sports physicals, one sister was found to have a QTc of 490 ms. The other sister's QTc is normal. Neither girl has ever had a cardiac arrest or syncopal episode. Both girls were subsequently tested and found to be positive for LQT1 mutation. Which of the following is your recommendation regarding sports participation?

   A. Neither girl should participate in competitive swimming
   B. Both girls may take part in any sport without restrictions, including swimming
   C. The girl with prolonged QTc should be restricted to class IA (low static and dynamic component) sports; her sister (normal QTc) may take part in any sport without restrictions
   D. The sister with prolonged QTc should not take part in any competitive sport; her sister (normal QTc) may take part in only class IA (low static and dynamic component) sports
   E. Both girls should have an ICD placed. After ICD placement, they may continue competitive swimming

36. In a 6 year old with double-chambered right ventricle (DCRV), which of the following would NOT be expected?

   A. Membranous VSD
   B. Subaortic VSD
   C. No VSD
   D. Branch pulmonary artery stenosis
   E. Discrete subaortic stenosis

37. A 16 year old presents after two episodes of vasovagal syncope. These symptoms never occur during exercise. The symptoms usually occur in the midmorning, especially after not eating breakfast. There is no family history of sudden death. She had no prior evaluation. What is the next appropriate test to order?

   A. Echocardiogram
   B. 24-Hour Holter monitor
   C. 30-Day event monitor
   D. ECG
   E. Tilt-table test

38. What is the most common cause of chest pain in children?

   A. Musculoskeletal chest wall pain
   B. Asthma
   C. Pneumonitis
   D. Coronary artery disease
   E. Gastroesophageal reflux/esophagitis

39. In which of the following situations would one expect to observe pulsus paradoxus?

   A. Severe aortic valve regurgitation
   B. Severe aortic valve stenosis
   C. Hypovolemia
   D. Acute pericarditis
   E. Coronary artery aneurysms from Kawasaki disease

40. A 16-year-old boy has a high-pitched early diastolic murmur heard best with the diaphragm of the stethoscope at the left midsternal border with radiation toward the apex. When the patient leans forward and exhales, the murmur is accentuated. Which of the following is the most likely cause of this murmur?

   A. Pulmonary valve regurgitation
   B. Aortic valve regurgitation
   C. Mitral valve regurgitation
   D. Tricuspid valve stenosis
   E. Mitral valve stenosis

CHAPTER 9

41. You are evaluating a teenage athlete who has complained of chest pain with exercise. On further questioning, she recalls that she had a syncopal episode during a basketball game earlier this year. Which of the following is the most common cause of sudden cardiac death in young athletes?

    A. Prolonged QT syndrome
    B. Arrhythmogenic RV cardiomyopathy
    C. Anomalous origin of the right coronary artery from the left sinus of Valsalva
    D. Anomalous origin of the left main coronary artery from the right sinus of Valsalva
    E. Hypertrophic cardiomyopathy

42. In a patient with an anomalous left coronary artery from the pulmonary artery (ALCAPA), what associated defect may protect the patient from LV dysfunction?

    A. Pulmonary valve stenosis
    B. Large PDA with large left-to-right shunt
    C. Tricuspid regurgitation
    D. Mitral regurgitation
    E. LVH

43. What is the most likely etiology of restrictive cardiomyopathy (RCM) in a 7 year old?

    A. Glycogen-storage disease
    B. Thiamin deficiency
    C. Amyloidosis
    D. Muscular dystrophy
    E. Collagen vascular disease

44. A 12 year old has an early systolic click at the apex and a 2/4 blowing diastolic decrescendo murmur heard best at the upper sternal border radiating toward the apex. The bilateral radial and femoral pulses are equal. Which of the following would be expected?

    A. Severe pulmonary valve regurgitation on echo
    B. Large PDA on echo
    C. Prolongation of the PR interval on ECG
    D. Prominent pulmonary vascularity on chest radiograph
    E. Blood pressure in the right arm of 140/50 mm Hg

45. A 17 year old with a history of chronic cough undergoes a chest CT. It incidentally detects that the patient has an anomalous origin of the right coronary artery from the left sinus of Valsalva (AORCA). Which of the following is the next best course of action?

    A. Surgical referral for coronary artery bypass grafting
    B. Obtain a stress echo
    C. Restrict immediately from all contact sports
    D. Start aspirin 81 mg once daily

46. A 10-year-old boy with a bicuspid aortic valve is scheduled for repair of a dental cavity. Based on the 2007 ACC/AHA endocarditis guideline statement, administration of which of the following antibiotics for this boy would be in closest accordance with current recommendations for endocarditis prophylaxis?

    A. None
    B. Procaine penicillin, 1 million units intramuscularly (IM), immediately prior to the procedure
    C. Amoxicillin, 50 mg/kg orally, 1 hour prior to the procedure
    D. Amoxicillin, 50 mg/kg orally, immediately after the procedure
    E. Clindamycin, 20 mg/kg IM, immediately prior to the procedure

47. According to the 2007 ACC/AHA endocarditis guidelines, which of the following conditions (all 5 years after intervention or infection) would warrant antibiotic prophylaxis against infective endocarditis (IE) before a dental procedure?

    A. Small residual VSD after primary surgical closure
    B. Heart transplantation
    C. Bicuspid aortic valve with mild aortic regurgitation and a history of endocarditis
    D. Device closure of a secundum ASD
    E. Extended end-to-end coarctation repair with a 10-mm Hg residual gradient

48. A 13 year old presents because a recent echo performed due to murmur demonstrated an 18-mm secundum ASD with left-to-right shunt. The family requests clearance for high school sports participation. In which of the following sports can he participate competitively?

    A. He cannot participate in sports
    B. Baseball
    C. Football
    D. Golf
    E. Soccer

49. A local primary care physician asks you about a recent ECG performed on a teenage male who is a state champion high school football player. Which of the following ECG findings would be most concerning in this patient?

    A. PR prolongation
    B. T-wave inversion in leads V4–V6
    C. Incomplete RBBB
    D. Early repolarization
    E. QRS voltage criteria for LVH in lead V6

50. A 13-year-old patient with newly diagnosed SLE is referred for cardiac evaluation. An echocardiogram was performed prior to the visit. What is the most likely abnormal finding on this patient's echocardiogram?

    A. LV systolic dysfunction
    B. Pericardial effusion
    C. Tricuspid regurgitation
    D. Tricuspid valve vegetation
    E. Coronary artery dilation

51. A 15-year-old boy is being seen for a pre-participation evaluation for football. He had one episode of syncope, which happened when he stood quickly after taking a nap. He has a history of mild asthma, and occasional shortness of breath after intense training, which resolves with albuterol. His paternal grandfather died of a heart attack at age 61, and his older brother drowned while swimming competitively last year. On cardiac examination, he has a 2/6 systolic vibratory murmur that is more prominent when supine. Which of the following features of his examination and history is most concerning and requires further workup?

    A. Episode of syncope
    B. Shortness of breath with exercise
    C. Grandfather's heart attack
    D. Brother's death
    E. Murmur

52. A 4-week-old infant, with a murmur, has an echocardiogram performed that identifies a 4-mm secundum ASD. The mother wants to know if this means her baby will need heart surgery. What should you tell her?

    A. ASD will get larger as she grows
    B. ASD will likely close on its own
    C. ASD should be closed via a device in the cath lab soon to prevent symptoms
    D. ASD will probably need surgical closure by age 1 year

53. A 20-year-old man had successful repair of coarctation of the aorta when he was 13 years old. This was immediately after diagnosis when he presented with hypertension. He has done well since then aside from occasional difficulty with blood pressure control. He is otherwise healthy and has a normal aortic valve. He asks if he is at risk for other complications. Which of the following is he at higher risk for developing?

    A. Renal injury
    B. Intracranial aneurysm
    C. DVT
    D. Liver damage
    E. Retinal hemorrhage

54. A 9-year-old boy with a history of HLHS status post a Fontan operation has been doing well but has been struggling with school performance. His parents are concerned and feel that he is falling behind his peers. Which of the following is true regarding neurodevelopmental outcomes in children with congenital heart defects?

    A. Children with cyanotic and acyanotic lesions have the same degree of learning difficulties
    B. If a child has complete repair of a cyanotic lesion, developmental outcomes will normalize
    C. Longer duration of cyanosis is associated with greater decline in cognitive ability
    D. Visual–spatial skills are often intact, even if there are other learning difficulties
    E. Children with a VSD have the highest risk of adverse developmental outcomes

55. An 11 year old presents with left-sided chest pain that is nonexertional and has been occurring periodically for the last several weeks. His physical examination is completely normal. There is no family history of sudden death or cardiomyopathy. He originally presented to a local urgent care center where a normal ECG was performed. In this clinical scenario, ordering an echocardiogram at this point would be classified by the 2014 American Society of Echocardiography (ASE) Appropriate Use Criteria to be:

    A. Appropriate
    B. May be appropriate
    C. Rarely appropriate
    D. This clinical scenario is not addressed by these guidelines

56. A 3 year old has left-axis deviation (LAD) on ECG. Which diagnosis is most likely?

    A. Bicuspid aortic valve
    B. Secundum ASD
    C. Tricuspid atresia
    D. Coarctation of the aorta
    E. Muscular VSD

57. A 12 month old, who recently transitioned from formula feedings, is being treated with a sodium channel blocker for AVNRT that was diagnosed as a neonate. Mom states that the baby is doing well and she has no concerns. What findings on ECG would be of most concern to you?

    A. Inverted T waves in leads V1–V3
    B. Prolonged PR interval
    C. RSR′ pattern in V1
    D. Heart rate = 140 bpm
    E. S > R wave in lead I

58. A 2-week-old male infant with a history of poor prenatal care now presents with somnolence, poor feeding, frequent emesis, and failure to gain weight. The infant is tachycardic with a prominent RV impulse, liver edge is 2 cm below the right costal margin, and there is a bruit over the anterior fontanelle. Cranial ultrasound is suspicious for a vein of Galen malformation. Which of the following is true regarding this lesion?

    A. Structural cardiac defects are not associated with this lesion
    B. Presentation is delayed until pulmonary vascular resistance drops
    C. Intracranial hemorrhage is common
    D. Holodiastolic flow reversal can be seen in the abdominal aorta on echocardiography
    E. Surgical ligation of anomalous vessels is the preferred therapy

59. A 6 year old is referred by a primary care physician for lipid screening. The patient's uncle had a myocardial infarction (MI) at the age of 56 and the grandmother had an MI at the age of 67. The patient's mother recently had a cholesterol panel checked and total cholesterol level was 230 mg/dL. There is no other pertinent family history. On examination, the patient appears well with a BMI at the 62nd percentile. The remainder of the examination is unremarkable. Based on these data, what do you recommend regarding cholesterol screening for this patient?

    A. No need to check a cholesterol level until the patient is 25 years old
    B. No need to check a cholesterol level until the patient is 17 years old
    C. Check a fasting lipid profile now
    D. Check a nonfasting lipid profile at age 9 years and calculate a non-HDL cholesterol
    E. Check a fasting lipid profile now and again in 4 weeks

60. You are asked to manage the anticoagulation for a noncardiac surgical procedure in a patient who receives warfarin for a mechanical valve and has no history of thrombosis. You recommend that the patient check their INR 72 hours prior and if it is in the usual therapeutic range, stop warfarin 48 hours prior to the procedure. You recommend no bridging with heparin and restarting warfarin on the evening of the procedure. This management plan is most appropriate for which of the following situations:

    A. A 13 year old with a bileaflet mechanical mitral prosthesis
    B. A 15 year old with a bileaflet mechanical aortic prosthesis
    C. A 14 year old with a bileaflet mechanical tricuspid prosthesis
    D. A 13 year old with a bileaflet mechanical pulmonary prosthesis

61. You are counseling a family regarding their infant with a complete atrioventricular (AV) septal defect. The child is scheduled to undergo cardiac surgery, and the family asks if additional cardiac surgeries will be needed in the future. What is the most common indication for reoperation in this patient?

    A. Right AV valve regurgitation
    B. Left AV valve regurgitation
    C. Left AV valve stenosis
    D. Residual VSD
    E. Left ventricular outflow tract obstruction

62. During the physical examination of a 15 year old with known pulmonary valve stenosis (PS), you note a prominent "a" wave when inspecting the neck veins. Which of the following physical examination findings would you also expect?

    A. Early systolic click at the apex in the supine position
    B. Systolic click that moves earlier in systole in the standing position
    C. Normal splitting of S_2
    D. Thrill at the left upper sternal border
    E. Severe tricuspid regurgitation demonstrated on echo

63. Which of the following is true regarding Brugada syndrome?

    A. Testosterone is contributory, and arrhythmic events are more common in males
    B. Inheritance is autosomal recessive
    C. ICD implantation is indicated in asymptomatic patients with a drug-induced type I ECG if there is a family history of sudden cardiac death
    D. Symptoms are exercise induced

64. A 17-year-old male is referred due to a history of Marfan syndrome (MFS) in his brother. An echocardiogram performed just prior to the visit shows a dilated aortic root with a Z-score of +3.2. He is otherwise healthy. Which of the following is NOT true?

    A. He has MFS based on the revised Ghent criteria
    B. He should undergo a repeat echocardiogram in 6 months
    C. No medical therapy should be initiated at this time
    D. Baseline CT or MRI is recommended
    E. He should be restricted from weight lifting

65. In a patient with Marfan syndrome and mitral valve prolapse (MVP), a systolic murmur and a midsystolic click are auscultated. Which of the following is true regarding these findings?

    A. Squatting will result in the click moving closer to S_1
    B. Decreased left ventricular contractility will result in the click moving closer to S_1
    C. Standing will result in the click moving closer to S_1
    D. Standing will accentuate a diastolic murmur
    E. The click may be followed by a low-pitched diastolic murmur

66. A 4-year-old boy with tetralogy of Fallot and peripheral pulmonary artery stenoses has a history of a Kasai procedure and butterfly vertebrae noted on x-ray. On examination, the child has a broad forehead, deep-set eyes, and a small, pointed chin. Which of the following syndromes is likely?

    A. DiGeorge
    B. Alagille
    C. Noonan
    D. Down
    E. Kabuki

67. You are explaining the diagnosis of hypertrophic cardiomyopathy (HCM) to an adolescent and his family. Which of the following is true regarding HCM?

    A. ECG abnormalities may precede 2D echocardiographic abnormalities
    B. During high school, echocardiographic screening is recommended every 3 years
    C. LVH on ECG is usually present at birth
    D. Genetic testing is less likely to detect abnormalities in young compared to elderly patients

68. An elite collegiate hockey player seeks a second opinion after being disqualified from sports because of the finding on a recent echocardiogram of a septal wall thickness = 14 mm. The patient was told this is consistent with hypertrophic cardiomyopathy (HCM). Which of the following supports a diagnosis of "athlete's heart" instead of HCM?

    A. Transmitral Doppler waveform consistent with abnormal LV filling
    B. LV end-diastolic dimension >55 mm
    C. History of HCM in a first-degree relative
    D. Abnormal genetic testing for HCM
    E. Female sex

69. A 16-year-old boy is currently on dual diuretic therapy for chronic congestive heart failure. He presents to your office with complaints of a new onset of palpitations and muscle weakness. ECG is notable for widened QRS complexes and diffuse ST elevation with no discernable P waves. Which combination of medications has most likely led to the electrolyte disturbance associated with these side effects and ECG findings?

    A. Furosemide and hydrochlorothiazide
    B. Spironolactone and hydrochlorothiazide
    C. Furosemide and lisinopril
    D. Spironolactone and lisinopril
    E. Hydrochlorothiazide and lisinopril

70. A routine chemistry panel is obtained on a patient receiving single diuretic therapy. It reveals a hypokalemic, hypochloremic, metabolic alkalosis and hypocalcemia. Which diuretic is most likely to have caused these metabolic disturbances?

    A. Furosemide
    B. Hydrochlorothiazide
    C. Lisinopril
    D. Spironolactone
    E. Losartan

71. In a 19 year old with hypertrophic cardiomyopathy, which of the following factors is LEAST predictive for risk of sudden cardiac death?

    A. Unexplained syncopal episodes
    B. Significant left ventricular outflow tract (LVOT) obstruction
    C. Left ventricular wall thickness >30 mm
    D. Family history of sudden cardiac death related to hypertrophic cardiomyopathy
    E. Hypotension in response to exercise

72. An 18-year-old female is roller-skating with her boyfriend when she develops chest pain and suddenly collapses. Cardiopulmonary resuscitation is quickly started, and she is transported to the emergency room. The boyfriend reports that she has Turner syndrome and had heart surgery as a newborn. Tragically, resuscitation is unsuccessful. Her sudden cardiac death was MOST LIKELY a result of:

    A. Myocardial infarction
    B. Aortic dissection
    C. Right heart failure
    D. LVOT obstruction
    E. Long QT syndrome

CHAPTER 9

73. A neonate is diagnosed with supravalvar aortic stenosis. Which of the following is MOST LIKELY also to be present in this neonate?

    A. A mutation in the NOTCH2 gene
    B. Butterfly vertebrae
    C. Hypercalcemia
    D. Primary ovarian insufficiency
    E. Hypoplastic thymus

74. Which of the following class of medications is NOT recommended in the acute treatment of myocarditis?

    A. Nonsteroidal anti-inflammatory drugs (NSAIDs)
    B. Angiotensin-converting enzyme inhibitors
    C. β-Blockers
    D. Aldosterone receptor antagonists
    E. Calcium channel blockers

75. Which of the following statements is true concerning the diagnosis of pericarditis and cardiac tamponade?

    A. Absence of a pericardial effusion excludes pericarditis
    B. Respiratory distress is uncommon in the absence of cardiac tamponade
    C. Pulse pressure widens in cardiac tamponade
    D. An increase in systolic blood pressure by more than 10 mm Hg with inspiration is suggestive of cardiac tamponade
    E. Earliest sign of tamponade on echocardiogram is a dilated right ventricle

76. When are abnormalities in brain development first recognizable on neuroimaging in patients with hypoplastic left heart syndrome?

    A. Prenatally
    B. Prior to first surgery
    C. Immediately after first surgery
    D. 3 years of age
    E. 5 years of age

77. An American Heart Association (AHA) Scientific Statement from 2012 outlines criteria for identifying pediatric congenital heart disease patients who are at "high risk" for developmental disorders or disabilities. According to the criteria specified in the 2012 AHA Scientific Statement, which of the following patients would be considered "high risk" for a developmental disorder or disability?

    A. A 2-month-old infant with a moderate-sized ASD that was discovered shortly after birth
    B. A 5-month-old infant with a large VSD that was discovered shortly before birth
    C. A 12-month-old infant with prenatally diagnosed tricuspid atresia
    D. A 7-month-old infant with prenatally diagnosed AVSD
    E. A 9-month-old infant with AVSD diagnosed shortly after birth

78. On average, children with hypoplastic left heart syndrome (HLHS) have full-scale intelligence quotient (IQ) scores that are:

    A. 2 points below the population mean
    B. 5 points below the population mean
    C. 7 points below the population mean
    D. 10 points below the population mean
    E. 12 points below the population mean

79. A 12-year-old boy with d-TGA, status post neonatal arterial switch operation, presents to your outpatient cardiology clinic with his mother for a routine follow-up visit. During the visit, the mother expresses concerns that her son's school grades have begun slipping lately. She further notes that he seems more distractible, he is forgetting to turn in homework assignments, and he seems to be getting increasingly frustrated with school. What should you do?

    A. Order an ECG and start the patient on a trial of guanfacine
    B. Assure the mother that concerns like hers are common and nothing to worry about
    C. Refer the patient to a child psychiatrist for a medication consult
    D. Refer the patient for neuropsychological assessment
    E. Call the patient's school and recommend that they seat him closer to the teacher

80. A 15 year old is 2 years status post mitral valve replacement with a mechanical prosthesis and he receives chronic warfarin therapy. His goal INR range is 2.5 to 3.5. He usually takes 5 mg of warfarin daily to achieve this INR goal. He has been trying to eat a healthier diet. In advising him regarding food choices, which of the following is true?

    A. He should avoid green or red peppers because they will increase his INR
    B. If he eats fresh kale, his INR will likely increase
    C. If he eats frozen, cooked, drained kale, his INR will likely increase
    D. Spinach would be expected to decrease his INR
    E. Bananas should be limited to one daily, since they will increase his INR

Answers

1. (A) The current AAP guidelines recommend lifestyle modifications for 6 months prior to pharmacotherapy. ACE inhibitors and calcium channel blockers are some of the recommended first-line agents, but β-blockers and thiazide diuretics are no longer considered first-line agents.

2. (C) The history is concerning for LQTS 2 where arrhythmia can be precipitated by auditory stimuli and strong emotions. Begin evaluation with a baseline ECG. Reassurance only is inappropriate in this case. Echocardiogram is likely to be normal. Exercise testing is reasonable in the workup but after a baseline ECG. Medication may be started after the diagnosis is established.

3. (B) A pulmonary flow murmur is the most common benign murmur in teenagers. Answer A describes the murmur associated with mitral valve prolapse. C is likely a PDA murmur, D describes the classic Still murmur, and E describes a typical small VSD murmur.

4. (C) Aortic regurgitation is associated with bounding peripheral pulses with rapid upstroke and descent (often referred to as a "water hammer pulse") and wide pulse pressure. Narrow pulse pressure is associated with severe aortic stenosis. Radial-femoral delay is a pulse discrepancy noted in coarctation of the aorta. Prominent jugular venous V waves are present with severe tricuspid valve regurgitation. Prominent hepatojugular reflex is a sign of right heart failure.

5. (C) Genetic testing for Turner syndrome should be performed in all girls diagnosed with coarctation because of the increased association rate (5% to 15%) and because clinical findings suggestive of Turner syndrome may be absent in girls with mosaicism. The patient is hypertensive and the gradient is high, so repeat echocardiography is not indicated. At some point a fasting lipid profile is necessary since patients with coarctation are at risk for early-onset coronary disease, but that is not needed at initial presentation of a 10 year old.

6. (C) Glycogen-storage diseases are associated with short PR interval. An example of a straight memory question that may appear on a board examination.

7. (D) Per the most recent Kawasaki disease guidelines, since he did not have coronary artery aneurysms, there are no physical activity restrictions beyond 6 to 8 weeks from the date of diagnosis if echo remains normal.

8. (C) He had myocarditis/myocardial dysfunction associated with MIS-C. According to the 2017 AHA/ACC guidelines on myocarditis, before returning to competitive sports, athletes who initially present with an acute clinical syndrome consistent with myocarditis should undergo a resting echocardiogram, 24-hour Holter monitoring, and an exercise ECG no less than 3 to 6 months after the initial illness (Class I; Level of Evidence C).

9. (E) In multiple case series, as many as 50% to 80% of the children with MIS-C developed signs of systemic hypoperfusion or shock. In contrast, in patients with KD, <5% of cases require vasopressor support. Coronary artery aneurysms and desquamation occur in both. Steroids may be used early in the course of MIS-C, but rarely in KD. GI symptoms are more common in MIS-C.

10. (E) The supplemental laboratory criteria used in the diagnosis of suspected Kawasaki disease include hypoalbuminemia ≤3.0 g/dL, anemia for age, elevation of alanine aminotransferase, platelet count after 7 days ≥450,000/mm^3, white blood cell count ≥15,000/mm^3, and urinalysis with ≥10 white blood cells/high-power field and no bacteria.

11. (B) Regardless of the physical examination or symptoms, the sudden death of a first-degree relative should prompt further cardiac testing. The dynamic outflow murmur caused by obstructive hypertrophic cardiomyopathy (HCM) is typically loudest in the standing position, especially when moving from squatting to standing. Although the ECG may eventually be abnormal in most patients with HCM, in a young child it may be normal. The other answers describe features of benign or "physiologic" murmurs frequently heard in young children.

12. (E) Cholesterol screening should be performed on all children with a positive family history of dyslipidemia or premature coronary vascular disease. Screening should also be performed on all children with unknown family history or the following risk factors: overweight or obese, hypertension, cigarette smoking, or diabetes mellitus. This child was appropriately screened given his positive family history of premature coronary vascular disease. Pharmacotherapy should not be started until the child is 8 years of age. At this age, weight management should be the focus to lower the LDL level.

13. (B) More information is needed for a conclusive diagnosis, but the patient has history and physical examination findings consistent with Marfan syndrome, in addition to a family history of aortic aneurysm. *FBN1* has been identified as the causal gene in Marfan syndrome. It is also associated with Shprintzen–Goldberg syndrome, Weill–Marchesani syndrome, and ectopia lentis syndrome. *TGFBR1* is associated with Loeys–Dietz syndrome and familial thoracic aortic aneurysm syndrome. *COL3A1* is associated with Ehlers–Danlos syndrome. *ADAMTS10* is associated with Weill–Marchesani syndrome. *ACTA2* is associated with familial thoracic aortic aneurysm syndrome.

14. (C) β-Blockers are generally given to most patients with Marfan syndrome and aortic root dilation. Use of losartan has increased in recent years. ACE inhibitors, ARBs, and calcium channel blockers are also used in patients with β-blocker intolerance. Digoxin usually has no role in this disease process.

CHAPTER 9

15. (A) To confirm a diagnosis of hypertension, three blood pressure measurements are needed. This patient has two blood pressures that place him >95%, and the concern is that he has stage 1 hypertension. A single third blood pressure measurement could be performed at a later date. Alternatively, ambulatory blood pressure monitoring could be used. This is especially useful if there is any concern of "white coat" hypertension. In addition, a thorough history and physical examination should be performed to identify any possible causes. If the patient does have stage 1 hypertension, then he needs a diagnostic workup.

16. (D) Prehypertension is defined as average systolic or diastolic blood pressure levels that are ≥90th percentile but <95th percentile. A thorough history and physical examination should be performed, and further testing performed if indicated. It is reasonable to start with lifestyle changes, and blood pressure check should be repeated in 6 months.

17. (B) The patient has auscultation findings consistent with aortic regurgitation. The systolic ejection murmur is secondary to increased stroke volume. The blowing diastolic murmur is the aortic regurgitation. Widened pulse pressure is often found in aortic regurgitation, especially if it is moderate or severe. Widened pulse pressure occurs because there is an increased stroke volume that causes distension of the peripheral arteries and elevation in systolic blood pressure. Diastolic blood pressure is reduced because the regurgitation into the left ventricle leads to a rapid fall in pressure. A systolic ejection click is typically associated with the presence of a bicuspid aortic valve, which would be expected in a patient with physical findings of aortic stenosis/regurgitation.

18. (E) Rheumatic fever is diagnosed based on the Jones criteria. The probability is high if there is group A streptococcal infection as well as two major criteria or one major and two minor criteria. The five major criteria are migratory arthritis, carditis and valvulitis, central nervous system involvement/Sydenham chorea, erythema marginatum, and subcutaneous nodules. The four minor criteria are arthralgia, fever, elevated ESR or CRP, and prolonged PR interval. The patient has one major criterion—valvulitis. To confirm the diagnosis, one more major criterion would need to be present. Otherwise, two minor criteria would be required to make the diagnosis.

19. (A) According to the 2009 guidelines for the diagnosis and management of syncope, there are several high-risk criteria that require hospitalization or intense evaluation (**Table 9.1**).

20. (D) This patient is at high risk for major cardiovascular events based on her episodes happening with exercise and having palpitations prior to the syncope. Therefore, it is reasonable to admit her to the hospital and do inpatient monitoring while a thorough workup is performed.

21. (C) Endomyocardial biopsy is the gold standard for establishing the diagnosis of myocarditis, although it only yields diagnostic information in 10% to 20% of cases.

TABLE 9.1 Risk Stratification for Patients With Syncope

Short-term high-risk criteria that require prompt hospitalization or intensive evaluation:

Severe structural or coronary artery disease (heart failure, low LVEF, or previous myocardial infarction)

Clinical or ECG features suggesting arrhythmic syncope:
- Syncope during exertion or supine
- Palpitations at the time of syncope
- Family history of SCD
- Nonsustained VT
- Bifascicular block (LBBB or RBBB combined with left anterior or left posterior fascicular block) or other intraventricular conduction abnormalities with QRS duration ≥120 ms
- Inadequate sinus bradycardia (<50 bpm) or sinoatrial block in the absence of negative chronotropic medications or physical training
- Pre-excited QRS complex
- Prolonged or short QT interval
- RBBB pattern with ST elevation in leads V1–V3 (Brugada pattern)
- Negative T waves in right precordial leads, epsilon waves, and ventricular late potentials suggestive of ARVC

Important comorbidities:
- Severe anemia
- Electrolyte disturbance

LVEF, left ventricular ejection fraction; SCD, sudden cardiac death; VT, ventricular tachycardia; LBBB, left bundle branch block; RBBB, right bundle branch block; bpm, beats per minute; ARVC, arrhythmogenic right ventricular cardiomyopathy.

Endomyocardial biopsy is a class IIb recommendation in the ACC/AHA guidelines for the treatment of heart failure.

22. (A) Patients with sickle cell anemia have chronic anemia and therefore have increased cardiac output. This causes the heart to become enlarged, as can be seen on chest x-ray. Increased cardiac output can cause a flow murmur heard over the left parasternal area. Thrombotic crisis will cause acute chest syndrome, but this is usually not cardiac in nature. A patient with sickle cell anemia may have prolonged PR interval and nonspecific ST changes seen on ECG, but it is rare for arrhythmias to develop. Iron overload causes the cardiac abnormalities seen with thalassemia major.

23. (A) The American Heart Association (AHA) recommends using a blood pressure cuff with a bladder that is at least 80% of the arm circumference. Utilizing a blood pressure cuff with measurements less than this can lead to falsely elevated measurements. Given the recent increase in pediatric obesity rates, it is important to remember that a child-size blood pressure cuff may not be appropriate for all children. While he may have a coarctation, his blood pressure should be accurately measured before undertaking further evaluation. Whether or not this child's blood pressure is elevated, his obesity should be addressed. When taking an auscultatory blood pressure, patients should be positioned in a seated position with their back flat to a firm surface. The arm should be at the level of the heart. Positioning the arm below the heart may lead to venous congestion and falsely elevated readings. There are a total of five Korotkoff sounds described. Phase 1 is considered to be the SBP and is the first appearance of faint clear tapping sounds that gradually increase and are heard for at least two consecutive beats. Phase 2 is the softening of sounds, which may have a swishing nature. During phase 3, the sounds become more sharp and crisp again compared to phase 2, but less intense than phase 1. There is no described clinical significance of phase 2 or phase 3. Phase 4 is the distinct abrupt muffling of sounds, which become soft and blowing. Phase 5 is the point at which all sounds disappear. There has been debate over the years as to whether phase 4 or 5 should be used for determining DBP. Currently, the AHA recommends using phase 5.

24. (B) Patients with an isolated ASD typically will exhibit left-to-right shunting. Given that the difference in atrial pressures is relatively small, the velocity of shunting across the defect is not high enough to cause a murmur. The increased volume in the right atrium may cause a diastolic flow murmur across the tricuspid valve (if the $Q_p:Q_s$ is >2:1). The systolic ejection murmur is caused by increased stroke volume across a normal pulmonary valve.

25. (C) The constellation of symptoms in this patient is consistent with pulmonary hypertension and little residual left-to-right shunting across the ASD. The prominent S_2 and paradoxical splitting indicate that the pulmonary pressures are high. As the child breathes in, RV outflow increases and the splitting resolves, but with expiration, the RV outflow decreases and the increased pulmonary pressures result in faster and louder closure of the pulmonary valve. If the decrease in left-to-right shunt was from the ASD becoming smaller, then you would expect the splitting to be physiologic and the P2 to be of normal intensity. There is no diastolic murmur because the decreased left-to-right shunt has reduced the flow across the tricuspid valve.

26. (D) This infant has signs of pulmonary overcirculation: poor feeding, tachypnea, and poor weight gain. The appropriate dose of furosemide for this patient is 1 mg/kg/dose given twice daily. One can make the case that surgical repair should be entertained in the near future but that is not one of the options. In this "patient management" type of question, always note patient age, vital signs, and lesion. Management questions will be fairly straightforward if one notes these details in the question stem.

27. (C) The murmur described in this vignette is consistent with a Still's murmur. It is a common innocent murmur and intermittently found in 75% to 85% of school-aged children. The musical nature and typical qualities are listed in the question stem. The etiology of this murmur is unknown, but there are many theories including physiologic narrowing of the left ventricular outflow area, systolic/diastolic hypermobility of the mitral valve chordae, small aortic diameter, the presence of left ventricular false tendons, or increased aortic flow volume and velocity. Given its position, it is important to differentiate a Still murmur from that of HCM or a VSD. The murmur of HCM would be expected to get louder with Valsalva or standing (maneuvers that decrease

venous return). A small VSD would not be affected by physiologic maneuvers and has a harsher quality, frequently begins coincident with the S_1. Reassurance only is sufficient in this patient.

28. (B) The murmur described in the vignette is most consistent with a neonatal transitional murmur of peripheral pulmonary stenosis. Infants born prematurely and of low birth weight are more likely to have this murmur. In about two-thirds of infants, this will disappear by 6 weeks of age. The location of this murmur with radiation to the axilla and the back is the hallmark of peripheral pulmonary stenosis. Persistence beyond 9 months of age warrants further evaluation for branch pulmonary artery or pulmonary valve stenosis. A murmur of pulmonary valve stenosis would best be heard at the left upper sternal border. A right-to-left shunt at the ventricular level or across a PDA would typically be silent and result in systemic desaturation. Classically a PDA with a left-to-right shunt has a continuous murmur. A pulmonary artery to pulmonary vein fistula is low velocity and silent. A systemic artery to pulmonary artery collateral vessel would create a continuous murmur, similar to a PDA with left-to-right shunt.

29. (A) The 2007 AHA guidelines for infective endocarditis (IE) prophylaxis state that the highest-risk patients include:

1. Patients with prosthetic heart valves, including bioprosthetic and homograft valves.
2. Patients with prosthetic material used for cardiac valve repair.
3. Patients with a prior history of IE.
4. Patients with unrepaired cyanotic congenital heart disease, including palliative shunts and conduits.
5. Patients with completely repaired congenital heart defects with prosthetic material or device, whether placed by surgery or by catheter intervention, during the first 6 months after the procedure.
6. Patients with repaired congenital heart disease with residual defects at the site or adjacent to the site of the prosthetic device.
7. Patients with "valvulopathy" in a transplanted heart. Valvulopathy is defined as documentation of substantial leaflet pathology and regurgitation.

It is recommended that prophylaxis be given for procedures that will likely result in bacteremia. These include dental procedures involving manipulation of gingival tissue or the periapical region of the teeth or perforation of the oral mucosa. In regard to respiratory procedures, there is little direct evidence that bacteremia caused during these procedures leads to IE. The AHA does not recommend routine prophylaxis for respiratory procedures unless they involve incision or biopsy of the respiratory tract mucosa. Procedures in which prophylaxis would be indicated include tonsillectomy, adenoidectomy, or bronchoscopy with biopsy. The guidelines no longer recommend prophylaxis for any GI (including diagnostic colonoscopy or esophagogastroduodenoscopy) or GU procedures, even in those patients with the highest-risk lesions unless there is an active or ongoing infection of the GI or GU tract. Routine prophylaxis for either vaginal delivery or caesarian section is not indicated unless there is an active infection that may increase the risk of IE, such as chorioamnionitis. Additional high-risk procedures would be those involving infected skin or musculoskeletal structure.

30. (B) Gram-positive cocci, particularly viridans group streptococci, are responsible for the vast majority of IE. Antibiotic choice should be tailored and directed against these pathogens. The first-line therapy for high-risk patients undergoing high-risk procedures (see Question 29 explanation) is amoxicillin. For patients with penicillin allergy who can take oral medications, cephalexin, clindamycin, azithromycin, and clarithromycin are appropriate. The medication is typically given as a single dose 30 to 60 minutes before beginning the procedure.

31. (B) There are three phases of anthracycline-related cardiotoxicity. The greatest risk factor for all phases is the total cumulative anthracycline dose. The *acute phase* occurs within 1 week of the infusion (high dose correlates with early cardiac dysfunction). This is often a transient phenomenon and can have a wide spectrum of findings from minor ECG abnormalities and sinus tachycardia to severe ventricular dysfunction and fulminant heart failure. Acute toxicity occurs in 1% of pediatric patients. *Early-onset, chronic progressive cardiomyopathy* occurs within the first year of treatment. This is a nontransient depression in myocardial function that is due to damage or death of myocytes. It occurs in ~2% of patients. *Late-onset toxicity* occurs at least 1 year after treatment. Within 6 years of treatment, 65% of children who received 228 to 550 mg/m^2 of an anthracycline have cardiac dysfunction. The risk of clinical heart failure 15 to 20 years following chemotherapy is 4% to 5%.

32. (C) Studies in children with idiopathic pulmonary arterial hypertension (IPAH) and hereditary PAH (HPAH) have shown that the survival of those treated prior to the advent of targeted therapies (1950s to 1990s) was 66%, 52%, and 35% for 1, 3, and 5 years, respectively. Studies utilizing targeted therapies such as sildenafil, bosentan, and IV prostacyclin have shown considerable improvement in morbidity and mortality associated with PAH. The 1-, 3-, and 5-year survival rates improved to 94%, 88%, and 81% in a number of studies. The most likely presenting symptoms in children with PAH are dyspnea, fatigue, syncope, or near-syncope. Children are unlikely to present with right heart failure as an initial finding as they are often quite active. Dyspnea on exertion is an early symptom. Children or adults who develop PAH as a result of unrepaired congenital heart disease such as a large VSD typically have a lower mortality than those with IPAH or HPAH as it takes more time for secondary PAH to develop.

33. (D) According to the 2008 AAP Committee on Nutrition guidelines, patients with diabetes mellitus are at particular risk of coronary complications from hyperlipidemia. The most appropriate next step would be to start a statin at this time since the LDL is markedly elevated. The ADA recommends starting a statin in children >10 years of age if the LDL is >160 after lifestyle changes. Goal LDL is <100 mg/dL.

34. (C) This patient's examination is most consistent with someone who has pulmonary vascular disease. After long-standing left-to-right shunting through a large VSD, the patient has now developed elevated pulmonary vascular resistance and elevated RV pressure. The shunt has reversed and is now right to left, hence the systemic desaturation. The right and left ventricular pressures are likely equal, and there is low-velocity flow across the VSD that is inaudible. As a result of the increased pulmonary pressures, she has developed right ventricular hypertrophy (RVH) resulting in the parasternal lift. LVH would present as a lift or heave along the apex. As a result of the RVH and the increased pulmonary pressures, she has developed audible tricuspid regurgitation. As a result of the RVH, the murmur is displaced more rightward than normal. If the murmur were from increased pulmonary flow, it would be expected along the upper left sternal border and would likely be ejection in quality.

35. (A) The sister with a long QT should be restricted to class IA activities. She is asymptomatic but has baseline QT prolongation (QTc >470 ms or more in males, >480 ms or more in females), so she should be restricted to class 1A sports. If she had genetically proven type 3 LQTS, the restriction limiting participation to class IA activities may be liberalized. But the sisters have LQT1.

The sister with genotype-positive/phenotype-negative LQTS (i.e., identification of an LQTS-associated mutation in an asymptomatic individual with a nondiagnostic QTc) may be allowed to participate in competitive sports. The risk of sudden cardiac death is not zero, but there are no compelling data available to justify restricting these individuals from competitive activities.

Because of the strong association between swimming and LQT1, both sisters should refrain from competitive swimming.

The presence of an ICD would restrict both sisters to class IA activities.

36. (D) DCRV is a progressive lesion and may present in older children and in adulthood. It is caused by a pyramidal mass of muscle that divides the RV cavity into two chambers, higher and lower pressure zones. VSDs occur in 60% to 90% of patients, and are usually membranous, but occasionally subarterial. A VSD may have closed spontaneously before the age that a patient presents with this lesion. It is postulated that inadequate bulbar incorporation is the etiology of DCRV, hence discrete subaortic stenosis has also been reported. Branch pulmonary artery stenosis is not typically associated with DCRV.

37. (D) Neurocardiogenic (vasovagal) syncope is very common in the teenage population. The most cost-effective initial evaluation includes taking a detailed history to ensure that there is no family history of sudden death. After the history and physical examination, the next appropriate test is an ECG if the patient has had no previous evaluation. The other tests listed may be considered if further evaluation is needed or the examination and history raise suspicion of specific pathology.

38. (A) Chest wall pain is the most common cause of chest pain in children. Types of chest wall pain include costochondritis, Tietze syndrome, nonspecific (idiopathic) chest wall pain, precordial catch syndrome, slipping rib syndrome, hypersensitive xiphoid syndrome, trauma and muscle strain, and sickle cell disease. Other, less common causes of chest pain include asthma, infection, pericarditis, gastrointestinal, and pneumothorax. Least common are cardiac causes of chest pain that include HCM, aortic stenosis, pericarditis, arrhythmias, coronary insufficiency, dissecting aortic aneurysm, and mitral valve prolapse. The most common causes of coronary insufficiency in children are Kawasaki disease, Williams syndrome, anomalous origin of the coronary arteries, and coronary arteriovenous and coronary cameral fistulae.

39. (D) Pulsus paradoxus is defined as an exaggeration of the normal variation during the inspiratory phase of respiration, in which the blood pressure declines as one inhales and increases as one exhales. It is one of the hallmarks of cardiac tamponade. It is also a sign that is indicative of several other conditions including pericarditis, chronic sleep apnea, croup, and obstructive lung disease such as asthma or COPD.

Normally, inspiration results in negative intrathoracic pressure, which causes an increase in systemic venous return to the right heart; it increases the capacity of the pulmonary vascular bed to a greater degree. This ultimately leads to a decrease in left-sided output even though there is increased systemic venous return to the right. In cardiac tamponade, right ventricular filling causes restriction to left ventricular filling. With inspiration, this decreased left ventricular filling, coupled with the increased capacity of the pulmonary vascular bed, results in a greater reduction in systemic output and therefore a greater decline in systolic pressure (>10 mm Hg). To measure pulsus paradoxus, one should listen for the difference between the first Korotkoff sound (intermittent and heard only during exhalation) and the second Korotkoff sound (a constant sound not dependent on respiratory cycle) as a reflection of the pulsus paradoxus; this is best accomplished by slow deflation of the BP cuff, but can also be observed by a difference in systolic BP recorded on an invasive arterial pressure monitoring line in relationship to respiration.

Severe aortic regurgitation or a "run-off" lesion, such as a PDA, result in a wide pulse pressure. Severe aortic stenosis results in a narrow pulse pressure with delayed upstrokes. Hypovolemia results in low BP. Kawasaki disease would not be expected to cause a pulsus unless there also was inflammation of the pericardium causing pericarditis.

40. (B) Early diastolic murmurs begin immediately after S_2 and are decrescendo in nature. High-pitched early diastolic murmurs are due to aortic regurgitation with higher diastolic pressure in the aorta. They are heard best with the diaphragm at the left midsternal border. This murmur radiates to the apex and is decrescendo in nature due to a decrease in the intensity of the murmur as the diastolic pressure gradient equalizes. This is also why the murmur is accentuated when the patient leans forward and exhales.

Pulmonary valve regurgitation also produces an early diastolic murmur that is generally low pitched, but can be high pitched if pulmonary hypertension is present. It is also heard at the left midsternal border or at the left upper sternal border; however, radiation of this murmur is down the left sternal border. Patients with significant pulmonary regurgitation have murmurs with to-and-fro qualities due to increased forward volume load during ejection across the pulmonary valve.

Tricuspid and mitral valve stenosis cause mid-diastolic or late diastolic murmurs. These murmurs are produced during the early filling phase of diastole when blood crosses a narrow or thickened AV valve (mid-diastolic) or with atrial contraction (late diastolic). These murmurs are low pitched and are heard best with the bell of the stethoscope.

Mitral valve regurgitation results in a high-pitched holosystolic murmur at the apex with radiation to the back, left axilla, or clavicular area.

41. (E) All of these entities have been implicated as a cause of sudden cardiac death in the young. Many studies have described hypertrophic cardiomyopathy as the most common cause of sudden cardiac death in young athletes.

42. (B) After birth, as pulmonary artery pressures fall below systemic pressures and the pulmonary artery contains desaturated blood, left ventricular perfusion is compromised. Collateral flow is initially low, as collaterals do not form in fetal life when the pressures in the aorta and pulmonary arteries are essentially equal. As the left ventricle's demand for oxygen is not met, the left ventricular myocardial vessels dilate to reduce resistance and increase flow. When coronary vascular reserve is exhausted, the result is myocardial ischemia. In response to ischemic stimuli, collateral vessels form and enlarge between the normal right and the abnormal left coronary arteries. However, with the left coronary artery connected to the low-pressure pulmonary artery, there is pulmonary–coronary steal as blood tends to flow into the pulmonary artery rather than into the high-resistance myocardial vessels. This results in a left-to-right shunt, which is not significant in terms of cardiac output but which can be critical in terms of coronary flow and creating a "steal" phenomenon and resultant myocardial ischemia.

Any lesion that increases pressure in the pulmonary artery will help to decrease the pulmonary–coronary steal. If there is pulmonary hypertension, as may result with a large VSD or PDA, there may be adequate pulmonary artery pressure to drive left ventricular perfusion and to prevent left ventricular ischemia. In these cases, closure of the VSD or PDA results in a decrease in pulmonary arterial pressure, an effect that may decrease perfusion of the anomalous left coronary artery.

43. (A) There are several metabolic disorders resulting from specific enzyme deficiencies that cause RCM. These include Hurler syndrome, Gaucher disease, Fabry disease, and glycogen-storage diseases that can be lysosomal disorders or cytoplasmic enzyme deficiencies. Amyloidosis does result in RCM; however, this disease is seen almost exclusively in the adult population. Thiamin deficiency, muscular dystrophy, and collagen vascular diseases all cause dilated cardiomyopathy (DCM), not RCM.

44. (E) The physical examination described in the stem is consistent with a bicuspid aortic valve and aortic valve regurgitation. Of the choices offered, only the widened pulse pressure is consistent with aortic regurgitation. Coarctation of the aorta is an associated lesion but is less likely in this patient with normal femoral pulses.

45. (B) Most people with AORCA are asymptomatic. There may be a risk of sudden death with this anomaly, although the exact incidence is unknown. It occurs six times more commonly than anomalous origin of the left coronary artery from the right sinus of Valsalva (AOLCA). Therefore, surgical intervention remains controversial, as do sports participation recommendations. When surgery is performed, unroofing of the coronary origin is usually performed, not revascularization procedures. A stress echo will likely be normal, but serves as reassurance that there are no ECG or wall motion abnormalities detected with exercise.

46. (A) See Answer 29.

47. (C) See guideline statement and Answer 29.

48. (D) According to the 2015 AHA/ACC guidelines regarding competitive athletic participation in patients with cardiovascular abnormalities, in children with a large, unrepaired ASD, only low-intensity 1A sports are recommended. See **Figure 9.1** for sports intensity classification. Six months after successful ASD repair (or device closure), sports participation is unrestricted.

49. (B) Several ECG changes can be attributed to athletic training. These include sinus bradycardia, first-degree AV block, incomplete RBBB, early repolarization, and isolated QRS voltage criteria for LVH. These findings require no further investigation in an asymptomatic individual. Uncommon changes should warrant further investigation, such as T-wave inversions in the left precordial leads.

50. (B) Cardiovascular manifestations are common in SLE; 50% to 80% of patients report some cardiovascular complication in their lifetime. The most frequent clinically apparent cardiovascular complication is pericarditis with a frequency of ~25% and a pericardial effusion may be detected in as many as 50% of patients.

While necropsy studies have found evidence of myocarditis in as many as 40% of SLE cases, the rate of clinically evident myocarditis has been reported in <25% of patients. While less common, lupus myocarditis is an important cardiovascular complication because it has the potential to precipitate heart failure and arrhythmia and may contribute to the insidious development of cardiomyopathy. Libman–Sacks endocarditis is found in approximately 10% of SLE patients, usually on the mitral valve. It can also occur on the tricuspid or aortic valve. Angina is a complication of SLE, especially in the adult population, though not as common as pericarditis. Angina results from extra- and intramural coronary arteritis, accelerated atherosclerosis, embolism, thrombosis, spasm, or any combination thereof. These complications may be secondary to prolonged corticosteroid therapy and/or related to other lupus nonsteroid-related

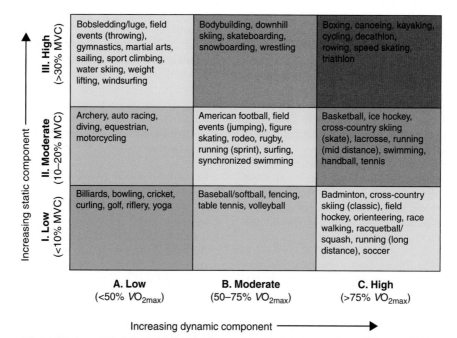

FIGURE 9.1 Classification is based on peak static and dynamic components achieved during exercise. Dynamic component is based on estimated percentage of maximal oxygen uptake (VO_{2max}), and static component is based on estimated percentage of maximal voluntary contraction (MVC). Sport classifications are consistent with 2015 AHA/ACC Eligibility and Disqualification Recommendations for Competitive Athletes With Cardiovascular Abnormalities.

mechanisms such as lupus-induced lipid disturbances, lupus-related antiphospholipid antibodies, and lupus-related intimal damage.

51. (D) The brother's death during swimming last year is concerning for a possible fatal arrhythmia, and this may be an indication of an underlying inheritable abnormality such as long QT syndrome. This should be worked up further, with an ECG and additional family history at a minimum, and potentially with genetic testing as well.

The other answers are all explainable. The syncope is very consistent with vasovagal syncope and is not associated with exercise. The shortness of breath is attributable to asthma and is confirmed by the response to albuterol. The grandfather's heart attack would be concerning if it occurred at an age <50 years old. Finally, the heart murmur is consistent with a benign Still murmur. It may still be worthwhile to work up if you're not completely sure that it is a benign murmur, but it is still not as concerning as the unexplained death in an immediate family member.

52. (B) ASDs found in infants <6 mm in size have an 80% to 90% chance of closing spontaneously.

53. (B) Patients with coarctation of the aorta have a roughly 10% incidence of intracranial aneurysms, which is about five times greater than the general population. They can still occur after repair, and they are not always associated with hypertension (though uncontrolled hypertension may be a risk factor). Most patients that develop aneurysms do so in adulthood, but they can occur at younger ages as well. Screening for aneurysms with head imaging is still controversial, though it could be considered.

54. (C) Children with congenital heart disease have well-recognized deficits in neurodevelopmental outcomes. They may have lower IQ scores, inferior achievement testing, and worse gross and fine motor functions. Children with cyanotic lesions are affected more than those with acyanotic lesions. The duration of cyanosis is also associated with a greater decline in cognitive function. Visual–spatial skills are an area of specific weakness in children with congenital heart disease. Children with single ventricle physiology are at highest risk of adverse developmental outcomes. Children with simple repaired lesions, such as those with an isolated ASD, often have normal neurodevelopmental outcomes.

55. (C) In 2014, the ASE published appropriate use criteria for ordering echocardiograms in pediatric patients. In this clinical scenario with nonexertional chest pain with a normal ECG or no other signs or symptoms of cardiac disease, an echo would be considered "Rarely Appropriate." Prior to taking the test, review of these criteria is recommended.

56. (C) A patient with tricuspid atresia frequently will have the ECG finding of LAD. Other diagnoses to consider in patients with LAD include partial and complete AV septal defects and WPW.

57. (B) The patient is likely being treated with flecainide, which is a sodium channel blocker. Flecainide levels increase once a patient stops breastfeeding or stops receiving formula. Given the patient's age of 12 months, it is likely that he is weaning off formula and one should be concerned about flecainide toxicity. Findings of toxicity include PR prolongation and possible signs of heart failure. The other answer options may all be normal findings on ECG in a 12 month old.

58. (D) Vein of Galen malformation (VGAM) is a rare embryonic arteriovenous shunt seen in 1:25,000 live births and more common in males. Intracardiac anatomy may be normal, but there is an association of VGAM with sinus venosus defects or coarctation. Fetal presentation can range from mild cardiac failure to fetal hydrops. VGAM is commonly diagnosed after birth with rapid deterioration and cardiac failure with large shunts and pulmonary hypertension. High-output cardiac failure is the primary clinical concern. Intracranial hemorrhage is uncommon. Smaller shunts may present later in life, with macrocephaly and prominent facial veins. Initial assessment includes cranial ultrasound in an infant, followed by MRI or CT. Transcatheter chemical embolization approaches have been the most successful treatment method, but morbidity and mortality remain high.

59. (D) The patient outlined in the question stem has normal risk for an elevation of her cholesterol level. According to the 2011 NHLBI guidelines for cardiovascular health, all children should have a nonfasting lipid profile with a calculated non-HDL cholesterol performed once between the ages of 9 and 11 years. Children should be screened earlier (ages 2 to 8 years) if:

- A parent, grandparent, aunt/uncle, or sibling has an MI, angina, stroke, coronary artery bypass graft (CABG)/stent/angioplasty at <55 years in males and <65 years in females
- Parent with TC >240 mg/dL or known dyslipidemia
- Child has diabetes, hypertension, or BMI >95th percentile, or smokes cigarettes
- Child has a moderate- or high-risk medical condition:

  High risk:
  - Diabetes mellitus type 1 and type 2
  - Chronic kidney disease/end-stage renal disease/renal transplant
  - Post-orthotopic heart transplant
  - Kawasaki disease with current aneurysms

  Moderate risk:
  - Kawasaki disease with regressed coronary aneurysms
  - Chronic inflammatory disease (SLE, JRA)
  - HIV infection
  - Nephrotic syndrome

60. (B) Guidelines for anticoagulation in pediatric patients with mechanical prostheses are extrapolated from the adult guidelines. In a patient with a bileaflet aortic prosthesis and no other risk factors for thrombosis, bridging with heparin is not required. Warfarin can be stopped 48 to 72 hours prior to the procedure and restarted on the evening of the procedure if there are no postoperative bleeding issues. Mechanical prostheses in the mitral position and in right-sided valves are at increased risk for thrombosis, so bridging with heparin is usually recommended when stopping warfarin therapy.

61. (B) The most common indication for reoperation after repair of complete atrioventricular septal defect (AVSD) is left AV valve regurgitation; left AV valve stenosis is rare. Right AV valve regurgitation occurs less commonly and primarily in association with pulmonary hypertension or tetralogy of Fallot. Late LVOT obstruction due to subaortic stenosis is more common with partial AVSD than with the complete form.

62. (D) The prominent "a" wave implies severe PS. The murmur of pulmonary stenosis may vary with respiration. In severe PS, one can expect the ejection click at the left upper sternal border to become softer, the S_2 split becomes fixed with a softer P2, the ejection murmur may extend through the S_2, a thrill will be present unless the patient has low cardiac output. The ejection click of a bicuspid aortic valve is best at the apex and does not vary with respiration. The systolic click from mitral valve prolapse moves earlier when standing. Severe tricuspid regurgitation would cause a prominent "v" wave, except in young patients with Ebstein anomaly.

63. (A) Brugada syndrome is more common in men, and more arrhythmic events occur in men; higher testosterone levels are thought to have a role. Inheritance is autosomal dominant. ICD implantation is not indicated in asymptomatic Brugada patients with drug-induced type I ECG on the basis of family history of sudden cardiac death alone. Symptoms commonly occur during rest, sleep, febrile state, or vagotonic conditions. Symptoms during exercise are very rare.

64. (C) Based on the revised Ghent nosology, he meets criteria for diagnosis of MFS based on a positive family history and aortic root Z-score ≥3.0 (below 20 years old). Following diagnosis, an echo should initially be performed at 6-month intervals to assess the progression of aortic involvement. Baseline imaging with MRI or CT of the thoracic aorta is reasonable in children who are fully grown. Medical therapy with a β-blocker or an angiotensin receptor blocker therapy should be initiated at diagnosis in the presence of significant aortic dilation.

65. (C) Squatting will increase preload and delay prolapse, moving the click closer to S_2. Decreased left ventricular contractility and increased afterload will delay the click, moving it closer to S_2. Standing moves the click closer to S_1. The regurgitant murmur of MVP follows the click. When mitral regurgitation is severe, an inflow murmur in diastole may occur.

66. (B) Alagille syndrome is an autosomal dominant disorder with bile duct paucity, heart disease, skeletal and ocular abnormalities, and characteristic facies as described in the stem. DiGeorge is highly variable and includes heart

disease, palatal anomalies, hypocalcemia, immunodeficiency, speech and learning disabilities, renal anomalies, psychiatric problems, and distinct facial features. Down syndrome has other characteristic facial features and is associated with septal defects. Noonan syndrome can have pulmonary valve dysplasia and non-sarcomeric hypertrophic cardiomyopathy. Patients with Kabuki syndrome have distinct facial features and associated ASDs, VSDs, and left-sided obstructive lesions.

67. (A) The incidence of HCM is 1:500. Dissimilar patterns of LVH can occur in patients with the same genetic substrate, except in identical twins in which hearts have been shown to have the same patterns of LVH. Hypertrophy is usually not present at birth, and ECG abnormalities may be the initial clinical manifestation before increased wall thickness becomes evident on 2D echo. More than 90% of patients with HCM have ECG abnormalities. Echocardiographic screening is recommended annually when teens are in high school (especially those participating in sports). Yield for genetic testing is higher in younger patients (<45 years old), those with reverse curve morphology, wall thickness >20 mm, and family history of HCM or sudden death.

68. (B) See **Figure 9.2** regarding the differential diagnosis of HCM versus physiologic athlete's heart. Maximal LV wall thickness within the shaded gray area is consistent

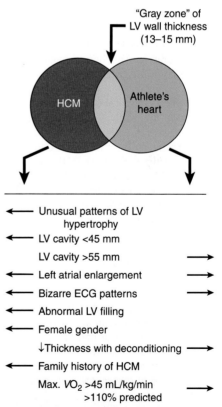

FIGURE 9.2 Differential diagnosis of hypertrophic cardiomyopathy (HCM) versus physiologic athlete's heart. (Adapted from Maron BJ, Pelliccia A. The heart of trained athletes: cardiac remodeling and the risks of sports, including sudden death. *Circulation.* 2006;114[15]:1633–1644.)

with both diagnoses. Clinical criteria used to distinguish nonobstructive HCM from athlete's heart are listed in the figure.

69. (D) Hyperkalemia is an electrolyte disturbance that may cause the ECG findings and symptoms found in this patient. Of the answer choices, spironolactone (a potassium-sparing diuretic) and lisinopril (an angiotensin-converting enzyme inhibitor) both decrease the effects of aldosterone and together have a high propensity to cause hyperkalemia. Hydrochlorothiazide (a thiazide) and furosemide (a loop diuretic) each have potassium-losing properties.

70. (A) Furosemide (a loop diuretic) may cause hypokalemia, hyponatremia, hypocalcemia, hypomagnesemia, and *hyper*chloremic metabolic alkalosis. Hydrochlorothiazide can cause hypokalemia, hyperuricemia, and hypercalcemia. Lisinopril can induce neutropenia, proteinuria, and hyperkalemia. Spironolactone (a potassium-sparing diuretic) may cause hyperkalemia. Losartan is also associated with hyperkalemia.

71. (B) LVOT obstruction is a strong determinant of progressive heart failure. However, LVOT obstruction has a weak relationship to sudden cardiac death with a low positive predictive value. All of the other factors have been linked to increased risk for ventricular arrhythmia and/or sudden death in HCM.

72. (B) Aortic dissection or rupture is an increasingly recognized cause of death in young women with Turner syndrome. Other risk factors for aortic dissection include a history of coarctation, the presence of a bicuspid aortic valve, and/or hypertension. However, not all women with Turner syndrome who develop aortic dissection have one of these risk factors, and dissection is not always preceded by progressive dilation.

73. (C) Supravalvar aortic stenosis is a congenital heart defect associated with Williams syndrome, which is also associated with hypercalcemia. Mutations in the NOTCH2 gene and butterfly vertebrae are present in Alagille syndrome (associated with peripheral pulmonary artery stenosis). Primary ovarian insufficiency is present with Turner syndrome (associated with bicuspid aortic valve and coarctation). A hypoplastic thymus is present with DiGeorge syndrome (tetralogy of Fallot and *hypo*calcemia).

74. (A) NSAIDs are not recommended during the acute or subacute phase of myocarditis due to several animal studies that demonstrate worsening of myocardial inflammation, necrosis, and mortality compared to placebo. ACE inhibitors and ARBs have been associated with decreasing myocardial fibrosis, inflammation, and autoantibody protection. Similarly, aldosterone receptor antagonists have been associated with less fibrosis. Calcium channel blockers have also been associated with a decrease in inflammatory cytokines and improved survival.

75. (B) The diagnosis of pericarditis does not require presence of an effusion on echocardiogram. Pericarditis with or without effusions typically present as chest pain without respiratory distress. However, respiratory distress may develop in large effusions with tamponade physiology. In tamponade, pulse pressure narrows and pulsus paradoxus develops. Pulsus paradoxus is defined as a decrease in systolic blood pressure by more than 10 mm Hg with inspiration. The earliest sign of tamponade on echocardiogram is collapse of the right ventricular free wall.

76. (A) This question is asking about when brain development begins to deviate from expected trajectories in children with HLHS. Fetal neuroimaging studies of fetuses with HLHS (and also fetuses with TGA) have documented abnormalities in axonal/neuronal health, total brain volume, white matter volume, and cortical plate volume during the third prenatal trimester. Delays in cortical gyrification (folding) have been documented even earlier in gestation, as early as around 25 weeks gestation. Brain imaging abnormalities have also been documented in patients with HLHS during childhood, adolescence, and adulthood.

77. (C) According to the AHA guidelines published by Marino et al. in 2012, neonates or infants requiring open heart surgery should be considered at "high risk" for developmental disorder or disability. This would include children diagnosed with tricuspid atresia. Children with relatively milder forms of CHD such as atrial septal defect, ventricular septal defect, or atrioventricular septal defect may also be at risk for developmental disorder or disability, particularly if they fall within any of the following risk categories:

- Neonates or infants requiring open heart surgery (cyanotic and acyanotic types) HLHS, IAA, PA/IVS, Truncus arteriosus, TAPVC, TGA, TOF, tricuspid atresia
- Children with other cyanotic heart lesions not requiring open heart surgery during the neonatal or infant period, for example, TOF with PA and MAPCA(s), TOF after systemic to PA shunt without use of CPB, Ebstein anomaly
- Any combination of CHD and the following comorbidities:
  - Prematurity (<37 weeks)
  - Developmental delay recognized in infancy
  - Suspected genetic abnormality or syndrome associated with developmental delay
  - History of mechanical support
  - Heart transplantation
  - Need for CPR
  - Postoperative hospitalization >14 days
  - Perioperative seizures related to CHD surgery
  - Significant abnormalities on neuroimaging or microcephaly
- Other conditions determined at the discretion of the medical home providers

78. (E) According to two meta-analyses, children with critical forms of CHD are at risk for relative deficits in general cognitive ability or "IQ" (intelligence quotient). However, the magnitude of deficit in IQ seems to depend on the type of CHD. Whereas children with TGA or TOF, on average, tend to have IQ scores that are about 2 or 3 points lower than the population mean of 100, children with HLHS are more severely affected with average IQ scores approximately 12 points lower than the population mean.

79. (D) While it is true that problems with distractibility, attention, forgetfulness, and school-related frustration are common among school-age children with critical CHD, they are not necessarily "nothing to worry about." Many children with critical CHD meet criteria for attention-deficit/hyperactivity disorder (ADHD), and many do seem to benefit from psychopharmacological treatment of their ADHD. However, in this case, prior to initiating treatment, more information is needed to better understand the nature of this child's concerns. Referring the child for comprehensive neuropsychological assessment is recommended to understand this child's profile of neurobehavioral strengths and

weaknesses, and to obtain recommendations for treatment/management. Recommendations may include child psychiatry and/or pediatric neurology consults, as well as a range of behavior management and cognitive strategies, as needed, to address this child's particular difficulties at home, school, and within the community.

80. (D) Brussel sprouts, collard greens, and spinach are rich in vitamin K and could decrease the INR. Kale (fresh, frozen, cooked, drained) is a very high vitamin K food and would be expected to decrease one's INR. These are healthy foods and patients who eat a diet rich in these foods and take warfarin therapy may need higher warfarin doses to achieve their goal INR. Bananas, avocados, corn, most fruits, and green and red peppers are examples of low vitamin K foods and would not typically affect the INR.

SUGGESTED READINGS

American Heart Association. Dietary recommendations for children and adolescents. *Circulation*. 2005;112:2061–2075.

Barst RJ, Ertel SI, Beghetti M, et al. Pulmonary arterial hypertension: A comparison between children and adults. *Eur Res J*. 2011;37(3):665–677.

Basso C, Maron BJ, Corrado D, et al. Clinical profile of congenital coronary artery anomalies with origin from the wrong aortic sinus leading to sudden death in young competitive athletes. *J Am Coll Cardiol*. 2000;35(6):1493–1501.

Bos JM, Will ML, Gersh BJ, et al. Characterization of a phenotype-based genetic test prediction score for unrelated patients with hypertrophic cardiomyopathy. *Mayo Clin Proc*. 2014;89(6):727–737.

Committee on Nutrition; Daniels SR, Greer FR. Lipid screening and cardiovascular health in childhood. *Pediatrics*. 2008;122(1):198–208.

Driscoll DJ. History and physical evaluation. In: Shaddy RE, Penny DJ, Feltes TF, et al., eds. Moss and Adams' Heart Disease in Infants, Children and Adolescents: Including the Fetus and Young Adult. 10th ed. Wolters Kluwer; 2021.

Gerber MA, Baltimore RS, Eaton CB, et al. Prevention of rheumatic fever and diagnosis and treatment of acute streptococcal pharyngitis: A scientific statement from the American Heart Association Rheumatic Fever, Endocarditis, and Kawasaki Disease Committee of the Council on Cardiovascular Disease in the Young, the Interdisciplinary Council on Functional Genomics and Translational Biology, and the Interdisciplinary Council on Quality of Care and Outcomes Research: endorsed by the American Academy of Pediatrics. *Circulation*. 2009;119(11):1541–1551.

Godfrey M. Congenital contractural arachnodactyly. GeneReviews. NCBI Bookshelf Online. 2011.

Lipshultz SE, Colan SD, Gelber RD, et al. Late cardiac effects of doxorubicin therapy for acute lymphoblastic leukemia in childhood. *N Engl J Med*. 1991;324(12):808–815.

Loeys BL, Dietz HC, Braverman AC, et al. The revised Ghent nosology for the Marfan syndrome. *J Med Genet*. 2010;47(7):476–485.

Magnani JW, William G. Myocarditis: Current trends in diagnosis and treatment. *Circulation*. 2006;113(6):876–890.

Marino BS, Lipkin PH, Newburger JW, et al. Neurodevelopmental outcomes in children with congenital heart disease: evaluation and management: A scientific statement from the American Heart Association. *Circulation*. 2012;126(9):1143–1172.

McCrindle BW, Rowley AH, Newburger JW, et al. Diagnosis, treatment and long-term management of Kawasaki disease: A scientific statement for health professionals from the American Heart Association. *Circulation*. 2017;135(17):e927–e999.

National High Blood Pressure Education Program Working Group on High Blood Pressure in Children and Adolescents. The fourth report on the diagnosis, evaluation, and treatment of high blood pressure in children and adolescents. *Pediatrics*. 2004;114(2): 555–576.

Niaz T, Hope K, Fremed M, et al. Role of a pediatric cardiologist in the COVID-19 pandemic. *Pediatr Cardiol*. 2020:1–17. doi:10.1007/s00246-020-02476-y

Nishimura RA, Otto CM, Bonow RO, et al. 2017 AHA/ACC focused update of the 2014 AHA/ACC guideline for the management of patients with valvular heart disease: A report of the American College of Cardiology/American Heart Association Task Force on Clinical Practice Guidelines. *J Am Coll Cardiol*. 2017;70(2):252–289.

O'Brien ET, O'Malley K. ABC of blood pressure measurement: Technique. *Br Med J*. 1979;2(6196):982–984.

Ogedegbe G, Pickering T. Principles and techniques of blood pressure measurement. *Cardiol Clin*. 2010;28(4):571–586.

Ruggiero A, Ridola V, Puma N, et al. Anthracycline cardiotoxicity in childhood. *Pediatr Hematol Oncol*. 2008;25(4):261–281.

Smith LA, Cornelius VR, Plummer CJ, et al. Cardiotoxicity of anthracycline agents for the treatment of cancer: Systematic review and meta-analysis of randomized controlled trials. *BMC Cancer*. 2010;10:337.

Task Force for the Diagnosis and Management of Syncope; European Society of Cardiology (ESC); European Heart Rhythm Association (EHRA); Heart Failure Association (HFA); Heart Rhythm Society (HRS); Moya A, Sutton R, Ammirati F, et al. Guidelines for the diagnosis and management of syncope (version 2009). *Eur Heart J*. 2009;30(21):2631–2671.

Van Hare GF, Ackerman MJ, Evangelista JA, et al. Eligibility and disqualification recommendations for competitive athletes with cardiovascular abnormalities: Task Force 4: congenital heart disease—a scientific statement from the American Heart Association and American College of Cardiology. *Circulation.* 2015;132(22):e281–e291.

Wilson W, Taubert KA, Gewitz M, et al. Prevention of infective endocarditis: Guidelines from the American Heart Association: A guideline from the American Heart Association Rheumatic Fever, Endocarditis, and Kawasaki Disease Committee, Council on Cardiovascular Disease in the Young, and the Council on Clinical Cardiology, Council on Cardiovascular Surgery and Anesthesia, and the Quality of Care and Outcomes Research Interdisciplinary Working Group. *Circulation.* 2007;116(15):1736–1754.

Zipes DP, Ackerman MJ, Estes NAM, et al. Task Force 7: Arrhythmias. *J Am Coll Cardiol.* 2005;45(8):1354–1363.

Cardiac Intensive Care

Anthony C. Chang, Sheri S. Crow, and Sylvia Del Castillo

Questions

1. Two hours after returning from a bidirectional Glenn procedure, a 10-month-old male with a history of pulmonary atresia with intact ventricular septum (PA/IVS) is intubated with SaO_2s (oxygen saturations) persistently 66% to 68%.

   Which of the following is <u>most</u> likely responsible for the hypoxemia?

   A. Venovenous collateral vessel
   B. Systemic hypertension
   C. $PaCO_2$ of 38 mm Hg
   D. PA pressure 14 mm Hg
   E. Moderate atrioventricular valve regurgitation

2. An 11-month-old male with a history of tetralogy of Fallot (TOF) on propranolol at home is now immediately status post a valve-sparing complete TOF repair. Vital signs: core temperature 38.7°C, HR 178 bpm, CVP 11 mm Hg, BP 72/46 mm Hg, SaO_2 97% on FiO_2 0.35 on minimal ventilatory support. Regular and atrial ECG is shown in **Figure 10.1**.

3. A 4-year-old male with a history of HLHS is now immediately status post an 18-mm nonfenestrated extracardiac Fontan procedure. He is intubated and on inotropes. Which of the following vital signs would NOT support a diagnosis of postoperative low cardiac output state?

   A. Sinus tachycardia with HR 172 bpm
   B. Core temperature 38.8 °C
   C. Pulmonary artery pressure 18 mm Hg
   D. SaO_2 99% on FiO_2 0.6
   E. Arterial line BP 68/43 mm Hg

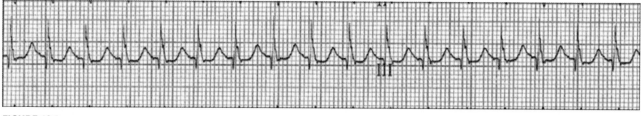

FIGURE 10.1

The <u>most</u> likely diagnosis is:

A. Sinus tachycardia
B. Ectopic atrial tachycardia
C. Junctional ectopic tachycardia
D. Supraventricular tachycardia (AVNRT)
E. Complete AV block

4. A 1-week-old male with d-TGA/ASD/VSD is now 4 hours after an arterial switch operation with ASD and VSD closure, PDA ligation, and a LeCompte maneuver. He is intubated, with a closed sternum, on the following inotropes: epinephrine 0.05 mcg/kg/min, milrinone 0.25 mcg/kg/min.

   Vital signs are as follows: core temperature 37.4 °C, HR 173 bpm, BP 46/19 (28) mm Hg, LA pressure 14 mm Hg, CVP 13 mm Hg, SaO_2 98% on FiO_2 0.4.

   Which of the following would likely NOT be a cause of the above vital signs?

   A. Moderate mitral valve regurgitation
   B. Hypovolemia
   C. Coronary artery ischemia
   D. Left ventricular systolic dysfunction
   E. Pericardial tamponade

5. A 16-year-old previously healthy male is admitted to the CVICU after presenting to the emergency department with a 2-week history of intermittent fever, rhinorrhea, cough, SOB, and orthopnea. Vital signs: temperature 37.4 °C, HR 135 bpm with S_3 gallop heard, respiratory rate 30 breaths per minute, cuff BP 111/62 mm Hg, and SaO_2 95% on room air. Rales heard on lung examination and hepatomegaly palpated.

   The CXR in **Figure 10.2** is obtained.

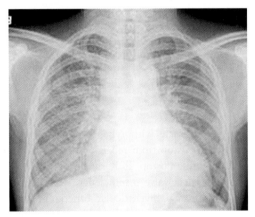

FIGURE 10.2

   Which of the following therapies is the BEST initial therapy?

   A. Furosemide IV
   B. Dopamine
   C. Digoxin PO
   D. Milrinone
   E. Carvedilol

6. A 1-week-old female with HLHS just returned from the OR following a Norwood procedure with a 3.5-mm Blalock–Taussig (BT) shunt. She is intubated with an open sternum, on inotropic support, bleeding, and requiring volume resuscitation with several blood products. During resuscitation, she has an acute drop in her SaO_2 from the low 80%s to the low 60%s with significant drop in $ETCO_2$ followed by hypotension. The <u>most</u> likely cause of this is:

   A. Accidental extubation
   B. Acute tension pneumothorax
   C. Right mainstem endotracheal tube displacement
   D. Acute pulmonary hypertensive crisis
   E. Acute occlusion of the systemic to pulmonary artery shunt

7. A 2-day-old male with HLHS has a systemic SaO_2 of 92% on room air. SvO_2 via an umbilical venous catheter with the end in the IVC/RA junction is 65%. Based on this data, the ratio of pulmonary to systemic blood flow is approximately:

   A. 2:1
   B. 1:1
   C. 4:1
   D. 5:1
   E. 0.8:1

8. Which of the following congenital heart lesions is NOT associated with postoperative junctional ectopic tachycardia (JET)?

   A. VSD
   B. Tetralogy of Fallot
   C. Total anomalous pulmonary venous return
   D. ASD
   E. d-TGA status post arterial switch operation

9. A 15-year-old previously healthy male with no significant past medical history is admitted with a diagnosis of acute viral myocarditis with an LV ejection fraction of 25% on a transthoracic echocardiogram. He is peripherally cannulated emergently to venoarterial extracorporeal membrane oxygenation (ECMO) support. Shortly after cannulation, copious pink frothy secretions are noted from his endotracheal tube. The <u>best</u> therapy to address this event is:

   A. Furosemide 20 mg IV × 1
   B. STAT cardiac catheterization for balloon atrial septostomy
   C. Increase PEEP on the ventilator from 10 mm Hg to 15 mm Hg
   D. Increase ECMO flows from 100 cc/kg/min to 130 cc/kg/min
   E. Start an epinephrine infusion to aid with myocardial contractility

10. Preoperative management of an 8-week-old male with newly diagnosed anomalous left coronary artery from the pulmonary artery (ALCAPA) who presented with CHF with severe MR, a dilated LV with poor systolic function, but with stable blood pressure, would include all EXCEPT:

    A. Epinephrine infusion
    B. Milrinone infusion
    C. Supplemental oxygen therapy
    D. PRN lorazepam
    E. Furosemide

11. Factors that increase endothelial-derived nitric oxide (EDNO) production include all of the following EXCEPT:

    A. Bradykinin
    B. Serotonin
    C. Vasopressin
    D. NG-monomethyl-L-arginine (L-NMMA)
    E. Histamine

12. The Law of Laplace, as it relates to wall stress of the left ventricle states:

    A. Wall stress is directly proportional to the thickness of the ventricle
    B. Wall stress is indirectly proportional to the transmural pressure of the ventricle
    C. Wall stress is directly proportional to the change in radius of the ventricle
    D. Wall stress is increased with positive pressure ventilation
    E. Wall stress is decreased with upper airway obstruction

13. A 5-month-old male with a history of tetralogy of Fallot and pulmonary stenosis who is on propranolol at home is admitted to the cardiac ICU for severe hypoxemia. His VS: temperature 37.5 °C, HR 155 bpm, BP 70/46 mm Hg, RR 32, SaO_2 66% on 4 LPM nasal cannula. All of the following therapies are indicated EXCEPT:

    A. Initiation of milrinone infusion
    B. Consider intubation if hypoxemia persists
    C. Initiation of an esmolol infusion
    D. Sedation with morphine 0.1 mg/kg IV
    E. Initiation of phenylephrine infusion

14. A 3-week-old male is 5 hours following complete repair of type I truncus arteriosus with ASD and VSD closure. He is intubated on volume control ventilatory support with a PEEP of 4, with low peak pressures on the ventilator, tidal volumes of 6 cc/kg, with SaO_2 96% on FiO_2 0.6. Arterial blood pressure is 72/40 mm Hg on milrinone 0.5 mcg/kg/min and epinephrine 0.03 mcg/kg/min. He has an acute increase in his CVP from 8 mm Hg to 15 mm Hg and a drop in his $ETCO_2$ with hypoxemia to 76% followed by hypotension. All of the following are appropriate immediate therapies EXCEPT:

    A. Bolus of fentanyl 1 mcg/kg IV
    B. Initiation of iNO at 20 ppm
    C. Increase FiO_2 to 1.0
    D. Increase milrinone infusion to 0.75 mcg/kg/min
    E. Hyperventilate the patient

15. Which of the following postoperative complications is most anticipated following repair of a patient with a complete atrioventricular septal defect?

    A. Ventricular tachycardia
    B. Junctional ectopic tachycardia
    C. Aortic valve regurgitation
    D. Atrial flutter
    E. Ectopic atrial tachycardia

16. Expected complications following end-to-end anastomosis of a coarctation of the aorta (CoA) include:

    A. Systemic hypotension
    B. Pulmonary hypertension
    C. Acute kidney injury
    D. Phrenic nerve injury
    E. Feeding intolerance

17. A 2-week-old male with type I truncus arteriosus is immediately postop from repair with VSD closure and RV-PA conduit. Postop TEE showed moderate RVH, moderate truncal valve insufficiency, no residual ASD/VSD, and normal biventricular function. Vital signs: core temperature 38.6 °C, HR 178 bpm (junctional), BP 74/48 mm Hg, CVP 12 mm Hg, RR 30 with the ventilator, SaO_2 97%, FiO_2 0.4. Pressors include epinephrine 0.03 mcg/kg/min, milrinone 0.5 mcg/kg/min. Of the listed therapies, the least likely to benefit this patient would be:

    A. Increase epinephrine to 0.05 mcg/kg/min
    B. Cool patient to 36 °C
    C. Amiodarone 5 mg/kg IV bolus
    D. Maintain arterial pH >/ = 7.40
    E. Increase milrinone to 0.75 mcg/kg/min

18. A 10-week-old male with a history of HLHS, status post a Norwood procedure with a 3.5-mm modified BT shunt as a neonate, is admitted to the cardiac ICU after presenting in the emergency department with a history of poor feeding, lethargy, diaphoresis, and poor weight gain over the last 5 days. On examination, he is tachypneic to the 50s, with 1+ pulses distally and a loud continuous shunt murmur heard at the right upper sternal border. Pulse oximetry reads 76% on room air. Which of the following is the most likely reason for his presenting symptoms?

    A. Pulmonary vein stenosis
    B. Distal aortic arch obstruction
    C. Shunt stenosis
    D. Anemia
    E. Pulmonary artery distortion

19. Each of the following scenarios would be expected in a newborn male with a diagnosis of infracardiac total anomalous pulmonary venous return (TAPVR) immediately postop following repair EXCEPT:

    A. Low left atrial filling pressures
    B. Decreased pulmonary compliance
    C. High pulmonary vascular resistance
    D. Pulmonary edema
    E. Junctional ectopic tachycardia

20. A term newborn male was just delivered at an outside hospital and intubated (without sedation) for persistent hypoxemia. An echocardiogram done by an adult sonographer was suspicious for hypoplastic left heart syndrome. The patient had umbilical venous and arterial lines placed. He has had minimal urine output since birth. Prostaglandin infusion was started at 0.025 mcg/kg/min. He was transferred to your CICU and upon arrival his vital signs are as follows: axillary temperature 36.8 °C, HR 188 bpm, BP via UAC 68/36 (47) mm Hg, RR 72 breaths per minute, SaO_2 90% on pressure control 14 mm Hg, PEEP 4 mm Hg, ventilator rate 16 breaths per minute, inspiratory time 0.4 seconds, FiO_2 0.45.

    On examination, he is agitated, mottled, tachycardic, tachypneic, with a murmur along the midsternal border. Pulses are 1+ distally. Initial ABG: 7.48/20/48/18/-6/88%. Serum lactate was 2.8 mmol/L.

    All of the following are possible therapies for this patient EXCEPT:

    A. Sedate the patient with morphine 0.05 mg/kg IV ×1
    B. Paralyze the patient, then increase the ventilator rate to 30 breaths per minute
    C. Give a bolus of normal saline 10 cc/kg IV ×1
    D. Give a bolus of sodium bicarbonate 1 mEq/kg IV ×1
    E. Wean the FiO_2 to 0.21

21. In a patient with complete heart block (CHB), what is the safest pacemaker mode to check the underlying ventricular escape rhythm?

    A. DDD
    B. AAI
    C. VOO
    D. VVI
    E. AOO

22. Left-to-right intracardiac shunts can result in excessive pulmonary blood volume and increased pulmonary vascular pressures. Over time, children with large left-to-right shunts may develop tachypnea secondary to:

    A. Increased pulmonary blood volume leading to increased lung weight and increased compliance
    B. Pulmonary edema: increased pulmonary blood flow → increased pulmonary artery, capillary, and venous pressures → increased extravascular lung water
    C. Extravascular fluid accumulation → atelectasis → decreased lung volume → decreased lung compliance → increased tidal volume → increased respiratory frequency
    D. Increased pulmonary vascular resistance, that is, pulmonary hypertension
    E. Decreased left ventricular volume (preload) and cardiac output

23. Positive pressure ventilation (PPV) (mechanical ventilation):

    A. Increases LV afterload
    B. Increases systemic venous return
    C. Increases right heart afterload
    D. Generates negative intrathoracic pressure
    E. Has no direct interaction with coronary blood flow

24. A 4-month-old male status post complete tetralogy of Fallot repair arrives from the OR intubated and mechanically ventilated. An hour after arrival the baby becomes increasingly agitated and the ventilator begins intermittently alarming due to high peak inspiratory pressures. Arterial blood gas demonstrates respiratory acidosis: pH 7.25, PCO_2 60, PO_2 110. Lactate 0.7. CXR demonstrates clear lung fields without pneumothorax or effusion. ETT is in good position. Which of the following interventions has the potential to achieve the quickest decrease in carbon dioxide levels?

    A. Chest physiotherapy
    B. Bronchodilator nebulization
    C. Increase the respiratory rate on the ventilator from 24 to 28
    D. Decrease the tidal volume in order to decrease the peak inspiratory pressure
    E. Administer a muscle relaxant/paralytic

25. A repeat blood gas is obtained after increasing the ventilator rate in the previous question: pH 7.28, CO_2 52, PO_2 110. Lactate 0.5. On examination, the patient continues to have significant work of breathing with accessory muscle use and a prolonged expiratory phase. Wheezes are auscultated throughout both lung fields. All the following can contribute to a persistent respiratory acidosis in this patient EXCEPT:

    A. Patient–ventilator asynchrony
    B. Bronchospasm
    C. Airway secretions
    D. Endotracheal tube malposition, dislodgement
    E. Increased pulmonary vascular resistance

26. A 6-month-old female with single ventricle physiology is status post a bidirectional Glenn operation. Her postoperative course has been uncomplicated. She is on room air with oxygen saturations of 85%. Full enteral feeds were achieved by POD #2 and chest tubes were removed on POD #3. The morning of POD #4, the patient develops increased work of breathing and requires supplemental oxygen to maintain saturations above 75%. Which of the following investigations is <u>most</u> likely to identify the cause of her acute respiratory decompensation?

    A. Right atrial pressure monitoring
    B. Ultrasound of upper extremity vessels
    C. Echocardiogram to evaluate ventricular function
    D. Cardiac catheterization to identify the presence of venous collaterals
    E. CXR to evaluate for pleural fluid

27. In the previous question, the diagnosis of pleural effusion is made. A chest tube is placed and fluid is sent for analysis which confirms that the fluid is chyle. Initial strategies for managing chylous effusions in the acute postoperative setting include all of the following EXCEPT:

    A. Change the formula to one that is high in medium-chain triglycerides
    B. Pleurodesis
    C. Make patient NPO and start parenteral nutrition
    D. Ultrasound evaluation of bicaval anastomosis and head and neck vessels looking for thrombosis or obstruction to flow
    E. Ensure continued evacuation of pleural fluid and maintain lung recruitment to avoid atelectasis

28. Postoperative principles of respiratory management of patients following the bidirectional Glenn and Fontan operation include which of the following:

    A. Utilize a higher PEEP strategy to ensure optimal lung recruitment
    B. Target early extubation or spontaneous breathing if the child cannot be liberated from mechanical ventilation
    C. Avoid noninvasive pressure ventilation
    D. Use caution when providing supplemental oxygen to avoid acute changes in pulmonary vascular resistance that will preferentially shunt blood to the pulmonary circulation at the expense of the systemic/coronary circulations
    E. Increase sedation/analgesia as needed to prevent patient/ventilator asynchrony

29. A 1-week-old male status post a Norwood Sano palliation for HLHS develops rhythmic twitching of his upper extremities with eye deviation to the right. The movement stops following intravenous lorazepam administration. Risk factors for seizures in the cardiac surgical perioperative period include which of the following:

    A. Older age at the time of surgery
    B. Deep hypothermic circulatory arrest (DHCA)
    C. Absence of preoperative CNS pathology
    D. Vasopressor requirements
    E. Fontan physiology

30. End-tidal CO_2 measurement is a reliable method for evaluating all of the following parameters EXCEPT:

    A. Effectiveness of alveolar ventilation for carbon dioxide removal
    B. Changes in pulmonary blood flow
    C. Endotracheal tube dislodgement
    D. Effectiveness of cardiopulmonary resuscitation (CPR)
    E. Noninvasive monitoring of arterial CO_2 level after congenital cardiac surgery in cyanotic heart disease

31. Near-infrared spectroscopy (NIRS) provides noninvasive continuous estimation of tissue oxygen saturation. Regarding NIRS utilization in the ICU, which of the following statements is correct?

    A. NIRS readings represent continuous bedside application of the Fick principle
    B. NIRS assesses tissue oxygenation by detecting light wave absorption within venous blood
    C. For children weighing less than 10 kg, there is poor correlation between cerebral NIRS and jugular bulb venous saturation
    D. Abnormal NIRS values in the postoperative period are predictive of short- but not long-term cognitive deficits
    E. Cerebral NIRS values are similar for children with and without left-to-right shunts

32. All of the following patient populations are at risk for thrombosis in the postoperative period EXCEPT:

    A. Mechanical prosthetic valve
    B. Severely reduced ejection fraction
    C. Children with synthetic shunt–dependent circulation
    D. Central venous catheters
    E. Paroxysmal supraventricular tachycardia

33. Hemodynamic changes after cardiac surgery are common. Choose the answer that correctly describes the hemodynamic changes associated with patterns of cardiac decompensation during the acute postoperative period.

    A. Low cardiac output syndrome: Decreased HR and mean arterial pressure (MAP), increased or decreased CVP, delayed capillary refill, poor urine output, and narrowed pulse pressure
    B. Cardiac tamponade: Increased HR, MAP, and CVP. Narrow pulse pressure, delayed capillary refill, and decreased urine output
    C. Hypovolemia: Increased HR, decreased MAP, delayed capillary refill, poor urine output, and decreased CVP
    D. Low cardiac output syndrome: Increased HR, decreased MAP, increased CVP, widened pulse pressure, brisk capillary refill
    E. Hypovolemia: Increased HR, increased MAP, brisk capillary refill, poor urine output, normal CVP

34. A 5-year-old female arrives in the ICU extubated following uncomplicated ASD repair. In addition to a right IJ central venous catheter and right radial arterial line, she has a mediastinal chest tube. During the first postoperative hour, she has >10 mL/kg/hr of serous output from her mediastinal chest tube. Coagulation studies show an INR of 2.2, aPTT of 30, and platelet count of 115,000. Which of the following answers describes the best assessment and management of this problem:

    A. The child is experiencing acute postoperative bleeding due to a coagulopathy. Following administration of fresh frozen plasma (FFP) and heparin reversal with protamine, coagulation factors should be reanalyzed to confirm resolution of coagulopathy
    B. The child is experiencing surgical bleeding and requires immediate transfer to the OR to identify and manage the bleeding source
    C. The volume of chest tube output is concerning for surgical bleeding. Immediate administration of FFP and reevaluation of coagulation studies and chest tube output can precede surgical exploration provided hemodynamic stability can be maintained
    D. The child is experiencing surgical bleeding in the context of a coagulopathy. Appropriate interventions include FFP and protamine administration while transporting to the operating room for surgical exploration
    E. The child is bleeding secondary to thrombocytopenia. Rapid platelet transfusion is indicated followed by reevaluation of coagulation studies and platelet count

35. The child in Question #34 receives FFP and her repeat INR is 1.4. Mediastinal chest tube output decreases significantly to 1 cc/kg/hr. Thirty minutes later the nurse calls you back to the bedside. Heart rate is 190 and the child is now hypotensive, with a CVP of 14, and poor urine output despite having just received 20 cc/kg of FFP. Which of the following answers correctly identifies the problem and appropriate treatment?

    A. Hypovolemic shock secondary to inadequate replacement of high-volume chest tube output. Administer 10 cc/kg of 5% albumin and monitor for a decrease in heart rate and improvement in blood pressure to confirm intravascular volume has been adequately repleted
    B. Cardiogenic shock caused by volume overload following rapid infusion of 20 cc/kg of FFP. Administer furosemide and push diuresis until CVP decreases and hemodynamics normalize
    C. Hemodynamically significant arrhythmia has developed. Obtain stat ECG and perform vagal maneuvers. If unsuccessful in converting to sinus rhythm, prepare for cardioversion
    D. Tension pneumothorax. Obtain a stat CXR and strip pleural chest tubes to attempt evacuation of intrathoracic air while waiting for CXR. Prepare for needle decompression if no improvement
    E. Cardiac tamponade. Strip mediastinal chest tube, administer volume, obtain stat echo to evaluate for pericardial effusion, and notify surgeon to prepare for emergent surgical exploration

36. A 3-year-old female with HLHS is POD #1 status post a fenestrated Fontan. The parents and bedside nurse are concerned because she doesn't appear to be moving her right arm and leg. Comprehensive neurologic examination reveals right-sided hemiparesis. The patient is taken for an emergent head CT scan. Regardless of the cause for her neurologic deficits, supportive care should include all of the following EXCEPT:

    A. Target normal blood glucose levels
    B. Initiate hypothermia protocol
    C. Transfuse to correct anemia in order to optimize oxygen delivery
    D. Monitor for and treat seizures
    E. Consider anticoagulation to prevent further thrombosis

37. Acute kidney injury (AKI) following pediatric congenital cardiac surgery is common. Risk factors for AKI in the perioperative period include all of the following EXCEPT?

    A. Cardiopulmonary bypass
    B. Deep hypothermic circulatory arrest
    C. Low cardiac output syndrome
    D. Nephrotoxic medications
    E. Fluid overload

CHAPTER 10

38. Postoperative management of the patient with AKI should include which of the following?

    A. Administration of diuretics as needed to achieve a net negative fluid balance
    B. Frequent laboratory analysis of BUN and creatinine to detect progression in renal failure
    C. Careful monitoring of electrolyte levels
    D. Review all patient medications and increase doses of those with renal clearance
    E. Target diuresis toward reduction in body wall edema

39. During the neonatal period, which of the following congenital cardiac defects is associated with a higher risk of necrotizing enterocolitis (NEC) during the perioperative period?

    A. Tetralogy of Fallot
    B. Ventricular septal defect with large left-to-right shunt
    C. Transposition of the great arteries
    D. Total anomalous pulmonary venous return
    E. Truncus arteriosus

40. A 2-week-old male status post coarctation of the aorta surgical repair develops abdominal distention and high gastric residuals with the initiation of enteral feeds. Which one of the following clinical signs are least likely to be associated with NEC?

    A. Thrombocytopenia
    B. Bradycardia
    C. Apnea
    D. Normal lactate
    E. Watery stool output

41. Central venous access is an essential tool to optimally support critically ill children after congenital cardiac surgery. Although not always symptomatic, the incidence of pediatric catheter-related venous thrombosis is estimated to be approximately 20%. Which of the following interventions has been shown to decrease the incidence of pediatric catheter-related venous thrombosis:

    A. Unfractionated heparin infusion through the line
    B. Low–molecular-weight heparin
    C. Nitroglycerin
    D. Heparin-bonded catheters
    E. Removal of central venous catheter

42. A 4-month-old female status post uncomplicated VSD repair develops a pneumothorax after chest tube removal that progresses to tension physiology and subsequently a pulseless electrical activity (PEA) cardiac arrest. Needle decompression followed by chest tube placement leads to return of spontaneous circulation. Postresuscitation care for this child should include all of the following EXCEPT:

    A. Post-cardiac arrest debriefing with all team members involved in the resuscitation
    B. Identify, and intervene if possible, precipitating factors that led to instability and arrest
    C. Maintain continuous cardiopulmonary monitoring and consider Foley catheter placement
    D. Consider placement of arterial and central venous lines to optimize monitoring and treatment abilities
    E. Provide subambient oxygen to the patient

Answers

1. (A) Hypoxemia is the most common short- and long-term complication following the bidirectional Glenn connection. Etiologies include decreased cerebral blood flow from hypocapnia or hypotension, decreased pulmonary blood flow from elevated PVR, venovenous collateral vessels, stenosis of cavopulmonary junction, and ventilation/perfusion mismatch (pleural effusion/pneumothorax). The PA pressure listed is normal.

2. (C) Junctional ectopic tachycardia is believed to be a result of direct trauma to the AV node and bundle of His, most commonly seen after TOF repair. Diagnosis is based on ECG evidence of narrow complex tachycardia with heart rates ranging from 170 to 260 bpm and a regular rhythm with AV dissociation. The QRS is usually narrow but can be wide with RBBB. P waves can be hidden, dissociated, or retrograde, as demonstrated by the two ECGs shown.

3. (D) After the Fontan operation, cardiac output is determined by pulmonary blood flow (PBF). Any reduction of PBF will reduce systemic oxygen delivery and cardiac output.

All of the vital signs listed are seen in a low cardiac output state in a nonfenestrated extracardiac Fontan except for hypoxemia.

4. (B) All of the listed options are examples of low cardiac output state following arterial switch operation. Elevated CVP is not consistent with a hypovolemic state.

5. (A) The presence of cardiomegaly, hepatomegaly, tachypnea, and a gallop rhythm are all consistent with volume overload from congestive heart failure (CHF) and loop diuretics are essential first-line therapy, particularly with stable pressures. The use of inotropes may be necessary to improve contractility, but diuresis is an important hallmark of initial therapy for CHF.

6. (E) Acute hypoxemia in a patient with a modified BT shunt must be evaluated promptly and suspicion for occlusion of the shunt must be high, especially in a patient who is bleeding postoperatively and actively being resuscitated with blood products. All of the other options could possibly explain an acute episode of hypoxemia, however, are less likely given the scenario of postoperative bleeding with blood product administration.

7. (C) The ratio of pulmonary to systemic blood flow can be easily calculated in *single ventricle physiology* patients by using the Fick method, which states Cardiac output = Oxygen consumption divided by arteriovenous oxygen difference. There are assumptions that allow the Fick equation to be derived to incorporate systemic and pulmonary saturations to calculate Qp:Qs. First, there is no significant pulmonary venous desaturation so that the pulmonary venous saturation is 95% to 100%. Second, the aortic and pulmonary artery saturations are equal as measured by pulse oximetry. The equation Qp:Qs is [SaO_2 – SvO_2]/[pulmonary venous saturation – pulmonary artery saturation]. In this case, the equation is [92% – 70%]/[99% – 92%] or about 4:1.

8. (D) All of the lesions listed are commonly associated with postop JET except for ASDs. The mechanism of JET is not proven but thought to be related to a combination of traction or trauma to the AV node and His bundle or ischemia during surgery.

9. (B) Pulmonary edema following ECMO cannulation is a clear indicator of severe left ventricular (LV) dysfunction. The best therapy to ultimately address the inability of the LV to decompress until it can regain function is a balloon atrial septostomy thus creating an LV/LA vent to further prevent myocardial ischemia. The other therapies are useful adjunctive therapies to address the pulmonary edema but will not resolve the underlying issue of poor LV function.

10. (A) The goal of preoperative management of patients with severe CHF is focused on optimizing myocardial oxygen supply and reducing myocardial oxygen demand. Of all of the therapies listed, epinephrine would be the most likely to increase myocardial oxygen demand based on the chronotropic effect, while all other therapies would either increase oxygen supply or reduce demand.

11. (D) Of all the factors listed, L-NMMA is known to decrease the synthesis of EDNO.

12. (C) Laplace law states the circumferential wall stress (T) is equal to the pressure (P) times the radius (r) divided by twice the wall thickness (t): $T = (P \times r)/2t$. Positive pressure ventilation decreases LV wall stress by decreasing LV transmural pressure. Upper airway obstruction increases LV wall stress by causing huge increases in transmural pressure.

13. (A) All of the therapies listed are known to aid acute Tet spells except the initiation of milrinone.

14. (D) All of the therapies listed would provide immediate benefit to a patient during an acute pulmonary hypertensive crisis except increasing the milrinone, as the effect would not be seen immediately.

15. (B) The most common dysrhythmias seen after repair of complete atrioventricular canal (CAVC) defect include junctional ectopic tachycardia and complete or transient AV block due to repair around the AV node. The other dysrhythmias are not commonly seen after CAVC repair.

16. (D) Surgical morbidity after repair of CoA includes anastomotic bleeding, cardiac arrest, chylothorax, GI bleeding, phrenic nerve or recurrent laryngeal nerve injury, postcoarctectomy hypertension, seizures, and spinal cord injury. None of the other complications listed are expected after end-to-end repair of CoA.

17. (A) Common postoperative complications following repair of truncus arteriosus include arrhythmias such as JET, pulmonary hypertension, and truncal valve insufficiency. Based on the patient's postoperative TEE showing moderate truncal insufficiency, and current JET, all the therapies listed are geared toward reducing pulmonary vascular resistance (arterial pH 7.40 and increasing milrinone) or treatment of JET (cooling patient and amiodarone bolus). Increasing epinephrine infusion would potentially increase SVR, worsening truncal valve insufficiency and cardiac output.

18. (B) In a patient following a Norwood procedure with arch reconstruction who presents with CHF symptoms, distal aortic arch obstruction should be high on the differential diagnosis as this is a common late complication. All the other choices would have presented with hypoxemia as the primary symptom.

19. (A) Infracardiac TAPVR is the second most common type of TAPVR and is characterized by severe hypoxemia, acidosis, and hypotension. A low cardiac output state results from decreased left atrial and left ventricular (LV) compliance due to abnormal preoperative filling. Underfilling of the LV can be exacerbated by pulmonary hypertension (PHTN) and right ventricular (RV) dilation. Often, the removal of the pulmonary venous obstruction with a subsequent increase in blood return to the LA further increases LAP, causing the cycle of worsening pulmonary edema, PHTN, and subsequent RV and LV dysfunction.

20. (D) In a preoperative patient with HLHS, the balance between Qp:Qs is of utmost importance. A systemic SaO_2 of 90% tells the clinician the Qp:Qs is weighted toward the pulmonary circulation, which could be contributing to the development of lactic acidosis. The patient is agitated and tachypneic, contributing to the alkalotic arterial pH, which along with the FiO_2 of 0.45 increases pulmonary blood flow through decreasing pulmonary vascular resistance. The patient should be appropriately sedated and paralyzed to take control of the hyperventilation and bring the $PaCO_2$ up to normal levels, while weaning the FiO_2 to 0.21 and increasing circulating volume with a fluid bolus. Sodium bicarbonate alone as a therapy would NOT be indicated as it wouldn't treat the underlying process.

21. (D) In patients with CHB but normal atrial rate, AV conduction can be tested in DDD mode by gradually prolonging the AV interval. However, VVI mode can also be used by gradually turning down the ventricular rate until either a minimum safe ventricular rate is reached or until the intrinsic rhythm emerges. The other modes will not test for underlying ventricular escape rhythm.

22. (B) In a patient with a large left-to-right intracardiac shunt, pulmonary edema develops due to increased pulmonary blood flow, increased pulmonary artery, capillary, and venous pressures, and increased extravascular lung water (pulmonary edema). This process increases lung weight which DECREASES lung compliance (A) and DECREASES tidal volume (C). The child's minute ventilation (Tidal volume × Respiratory rate) and CO_2 removal are maintained by increasing the respiratory rate to compensate for the decrease in tidal volume. Longstanding left-to-right intracardiac shunting can lead to increased pulmonary vascular resistance (D) thereby reducing left-to-right shunting and improvement in symptoms of pulmonary overcirculation like tachypnea. Left untreated, PVR continues to increase putting patients at risk for developing Eisenmenger complex and death. (E) Left-to-right shunts increase pulmonary blood flow, which increases preload and volume overloads the left ventricle, eventually creating congestive heart failure.

23. (C) The mean airway pressure generated by PPV increases intrathoracic pressure and right heart afterload while decreasing systemic venous return (B) and right ventricular preload. In contrast, PPV decreases LV afterload (A) through a combination of increased LV transmural and intrathoracic arterial pressures. Subsequent baroreceptor stimulation decreases aortic pressure and therefore LV afterload (D). (E) The increased intrathoracic pressures generated by PPV decrease the RV/aortic pressure gradient, which decreases RV coronary blood flow.

24. (C) CO_2 removal is determined by minute ventilation (Respiratory rate × Tidal volume). Therefore, the most effective strategy for immediately increasing CO_2 removal is to increase the respiratory rate and/or tidal volume.

25. (E) Although respiratory acidosis can lead to elevations in pulmonary vascular resistance, clinical signs of pulmonary hypertension are hypoxia, tachycardia, and hypotension, not respiratory acidosis (CO_2 retention). All of the other scenarios mentioned can contribute to alveolar hypoventilation manifested as CO_2 retention and respiratory acidosis.

26. (E) Children are at risk for chylous effusions following intrathoracic surgery due to thoracic duct injury. Physiologic changes that increase central venous pressure, such as the bidirectional Glenn and Fontan operations, or internal jugular and subclavian vessel thrombosis following central line insertion are associated with chylous effusions. Although all of the options listed can be helpful in identifying factors that might contribute to hypoxia and/or the development of a chylous effusion, a CXR (or bedside ultrasound) permits rapid detection of pleural fluid while simultaneously evaluating for other causes of hypoxia that would necessitate urgent intervention (pneumothorax, atelectasis).

27. (B) Management of chylous effusions involves drainage of pleural fluid, investigation for and treatment of venous thrombosis and obstruction, and adjustments in nutrition management to reduce lymphatic flow while lymphatic vessels heal. Enteral formulas that are low in long-chain triglycerides and high in medium-chain triglycerides are typically tried first. If chylous output persists, switching to parental nutrition and keeping the child NPO may become necessary. Pleurodesis with talc/tetracycline or fibrin glue and surgical thoracic duct ligation are utilized only after persistent failure of medical management.

28. (B) Pulmonary blood flow is passive following the Glenn and Fontan procedures. Therefore, anything that increases intrathoracic pressure or obstructs SVC or IVC drainage into the pulmonary arteries will impede pulmonary blood flow. Lower PEEP, early extubation, or attempts to achieve spontaneous breathing while mechanically ventilated will optimize pulmonary blood flow. Noninvasive pressure ventilation can be utilized in the Fontan and Glenn circulations provided the pressures delivered don't significantly increase intrathoracic pressure. Supplemental oxygen must be used with caution in the unpalliated or stage 1 Norwood to avoid acute changes in Qp/Qs. Conversely, after the Glenn and Fontan procedure, supplemental oxygen and even inhaled NO may be helpful in the acute postoperative period to decrease PVR with the objective of increasing the now passive pulmonary blood flow. Avoiding patient/ventilator asynchrony is important as this can generate high peak and mean airway pressures that will impede pulmonary blood flow. However, the best strategy would be to attempt extubation or spontaneous breathing rather than increasing sedation/analgesia that might prolong mechanical ventilation requirements.

29. (B) Cardiopulmonary bypass and specifically prolonged periods of DHCA are known risk factors for postoperative seizures. Younger age and preexisting CNS abnormalities are additional risk factors. Fontan physiology is not a specific risk factor for seizures; however, these patients are at increased risk for postoperative stroke which can present with seizures. Vasopressor requirements do not intrinsically increase seizure risk.

30. (E) End-tidal carbon dioxide monitoring or capnography underestimates arterial carbon dioxide levels in children with right-to-left shunts. The end-tidal and arterial carbon dioxide gradient increases as oxygen saturations decrease. Right-to-left shunts introduce deoxygenated hypercarbic blood into the systemic circulation, increasing alveolar dead space and reducing pulmonary blood flow.

31. (A) NIRS provides a continuous noninvasive measurement of cardiac output using the Fick principle. NIRS measures tissue oxygenation by quantitatively assessing the color of hemoglobin in the blood beneath the probe (B). The strongest correlation between NIRS and jugular bulb saturations is observed in children less than 10 kg (C). Abnormal NIRS values are associated with poor short- and long-term outcome including prolonged mechanical ventilation and hospital stay, and neurodevelopmental delay (D). Cerebral NIRS values are lower in children with left-to-right shunts (E).

32. (E) Paroxysmal supraventricular tachycardia or SVT does not increase the risk for thrombosis. In contrast, atrial arrhythmias such as atrial flutter or fibrillation that persist for greater than 48 hours warrant consideration of imaging to rule out intracardiac thrombus.

33. (C) Hypovolemia in the postoperative period can be multifactorial and includes preoperative NPO status, blood loss, postbypass ultrafiltration, and aggressive attempts at diuresis. Low cardiac output syndrome is also common and typically characterized by increased HR, decreased MAP, delayed capillary refill, and poor urine output. CVP may be high, normal, or low depending on the underlying reason for cardiac failure. Cardiac tamponade that results from fluid collection in the pericardial space is important to recognize and treat before it leads to complete cardiac collapse. Characteristic signs include increased HR, increased CVP, narrow pulse pressure, poor urine output, and delayed capillary refill.

34. (C) Chest tube output >10 mL/kg/hr in the first hour, or >5 mL/kg/hr after 2 hours is concerning for surgical bleeding. Provided hemodynamic stability can be maintained, medical management of bleeding precedes surgical reexploration, especially in the presence of documented coagulopathy or thrombocytopenia. Intervention seeks to keep up with ongoing blood loss while administering blood products that target the specific hematologic derangement. In this patient, the INR is elevated and FFP administration would be appropriate. Successful resolution of coagulopathy is confirmed by rechecking coagulation studies and observing an associated decrease in chest tube output. Protamine would not be the first line of therapy in this patient because the aPTT is only 30 suggesting minimum residual heparin effect. Platelet administration may be helpful if platelet count is <100,000 or bleeding does not improve with INR correction. However, unlike other blood components, platelets should be given slowly to avoid causing vasodilation and hypotension.

35. (E) Although all options provide potential explanations for the change in vital signs, this clinical scenario is most consistent with cardiac tamponade. A significant decrease in mediastinal chest tube output that is associated with tachycardia, hypotension, narrow pulse pressure, and an elevated CVP suggests chest tube obstruction and collection of fluid in the mediastinal/pericardial space resulting in tamponade.

36. (B) Hypothermia is not indicated for acute ischemic stroke. Clinical trials have failed to demonstrate a consistent benefit for the application of hypothermia in pediatric neurologic injury. Recommendations are to avoid hyperthermia surrounding any neurologic insult.

37. (E) Cardiopulmonary bypass induces a systemic inflammatory response syndrome that can be associated with low cardiac output and capillary leak, thereby compromising renal perfusion pressure and intravascular volume. Although clinical evidence of fluid overload is common with AKI, it is usually a reflection of the ongoing inflammatory response and capillary leak rather than the cause of kidney injury.

38. (C) Electrolyte abnormalities are common in AKI. Normal anion gap metabolic acidosis, hypo- and hyperkalemia, hypomagnesemia, hyponatremia, and hypochloremia are typical derangements. Although postoperative fluid management generally targets a net negative fluid balance, maintaining intravascular volume is critical to avoid further prerenal insult (A). Elevated BUN and creatinine can confirm and describe severity of renal injury. However, bedside assessment of hemodynamics, capillary refill, and urine output provide real-time evidence for the adequacy of renal perfusion (B). Patient medications should be reviewed, and doses DECREASED for renally cleared medications (D). A child can have significant edema due to capillary leak and third spacing while being intravascularly underfilled. Maintaining intravascular volume and renal perfusion during postoperative diuresis is critical to avoid further prerenal insult (E).

39. (E) A higher incidence of NEC has been observed in cardiac lesions with diastolic run-off (truncus arteriosus, aortopulmonary window, and ductal-dependent single ventricle circulations).

40. (E) Watery stool output is more suggestive of malabsorption than enteric ischemia. Thrombocytopenia, temperature instability, bradycardia, lethargy, and apnea should raise suspicion for NEC in this patient (A, B, C). Although bowel ischemia should be in the differential for any child with a high lactate level, a normal lactate level does not rule out underlying bowel pathology (D).

41. (E) Central line removal is the only intervention that has been shown to reduce catheter-associated thrombosis.

42. (E) Oxygen administration is a critical component to cardiac resuscitation. However, once spontaneous circulation is reestablished, oxygen should be titrated to avoid hypoxemia or hyperoxemia, as both are associated with worse outcomes following cardiac arrest. AHA recommendations are to target normoxia (PaO_2 level 60 to 300 mm Hg). When PaO_2 is unavailable, target saturations of 94% to 100%. Physiologically individualized PaO_2 and oxygen saturation ranges should be determined for children with cyanotic heart disease.

SUGGESTED READINGS

Abdelaziz O, Deraz S. Anticipation and management of junctional ectopic tachycardia in postoperative cardiac surgery: Single center experience with high incidence. *Ann Pediatr Cardiol.* 2014;7(1):19–24.

da Cruz EM, Ivy D. Chapter 42: Acute pulmonary hypertension. In: Munoz RA, Morell VO, da Cruz EM, et al., eds. *Critical Care of Children with Heart Disease.* 2nd ed. Springer Nature Switzerland AG; 2020:459–460.

da Cruz EM, Kaufman J, Fonseca B, et al. Chapter 30: Single ventricle: General aspects. In: Munoz RA, Morell VO, da Cruz EM, et al., eds. *Critical Care of Children with Heart Disease.* 2nd ed. Springer Nature Switzerland AG; 2020:338.

Del Castillo S, Shaddy RE, Kantor PF. Update on pediatric heart failure. *Curr Opin Pediatr.* 2019;31(5):598–603.

Domnina YA, Kerstein J, Johnson J, et al. Chapter 18: Tetralogy of Fallot. In: Munoz RA, Morell VO, da Cruz EM, et al., eds. *Critical Care of Children with Heart Disease.* 2nd ed. Springer Nature Switzerland AG; 2020:193–194.

Epstein D, Wetzel RC. Chapter 2: Cardiovascular physiology and shock. In: Nichols DG, Ungerleider RM, Spevak PJ, et al., eds. *Critical Heart Disease in Infants and Children.* 2nd ed. Mosby Elsevier; 2006:28.

Fan E, Brodie D, Slutsky AS. Acute respiratory distress syndrome: Advances in diagnosis and treatment. *JAMA.* 2018;319(7):698–710.

Follansbee CW, Arora G, Beerman L. Chapter 51: Arrhythmias in the intensive care unit. In: Munoz RA, Morell VO, da Cruz EM, et al., eds. *Critical Care of Children with Heart Disease.* 2nd ed. Springer Nature Switzerland AG; 2020:600.

Fraser CD. Chapter 30: Anomalous origin of the coronary arteries. In: Nichols DG, Ungerleider RM, Spevak PJ, et al., eds. *Critical Heart Disease in Infants and Children.* 2nd ed. Mosby Elsevier; 2006:679.

Hastings LA, Heitmiller ES, Nyhan D. Chapter 14: Perioperative monitoring. In: Nichols DG, Ungerleider RM, Spevak PJ, et al., eds. *Critical Heart Disease in Infants and Children.* 2nd ed. Mosby Elsevier; 2006:496.

Jaggers J, Cole CR. Chapter 55: Truncus arteriosus. In: Ungerleider RM, Meliones JN, McMillan KN, et al., eds. *Critical Heart Disease in Infants and Children.* 3rd ed. Mosby Elsevier; 2019:668.

Kanter RJ, Caroboni MP, Silka MJ. Chapter 8: Pediatric arrhythmias. In: Nichols DG, Ungerleider RM, Spevak PJ, et al., eds. *Critical Heart Disease in Infants and Children.* 2nd ed. Mosby Elsevier; 2006:222–223.

Karl TR, Kirshbom PM. Chapter 33: Transposition of the great arteries and the arterial switch operation. In: Nichols DG, Ungerleider RM, Spevak PJ, et al., eds. *Critical Heart Disease in Infants and Children.* 2nd ed. Mosby Elsevier; 2006:726.

Kaufman J, Goldberg SP, Ibrahim J, et al. Chapter 16: Complete atrioventricular septal defects. In: Munoz RA, Morell VO, da Cruz EM, et al., eds. *Critical Care of Children with Heart Disease.* 2nd ed. Springer Nature Switzerland AG; 2020:181–182.

Marino BS, Spray RL, Greeley WJ. Chapter 41: Separating the circulations: cavopulmonary connections (Bidirectional Glenn, Hemi-Fontan) and the modified Fontan operation. In: Nichols DG, Ungerleider RM, Spevak PJ, et al., eds. *Critical Heart Disease in Infants and Children.* 2nd ed. Mosby Elsevier; 2006:860.

Martin LD, Nyhan D, Wetzel RC. Chapter 3: Regulation of pulmonary vascular resistance and blood flow. In: Nichols DG, Ungerleider RM, Spevak PJ, et al., eds. *Critical Heart Disease in Infants and Children.* 2nd ed. Mosby Elsevier; 2006:79–83.

Nelson JS, Stone ML, Gangemi JJ. Chapter 45: Coarctation of the aorta. In: Ungerleider RM, Meliones JN, McMillan KN, et al., eds. *Critical Heart Disease in Infants and Children.* 3rd ed. Mosby Elsevier; 2019:556.

O'Laughlin MP, Ringel RE. Chapter 18: Diagnostic and therapeutic cardiac catheterization. In: Nichols DG, Ungerleider RM, Spevak PJ, et al., eds. *Critical Heart Disease in Infants and Children.* 2nd ed. Mosby Elsevier; 2006:472.

Quintessenza J, Desena HC, Justice L, et al. Chapter 66: Hypoplastic left heart syndrome. In: Ungerleider RM, Meliones JN, McMillan KN, et al., eds. *Critical Heart Disease in Infants and Children.* 3rd ed. Mosby Elsevier; 2019:780–794.

Short JA, Paris ST, Booker PD, et al. Arterial to end-tidal carbon dioxide tension difference in children with congenital heart disease. *Br J Anaesth.* 2001;86(3):349–353.

Spector ZZ, Meliones C, Idriss SF. Chapter 27: Arrhythmias and pacing. In: Ungerleider RM, Meliones JN, McMillan KN, et al., eds. *Critical Heart Disease in Infants and Children.* 3rd ed. Mosby Elsevier; 2019:348.

St. Louis J, Molitor-Kirsch E, Shah H, et al. Chapter 48: Total anomalous pulmonary venous return. In: Ungerleider RM, Meliones JN, McMillan KN, et al., eds. *Critical Heart Disease in Infants and Children.* 3rd ed. Mosby Elsevier; 2019:587–595.

Susheel Kumar TK, Knott-Craig CJ. Chapter 64: Ebstein anomaly. In: Ungerleider RM, Meliones JN, McMillan KN, et al., eds. *Critical Heart Disease in Infants and Children.* 3rd ed. Mosby Elsevier; 2019:759.

Ungerleider RM, Meliones JN, McMillan KN, et al. *Critical Heart Disease in Infants and Children.* 3rd ed. Mosby Elsevier; 2019.

Wearden PD, Manrique AM, Kelly K. Chapter 49: Mechanical circulatory support in pediatric cardiac surgery. In: Munoz RA, Morell VO, da Cruz EM, et al., eds. *Critical Care of Children with Heart Disease.* 2nd ed. Springer Nature Switzerland AG; 2020:566–567.

Heart Failure, Pulmonary Hypertension, and Cardiac Transplantation

Ezequiel Sagray, Charlotte Van Dorn, Jonathan N. Johnson, and Robert E. Shaddy

Questions

1. A 13-year-old male sees you in clinic for routine follow-up. He is 2 years post orthotopic heart transplantation for dilated cardiomyopathy. He reports that he has felt "jittery" lately. When he lifts his hand, he is unable to keep it still. Which of the following medications most likely is causing this degree of tremulousness in this patient?

   A. Prednisone
   B. Mycophenolate mofetil
   C. Azathioprine
   D. Tacrolimus
   E. Sirolimus

2. A 3-year-old male with normal intracardiac anatomy is undergoing a cardiac catheterization procedure with the following measurements:

Rest	Oxygen 100%	Nitric oxide 80 ppm
LVSP 68 mm Hg	LVSP 72 mm Hg	LVSP 74 mm Hg
LVEDP = 6 mm Hg	LVEDP = 5 mm Hg	LVEDP = 4 mm Hg
CI = 3.0 L/min/m^2	CI = 3.1 L/min/m^2	CI = 2.9 L/min/m^2
RPA = 41/17 mean 30 mm Hg	RPA = 32/13 mean 22 mm Hg	RPA = 29/12 mean 20 mm Hg
RPCW = mean 10 mm Hg	RPCW = mean 7 mm Hg	RPCW = mean 9 mm Hg

- LVSP: Left ventricular systolic pressure
- LVEDP: Left ventricular end-diastolic pressure
- RPA: Right pulmonary artery
- RPCW: Right pulmonary capillary wedge
- CI: Cardiac index

   Which of the following is the best treatment for this patient?
   A. Home oxygen therapy
   B. Amlodipine
   C. Treprostinil IV
   D. Enalapril
   E. Bosentan

3. A 15-month-old male infant is 4 weeks post orthotopic heart transplantation. His parents bring him in with new-onset fussiness over the past day. He has been refusing to eat or drink for the last 4 hours. Of the following new physical examination findings, which one is most concerning for allograft rejection?

   A. Petechiae on his right foot
   B. Splitting of the first heart sound
   C. Dry mucous membranes
   D. Gallop rhythm
   E. Soft 1/6 systolic murmur at the left upper sternal border

4. A 14-year-old patient, 2 years post orthotopic heart transplantation for dilated cardiomyopathy, presents with new-onset shortness of breath. An echocardiogram is performed as part of the workup. Which of the following echo findings is most concerning for rejection?

   A. Increase in the descending aorta flow velocity from 1.2 to 1.4 m/s
   B. Decrease in the left ventricular ejection fraction from 68% to 62%
   C. Increase in the lateral mitral valve e′ velocity from 0.08 to 0.12 m/s
   D. Decrease in the IVC diameter from 2.3 to 1.8 cm.
   E. Increase in the degree of mitral regurgitation from trivial to moderate

5. A 14-year-old female presents for routine follow-up. She had an orthotopic heart transplantation at age 7 months for hypoplastic left heart syndrome and ventricular dysfunction. On examination, she has a blood pressure in her right arm of 150/85 mm Hg. Echocardiography reveals the following abdominal aortic Doppler signal (see **Figure 11.1**). Which of the following is the next best step?

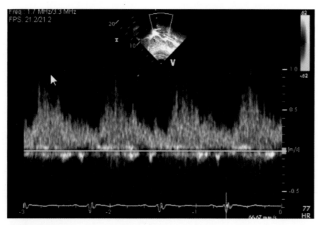

FIGURE 11.1

   A. ICU for administration of a steroid bolus (10 mg/kg/dose q24 hours × 3)
   B. Operating room for tricuspid valve repair
   C. Cardiac cath lab for balloon angioplasty or stenting
   D. Operating room for revision of IVC anastomosis
   E. Cardiac cath lab for coronary angiography with intravascular ultrasound (IVUS)

6. You are evaluating a 16-year-old male for a second opinion. He has a history of d-transposition of the great arteries and uneventful arterial switch operation at 3 days of life. He now complains of severe pulmonary hypertension, complicated by syncope and ascites. He underwent a cardiac catheterization procedure elsewhere. Which of the following is a theoretical advantage of the procedure pointed to by the arrow in **Figure 11.2** over atrial septostomy?

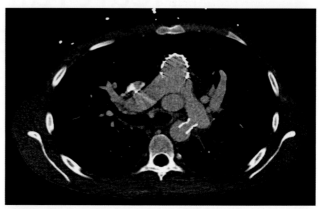

FIGURE 11.2

   A. Decreases central venous pressure
   B. Increases left ventricular preload
   C. Decreases left ventricular afterload
   D. Lower risk of stroke
   E. Higher peripheral arterial saturations

7. A 7-year-old female with a history of orthotopic heart transplantation 2 years ago presents with new-onset seizures. The seizures are controlled successfully with benzodiazepine administration. Laboratory evaluation reveals that the patient's tacrolimus level is 31.2 (goal range 6 to 8). Two weeks ago, the child's tacrolimus level was 7.9. The family reports that the child was started on a new medication 1 week ago by their primary care pediatrician. Which of the following is the most likely medication that was started?

   A. Trimethoprim/Sulfamethoxazole
   B. Phenytoin
   C. Loratadine
   D. Fluconazole
   E. Metoprolol

8. A 14-year-old female is referred for evaluation for orthotopic cardiac transplantation. In the teenage years, which of the following is the most common indication for orthotopic heart transplantation?

   A. Cardiomyopathy
   B. Congenital heart disease
   C. Retransplantation
   D. Malignancy
   E. Intractable arrhythmias

9. An 8-year-old male with restrictive cardiomyopathy is admitted to the hospital with shortness of breath. Which of the following examination or test findings portends a poor prognosis for this child?

   A. Pulmonary venous congestion on chest radiography
   B. Increased medial mitral valve annular E′ velocity on echo
   C. 2/6 low-pitched systolic murmur heard at the left lower sternal border
   D. Right atrial enlargement on echo
   E. Isolated PACs on 24-hour Holter monitoring

10. You are seeing a 2-year-old patient in clinic who is now 4 months post orthotopic heart transplantation. His mother recently has gone back to work, and the patient is cared for by maternal grandmother. For the past 2 weeks, the child's mother reports that he has been more irritable and has a poor appetite. The child's pediatrician saw him the day prior and noted no significant examination findings other than a potential gallop rhythm. There have been several recent ill contacts for the patient, all of whom have been diagnosed with upper respiratory viral illnesses.

    In this patient, which of the following tests is the best to rule out rejection?

    A. Chest radiography
    B. Plasma BNP
    C. Cardiac MRI
    D. Electrocardiogram
    E. Myocardial biopsy

11. A 14-year-old female is admitted to the intensive care unit for monitoring after elective surgery. She has a history of hypoplastic left heart syndrome and underwent orthotopic heart transplantation as a neonate. She has had a relatively uncomplicated course, with no arrhythmias or other complications. During monitoring overnight, her nurse noted intermittent premature ventricular contractions, with brief runs of ventricular tachycardia. Which of the following is the most likely cause of her new-onset arrhythmia?

    A. Myocarditis
    B. Coronary artery vasculopathy
    C. Posttransplant lymphoproliferative disorder (PTLD)
    D. EBV viremia
    E. Posterior reversible encephalopathy syndrome (PRES)

12. Which of the following is a contraindication to orthotopic heart transplantation to a pediatric patient?

    A. History of Fontan operation
    B. Pulmonary vascular resistance ≥ 12 Woods units after nitric oxide administration
    C. History of protein-losing enteropathy
    D. Prior alcohol addiction, has been sober for 1 year
    E. History of pulmonary embolism, resolved

13. A 5-year-old female comes to the emergency department after one episode of loss of consciousness and "heart fluttering" for the last 12 hours. She has a history of dilated cardiomyopathy (DCM) secondary to an episode of myocarditis 6 months ago; she is currently on enalapril and propranolol, and echocardiogram shows LV end-diastolic dimension Z score of 1.6 with LV ejection fraction of 15%. Which of the following is her strongest predictor of sudden cardiac death (SCD)?

    A. History of myocarditis
    B. Age
    C. LV end-diastolic diameter
    D. Use of propranolol
    E. Sex

14. A previously healthy 4-year-old female is referred due to fatigue. Echocardiogram shows normal LV systolic function (LV ejection fraction 60%). Physical examination is unremarkable, and cardiac catheterization reveals the following:

Cardiac index	4 L/min/m^2
Left ventricle	75/6 mm Hg
Left ventricular end-diastolic pressure	15 mm Hg
Ascending aorta	72/46 mm Hg
Right ventricle	28/2 mm Hg
Right ventricular end-diastolic pressure	9 mm Hg
Main pulmonary artery	25/10 mm Hg

    Which of the following is most likely to be present on echocardiography?

    A. Mitral inflow E:A ratio = 0.6
    B. LV end-diastolic diameter Z score = 2.5
    C. Septal bowing to the left with inspiration
    D. TAPSE = 11 mm
    E. Normal indexed left atrial size

15. An 8-year-old male with restrictive cardiomyopathy is admitted to the hospital with shortness of breath. He has pulmonary venous congestion on his chest radiogram. His echocardiogram shows normal ventricular systolic function, massively dilated atria, and an estimated right ventricular systolic pressure of 65 mm Hg (systemic systolic blood pressure 120 mm Hg). Which of the following is the next best step in management of this patient?

    A. Liver ultrasound
    B. Cardiac CT to rule out pulmonary vein stenosis
    C. Reassurance
    D. Begin ACE-inhibitor medication
    E. Begin evaluation for orthotopic heart transplantation

16. A 13-year-old male is admitted for initiation of tre-prostinil. Which of the following is true regarding this medication?

    A. Liver function should be monitored before and during treatment
    B. Discontinuation of IV infusion can lead to pulmonary hypertension crisis in minutes
    C. It exerts its effect through potentiation of nitric oxide
    D. It causes vasodilation through increased cyclic AMP signaling
    E. Head imaging is recommended within 24 hours of initiation of the medication

17. A 7-year-old patient is diagnosed with dilated cardiomyopathy. Two months later, he is seen in heart failure clinic. At the time of his evaluation, the patient is on appropriate doses of enalapril, carvedilol, spironolactone, and furosemide. The patient's symptoms have improved since the initiation of the medications, though he does continue to have some dyspnea with exertion. He has been able to attend school full time. His echo reveals a left ventricular ejection fraction of 15% to 20%, unchanged compared to his echo at the time of diagnosis. Which of the following is the next best step in management?

    A. Wean enalapril
    B. Start digoxin
    C. Start verapamil
    D. Start amlodipine
    E. Wean carvedilol

18. A 14-year-old female is evaluation due to a syncopal event. She participates in competitive track running. She lost consciousness for 2 minutes after standing for over an hour during a hot morning in church. Physical examination was normal and resting ECG shows an rsR' pattern in lead V1. Family history is significant for heart disease secondary to Plakophilin 2 (PKP2) mutation in her older brother. What is the best next step?

    A. Increase hydration and no further testing
    B. Discontinue all competitive sports participation
    C. Refer for EP study
    D. Obtain 24-hour Holter
    E. Proceed with tilt table

19. You are taking care of a 3-month-old, 3.2-kg female infant with trisomy 21 and a complete AV canal defect, who is now status post complete repair and PFO closure. Intraoperatively, she is noted to have ¾ systemic right ventricular pressures with excellent biventricular function and no significant AV valve regurgitation or residual lesions. She was started on inhaled nitric oxide at 20 parts per million (ppm) in addition to Milrinone at 0.5 mcg/kg/min and returned to the CVICU on the following ventilator settings: SIMV respiratory rate 24 bpm, TV 20 cc, PEEP 5, PS 8, FiO$_2$ 60%. On postoperative day two, she is noted to have an acute decrease in her systolic pressure from 78 to 55 mm Hg with awakening, but without evidence of desaturation while on inhaled nitric oxide. Her hypotensive event lasted for 1 to 2 minutes and resolved with a dose of IV fentanyl. You are planning to extubate in the next 24 hours. Given this, what would be the next best step in management?

    A. Increase the inhaled nitric oxide to 40 ppm
    B. Start epinephrine at 0.05 mcg/kg/min
    C. Start sildenafil at 0.5 mg/kg and increase to 1 mg/kg PO every 6 hours
    D. Increase the fentanyl infusion from 1 to 2 mcg/kg/hr
    E. Start dexmedetomidine 0.2 mcg/kg/hr

20. A previously healthy 12-year-old male is admitted from the ED to the cardiac ICU because of a 3-day history of worsening fatigue, GI distress, and increased respiratory effort. An echocardiogram in the ED showed an estimated LVEF of 15% with moderate mitral regurgitation. The patient was started on milrinone in the ED and required intubation upon arrival to the ICU. Inotropic medications were escalated to dopamine and eventually epinephrine, with the patient ultimately requiring ECMO. Which of the following is the most appropriate next step for this patient?

    A. List immediately for orthotopic heart transplantation
    B. Atrial septostomy in the catheterization laboratory
    C. Extubation
    D. Left ventricular assist device
    E. Deep hypothermia

21. A 16-year-old male undergoes myocardial biopsy as part of a routine post–heart transplant protocol. The pathologist reports that the biopsy samples have several areas of lymphocytic infiltration with associated myocyte damage. The next best step in management for this patient is:

    A. Administration of IVIG
    B. Administration of antibiotics
    C. List for retransplantation
    D. Renal dialysis
    E. Administration of steroids

22. A 15-year-old otherwise normal female is diagnosed with dilated cardiomyopathy. The family asks whether other members of the family may develop dilated cardiomyopathy. You inform them that many cases are sporadic; however, in familial/inherited cases, the most common pattern of inheritance is:

    A. X-linked recessive
    B. X-linked dominant
    C. Autosomal recessive
    D. Autosomal dominant
    E. Mitochondrial

23. A 3-year-old male sees you in clinic for routine follow-up. He is 1 year post orthotopic heart transplantation for congenital heart disease. On laboratory evaluation, he is found to have a white blood cell count of 1.2, with an absolute neutrophil count of 0.4. Which of the following medications is likely causing his leukopenia?

    A. Prednisone
    B. Mycophenolate mofetil
    C. Amlodipine
    D. Tacrolimus
    E. Aspirin

24. A 7-year-old female undergoes orthotopic heart transplantation for restrictive cardiomyopathy. Her serologic testing shows:
    Donor: CMV positive, EBV positive, toxoplasma positive
    Recipient: CMV negative, EBV negative, toxoplasma negative

    The patient received induction therapy with antithymocyte globulin in the operating room. Considering the results of the serologic testing, which of the following would be recommended to reduce the likelihood of the patient developing posttransplant lymphoproliferative disorder (PTLD)?

    A. Safely minimize immunosuppression therapy due to EBV mismatch
    B. Start antiviral therapy directed at CMV immediately post transplant
    C. Identify and treat early rejection
    D. Close monitoring of CMV titers in the first year following transplant
    E. Early transition of the primary immunosuppressant medication from a calcineurin inhibitor to mTOR inhibitor

25. A newborn male infant is diagnosed with dilated cardiomyopathy via echocardiography. The neonatologist notes a mild degree of hypotonia as well as proximal muscle weakness. Genetic evaluation reveals increased levels of 3-methylglutaconic acid in the blood and urine. Laboratory evaluation reveals normal hemoglobin but low neutrophil count. Further genetic testing reveals a mutation in the *TAZ* gene. You counsel the family that the patient has a genetic syndrome with which of the following modes of inheritance?

    A. Autosomal recessive
    B. Autosomal dominant
    C. X-linked recessive
    D. Mitochondrial
    E. None of the above

26. A 16-year-old male with dilated cardiomyopathy (DCM) presents for evaluation of new-onset cough. The patient had been diagnosed with DCM 2 months prior, and treatment was begun with enalapril, spironolactone, furosemide, and digoxin. He describes the cough as dry, hacking, and persistent. Which of the following is the most appropriate next step in management?

    A. Discontinue furosemide and initiate bumetanide
    B. Discontinue enalapril and initiate losartan
    C. Discontinue digoxin
    D. Evaluate for heart transplantation
    E. Make no changes to the medical regimen

27. An 11-year-old female undergoes myocardial biopsy and coronary angiography as part of a routine post–heart transplant protocol. She is 10 years post orthotopic heart transplantation for congenital heart disease. The pathologist reports that the biopsy samples showed no evidence of rejection. On coronary angiography, areas of diffuse coronary luminal narrowing are noted in multiple branches. The left ventricular end-diastolic pressure is measured at 25 mm Hg. The patient's current medications include tacrolimus and mycophenolate mofetil. The most appropriate next step in management for this patient is:

    A. Administration of antibiotics
    B. Administration of pulsed steroids
    C. Conversion of tacrolimus to cyclosporine
    D. Plasmapheresis
    E. Evaluate the patient for cardiac retransplantation

28. An 18-month-old male infant with hypoplastic left heart syndrome (post Norwood and Glenn operations) undergoes orthotopic heart transplantation. Six months posttransplant, his family notes increased irritability. On examination, you note prominent veins in his neck and forehead. An echocardiogram is obtained (**Figure 11.3**). Which of the following is the most appropriate next step in management?

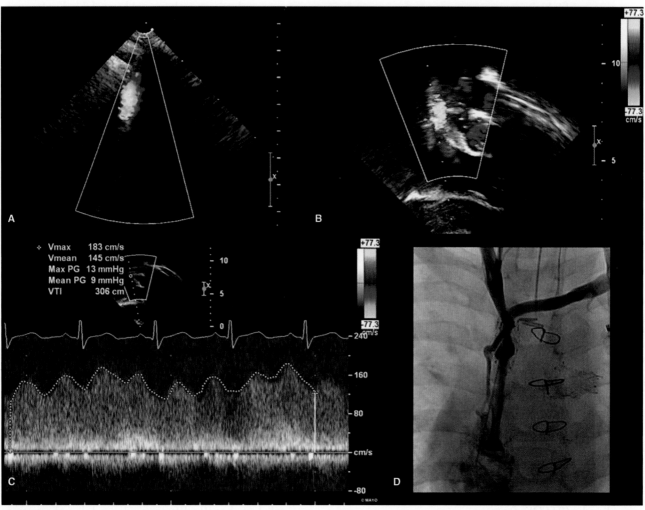

FIGURE 11.3

A. Admission to the intensive care unit for pulsed steroids

B. Cardiac catheterization with stenting of the aorta

C. Operating room for revision of the biatrial anastomosis

D. Cardiac catheterization with stenting of his superior vena cava (SVC)

E. Cardiac catheterization for myocardial biopsy to rule out rejection

29. A 2-week-old male is admitted with cardiogenic shock in the context of sepsis, with PCR+ for influenza virus. Echocardiogram shows severely reduced global LV function, and MRI confirms extensive subendocardial late gadolinium enhancement, consistent with ischemia. Viremia resolves but LV function remains globally reduced, so the patient undergoes cardiac transplantation at 3 weeks of life. Which of the following is true regarding his posttransplant management and outcome?

A. Graft ischemia time must be less than 4 hours

B. Donor must be ABO compatible

C. Long-term survival is better now than if transplant was performed as a teenager

D. Induction with thymoglobulin is highly recommended

E. Transplant cannot be performed before 2 months of age

30. A 4-year-old female presents with poor left ventricular function, estimated ejection fraction of 20%. There is a positive family history of cardiomyopathy, including her father who required cardiac transplantation at the age of 27. You decide to begin a heart failure regimen including carvedilol, enalapril, spironolactone, and furosemide. Which of the following best describes the mechanism of action of carvedilol in this patient?

   A. Selective blockade of β-1 adrenergic receptors, little or no effect on β-2 receptors
   B. Inhibition of angiotensin-converting enzyme, preventing conversion of angiotensin I to angiotensin II
   C. Direct vasodilation of arterioles with subsequent decrease in systemic resistance
   D. Nonselective β-adrenergic receptor blockade (β-1 and β-2) and α-adrenergic receptor blockade
   E. Blocks epithelial sodium channels in the late distal convoluted tubule and collecting duct, inhibiting sodium reabsorption from the lumen

31. An asymptomatic 2 year old is referred for cardiac evaluation because of a family history of dilated cardiomyopathy. Her physical examination is entirely normal. Her echocardiogram shows a dilated left ventricle with mild mitral regurgitation and an LV SF of 18% with an LVEF of 35%. You admit the patient to start therapy. Based on current recommended guidelines, which of the following therapies would be the most appropriate to initiate **first**?

   A. Milrinone
   B. Diuretic
   C. ACE inhibitor
   D. Digoxin
   E. Oxygen

32. A 16-year-old female is admitted to the ICU with acute decompensated heart failure. After stabilization, she underwent endomyocardial biopsy that showed acute lymphocytic myocarditis. Which of the following has been proven to be effective in the treatment of acute lymphocytic myocarditis?

   A. Intravenous immune globulin
   B. Corticosteroids
   C. Immunosuppression
   D. Antiviral drugs
   E. Supportive care

33. Endothelin receptor antagonists (ERAs) have been known to cause adverse drug reactions. Which of the following is a drug reaction that can be seen when using high-dose ERAs?

   A. Vision changes including the inability to distinguish blue from green
   B. Urinary retention
   C. Thrombocytopenia
   D. Hepatic dysfunction
   E. Leukopenia

Answers

1. (D) Irritability and tremulousness are common side effects of tacrolimus which tend to happen when serum levels are high. At high enough levels, tacrolimus toxicity can cause seizures to occur. The most common complication of azathioprine and mycophenolate is leukopenia, though many patients may have gastrointestinal side effects as well (constipation, diarrhea, nausea). The most common side effects of sirolimus are diarrhea and the development of mouth sores. The side effects of prednisone are well documented, including mood changes, increased appetite, increased blood glucose, weight gain, and a Cushingoid appearance. Long-term use is associated with the development of osteoporosis.

2. (B) Patient presents mild pulmonary hypertension (mean PAP = 30 mm Hg) with moderately elevated pulmonary resistance (PVR = 6.7 WU) at baseline, with decreased PVR to 4.8 and 3.8 with 100% oxygen and NO, respectively. According to the latest Pediatric Pulmonary Hypertension guidelines (Abman et al., 2015), for patients with idiopathic pulmonary arterial hypertension (IPAH) (and no CHD), a positive response to acute vasoreactivity testing (AVT) (to either oxygen and/or nitric oxide) is defined as (1) a decrease in mPAP of at least 10 mm Hg to <40 mm Hg with a normal or increased cardiac output; and/or (2) a decrease in mPAP of ≥20%, an increase or no change in CI, and a decrease or no change in PVR/SVR ratio. For IPAH patients, responsive PVR carries increased likelihood to long-term response to calcium channel blockers and better prognosis.

3. (D) Of all examination findings listed above, the presence of a new gallop rhythm is the most sensitive for rejection, though there typically are a constellation of findings. There may also be tachycardia, new murmurs of mitral regurgitation or tricuspid regurgitation, or evidence of congestion (hepatomegaly, jugular venous distension, abnormal chest x-ray, etc.). Early after transplant, the patient may be anemic resulting in the soft flow murmur as in answer (**E**).

4. (E) There is no single echocardiographic finding that, by itself, has been shown to have perfect sensitivity or specificity for rejection in transplant patients. This being said, the most common findings seen in patients with active rejection include new effusions, increased wall thickness and ventricular mass, and increased mitral or tricuspid valve regurgitation. Recent studies have shown that *decreases* in mitral valve tissue Doppler velocities may be very sensitive at detecting potential rejection episodes. The remainder of the findings listed are unlikely to be associated with rejection.

5. (C) The patient has evidence of diastolic continuation of forward flow in the abdominal aorta, consistent with upstream obstruction, most likely recoarctation. Patients with a history of hypoplastic left heart syndrome are at a particular risk for this complication after heart transplant.

6. (D) Reversed Potts shunt is a surgical or interventional alternative in the management of severe PH with intractable right heart failure. It involves the anastomosis of the left pulmonary artery and the descending aorta, with systolic right-to-left shunt, leading to decreased right afterload and improved function. As opposed to atrial septostomy, it does not decrease central venous pressure or increase left ventricular preload, although it does increase left ventricular afterload. As right-to-left shunt occurs at the descending aorta, there is lower risk of stroke, and central saturation is maintained (at the expense of peripheral cyanosis).

7. (D) Antifungal medications are a consistent cause of increased calcineurin inhibitor levels in transplant patients. As such, any time any of these medications are considered being started, close monitoring of tacrolimus or cyclosporine is required. Other medications that may increase their levels include amiodarone, macrolide antibiotics, calcium channel blockers, and metoclopramide. Medications that may decrease calcineurin inhibitor levels include: octreotide, some anticonvulsants (phenytoin, phenobarbital, carbamazepine), and some antibiotics (nafcillin, IV Bactrim). Beta blockers have little effect on tacrolimus or cyclosporine levels. Patients who have tacrolimus toxicity have irritability and tremulousness and may have seizures if levels are high enough.

8. (A) For patients over the age of 1 year, especially in teenagers, the most common underlying diagnosis in patients undergoing orthotopic heart transplantation is cardiomyopathy (including dilated, restrictive, hypertrophic, and noncompaction cardiomyopathies). For infants, congenital heart disease is the most common indication, though this has been decreasing in the last several years. In the 1990s, almost 75% of infants having transplants had congenital heart disease; this has decreased to 53% in the most recent 5 years. The reasons behind this are multifactorial but are at least in part indicative of improved Norwood outcomes for patients with hypoplastic left heart syndrome.

9. (A) In patients with restrictive cardiomyopathy, the presence of significant cardiomegaly and pulmonary venous congestion on chest x-ray are poor prognostic indicators. Cath-measured left ventricular end-diastolic pressure and the degree of left atrial dilatation are also predictive of poor survival. Patients with restrictive cardiomyopathy have low tissue Doppler parameters, including the medial mitral valve annular E' velocity. Right atrial enlargement on echo and a murmur consistent with tricuspid regurgitation have not been shown to predict poor outcomes, though they may be indicative of the degree of right ventricular dysfunction.

10. (E) Despite advances in other imaging technologies in recent years, the gold standard test to "rule out" rejection in a patient remains a myocardial biopsy obtained in the cardiac catheterization laboratory. Cardiac MRI may be useful in certain situations; however, the lack of tissue diagnosis, the relative lack of availability in the acute setting, and lack of data in pediatric patients do not yet support its use. Electrocardiographic changes may be seen in patients with rejection, including low-voltage QRS signals, though this is rarely diagnostic in isolation. Plasma BNP has been shown in several studies to be indicative of potential rejection when compared to baseline, though this is more an adjunctive test than a diagnostic one. Echocardiography is used at many centers on an intermittent basis to rule out rejection and can be very useful at limiting the number of biopsies performed. However, biopsy remains the gold standard.

11. (B) New-onset arrhythmia in a cardiac transplant recipient should raise concern for either rejection or coronary artery vasculopathy. In this patient 14 years out from transplant, the most likely diagnosis is coronary artery vasculopathy. Early after transplant, arrhythmias or ectopy may be a sign of rejection, though this is relatively nonspecific.

12. (B) An elevated pulmonary vascular resistance is a contraindication for heart transplantation, primarily due to the inability of the donor right ventricle to tolerate pumping against the elevated pressure and resistance. If the pulmonary hypertension is somewhat reversible with pulmonary vasodilators, transplantation might be considered, recognizing that significant right ventricular support may be needed postoperatively. A history of Fontan operation, protein-losing enteropathy, or plastic bronchitis are not contraindications to transplant; however, they do increase the risk of transplant due to multiple factors (extracardiac organ dysfunction, poor nutrition and wound healing, increased infection risk, increased risk of antibody-mediated rejection, and difficulty assessing prior sensitization). Drug or alcohol addiction is a contraindication, unless the patient is able to fulfill a predetermined period of time of sobriety—the exact length of time is institution dependent. A history of resolved pulmonary embolism is not a contraindication, though an active pulmonary embolism is.

13. (B) Risk factors for SCD in pediatric DCM patients have been reported to include LV end-diastolic dimension Z score ≥2.6, age at diagnosis of cardiomyopathy <14 years, ratio of LV posterior wall thickness to LV end-diastolic dimension ratio <0.14, and presence of congestive heart failure at presentation of DCM. Sex, ethnicity, cause of DCM, and family history were not associated with SCD (impact of LVEF was not evaluated).

14. (A) Hemodynamic data are consistent with ventricular diastolic dysfunction. In the context of a previously healthy child, the likelihood of constrictive pericarditis is extremely low, so the most likely diagnosis is restrictive cardiomyopathy (RCM). The most sensitive finding in the pediatric population is a dilated left atrium. Other findings include clinical or subclinical (abnormal S' wave on tissue Doppler) left ventricular systolic dysfunction (LVEF <55%), left ventricular hypertrophy, abnormal mitral inflow Doppler with inversed E:A ratio, and increased pulmonary vein atrial reversal on pulsed-wave Doppler (remember that with mitral inflow Doppler, normal E:A ratio is between 1.0 and 3.0). Left ventricular dilation is not a feature of RCM. Septal bowing with inspiration is suggestive of constrictive pericarditis.

15. (E) In patients with restrictive cardiomyopathy, the presence of significant cardiomegaly and pulmonary venous congestion on chest x-ray are poor prognostic indicators. Current medical therapy options are ineffective, and thus cardiac transplantation is considered the definitive therapy. Without transplantation, some authors have reported up to 50% mortality within 2 to 3 years of diagnosis of restrictive cardiomyopathy. Outside of transplant, the only medical therapy that has been reported to be useful is limited diuresis to help improve symptoms. However, caution must be used in this situation, as these patients are very sensitive to preload, and over-diuresis can be problematic. ACE-inhibition has not been shown to be of benefit in pediatric patients with restrictive cardiomyopathy. Ultrasound of the liver will likely be performed as part of a transplant evaluation, as there is a risk of long-term hepatic congestion; however, this is very unlikely to change the ultimate course in a pediatric patient. Pulmonary vein stenosis should be ruled out in a patient with elevated right ventricular systolic pressure; however, the massive left atrial enlargement points to the ventricles being the problem rather than the pulmonary veins.

16. (D) Treprostinil is a prostacyclin analog, which causes pulmonary vasodilation through increased cyclic adenylate monophosphate and enhanced adenylate cyclase action in vascular smooth muscle cells. If administered intravenously, it is not associated with acute PH crisis given its half-life of 4 hours, unlike Epoprostenol which will cause an acute PH crisis if infusion is stopped. Treprostinil can also be administered via subcutaneous infusion, avoiding the need of a central catheter, and it is currently in trial phases for oral administration. Treprostinil is not associated with hepatotoxicity (endothelin receptor antagonists are).

17. (B) In the most recent guideline statements for pediatric heart failure (International Society of Heart and Lung Transplantation 2004 and 2014), digoxin is considered reasonable to add to a heart failure regimen in the presence of heart failure symptoms. Digoxin has not been advocated for patients who are otherwise asymptomatic. The guidelines do note that special attention may be needed for patients who are at risk of renal dysfunction and that lower doses may be needed in those patients concurrently on carvedilol or amiodarone. In the absence of improvement in ventricular function, none of the medications should be weaned at this point—if anything, care should be made to ensure doses are appropriately weight based, as the patients grow older and increase in size. Milrinone may be considered in the presence of ongoing symptoms, though the guidelines are careful to point out that use in the outpatient setting should be limited to bridging to transplant.

18. (D) Although the features of the episode would point toward a neurocardiogenic event, the clinical scenario of syncope with underlying RBBB and family history with PKP2 mutation should raise concern for possible arrhythmogenic cardiomyopathy (ACM) and eventual ventricular arrhythmia causing the fainting. According to the 2019 ACM expert consensus, all first-degree relatives of affected patients should undergo comprehensive cardiovascular evaluation, including 12-lead ECG, 24-hour Holter monitoring, cardiac imaging (Class I), and eventual exercise stress test (Class IIb). In the case of a confirmed ACM, discontinuation of competitive sports is indicated (Class III), and ICD should be implemented for secondary prevention of VT/VF arrest, sustained VT which is not hemodynamically tolerated (Class I), or syncope suspected to be related to ventricular arrhythmia (Class IIa).

19. (C) Pulmonary hypertension is common in infants with trisomy 21 and can be seen in the early postoperative period. This infant's decrease in SBP is a sign of low cardiac output due to an acute rise in pulmonary pressures resulting in less right ventricular output and thus less left ventricular preload. There is no evidence that 40 ppm of inhaled nitric oxide offers any benefit over 20 ppm. One could consider starting epinephrine if there is a concern for ventricular dysfunction; however, that will not help with weaning of nitric oxide prior to extubation. Increasing the fentanyl infusion may limit additional pulmonary hypertensive events, but it would hinder extubation in this infant. Starting sildenafil and increasing to full dose should allow for weaning of the inhaled nitric oxide prior to extubation. Dexmedetomidine can be used in anesthesia management in these patients, although it does not significantly alter the pulmonary vascular resistance.

20. (B). This patient who has acute onset and rapidly progressive heart failure due to left ventricular systolic dysfunction has ultimately required placement on ECMO. Since ECMO does not relieve left atrial hypertension, this patient is at risk for worsening pulmonary edema and even pulmonary hemorrhage. Thus, the most immediate next step for this patient is to open the atrial septum in the catheterization laboratory using a transcatheter approach. It would be reasonable to start evaluating this patient for possible orthotopic heart transplantation, but it would be inappropriate to immediately list for transplant until one sees whether there is evidence of stabilization and recovery. There is no indication for extubation, particularly since this patient has elevated left atrial and therefore pulmonary venous pressures. Although a left ventricular assist device may be necessary at some point, it is not indicated immediately. Finally, since this patient has not suffered a cardiac arrest, there is no indication for considering deep hypothermia.

21. (E) The biopsy findings are consistent with an International Society for Heart and Lung Transplantation (ISHLT) grade 2R rejection (cellular mediated). A finding of 2R rejection and greater should be treated, initially with pulsed steroids and further therapies as indicated. Treatment of grade 1R rejection is controversial; decisions on whether to treat a patient with 1R rejection include many factors including prior biopsy results, institutional protocols, and other comorbidities.

The American Board of Pediatrics (ABP) content specifications for the pediatric cardiology board examination include a section on knowledge of histologic findings of rejection. While it is unlikely that specific pathologic specimens will be presented on an examination, it may be worthwhile to understand the grading system used for cellular-mediated rejection.

Grade 1R (mild) = interstitial and/or perivascular infiltrates with up to one focus of myocyte damage.

Grade 2R (moderate) = two or more foci of infiltrate with associated myocyte damage.

Grade 3R (severe) = diffuse infiltrate with multifocal myocyte damage, with or without edema, hemorrhage, or vasculitis.

22. (D) In cases with identifiable familial origin, the pattern of inheritance in dilated cardiomyopathy is most commonly autosomal dominant. This confers a 50% risk of developing dilated cardiomyopathy for children of an individual who has dilated cardiomyopathy. There are rare forms of inherited cardiomyopathies inherited in an X-linked or autosomal recessive pattern, though these are often associated with neuromuscular disease or metabolic derangements.

23. (B) The most common complication of azathioprine and mycophenolate is leukopenia, though many patients may have gastrointestinal side effects as well (constipation, diarrhea, nausea). Irritability and tremulousness are common side effects of tacrolimus that tend to happen when serum levels are high. The side effects of prednisone are well documented, including mood changes, increased appetite, increased blood glucose, weight gain, and a Cushingoid appearance. Long-term use is associated with the development of osteoporosis.

24. (A) PTLD is a significant cause of graft loss and death after transplant. Safe reduction in immunosuppression early after transplant has been recommended and led to improved survival. The majority of lymphomas after heart transplant have been found to be related to EBV. Retransplantation for survivors of PTLD continues to be controversial and institution dependent.

25. (C) The patient has Barth syndrome, an X-linked condition characterized by dilated or noncompaction cardiomyopathy, hypotonia, and proximal muscle weakness, all of which may be evident in early neonatal life. Though many present in neonatal life, the age and severity of presentation can vary widely. Neutropenia is common and may contribute to the patients developing recurrent infections. Short stature is common. Barth syndrome is one of a group of metabolic disorders which present with 3-methylglutaconic aciduria. The specific gene implicated in Barth syndrome is the *TAZ* gene, which encodes a protein called tafazzin. Barth syndrome is inherited in an X-linked recessive pattern.

26. (B) The patient is presenting with a dry, hacking cough after initiation of heart failure medication, most likely due to the ACE-inhibitor enalapril. ACE-inhibitor–induced cough is well described in adults, but relatively rare in children. The mechanism is not fully determined, but thought to be related to increased local concentration of kinins and substance P, which may induce bronchial irritation. It may also be related to arachidonic acid pathway activation, leading to elevated levels of thromboxane and subsequent bronchoconstriction. Treatment involves discontinuation of the ACE-inhibitor, after which the cough typically improves within a week. There is a high rate of recurrence, up to 67%, if a second challenge of medication is given. In a patient with DCM, afterload reduction is highly desirable, and an angiotensin-receptor blocker (ARB) such as losartan should be considered to replace the ACE inhibitor.

27. (E) The patient is presenting with severe coronary artery vasculopathy. Options for management of the patient after this diagnosis are limited, but may include using aspirin, a statin drug such as pravastatin, and/or switching the patient from a calcineurin inhibitor (CNI) to an mTOR inhibitor such as sirolimus or everolimus. Stenting can be considered in certain situations, but typically does not have long-term benefit due to a very high incidence of restenosis. As such, listing the patient for retransplantation is the best option. Steroids or plasmapheresis are treatments for rejection; and in the absence of pathologic findings or other evidence of acute rejection, they are not indicated. This being said, many patients will often receive presumptive treatment for rejection in this setting, in the hope of clinical improvement, though it should not be done in lieu of listing for retransplantation.

28. (D) The patient is presenting with signs of SVC obstruction, including irritability and prominent venous distension in the head and neck. This may be seen acutely in patients with SVC thrombus or chronically in patients with obstruction at the SVC anastomosis. The risk of SVC obstruction increases in patients with prior intervention on their SVC, particularly the Glenn operation/bidirectional cavopulmonary anastomosis, and in those who have had a bicaval anastomosis for their transplant. The first line of treatment is angioplasty with or without stenting.

29. (C). Neonatal heart transplantation accounts for 20% of all orthotopic heart transplantations. Although waiting time tends to be quite long (waiting-list mortality 34%), neonatal heart transplantation may allow for longer cold ischemia, ABO incompatibility, and no need for steroids or induction therapy. Furthermore, neonates have less chronic rejection with better long-term survival than when transplant is performed in older patients.

30. (D) Carvedilol has both β-receptor and α-receptor activity. In adult patients with heart failure, carvedilol has been shown to improve left ventricular performance and clinical status. Limited studies in children (including one large randomized trial) have shown varied results; however, it is still used widely in pediatric patients with systemic left ventricular dysfunction. Answer A describes metoprolol, an effective beta blocker which is selectively active on β-1 receptors. Answer B describes ACE-inhibitors including lisinopril, enalapril, and captopril. Answer C describes hydralazine, which effectively dilates peripheral arteries and decreases afterload, increases cardiac output, and may decrease filling pressures. Answer E describes amiloride, which blocks epithelial sodium channels in the late distal convoluted tubule and collecting duct, inhibiting sodium reabsorption from the lumen. This reduces the net negative potential of the lumen of the tubule, reducing both potassium and hydrogen excretion.

31. (C) Asymptomatic left ventricular systolic dysfunction is a relatively common finding. The current recommendations for the initial treatment of asymptomatic left ventricular systolic dysfunction in adults include starting either an ACE inhibitor or a beta blocker. Although there are no evidence-based guidelines to that extent in children, the current recommendations in pediatrics are similar. There is really no indication for starting milrinone or any pressor in this patient. Since the patient has a totally normal physical examination, and thus there is no evidence of volume overload, there is no indication for starting diuretics. Both adult and pediatric guidelines for the management of asymptomatic ventricular dysfunction do not include digoxin. Digoxin is reserved for persistent symptoms of heart failure. Finally, since this patient's physical examination (and therefore oxygen saturation) is totally normal, there is no indication for oxygen therapy.

32. (E) Acute lymphocytic myocarditis remains a relatively common and potentially life-threatening disease. Although there have been many therapies that have been utilized in this disease, very few have been shown to be efficacious. Furthermore, the evidence base for any medical intervention are lacking. Thus, although many centers use intravenous immunoglobulin, corticosteroids, some form of immunosuppression, and/or antiviral drugs, the only current evidence-based therapy for acute myocarditis remains supportive acre.

33. (D) Vision changes can be seen with high dose sildenafil therapy and was a concern for commercial pilots. Urinary retention and thrombocytopenia can be seen with prostacyclin such as treprostinil. Hepatic dysfunction can be seen in patients being treated with Bosentan therapy, therefore liver function tests should be frequently monitored after initiation of therapy and with dose increases. Anemia has been described in association with ERAs, but not thrombocytopenia or leukopenia.

Acquired and Systemic Heart Diseases

M. Yasir Qureshi and Emily R. Levy

Questions

1. A 3-month-old female presented with 5 days of fever, bilateral conjunctivitis, maculopapular rash, cracked lips, and cervical lymphadenopathy. A diagnosis of Kawasaki disease (KD) was established. The initial echocardiogram showed diffuse coronary artery ectasia. The proximal right coronary artery dimension Z-score was 3.4, left main coronary artery Z-score was 3.0, and the proximal left anterior descending artery Z-score was 3.8. One dose of intravenous immunoglobulins was administered resulting in complete resolution of the clinical features of KD within 12 hours of treatment. High-dose aspirin was continued for 48 hours after the alleviation of clinical features, and low-dose aspirin was started after that. Which of the following is the next best step of management?

   A. Repeat echocardiogram twice a week until the coronary dimensions have stabilized or normalized
   B. Repeat IVIG due to significant coronary artery ectasia
   C. Start oral steroids to prevent coronary aneurysms
   D. Repeat echocardiogram in 1 to 2 weeks
   E. Repeat echocardiogram in 4 to 6 weeks

2. A 16-year-old female is recently diagnosed with systemic lupus erythematosus. Her initial echocardiogram as part of her workup was completely normal. While counseling the patient about cardiac involvement in systemic lupus erythematosus, pericarditis and valvulitis were discussed. Which of the following valves is most likely to be involved in valvulitis associated with systemic lupus erythematosus?

   A. Mitral valve
   B. Aortic valve
   C. Tricuspid valve
   D. Pulmonary valve
   E. Eustachian valve

3. A 32-year-old gravida 1 para 0 female presented for a fetal echocardiogram at 19 weeks of gestation. She has a history of Sjogren syndrome with positive SSA/SSB antibodies. The fetal echocardiogram showed normal sinus rhythm, normal biventricular function and no pericardial effusion. What is the risk of congenital complete atrioventricular block in this fetus?

   A. No risk as the fetal echocardiogram is normal
   B. 1% to 5% risk
   C. 10% to 20% risk
   D. 50% risk
   E. 80% risk

4. A 17-year-old female presents with a 1-year history of intermittent fevers, loss of appetite, and weight loss. On examination, she was noted to be hypertensive in her arms and had diminished femoral pulses with significant radiofemoral delay. An echocardiogram showed left ventricular hypertrophy with normal aortic valve function and a normal aortic arch. A magnetic resonance (MR) angiogram was obtained and is shown in **Figure 12.1**.

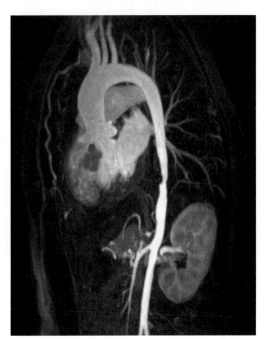

FIGURE 12.1

The most likely diagnosis in this patient is:

A. Systemic hypertension
B. Coarctation of aorta
C. Systemic lupus erythematosus
D. Takayasu arteritis
E. Infective endocarditis

5. A 4-month-old full-term male neonate was noted to be hypotonic on examination. Pulse oximetry showed an oxygen saturation of 99% in both the arms and legs. A chest x-ray showed significant cardiomegaly. A 12-lead electrocardiogram showed a short PR interval and biventricular hypertrophy. An echocardiogram was ordered and showed biventricular hypertrophy without any outflow tract obstruction. Which of the following therapies is most likely to benefit this infant?

A. Diuretics
B. Beta blocker
C. Implantable cardioverter-defibrillator
D. Surgical sympathectomy
E. Enzyme replacement therapy

6. A 15 year old with sickle cell anemia and a history of multiple blood transfusions is being evaluated for possible hemosiderosis. Which of the following is the best test to assess for hemosiderosis?

A. Transthoracic echocardiogram with tissue Doppler imaging
B. Cardiac catheterization and endomyocardial biopsy
C. Cardiac and liver MRI with T2* quantification
D. Magnetic resonance elastography of the liver
E. Liver biopsy

7. A 10 year old was diagnosed with Lyme disease 4 months ago. Which of the following is a clinical feature of late Lyme disease?

A. Erythema migrans
B. Large joint arthritis
C. Facial palsy
D. First-degree heart block
E. Conjunctivitis

8. A 7-year-old male presents with 4 days of fever, 3 weeks after being treated for acute pharyngitis with oral amoxicillin. He also reports right knee and right elbow swelling, erythema, and pain. On examination, tachypnea and increased work of breathing is noted. Cardiac examination revealed a 3/6 holosystolic murmur at the cardiac apex radiating to the left axilla. Chest x-ray showed mild cardiomegaly with increased pulmonary vascular markings and hazy lung fields. Laboratory evaluation showed elevated C-reactive protein and serum streptococcal antibody titers. The transthoracic echocardiogram is shown in **Figure 12.2**.

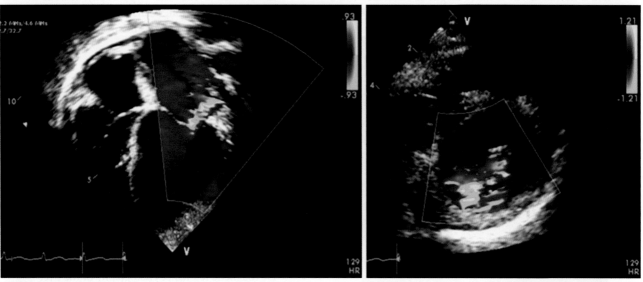

FIGURE 12.2

Which of the following options is the best treatment strategy for this patient?

A. Intramuscular penicillin G benzathine, naproxen, and furosemide
B. Intravenous immunoglobulin (IVIG) and high-dose aspirin
C. IVIG and low-dose aspirin
D. IVIG, prednisone, and high-dose aspirin
E. IVIG, amoxicillin, and aspirin

9. Which of the following is the most common presentation of chronic rheumatic heart disease?

A. Mitral valve regurgitation
B. Mitral valve stenosis
C. Aortic valve regurgitation
D. Aortic valve stenosis
E. Tricuspid valve disease

10. A 9-month-old infant is being seen in pediatric cardiology clinic for routine follow-up. He had a history of a large membranous ventricular septal defect for which he underwent surgical repair at 4 months of age. The postoperative course was complicated by junctional tachycardia which required treatment with amiodarone. One month after discontinuation of amiodarone, he had another episode of junctional tachycardia for which oral amiodarone was restarted. The infant has gaining weight but has severe constipation. The mother also reports some facial puffiness and dry skin. Some initial laboratory tests were ordered by the referring pediatrician prior to this visit. Which of the following laboratory findings can be expected in this infant?

A. Low thyroid-stimulating hormone (TSH) and low free T4
B. Normal TSH and low free T4
C. Low TSH and high free T4
D. High TSH and low free T4
E. High TSH and high free T4

11. A 17-year-old male is referred to pediatric cardiology for evaluation of claudication. His physical examination revealed decreased femoral pulses. A transthoracic echocardiogram showed a diffusely narrowed descending thoracic and abdominal aorta. Which of the following is associated with vasculopathy leading to stenosis of large vessels?

   A. Late syphilis
   B. Human immunodeficiency virus (HIV) disease
   C. Kawasaki disease
   D. Henoch-Schönlein purpura
   E. Rheumatic fever

12. An asymptomatic 22-year-old cancer survivor of thoracic lymphoma was previously treated with chemotherapy and radiation therapy. A surveillance echocardiogram showed calcification and thickening of the mitral valve annulus. This pattern of valvular involvement is typical of which of the following?

   A. Anthracycline exposure
   B. Radiation exposure
   C. Healed infective endocarditis
   D. Nonbacterial thrombotic endocarditis
   E. Rheumatic carditis

13. A 15-year-old female was diagnosed with systemic lupus erythematosus 2 years ago. She is completely asymptomatic from a cardiovascular standpoint. Her lupus is well controlled. Her echocardiogram shows vegetations on the mitral valve leaflets. Which of the following is true about these vegetations?

   A. Benign vegetations, no treatment needed
   B. Can get infected, prophylactic antibiotics are needed
   C. Need treatment with intravenous antibiotics
   D. Can embolize
   E. Need surgical resection

14. An 8-year-old is admitted to the hospital with abdominal pain, vomiting, fevers >102°F for 7 days, cracked red lips, and swollen hands and feet. The emergency room has obtained a CBC with differential and ESR. The absolute lymphocyte count (ALC) is noted to be 550 cells/uL (0.55). CRP is elevated at 102 mg/L. The family mentions that they all were mildly ill with cough, congestion, and pharyngitis approximately 1 month prior. The patient's mother had a "COVID19" test at the time which was a positive SARS-CoV-2 PCR. You suspect this child may have multisystem inflammatory syndrome in children (MIS-C). You plan to perform an echocardiogram. If there are *no* coronary artery aneurysms, the appropriate first-line therapy could include:

   A. IVIG and Tocilizumab (anti-IL6)
   B. IVIG and Methylprednisolone
   C. Anakinra (anti-IL1) monotherapy
   D. Tocilizumab (anti-IL6) monotherapy
   E. Doxycycline

15. A 7-day-old infant presents to the ICU in cardiogenic shock in early September. An echocardiogram demonstrates profoundly decreased biventricular systolic function with an LV ejection fraction of 10%, but no other abnormalities. The family describes that they all had fever and diarrhea 2 weeks ago, and both older siblings had perirectal rashes. The infant has had some mild diarrhea and poor feeding since birth. He has also had some upper right arm periodic twitching motions at times over the past couple of days. An LP is to be performed. In addition to cell count, glucose, protein, bacterial gram stain and culture, and HSV viral testing, you should request which of the following viral PCR testing be sent from the CSF?

   A. CMV
   B. EBV
   C. Enterovirus
   D. Hepatitis C
   E. HIV1

16. The infant in the question above develops multiple episodes of ventricular tachycardia and is placed on VA ECMO support for heart failure secondary to myocarditis. Although there is limited available data for treatment, you decide to proceed with first-line therapy for enteroviral myocarditis, which is:

   A. IVIG
   B. Zidovudine
   C. Remdesivir
   D. Acyclovir
   E. Ganciclovir

17. A 13 year old with a history of neonatal tetralogy of Fallot, repaired in infancy with RV to PA conduit, presents with 22 days of low-grade fevers, fatigue, weight loss, and headaches. She has a temperature of 38.2 on examination, and appears gaunt and tired. She has a notable 3/6 midsternal murmur with radiation to the left axilla. Her heart rate is 92, but the remainder of vital signs are normal. The diagnostic test with the highest sensitivity is:

   A. Nasal respiratory pathogen panel
   B. Multiple blood cultures
   C. Echocardiogram
   D. Cardiac MRI
   E. Stool culture

18. Which infectious organisms is the most likely cause of subacute infective endocarditis?

   A. Histoplasma species
   B. *Pseudomonas aeruginosa*
   C. *Streptococcus bovis* (Group D Streptococcus)
   D. *Staphylococcus aureus*
   E. *Enterococcus faecium*

19. A 16-year-old presents with new fatigue and dyspnea. He complains of chest pain and has a fever of 38.3°C. He has a mild cough. The influenza A nasal PCR is positive. Transthoracic echocardiography shows hypokinesia in the inferior segment of the left ventricle. A cardiac MRI is obtained, images below. Inversion recovery images (**Figure 12.3**) 7 minutes after the administration of IV gadolinium in the short axis (left) and long axis (right) of the left ventricle show focal patchy areas of delayed postcontrast enhancement (*arrows*). This MRI is consistent with:

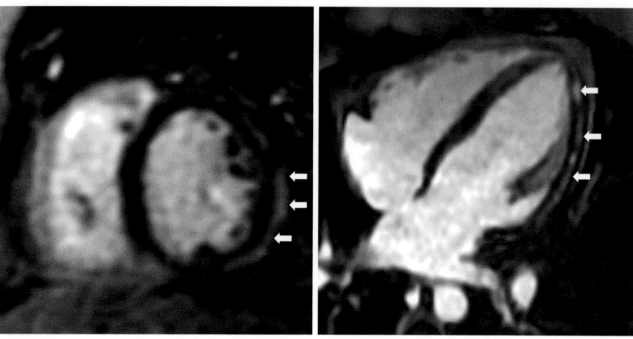

FIGURE 12.3

A. Endocarditis
B. Pericarditis
C. Tamponade secondary to pericardial effusion
D. Cardiac tumor
E. Myocarditis

20. A 12-year-old girl presents with syncope and is admitted to the hospital for persistent fatigue. She is found to have third-degree AV block on her 12-lead EKG. Lyme serologies are positive for 2 IgM bands and 5 IgG bands. She is diagnosed with Lyme carditis. Initial therapy should include:

A. IV meropenem
B. IV ceftriaxone
C. PO doxycycline
D. PO azithromycin
E. IV anti-Lyme IgG

21. A fully vaccinated 3-year-old girl from Minnesota presents with fever of 103°F, fatigue, cough, and tachypnea for several days. On examination, a friction rub is heard on auscultation and decreased breath sounds are present in the left lower lobe. A CXR shows left lower lobe consolidation. A transthoracic echocardiogram is obtained, and demonstrates a large pericardial effusion. Over the next 6 hours, she develops hypotension and progressive tachycardia. The medical team pursues diagnostic and therapeutic pericardiocentesis. The pericardial fluid appears purulent on direct examination. The most likely cause of this infection is:

A. Enterovirus
B. *Mycobacterium tuberculosis*
C. Toxoplasmosis
D. *Staphylococcus aureus*
E. *Haemophilus influenzae* type b

22. Gram stain and culture results are pending (previous question). While you await the bacterial culture result, the best empiric antibiotic regimen choice is:

A. Vancomycin and ceftriaxone
B. Oxacillin
C. Vancomycin, ceftriaxone, and clindamycin
D. Cefepime
E. Azithromycin and ceftriaxone

23. A 17-year-old boy with congenitally acquired HIV presents to cardiology clinic for a consultation ordered by his immunologist. His HIV has been well controlled since birth with antiretroviral therapy. He has a CD4 count of 600 cells/uL, and his HIV RNA quantitative PCR is undetected for the last several years. His current therapeutic regimen consists of ritonavir (ABT-538), zidovudine (AZT), and lamivudine (3TC). On history, he discloses he has felt like his heart is racing recently, and feels like he is getting easily short of breath. Dilated cardiomyopathy is diagnosed by a transthoracic echocardiogram. The best therapeutic intervention includes:

   A. Investigating lipid and cholesterol panel, followed by diet modifications if abnormal
   B. Trimethoprim-sulfamethoxazole PCP prophylaxis
   C. Changing HIV medication regimens
   D. High dose NSAIDs
   E. Methylprednisolone

24. A 5-day-old neonate who was born at home is brought to the emergency department. The infant is noted to have cataracts and microcephaly. Scattered petechiae are noted across chest, back, and face. Hepatosplenomegaly is discovered on abdominal examination. On further history, the mother tells you she has never had any vaccines "except DTAP and influenza." You are called to the ED to perform a transthoracic echocardiogram. The congenital heart abnormality most commonly associated with this infectious syndrome is:

   A. Patent ductus arteriosus
   B. Tetralogy of Fallot
   C. Hypoplastic left heart syndrome
   D. Pulmonary atresia
   E. Transposition of the great arteries

25. A 2-year-old previously unvaccinated child is adopted from Ghana. She is in the 10th percentile for weight and appears chronically malnourished. She had intermittent fevers for her first few weeks after adoption. On her initial physical examination to establish primary care, a pericardial rub is detected. A subsequent echocardiogram demonstrates a moderate pericardial effusion with no evidence of tamponade. Her PPD is negative, but her T-spot (tuberculosis interferon gamma release assay) is positive. A comprehensive diagnostic work-up is performed including pericardiocentesis. Fluid is noted to be blood tinged. In addition to cell count and differential, what diagnostic tests would be most helpful to send on this pericardial fluid?

   A. Myobacterial culture
   B. Acid-fast bacilli staining
   C. Adenine deaminase levels
   D. HIV PCR
   E. HIV viral culture

26. A 4-week-old who is status post a Norwood procedure for HLHS is ready for initial ICU discharge in November. In addition to hepatitis B vaccination which he received at birth, what other infectious prevention intervention may be appropriate to consider prior to hospital discharge?

   A. Early PCV13 vaccination
   B. Seasonal influenza vaccination
   C. COVID-19 mRNA vaccination
   D. Daily penicillin (oral) prophylaxis
   E. Palivizumab

27. A 12-year-old who immigrated from rural Mexico as a toddler is diagnosed with ALL, and begins to undergo induction chemotherapy. During her first week of chemotherapy with daunorubicin, vincristine, prednisone, and cyclophosphamide, she develops intermittent fevers. A 12-lead EKG also notes a new right bundle branch block, for which she is referred to pediatric cardiology. Her oncologists are concerned about daunorubicin toxicity. An echocardiogram demonstrated a dilated LV with mild mitral regurgitation and a reduced LV ejection fraction of 50%. You are concerned about Chagas disease reactivation. This disease is caused by:

   A. *Borrelia burgdorferi*
   B. *Trypanosoma cruzi*
   C. *Plasmodium falciparum*
   D. *Trypanosoma brucei*
   E. *Plasmodium vivax*

28. Given her immigration history, this patient could have undergone "chronic" Chagas disease screening prior to chemotherapy induction. The best diagnostic test to screen for chronic Chagas disease is:

   A. Blood smear with parasite examination
   B. *T. cruzi* PCR from blood
   C. *T. cruzi* PCR from stool
   D. Blood cultures, at least three sets
   E. IgG *T. cruzi* serologic testing

Answers

1. (A) KD guidelines of 2017 recommend repeating echo-cardiograms twice a week in patients with important or evolving coronary artery abnormalities (Z-score >2.5) noted during the acute phase of KD, until the coronary dimensions have stopped progressing. As the clinical features of inflammation have resolved with the 1st dose of IVIG, a repeat dose of IVIG or oral steroids is not needed.

2. (A) The mitral valve is the most commonly involved cardiac valve in systemic lupus erythematosus. The aortic valve is the 2nd most common, followed by the tricuspid valve and finally the pulmonary valve.

3. (B) The risk in the 1st child in mothers with positive SSA/SSB antibodies is 1% to 5%. If the 1st child has congenital complete heart block, the risk in 2nd child goes up to 11% to 19%. Complete heart block can manifest any time between 16 and 28 weeks of gestation; therefore, a normal fetal echocardiogram at 19 weeks of gestation does not alleviate the risk.

4. (D) The MR angiogram shows coarctation of the abdominal aorta. This image along with the clinical picture is consistent with the diagnosis of Takayasu arteritis.

5. (E) The clinical picture is consistent with Pompe disease, which is a lysosomal storage disease due to acid alpha-glucosidase deficiency. Enzyme replacement therapy with alglucosidase alfa given intravenously every 2 weeks is the most effective treatment for cardiomyopathy and developmental delays.

6. (C) Magnetic resonance imaging with T2* quantification is the best test to quantitate iron load in myocardium and the liver. Echocardiography and tissue Doppler may show restrictive pattern in hemosiderosis. Cardiac catheterization, liver magnetic resonance elastography, and liver biopsy are not needed for this purpose.

7. (B) Large joint arthritis is a feature of late Lyme disease. All other options are features of early localized and early disseminated Lyme disease.

8. (A) The patient has acute rheumatic fever with carditis. The echocardiogram shows severe mitral valve regurgitation, which is the most common manifestation of acute rheumatic carditis. Left heart enlargement and a small amount of pericardial effusion along the right atrium and right ventricle can also be noted. The treatment includes (1) antibiotics against group A streptococcal infection, (2) anti-inflammatory therapy with NSAIDs or high-dose aspirin, and (3) treatment of congestive heart failure. Penicillin G benzathine is a long-acting intramuscular injection that serves as prevention of group A streptococcal infection. Naproxen has favorable side effect profile compared to high-dose aspirin and is a preferred choice as an anti-inflammatory agent. Furosemide is needed in this child as there is evidence of respiratory distress and pulmonary edema from mitral regurgitation. IVIG and high-dose aspirin are first-line treatment for Kawasaki disease. IVIG is typically not used in acute rheumatic fever unless there is severe Sydenham chorea which is not responding to other therapy.

9. (B) Mitral valve stenosis in isolation and in combination with aortic valve disease is the most common manifestation of chronic rheumatic heart disease.

10. (D) Amiodarone exposure can cause hypothyroidism which will cause low TSH and high free T4. An elevated TSH with normal free T4, indicative of subclinical hypothyroidism, can also be seen after amiodarone exposure.

11. (B) HIV disease can cause vasculitis of the aorta and pulmonary arteries that can lead to diffuse stenosis. Late syphilis causes occlusion of vasa vasorum of large vessels resulting in aneurysmal dilation, not stenosis, of aorta. Other options are not associated with large vessel vasculopathy.

12. (B) Thoracic radiation exposure can lead to a degenerative process of the mitral valve which typically starts from the annulus and progresses toward the leaflet tips. Anthracycline exposure is more commonly associated with cardiomyopathy. Infective and nonbacterial thrombotic endocarditis typically do not involve the valve annulus primarily.

13. (D) Nonbacterial thrombotic endocarditis in systemic lupus erythematosus is not infective and does not need antibiotic prophylaxis. However, these vegetations can embolize and are not completely inconsequential. Rarely, surgical resection is needed for large vegetations.

14. (B) While still in the early phases of description and evidence-based therapy development, current recommendations for first-line therapy in patients hospitalized with MIS-C may include both IVIG and steroids. Most therapeutic regimens include IVIG. Tocilizumab and Anakinra, while potential treatments, are not typically used as initial therapies.

15. (C) The enterovirus family includes nearly 70 serotypes of closely related single-stranded RNA viruses that cause a wide spectrum of human illness. Disseminated neonatal enterovirus is a common cause of acquired neonatal myocarditis and encephalitis. There is often a family history of diarrheal type illness. The nonpolio enteroviruses include coxsackieviruses (one subtype of which may present in older children as "Hand, Foot, Mouth Disease"). Most enterovirus infections are mild and self-limited, but enterovirus strains which may cause mild illness in older children and adults may disseminate in neonates resulting in severe systemic disease. CMV and EBV may cause disseminated disease but are more rare causes of encephalitis and myocarditis than enterovirus in neonates. While patients with AIDS can present with both encephalitis and myocarditis, this would be an unlikely presentation for a neonate who had vertically acquired HIV. Both neonatal HIV and hepatitis are typically asymptomatic in the neonatal period.

16. (A) Treatment of the infant and child with myocarditis is specific for the causative agent. IVIG is commonly used for severe enteroviral myocarditis, although there is limited supportive data. None of the other antivirals listed would be appropriate to treat enteroviral disease.

17. (B) This child's presentation is consistent with subacute infective endocarditis. Although an echocardiogram is also indicated, endocarditis may be difficult to diagnose by imaging alone, particularly earlier in the course without large vegetations or in patients with conduit or valve replacements. Serial blood cultures remain the gold standard with the highest sensitivity test for endocarditis diagnosis.

18. (C) Of the organisms listed, the most common cause of subacute infective endocarditis is *Streptococcus Bovis*, a Group D Streptococci (viridans group). Approximately 80% of infective endocarditis cases are caused by Streptococci and Staphylococci. Acute bacterial endocarditis is usually caused by *Staphylococcus aureus*. Subacute bacterial endocarditis is often caused by Group D Streptococci. The third most common bacterial cause is enterococci. Although rare, gram-negative and fungal infections may occur.

19. (E) The MRI shows focal delayed enhancement within the myocardium of the left ventricular inferolateral wall which is most consistent with myocarditis.

20. (B) Lyme carditis is a manifestation of early disseminated Lyme disease. For Lyme carditis with symptomatic high-grade AV block, IV ceftriaxone is first-line therapy for both children and adults. Treatment duration is typically 14 to 21 days. Therapy can be completed as an outpatient with oral doxycycline.

21. (D) *S. aureus* is the most common cause for acute purulent pericarditis in the United States in vaccinated children. Typically, it accompanies sepsis, pneumonia, septic arthritis, or osteomyelitis. Another common cause is *Streptococcus pneumoniae*. Tuberculosis is a common cause of pericarditis in the developing world, but is likely to present as subacute or chronic, and less likely with tamponade. Effusions may be bloody. *Hib* was a more common cause of purulent pericarditis prior to vaccination. Toxoplasmosis is unlikely to cause purulent pericarditis.

22. (A) Empiric antibiotic regimens should include coverage for MRSA, MSSA, Streptococcus species, and gram-negative rods which may cause pneumonia like nontypeable *Haemophilus influenzae*. In a previously healthy child, anaerobic coverage (Flagyl) and antipseudomonal activity (cefepime) are unlikely to be necessary. However,

consideration should be given to *Pseudomonas* in the post-surgical pericarditis population.

23. (C) Although the patient's HIV infection is under very good control with his current regimen, antiretroviral therapy is one of probable causes for HIV-related dilated cardiomyopathy. Zidovudine (AZT) has specifically been associated with early cardiomyopathy in teenagers and young adults, although the mechanism remains unclear. While dyslipidemia is also a common side effect of many medications used to treat HIV, and should be screened for, it is not as likely to be contributing to the cardiomyopathy.

24. (A) This infant seems to be presenting with congenital rubella syndrome which may include cataracts, "blueberry muffin rash" secondary to petechiae or purpura, and hepatosplenomegaly. While postnatal rubella is usually a mild illness, congenital rubella syndrome (secondary to maternal infection during the first trimester) often has devastating consequences. Patent ductus arteriosus and peripheral pulmonary artery stenosis are the most common congenital heart deficits associated with the syndrome.

25. (C) Adenine deaminase (ADA) level is very high in patients with tuberculous pericarditis. Studies have estimated that ADA levels above 40 U/l may have nearly 90% sensitivity and specificity. Pericardial effusions associated with neoplasm may also have elevated ADA. Additional studies which may be helpful for diagnosing tuberculosis pericarditis include cell count and differential (specifically lymphocyte to neutrophil ratio) and pericardial IFN-gamma. Although AFB stain and mycobacterial culture should be sent, they are unlikely to be positive from pericardial fluid. HIV qualitative PCR should also be sent in this clinical scenario, but should be sent from blood samples.

26. (E) Children with congenital heart disease have a rate of hospitalization for RSV infection that is 3 to 5 times higher than age-matched controls. They are also more likely to require mechanical ventilation for RSV+ bronchiolitis. Children with congenital heart disease who are in the first year of life may benefit from monthly palivizumab (anti-RSV; "Synagis®") during the winter months, typically beginning in November. This infant is too young for PCV13, influenza, or COVID-19 vaccination. Daily penicillin is not indicated for Norwood repair prophylaxis.

27. (B) Chagas disease is caused by a trypanosome (blood parasite). The acute phase of parasitemia typically lasts 2 to 3 months and is characterized by mild flu-like symptoms. Meningoencephalitis and/or acute myocarditis can rarely occur, particularly in young children. The acute phase is followed by a chronic phase which is typically lifelong and involves low-level parasitemia. Most people are asymptomatic. In 20% to 30% of cases, serious progressive sequelae may develop years to decades after the initial infection. This may involve cardiomyopathy and ventricular arrhythmias, and can progress to congestive heart failure. Digestive diseases including esophageal or colonic dilation may occur. Reactivation parasitemia may be life threatening and may occur in immunocompromised people including those with new HIV, post solid organ transplantation, or undergoing chemotherapy.

28. (E) The best assessment for chronic *T. cruzi* infection is serologic testing, as circulating parasite levels are very low during the chronic phase. Unfortunately, no single serologic test is sufficiently sensitive or specific to confirm a diagnosis of chronic *T. cruzi* infection. The CDC and WHO both recommend samples be tested using two different serologic assays of different formats before treatment decisions are made. Acute infections can be diagnosed by parasitology methods, including identification of trypomastigotes in blood by microscopy.

Genetics and Congenital Heart Disease

Talha Niaz, Katherine Agre, and Jonathan N. Johnson

Questions

1. A 2-year-old male is referred after the finding of left ventricular noncompaction on cardiac MRI. The patient's mother reports a family history of left ventricular noncompaction, intellectual disability, and hypotonia in her now deceased brother. The patient's mother is currently 6 weeks pregnant with her second child. What is the likelihood the fetus is affected by the same genetic disorder?

   A. 75% (3/4)
   B. 50% (1/2)
   C. 25% (1/4)
   D. 3% to 5%
   E. 0%

2. A 30-year-old healthy male is referred due to a family history of infantile onset dilated cardiomyopathy in two of his siblings. There is no other family history of cardiac disease and he himself has a normal echo. Genetic testing in his siblings revealed homozygous pathogenic mutations in the DNAJC19 gene, associated with 3-methylglutaconic aciduria, type V. This condition has 100% penetrance. What is the likelihood your patient is a carrier of this condition?

   A. 100% (1)
   B. 66.7% (2/3)
   C. 50% (1/2)
   D. 25% (1/4)
   E. None of the above

3. The pedigree in the image is most consistent with what inheritance pattern (**Figure 13.1**)?

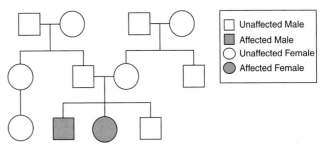

FIGURE 13.1 Three-generation family pedigree chart.

   A. Autosomal dominant
   B. Autosomal recessive
   C. X-linked recessive
   D. De novo
   E. Mitochondrial

4. A 7-month-old female dies suddenly of sudden infant death syndrome (SIDS). Autopsy is negative for cardiac anomalies. The decedent's family is motivated to determine cause of death to better understand risk to future children and other family members. Genetic testing on postmortem tissue reveals a variant of uncertain significance in the KCNH2 gene. What do you estimate the risk for future children to also suffer cardiac arrest based on this genetic finding?

   A. 100% (4/4)
   B. 50% (1/2)
   C. 25% (1/4)
   D. 3% to 5%
   E. Cannot estimate based on genetic finding

5. A 33-year-old male with hypertrophic cardiomyopathy, epilepsy, and hearing loss is found to have a pathogenic mutation in MT-TL1, causative of mitochondrial encephalopathy, lactic acidosis, and stroke-like episodes syndrome (MELAS). He has a healthy 3-year-old son and 1-year-old daughter. What do you estimate the likelihood his daughter is also affected by MELAS?

A. 100%
B. 50% (1/2)
C. 25% (1/4)
D. 0%
E. Cannot be determined with data provided

6. A 2-year-old female is diagnosed with Jervell and Lange-Nielsen syndrome due to an abnormal electrocardiogram and profound bilateral sensorineural hearing loss. Based on this diagnosis, you can conclude that:

A. Any siblings of the patient will also be affected by Jervell and Lange-Nielsen
B. The patient's parents would be unaffected carriers of this condition
C. The patient's parents are at risk for prolonged QT
D. This condition is most likely de novo in the patient
E. The patient will also have visual impairment

7. An 18-year-old male is seen due to diagnosis of hypertrophic cardiomyopathy (HCM). His family history is significant for his paternal aunt, paternal uncle, and paternal grandmother with HCM. The patient's father has had normal echocardiograms. What is the most likely inheritance pattern in this family?

A. X-linked recessive
B. Autosomal recessive
C. Autosomal dominant, full penetrance
D. Autosomal dominant, reduced penetrance
E. Mitochondrial pattern

8. A 2-month-old male infant is referred for failure to thrive and is diagnosed with supravalvar pulmonary stenosis and supravalvar aortic stenosis on echocardiography. The child is described as having an "elfin" face, with flared eyebrows, bright stellate irides, and a wide mouth. A deletion on which of the following chromosomes can lead to this presentation?

A. 11q
B. 22q
C. 7q
D. 1p
E. 8p

9. A 10-month-old male infant is referred to you with a history of atrial septal defect. On examination, you note that the patient has a missing thumb on his right hand. The patient's father also has a similar missing thumb. On further evaluation, all laboratory values, including CBC and electrolytes, are normal. Genetic analysis reveals a mutation in the *TBX5* gene. Which of the following is the most likely diagnosis?

A. Thrombocytopenia-absent radii (TAR) syndrome
B. LEOPARD syndrome
C. Holt–Oram syndrome
D. CHARGE association
E. Rubenstein–Taybi syndrome

10. A neonate is diagnosed with truncus arteriosus. Which of the following genetic syndromes is most likely in this patient?

A. Down syndrome
B. Turner syndrome
C. DiGeorge syndrome
D. Klinefelter syndrome
E. Holt–Oram syndrome

11. A 5-day-old female is diagnosed with a moderate-sized ventricular septal defect. On physical examination, she has hypotonia, microcephaly, hypertelorism, low set ears, and a high-pitched cry. There is no family history of any genetic disorders. Which of the following is the best diagnostic test from genetic standpoint?

A. No testing needed
B. Karyotype
C. Fluorescent in situ hybridization
D. Single gene sequencing
E. Gene panel testing

12. A 13-year-old female is seen for a heart murmur. Her parents note that she has numerous dark-brown freckle-like spots throughout her body, which seem to have increased in number as she has gotten older. She has a prior diagnosis of sensorineural deafness, as well as short stature. Her parents report that a murmur was heard in many well-child visits, but was always thought to be benign. An ECG is performed and shows first-degree AV block. Which of the following is most likely to be seen on echocardiography?

A. Coarctation of the aorta and bicuspid aortic valve
B. Atrial and ventricular septal defects
C. Pulmonary stenosis and left ventricular hypertrophy
D. Double aortic arch
E. Rhabdomyoma

13. A 14-year-old male is referred to your clinic. He has a history of recurrent sinusitis for which he has undergone numerous courses of antibiotics. A chest x-ray is performed which shows evidence of dextrocardia. In addition, the stomach bubble is located on the right side of the x-ray. A CT scan of the chest reveals bronchiectasis. Which of the following is the most likely diagnosis?

A. Carney complex
B. Kartagener syndrome
C. DiGeorge syndrome
D. Wiskott–Aldrich syndrome
E. Turner syndrome

14. A 5-year-old female presents with fatigue and is found to have complete heart block. Echocardiography reveals a moderate-sized secundum atrial septal defect. A mutation in which gene is most likely to be found in this patient?

A. *NKX2.5*
B. *TBX5*
C. *MLL2*
D. *JAG1*
E. *PTNP11*

15. A 17-year-old male basketball player is referred to you for a murmur. On examination, you note that he has significant scoliosis, pectus carinatum, and pes planus (flat feet). His height is 190 cm, and his arm span is 210 cm. He has positive "thumb" and "wrist" signs. His aortic root measures 45 mm in diameter (*Z*-score = 5.2). His carotid arteries, aortic arch, and descending aorta are normal. There is no significant family history. He admits to being admitted twice in the past with spontaneous pneumothoraces. Which of the following is true regarding this young man's diagnosis?

A. He has Loeys–Dietz syndrome
B. He should have a repeat echocardiogram in 5 years
C. He does not need an eye examination
D. He has Marfan syndrome
E. He needs an ECG to assess for a prolonged QT interval

16. An echo performed on a 2-day-old male infant demonstrates severe tricuspid and mitral valve dysplasia with prolapse. He is diagnosed with congenital polyvalvular dysplasia. Which of the following is the most likely genetic diagnosis in this patient?

A. Down syndrome
B. Noonan syndrome
C. Trisomy 18
D. DiGeorge syndrome
E. Alagille syndrome

17. Which of the following genetic syndromes are associated with an increased incidence of partial anomalous pulmonary venous return?

A. Trisomy 18 and trisomy 21
B. Holt–Oram and Marfan
C. Turner and trisomy 21
D. Turner and Noonan
E. Noonan and Alagille

18. A 5-year-old male has progressive limb ataxia and weakness, dysarthria, nystagmus, and loss of proprioception requiring a wheelchair for mobility. His molecular and genetic testing has revealed a mutation in the frataxin (FXN) gene. Which of the following is the likely cardiovascular phenotype?

A. High-grade atrioventricular block
B. Thickening of aortic and mitral valve
C. Concentric left ventricular hypertrophy
D. Dilation of the left ventricle
E. Reverse curve hypertrophy of the septum

19. A 9-year-old female presents to you for evaluation of a murmur. The patient is asymptomatic, but does not participate in any athletic activity. Her family history is significant for a paternal uncle, grandfather, and great grandfather who had "thick heart muscle." On examination, she has short stature, a triangular face, pectus excavatum, and a webbed neck. Her heart examination reveals an RV lift and a soft short systolic ejection murmur at the LUSB. What are you most likely to find on her echocardiogram?

A. Bicuspid aortic valve with or without coarctation
B. Thickened pulmonary valve with mild stenosis
C. Discrete supravalvular pulmonary stenosis
D. Bilateral pulmonary branch stenosis
E. Right aortic arch

20. As part of an evaluation for short stature, a 12-year-old female is noted to have streaked gonads on abdominal and pelvic ultrasound examination. A karyotype determines that she has Turner syndrome. Which of the following is most likely to be found on echocardiography?

A. Bicuspid aortic valve
B. Mitral valve stenosis
C. Subaortic membrane
D. Aortic root dilatation
E. Atrial septal defect

CHAPTER 13

21. A 6-week-old female infant with biliary atresia is found to have a murmur on examination. When you see the patient, you note that she has a broad forehead, deep-set eyes, and a pointed chin, which give her face a triangular appearance. She is significantly jaundiced. Auscultation reveals a 2/6 systolic murmur heard best at the left upper sternal border and radiating to the axillae bilaterally. Which of the following is the most likely diagnosis?

    A. CHARGE association
    B. Alagille syndrome
    C. Williams syndrome
    D. Noonan syndrome
    E. DiGeorge syndrome

22. You have been consulted on an 11-year-old male admitted to the pediatric intensive care unit after being diagnosed with Mobitz type II second degree heart block due to symptoms of dizziness and syncope. On echocardiographic evaluation, his left ventricle is severely dilated with reduced ejection fraction estimated at 25%. There is no mitral valve regurgitation and the intracardiac anatomy is normal without any shunt lesions. He has no recent history of any viral infections and has generally been healthy except symptoms of fatigue over the last few years. On physical examination, he has mild skeletal muscle weakness in lower extremities. The family history is positive for a pacemaker in patient's father and a paternal uncle who had sudden death with no known etiology. Which of the following mutations is most likely to be found in this patient?

    A. KCNQ1
    B. MYH7
    C. LMNA
    D. TTN
    E. MYBPC3

23. A 3-month-old male infant is referred to you for a murmur. The patient has already been referred to medical genetics for a history of low birth weight, hypotonia, and microcephaly. On examination, you note the patient has hypertelorism, epicanthal folds with down-slanting palpebral fissures, a flat nasal bridge, micrognathia, single palmar creases, and a high-pitched cry. Which of the following are you most likely to find on echocardiography?

    A. Coarctation of the aorta
    B. Transposition of the great arteries
    C. Double outlet right ventricle
    D. Ebstein anomaly
    E. Ventricular septal defect (VSD)

24. A 3-year-old patient is referred to you with postaxial polydactyly, large atrial septal defect, dwarfism, and fingernail dysplasia. Which of the following is the most likely genetic syndrome in this patient?

    A. Holt–Oram syndrome
    B. DiGeorge syndrome
    C. Alagille syndrome
    D. Ellis–van Creveld syndrome
    E. Down syndrome

25. A male neonate is diagnosed with tetralogy of Fallot. What is the inheritance pattern of the most frequently identified genetic cause of tetralogy of Fallot?

    A. X-linked dominant
    B. Mitochondrial
    C. Autosomal recessive
    D. X-linked recessive
    E. Autosomal dominant

26. A 6-month-old female is referred due to the finding of a pathogenic SCN5A mutation found incidentally on whole exome sequencing. There is no known family history of cardiac disease. Which of the following diagnosis is not associated with SCN5A?

    A. Dilated cardiomyopathy
    B. Brugada syndrome
    C. Long QT syndrome
    D. Atrial septal defect
    E. Sudden death

27. An 8-year-old, developmentally delayed male presents with shortness of breath. Echocardiography reveals a mitral valve arcade with severe stenosis (mean gradient = 14 mm Hg). On further questioning, his family reports a history of short stature and thrombocytopenia. Examination demonstrates wide-spaced eyes, mild ptosis, and small ears. A microarray is sent and reveals a deletion in chromosome 11q23. Which of the following is the diagnosis?

    A. Williams syndrome
    B. DiGeorge syndrome
    C. Turner syndrome
    D. Jacobsen syndrome
    E. Noonan syndrome

28. Which of the following chromosomal abnormalities portends the highest incidence of congenital heart disease (CHD) for affected patients?

    A. Trisomy 21
    B. Trisomy 18
    C. Turner syndrome
    D. DiGeorge syndrome
    E. 5p– syndrome

29. Which of the following patients is most likely to harbor a 22q11.2 deletion?

    A. 2-month-old male infant with tetralogy of Fallot
    B. 4 year old with a small ventricular septal defect (VSD)
    C. 4 month old with double outlet right ventricle and subaortic VSD
    D. 2-day-old infant with d-transposition of the great arteries and VSD
    E. 2-week-old infant with interrupted aortic arch type B

30. A 12-year-old male is referred to you from Genetics for cardiac screening. He has coarse facial features, hepatosplenomegaly, bone disease and deafness consistent with mucopolysaccharidoses type II, and Hunter syndrome. His genetic and molecular testing confirmed a deficiency of iduronate 2-sulfatase resulting in storage of heparan and dermatan sulfate in various tissues. Which of the following is the most common cardiovascular manifestation of the Hunter syndrome?

    A. Hypertrophic obstructive cardiomyopathy
    B. Atrial fibrillation
    C. Coronary artery aneurysms
    D. Dilated cardiomyopathy
    E. Thickened mitral or aortic valve

31. A 2-day-old newborn has facial dysmorphisms consisting of small ears, upslanting eyes with epicanthal folds, protruding tongue, transverse palmar creases, brachydactyly, a gap between first and second toes, and sparse hair. Which of the following is TRUE regarding this genetic syndrome?

    A. Echocardiogram should be performed only with clinical concern
    B. Almost 20% of the children with this syndrome have a congenital heart defect
    C. Tetralogy of Fallot is the most commonly associated congenital heart disease with this syndrome
    D. Children with this syndrome are at a higher risk of developing pulmonary hypertension
    E. The next step in the genetic evaluation is obtaining a chromosomal microarray

32. An 8-year-old male with a significant past medical history of repair of cleft lip/palate and tetralogy of Fallot is noted to have several dysmorphic facial features including a narrowed face with a small mouth, micrognathia, narrowed palpebral fissures, and a prominent nose. Additional clinical findings include short stature and developmental delay. Which of the following complications may occur in the newborn period in this genetic condition?

    A. Cardiac conduction abnormalities
    B. Pulmonary hypertension
    C. Prolonged QT interval
    D. Leukemia
    E. Hypocalcemia

33. A 5-year-old female with repaired coarctation of the aorta is referred to you for follow-up. She has no residual aortic arch gradient, normal biventricular function, and a normally functioning aortic valve with three cusps on echocardiogram. Her right upper and lower extremity blood pressures are 88/54 mm Hg and 83/50 mm Hg, respectively. On physical examination, there are no dysmorphic facial features, she has no murmurs and normal peripheral pulses with no radiofemoral delay. She is at 5th percentile for weight and height and has been very healthy with no other concerns. Which of the following is the most appropriate management?

    A. Obtain CT angiogram of the chest
    B. Obtain chromosomal karyotype
    C. Obtain TSH and T4
    D. Obtain CT angiogram of head
    E. No need for further testing

34. A 7-year-old female with Turner syndrome (45 XO) was referred by her primary care provider. She had an echocardiogram at birth that showed a normal aortic valve with three cusps, normal dimensions of the aorta, and no evidence of coarctation of the aorta. She has reassuring cardiovascular physical examination with no radiofemoral delay and normal blood pressure. Which of the following is the most appropriate management plan?

    A. No further testing is necessary considering normal echocardiogram at birth and reassuring physical examination
    B. Obtain an echocardiogram despite reassuring physical examination
    C. CT scan of the aorta should be obtained for cross-sectional imaging
    D. MRI should be obtained for cross-sectional imaging
    E. Patient can be discharged from Pediatric Cardiology follow-up

35. A 12-year-old previously healthy male is referred to you for a murmur. On examination he has a grade 2/6 systolic ejection murmur with an ejection systolic click. An echocardiogram was obtained that revealed a bicuspid aortic valve with mild stenosis and no regurgitation. Which of the following is TRUE regarding further management?

    A. All first-degree relatives should be evaluated by cardiology for a physical examination
    B. All first-degree relatives should have an echocardiogram regardless of normal physical examination
    C. Obtain genetic testing panel for bicuspid aortic valve
    D. Follow-up echocardiogram should be obtained in 5 years
    E. None of the above

CHAPTER 13

36. Which of the following morphologic forms of the hypertrophic cardiomyopathy (HCM) has the highest yield of genetic testing?

    A. Reverse curve
    B. Neutral
    C. Apical
    D. Sigmoid
    E. Concentric

37. You are seeing a 38-year-old male with a history of type A aortic dissection. On physical examination, you observe a bifid uvula. Which of the following genetic mutations is most likely in this patient?

    A. FBN1
    B. TGFBR1
    C. COL3A1
    D. ACTA2
    E. KCNQ1

38. A 14-year-old patient is referred for tall stature, high-arched palate, ectopia lentis with downward displaced lens, pectus deformity, and intellectual disability. He also has a history of recurrent thromboembolism but has a normal echocardiogram. Which of the following is the best test to arrive at a diagnosis for this patient?

    A. Measurement of homocysteine levels
    B. Alpha-galactosidase enzyme measurement
    C. Chromosomal microarray
    D. Brain MRI
    E. Measurement of frataxin level

39. A female patient with catecholaminergic polymorphic ventricular tachycardia (CPVT) is known to have a pathogenic mutation in the RYR2 gene. She wonders what would be the best way to evaluate her 9-year-old asymptomatic daughter. Which of the following is the best recommendation?

    A. 12-lead electrocardiogram
    B. Arrhythmia gene panel
    C. Site-specific analysis of RYR2
    D. No testing until adulthood
    E. Cardiac MRI

40. You are asked to consult on a newborn baby boy with tetralogy of Fallot. He is also found to have unilateral cleft lip and palate, choanal atresia, profound bilateral deafness, and micropenis. Ophthalmology is asked to consult. What ocular finding is most likely to be identified on further examination?

    A. Coloboma
    B. Ectopia lentis
    C. Corneal clouding
    D. Cherry-red spot
    E. Anophthalmia

41. A woman with Danon disease secondary to a pathogenic lysosome-associated membrane protein 2 (LAMP2) mutation recently gave birth to a baby boy. Genetic testing performed on cord blood reveals the familial pathogenic LAMP2 mutation. When discussing this diagnosis with your patient, you tell them that the most common cardiac abnormality in this condition is:

    A. Hypertrophic cardiomyopathy
    B. Arrhythmogenic right ventricular cardiomyopathy
    C. Ventricular septal defect
    D. Tetralogy of Fallot
    E. Atrial septal defect

42. A 28-year-old female presents after a history of uterine rupture during pregnancy. Family history is significant for the patient's mother who died suddenly at the age of 35 but did not have an autopsy. On examination, hypermobility and thin skin is noted. Which of the following is the most likely diagnosis?

    A. Marfan syndrome
    B. Long QT syndrome
    C. Ehlers–Danlos syndrome, vascular type
    D. Ehlers–Danlos syndrome, hypermobile type
    E. CHARGE syndrome

43. A 30-year-old female presents with pulmonary arteriovenous malformations (AVMs) and a history of recurrent epistaxis. Upon review of her history, she reports her father had pulmonary AVMs and history of early-onset colon cancer requiring total colectomy at age 28. She was found to have a familial pathogenic SMAD4 mutation. Which of the following is the likely diagnosis?

    A. Hepatic cirrhosis
    B. Hereditary hemorrhagic telangiectasia
    C. Thalassemia
    D. Large ventricular septal defect
    E. Klippel–Trenaunay syndrome

Answers

1. (C) The condition in this family is Barth syndrome which is an X-linked recessive condition that mainly affects males and causes syndromic left ventricular noncompaction, intellectual disability, and hypotonia. In the current case, 2-year-old male has Barth syndrome and his maternal uncle also had Barth syndrome, suggesting mother is a carrier of the disease. Therefore, likelihood the fetus is affected is based on the likelihood the mother (an obligate carrier) passes on the mutation (50%) multiplied by the likelihood that the fetus is male (50%), so 25% or ¼. Therefore, a carrier mother in X-linked disorders has a 25% chance of having an unaffected son, unaffected daughter, unaffected daughter who also is a carrier, and an affected son **(Figure 13.2).**

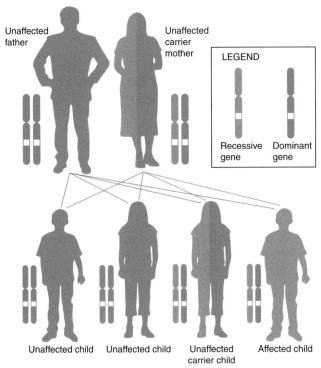

FIGURE 13.2 Pattern of inheritance in an X-linked recessive trait from unaffected carrier mother. (© Mayo Clinic Foundation)

2. (B) Homozygous pathogenic mutations in the DNAJC19 gene are associated with 3-methylglutaconic aciduria, type V which leads to dilated cardiomyopathy with ataxia (DCMA) syndrome. Since it is a homozygous condition, an affected individual has to inherit the identical mutant allele from both their biological mother and their biological father. In the current case as there is no other family history of cardiac disease other than his two siblings, it suggests that their biological mother and father are both carriers of the disease. There are four possibilities of inheritance if you do not know the patient's health status: 25% noncarrier, 50% carrier, 25% affected. Since the patient has a normal echo and the family history is consistent with infantile onset dilated cardiomyopathy which should have manifested by this age, there is 1/3 (33.3%) chance that he is a noncarrier and a 2/3 (66.7%) chance that he is a carrier.

3. (B) Autosomal recessive is the most likely answer considering the presence of affected siblings but no other affected family members. Autosomal dominant is less likely due to the unaffected status of parents; X-linked recessive is unlikely since a female is affected; de novo is unlikely given multiple affected siblings; and mitochondrial genes are maternally inherited which is unlikely due to unaffected status of mother.

4. (E) Variants of uncertain significance are inconclusive findings with genetic testing and should not be used to quote recurrence risk unless additional evidence reclassifies the variant to likely pathogenic or pathogenic.

5. (D) MELAS is a condition caused by mutations in the mitochondrial gene MT-TL1. Mitochondria are maternally inherited so only females can pass on the mitochondrial mutations to their children. Given the patient is a male, there is 0% likelihood his daughter inherited his mitochondria and thus, MELAS.

6. (C) Jervell and Lange-Nielsen syndrome is caused by biallelic mutations in the KCNQ1 gene. Heterozygous mutation in this gene cause Long QT Syndrome, so both of the patient's parents would be at risk for the manifestations of long QT syndrome. Siblings of the patient would have a 25% chance of also having Jervell and Lange-Nielsen; the patient's parents would be at risk for long QT syndrome. Autosomal recessive conditions, like Jervell and Lange-Nielsen, are rarely de novo due to the requirement of biallelic pathogenic mutation.

7. (D) HCM is typically inherited in an autosomal dominant fashion. This is evident in this family based on the presence of multiple affected individuals spanning multiple generations. X-linked recessive can be ruled out due to the presence of male-to-male transmission; autosomal recessive is unlikely given multiple affected generations; and autosomal dominant with full penetrance is less likely given the patient's father is unaffected. A person with an autosomal dominant disorder with full penetrance has a 50% chance of passing on the disease to a child **(Figure 13.3).**

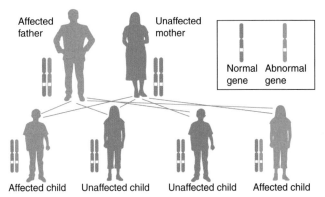

FIGURE 13.3 Pattern of inheritance in an autosomal dominant trait with full penetrance from affected father. (© Mayo Clinic Foundation)

8. (C) This child has Williams syndrome. Of patients with Williams syndrome, 90% have a deletion identifiable at chromosome 7q11. This may not be readily identifiable on routine karyotype but can be seen on FISH or microarray testing. Deletions on chromosome 11q23 cause Jacobsen syndrome. Deletions on chromosome 22q11.2 cause the constellation of disorders including DiGeorge syndrome and velocardiofacial syndrome. Both 1p36 and 8p23.1 are lesser recognized deletion syndromes that may result in patients with congenital heart disease.

9. (C) Holt–Oram syndrome is an autosomal dominant disorder caused by mutations of the *TBX5* gene. Patients most often present with abnormalities of the carpal bones of the wrist, which can include a malformed or missing thumb. Around 75% of patients have cardiac manifestations, the most common form being atrial septal defects.

10. (C) Patients with DiGeorge syndrome have an increased risk of conotruncal abnormalities compared to the other syndromes listed, particularly interrupted aortic arch and truncus arteriosus. The most common type of interrupted aortic arch in these patients is the type B interruption, between the second carotid and the ipsilateral subclavian artery.

11. (C) The patient has cri-du-chat syndrome (5p– syndrome) which is caused by deletion of part of the short arm of chromosome 5. Children with cri-du-chat syndrome have microcephaly, round face, hypertelorism, micrognathia, epicanthal folds, low-set ears, hypotonia, and severe psychomotor and mental retardation. One of the characteristic features is a high-pitched cat like cry. The best form of genetic testing for assessing deletion or duplication on the chromosome is microarray or fluorescent in situ hybridization (FISH). Karyotyping is obtained in chromosomal aneuploidies like Down syndrome or Turner syndrome. While Mendelian gene disorders like Noonan syndrome (PTPN1) may require single testing gene, gene panels, or even expanded whole exome sequencing.

12. (C) The vignette is describing a patient with LEOPARD syndrome, characterized by (L) lentigines, (E) electrocardiographic conduction defects, (O) ocular hypertelorism, (P) pulmonary stenosis, (A) abnormal genitals, (R) retarded growth with subsequent short stature, and (D) deafness. LEOPARD syndrome is an autosomal dominant disorder and overlaps in many features with Noonan syndrome. Similar to Noonan syndrome, mutations in PTPN11 and RAF1 have been implicated in LEOPARD syndrome.

13. (B) Kartagener syndrome is an autosomal recessive disorder including situs inversus, bronchiectasis, and immotility of cilia in the respiratory tract. As a result, these patients have poor mucociliary clearance, increasing their risk of having lower and upper respiratory infections, particularly sinusitis, bronchitis, pneumonia, and otitis. Patients with DiGeorge syndrome may have an increased risk of infection secondary to T-cell dysfunction. Wiskott–Aldrich is an X-linked disorder characterized by thrombocytopenia, eczema, and immune deficiency. Carney complex is an autosomal dominant syndrome of skin hyperpigmentation, endocrine overactivity, and myxomas of the skin and heart.

14. (A) The gene *NKX2.5* is located on chromosome 5q. Mutations in *NKX2.5* have been identified in familial cohorts of patients with atrial septal defects and conduction anomalies including heart block. Mutations in *TBX5* cause Holt–Oram syndrome, with associated large atrial septal defects and radial anomalies. Mutations in *MLL2* have been implicated in Kabuki syndrome. Mutations in *JAG1* cause Alagille syndrome. *PTNP11* is one of several genes which have been implicated in Noonan syndrome.

15. (D) The patient has Marfan syndrome, based on his enlarged aortic root/sinus of Valsalva and his systemic features. If he had a positive family history of Marfan syndrome, the aortic enlargement would be all that was needed to make a definitive diagnosis in him, even in the absence of systemic features. He should be followed with serial echocardiography for the remainder of his life (at least annually now that his aorta is dilated) and may be referred for surgery. He should have an eye examination to look for ectopia lentis. The normal extra-aortic vessels indicate that we are not likely dealing with Loeys–Dietz syndrome, though there is considerable overlap between all of the thoracic aortopathies.

16. (C) The patient has been diagnosed with congenital polyvalvular dysplasia, a valvular developmental disorder that results in thickened leaflets with significant regurgitation and prolapse. It typically involves two or more valves but can involve all four valves of the heart. This disorder most commonly occurs in patients with trisomy 18. In fact, at least 90% of patients with trisomy 18 have some form of valvular dysplasia. Many patients will have an associated ventricular septal defect or other congenital lesion.

17. (D) Patients with Turner syndrome and Noonan syndrome have a higher incidence of partial anomalous venous return. Additionally, patients with visceral heterotaxy, polysplenia, and asplenia have a high incidence of anomalous venous return.

18. (C) Friedreich ataxia is an inherited neuromuscular disorder caused by loss of function mutations in the FXN gene located on chromosome 9q13. Patients with Freidreich's ataxia have neurologic dysfunction that is generally characterized by progressive ataxia of limbs and gait. Patients with Freidreich's ataxia can also present with left ventricular hypertrophy which is generally symmetric and concentric.

19. (B) The family history is consistent with Noonan syndrome, of whom up to 85% of the patients may have congenital heart disease (most commonly pulmonary valvular stenosis, ASD, partial AV canal, coarctation, and hypertrophic cardiomyopathy). The right ventricular lift and short systolic ejection murmur suggest mild pulmonary valve stenosis, likely secondary to a thickened pulmonary valve. Noonan syndrome can affect both males and females. Bicuspid aortic valves and coarctation are common in Turner syndrome, and supravalvular pulmonary and aortic stenosis are common in Williams syndrome. Pulmonary branch stenosis is seen commonly in Alagille syndrome.

20. (A) Around 30% of patients with Turner syndrome have congenital heart disease, mostly involving the left-sided cardiac structures. Bicuspid aortic valve is the most common (15%), followed by coarctation (10%), and rarely mitral valve anomalies and hypoplastic left heart syndrome (<5%). Aortic root and ascending aorta dilatation are an issue as Turner patients get older, as there is a risk of aortic dissection and sudden death. As such, guidelines for management of patients with Turner syndrome advocate for routine screening with echocardiography, even in the absence of prior congenital heart disease.

21. (B) Alagille syndrome is an autosomal dominant disorder that presents with particular facial features including a triangular-shaped face, broad forehead, and deep-set eyes. They tend to have butterfly vertebrae, a paucity of bile ducts, and many will require liver transplantation. The most common cardiac manifestations include peripheral pulmonary stenosis and tetralogy of Fallot.

22. (C) Patients with familial dilated cardiomyopathy (DCM) due to mutations in LMNA can present with cardiac conduction disease and variable degrees of skeletal myopathy. LMNA is a gene that encodes lamin A and lamin C that are major components of the nuclear lamina. Mutations in LMNA are the most commonly identified cause of genetic DCM with prevalence of 5% to 8% among patients with familial DCM. LMNA mutations can manifest as isolated cardiomyopathy, skeletal myopathy, or both. The onset of LMNA associated DCM generally manifest with cardiac conduction disease often requiring pacemakers, supraventricular arrhythmias (atrial flutter or fibrillation), and with progressive ventricular arrhythmias.

23. (E) The clinical vignette is describing a patient with cri-du-chat syndrome (Lejeune syndrome), caused by a deletion of the short arm of chromosome 5 (5p–). The most common cardiac manifestations of cri-du-chat are VSDs, ASDs, PDAs, and tetralogy of Fallot.

24. (D) Ellis–van Creveld syndrome occurs most commonly among the Pennsylvania Amish community and includes skeletal and ectodermal dysplasias, including short stature, short limbs, hypoplastic or dysplastic fingernails, postaxial polydactyly, and neonatal or small teeth. It is caused by mutations in the *EVC* and *EVC2* genes on chromosome 4. Over half of these patients have congenital heart disease, of whom most have a large atrial septal defect or common atrium.

25. (E) While most patients with tetralogy of Fallot do not have an identifiable genetic cause, 22q11.2 is the most commonly *identified* genetic cause, occurring in 20% of patients. Most deletions are de novo, but the inheritance pattern is autosomal dominant. Up to 10% are familial, with variable expressivity and incomplete penetrance.

26. (D) SCN5A is not associated with congenital heart defects, like atrial septal defect. SCN5A-related disorders

can present with dilated cardiomyopathy, Brugada syndrome, Long QT Syndrome, and/or sudden death.

27. (D) This child has Jacobsen syndrome, characterized by distinctive facial features (wide-spaced eyes, ptosis, small ears, short stature) and thrombocytopenia. Patients have a tendency to have life-threatening hemorrhages and are often followed in hemophilia clinics. Patients with Jacobsen syndrome can have ventricular septal defects, left-sided lesions (primarily involving the mitral and aortic valve), and other forms of congenital heart disease. This syndrome has also been named the "11q23 deletion syndrome."

28. (B) Up to 95% of patients with trisomy 18 will have some form of CHD, including polyvalvular dysplasia, ventricular septal defects, outlet abnormalities (tetralogy of Fallot, double outlet right ventricle), and AV canal defects. Patients with Down syndrome have a 40% chance of having CHD. Around 25% of Turner syndrome patients will have CHD, as will 80% of patients with 22q11 deletion (DiGeorge syndrome, velocardiofacial syndrome). Patients with 5p–, or cri-du-chat syndrome, have a 20% risk of having CHD.

29. (E) At least 50% of patients with interrupted aortic arch type B have a 22q11.2 deletion, compared to 35% of patients with truncus arteriosus, 24% of patients with isolated arch anomalies, 15% of patients with tetralogy of Fallot, and 10% of patients with perimembranous VSDs. Of all patients with a 22q11.2 deletion, around 80% are estimated to have some form of congenital heart disease.

30. (E) Hunter syndrome is an X-linked disorder of metabolism of glycosaminoglycan due to deficiency of iduronate-2-sulfatase which is a lysosomal enzyme. Patients generally present around 2 to 4 years of age. Physical examination is consistent with coarse facial features, enlarged tongue leading to respiratory obstruction, hepatosplenomegaly, joint stiffness, and skeletal abnormalities. The most common cardiovascular finding in patients with Hunter syndrome is valve disease, generally left-sided valves, due to the thickening of the valves as a result of deposition of heparin and dermatan sulfate. This may lead to significant mitral or aortic valve regurgitation. Other less common manifestations are left ventricular hypertrophy, cardiomyopathy, arrhythmias, and myocardial ischemia due to coronary artery disease as a result of deposition and conduction disease.

31. (D) Almost half of the children born with Down syndrome have a congenital heart disease (CHD). The most common CHD associated with Down syndrome is atrioventricular septal defect (AVSD). Complete AVSD accounts for 40% of the CHD. All patients with Down syndrome require an echocardiogram due to the higher prevalence of CHD. Children with Down syndrome also have a higher risk of developing pulmonary hypertension which should be kept into account while managing complex CHDs in this group of patients. Diagnosis of Down syndrome is generally based on the characteristic phenotypic features, but diagnosis should be confirmed with a genetic test. Genetic testing for Down syndrome includes FISH which can confirm the diagnosis rapidly followed by karyotype to confirm and rule out translocation or mosaic forms of Down syndrome.

32. (E) The patient described in the question has 22q11.2 deletion syndrome. Individuals with 22q11.2 deletion syndrome can present with a wide range of clinical features including congenital heart disease (commonly ventricular septal defect, tetralogy of Fallot, interrupted aortic arch, and truncus arteriosus), palatal abnormalities, immune deficiency, learning difficulties, gastrointestinal, ophthalmologic, central nervous system, skeletal, and genitourinary anomalies. Hypocalcemia secondary to hypoparathyroidism is present in 17% to 60% of patients with 22q11.2 deletion and is generally most serious in the neonatal period. It is important to recognize hypocalcemia in the perioperative period among infants with 22q11.2 deletion undergoing surgery.

33. (B) Every female with coarctation of the aorta should undergo genetic testing for Turner syndrome (karyotype analysis) irrespective of the presence of clinical findings, due to high association of coarctation of the aorta with Turner Syndrome and the lack of overt clinical findings in girls with mosaicism. In several studies, 5.3% to 12.6% of female patients born with coarctation of the aorta had karyotype-confirmed Turner syndrome. Patients with mosaic Turner syndrome have variable phenotype and can lack classic phenotypic features of Turner syndrome; however, they generally have short stature.

34. (A) Females with Turner syndrome are at a higher risk of aortic dilation and dissection. Gravholt et al. reported aortic dissection occurring in approximately 40 per 100,000 person-years compared with 6 per 100,000 person-years in the general population, generally in patients older than 15 years of age. Therefore, in patients with Turner syndrome and normal-appearing aorta, periodic surveillance imaging is still recommended. In patients with Turner syndrome, the dimensions of aorta should be monitored in accordance with the Turner-specific z-score. American Heart Association has published a scientific statement on cardiovascular health of Turner syndrome patients that describes the suggested monitoring protocol for follow-up of patients with Turner syndrome.

35. (B) The incidence of bicuspid aortic valve among family members of a proband has been reported around 10% to 12% among various studies. Therefore American Heart Association (AHA) recommends echocardiographic screening of all the first-degree family members of a proband with bicuspid aortic valve. Generally, patients with bicuspid aortic valve are followed at variable intervals from every 1 to 3 years depending on the aortic valve function and aortic dimensions, based on the preference of the primary cardiologist. However, if there is some degree of stenosis or regurgitation, frequent follow-up may be warranted.

36. (A) The reverse curve form of the HCM has the highest yield of genetic testing among all the other morphologic forms. As estimated genetic yield in various morphologic subtypes of HCM is shown in **Figure 13.4**.

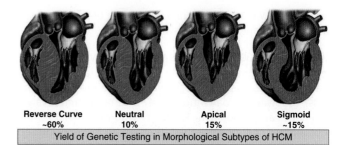

Reverse Curve ~60%	Neutral 10%	Apical 15%	Sigmoid ~15%

Yield of Genetic Testing in Morphological Subtypes of HCM

FIGURE 13.4 Morphologic subtypes of hypertrophic cardiomyopathy and their respective yield of genetic testing. HCM, hypertrophic cardiomyopathy. (Figure adapted from: O'Leary P. Hypertrophic cardiomyopathy. In: Eidem BW, Cetta F, Johnson JN, Lopez L, eds. *Echocardiography in Pediatric and Adult Congenital Heart Disease*. 3rd ed. Wolters Kluwer; 2021. Figure 23.6.)

37. (B) TGFBR1 mutation is associated with Loeys–Dietz syndrome. It is inherited in an autosomal dominant fashion; FBN1 is associated with Marfan syndrome; COL3A1 with Ehlers–Danlos syndrome, vascular type; and ACTA2 with familial thoracic aortic aneurysm and dissection (FTAAD). KCNQ1 gene is associated with long QT syndrome.

38. (A) The finding of Marfan-like features in a child with intellectual disability should raise concern for autosomal recessive homocystinuria, caused by biallelic mutations in the CBS gene. Patients with homocystinuria generally do not have progressive aortic dilation, they often have recurrent thromboembolism and the pattern of lens dislocation is generally downwards (in comparison to the Marfan syndrome where lens dislocation is generally upwards). Alpha-galactosidase deficiency can lead to Fabry disease that causes left ventricular hypertrophy, kidney disease, acroparesthesias, and other health concerns. It is not associated with aortic aneurysm or intellectual disability. Chromosomal microarray would not detect point mutations in the CBS gene, and brain MRI would not diagnose homocystinuria. Frataxin levels are obtained in patients with Friedreich's ataxia for diagnosis and monitoring of the disease.

39. (C) The best way to confirm affected status would be to genetically test for the presence of the RYR2 pathogenic mutation in the daughter. A 12-lead electrocardiogram is unlikely to detect CPVT. Ordering a comprehensive arrhythmia gene panel is not warranted given the presence of a known familial pathogenic mutation in RYR2. Moreover, CPVT can affect both children and adults so testing is warranted during childhood.

40. (A) The newborn likely has CHARGE syndrome (coloboma, heart defect, choanal atresia, retarded growth and development, genital hypoplasia, and ear anomalies) and coloboma is the most common ocular finding with this condition. Ectopia lentis is a common finding in Marfan syndrome; corneal clouding is often seen in Hurler syndrome; and cherry-red spot is a hallmark feature in Tay-Sachs disease.

41. (A) Danon disease or LAMP2 deficiency is an X-linked disorder due to mutations in the gene encoding LAMP2. It is characterized by hypertrophic cardiomyopathy, neuromuscular disease, ophthalmologic abnormalities, and variable intellectual disability.

42. (C) Uterine rupture and increased risk for sudden cardiac death secondary to arterial dissection are prominent features of Ehlers–Danlos syndrome, vascular type. Uterine rupture is less common in Marfan syndrome. Long QT syndrome can present with sudden cardiac death, but you would not expect to see connective tissue findings like uterine rupture, thin skin, and hypermobility. Ehlers–Danlos syndrome, hypermobile type, is not associated with uterine rupture or risk for arterial dissection.

43. (B) Hereditary hemorrhagic telangiectasia (HHT) or Osler–Weber–Rendu syndrome is an autosomal dominant vascular disorder. Patients with HHT may have a wide spectrum of clinical presentation including epistaxis, AVMs of the liver, lung, and central nervous system. Three major HHT genes are ENG, ACVRL1, and SMAD4 that have roles in the transforming growth factor beta (TGF-β) signaling pathway.

SUGGESTED READINGS

Silberbach M, Roos-Hesselink JW, Andersen NH, et al. Cardiovascular health in Turner syndrome: a scientific statement from the American Heart Association. *Circ Genom Precis Med.* 2018;11: e000048.

Cardiac Pharmacology

Justin M. Horner, Nathaniel W. Taggart, and Philip L. Wackel

Questions

1. An 11-year-old female is admitted to the hospital after cardiac arrest from which she was successfully defibrillated. Her baseline electrocardiogram (ECG) from 1 month earlier when she was not on any medication is shown in **Figure 14.1**. Later that evening she develops recurrent nonsustained polymorphic ventricular tachycardia. Which of the following intravenous medications may be useful in treating this patient's dysrhythmia?

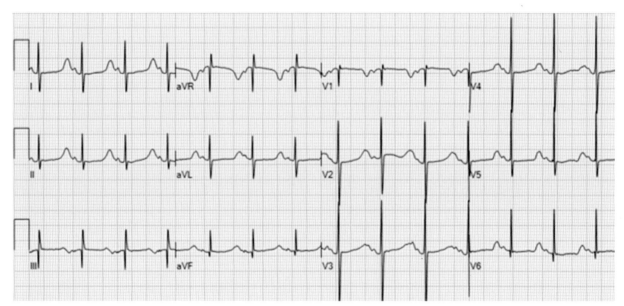

FIGURE 14.1

    A. Procainamide
    B. Magnesium sulfate
    C. Sotalol
    D. Quinidine
    E. Dofetilide

2. An 8-year-old male is diagnosed with long QT syndrome (LQTS) associated with a mutation in sodium channel gene *SCN5A* following an evaluation for unexplained syncope. His baseline QTc interval is 490 msec. He undergoes placement of an ICD/pacemaker. While in the ICU, he has frequent episodes of nonsustained polymorphic ventricular tachycardia, which are suppressed by intravenous lidocaine administration. Which of the following oral medications would be the best outpatient treatment for this patient?

   A. Quinidine
   B. Sotalol
   C. Dofetilide
   D. Procainamide
   E. Mexiletine

3. An 18-year-old man with a bileaflet aortic valve mechanical prosthesis that was placed 2 years ago is scheduled for an elective open urologic operation. He has no previous history of clots, arrhythmia, stroke, or transient ischemic attacks. On a recent echocardiogram, his left ventricular ejection fraction was 55%. Which of the following statements is most consistent with the 2020 recommendations from the American College of Cardiology for perioperative anticoagulation in this setting?

   A. Warfarin should be stopped 3 days prior to the procedure, and he should be bridged with unfractionated heparin
   B. Warfarin should be stopped 3 days prior to the procedure, and he should be bridged with subcutaneous heparin
   C. Warfarin should be stopped 3 days prior to the procedure, and he should be started on clopidogrel
   D. Warfarin should be stopped 3 days prior to the procedure, and no heparin bridging is necessary
   E. Warfarin should be stopped 3 days prior to the procedure, and he should be bridged with a direct factor Xa inhibitor such as rivaroxaban

4. A 16-year-old male with a previously repaired partial AV canal defect and cleft mitral valve undergoes mechanical bileaflet mitral valve prosthesis placement for symptomatic severe mitral valve regurgitation. His discharge echocardiogram shows a left ventricular ejection fraction of 60%. He has no history of thromboembolic events or thrombophilia. Based on the 2020 American College of Cardiology recommendations for postoperative anticoagulation, which of the following anticoagulation strategies is recommended for this patient?

   A. Warfarin only (goal INR of 2.5)
   B. Warfarin only (goal INR of 3.0)
   C. Warfarin only (goal INR of 3.5)
   D. Warfarin (goal INR of 3.0) and aspirin 325 mg
   E. Warfarin (goal INR of 2.5) and aspirin 325 mg

5. An 18-year-old woman with a history of parachute mitral valve and mechanical mitral prosthesis placement takes warfarin 4 mg/d. She has just learned that she is 14 weeks pregnant and wishes to continue with her pregnancy. Which of the following treatment options would you advise?

   A. Strongly recommend elective termination of the pregnancy
   B. Discontinue warfarin for the remainder of the pregnancy, then restart in the postpartum period
   C. Continue warfarin for the remainder of the pregnancy and through delivery
   D. Discontinue warfarin now and restart at 25 to 30 weeks gestation, treating with subcutaneous heparin in the interim
   E. Continue warfarin until 1 week prior to planned delivery, then treat with continuous intravenous heparin or LMWH

6. A 9-year-old patient with myocarditis, cardiomegaly, and reduced left ventricular systolic function develops a dry cough without other respiratory symptoms after starting oral heart failure therapy. Which of the following is the most likely mechanism of cough?

   A. Increased bradykinin
   B. Inhibition of Na^+–K^+ ATPase pump
   C. Inhibition of calcium entry into vascular smooth muscle cells
   D. Inhibition of activation of angiotensin II receptors
   E. Increased production of angiotensin II

CHAPTER 14

7. A 7-year-old well child with a recent history of palpitations is admitted to the ED with shortness of breath and tachyarrhythmia. He has no previous history of syncope or exercise-induced symptoms. His ECG is shown in **Figure 14.2**. Vagal maneuvers have failed. His blood pressure (BP) is 100/60 mm Hg. The patient has undergone electrical cardioversion three times, with transient return to sinus rhythm, after which the tachycardia recurs. Which of the following medications would be most likely to treat this patient's arrhythmia?

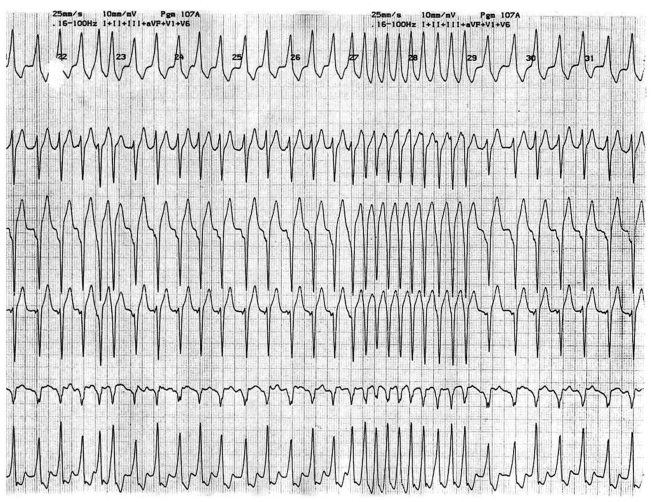

FIGURE 14.2

    A. IV adenosine
    B. IV digitalis
    C. IV amiodarone
    D. IV β-blocker
    E. IV diltiazem

8. A 10-month-old female infant presents 1 week after hospital discharge following repair of tetralogy of Fallot (TOF). Her parents describe a 3-day history of vomiting without diarrhea. She has not had a fever. Cardiac monitoring reveals the rhythm shown in **Figure 14.3**.

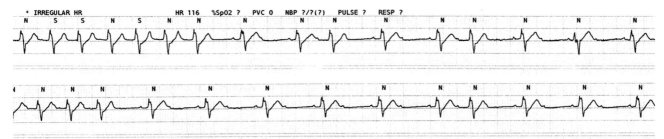

FIGURE 14.3

Which of the following medications is most likely to cause this patient's symptoms and electrocardiographic findings?

A. Digoxin
B. Propranolol
C. Furosemide
D. Amiodarone
E. Chlorothiazide

9. A 13-year-old male with a history of catecholaminergic polymorphic ventricular tachycardia (CPVT) is admitted to the ICU after an episode of syncope with exertion. In the ICU, he is noted to have frequent episodes of polymorphic ventricular tachycardia associated with hypotension. Which of the following is the best first-line antiarrhythmic therapy for this child?

A. Amiodarone
B. Lidocaine
C. β-Blocker
D. Calcium channel blocker (CCB)
E. Digoxin

10. A 13-month-old male infant referred to you for a heart murmur is diagnosed with a secundum atrial septal defect (ASD) measuring 6 mm. He was born at 38 weeks of gestation and has been thriving well without any symptoms. There is mild right heart enlargement on echocardiogram, and right ventricular systolic pressure is estimated to be 30 mm Hg. His mother is concerned about RSV and wants to know whether her son needs any palivizumab prophylaxis for the RSV season. Which of the following is the most appropriate answer?

A. RSV prophylaxis is not indicated, because he is over 1 year old
B. RSV prophylaxis is recommended for him until he is 2 years old
C. His heart disease does not qualify him for RSV prophylaxis
D. RSV prophylaxis would only be recommended if he had a prior history of RSV infection
E. RSV prophylaxis would be recommended for him if he were exposed to cigarette smoke at home

11. You are evaluating a 3-month-old female infant in the outpatient pediatric cardiology clinic. She was diagnosed with double-outlet right ventricle with normally related great arteries. She is receiving concentrated feedings (24 kcal/oz) and 1 mg/kg furosemide twice daily. She is growing well with mild tachypnea at rest. Her resting oxygen saturation is 94%. Surgery is scheduled in early December, one month away. Her mother wants to know whether palivizumab would be helpful during the current RSV season. Which of the following is the most appropriate response to her question?

A. Palivizumab prophylaxis has been shown to reduce the risk of RSV infection and is therefore beneficial
B. Palivizumab prophylaxis has been shown to reduce mortality rate from RSV in patients with congenital heart disease and therefore is recommended
C. Palivizumab would protect her from most viral infections including influenza A and B
D. Palivizumab would likely decrease her risk of hospitalization due to RSV and therefore is recommended
E. Palivizumab is not recommended in infants under 6 months of age

12. A 5-month-old female infant with dilated cardiomyopathy is started on furosemide. This medication acts by inhibiting which of the following ion channels?

A. Na^+–$2Cl^-$–K^+ cotransporter in the loop of Henle
B. Na^+–Cl^- cotransporter in the proximal tubule
C. Na^+–K^+ ATPase pump in the distal tubule
D. Na^+–H^+ cotransporter in the loop of Henle
E. Na^+–Ca^{2+} cotransporter in the proximal tubule

13. A 17-year-old previously healthy female presents to the ED with a 2-day history of chest pain. Her ECG shows diffuse ST-segment elevation and PR-segment depression suggestive of pericarditis. Echocardiogram shows normal biventricular size and function with a small pericardial effusion. There is no history of recent fever, rash, sore throat, or joint pains. Which of the following is the best treatment option for this patient?

A. Aspirin 325 mg four times/d for 4 weeks

B. Prednisone 1 mg/kg/d followed by tapering after 2 weeks once the patient is asymptomatic

C. Colchicine therapy for 4 to 6 days

D. Ibuprofen 600 to 800 mg three times a day for 7 to 10 days

E. Clopidogrel 75 mg daily for 2 weeks

14. A 5-day-old neonate with hypoplastic left heart syndrome is being cared for in the cardiac ICU 2 days after a Norwood operation with right modified Blalock–Taussig shunt. Arterial blood gas (on $FiO_2 = 21\%$) shows a pH of 7.2. PO_2 is 42 mm Hg, PCO_2 is 45 mm Hg, SpO_2 is 80%, and hemoglobin is 14 g/dL. Near-infrared spectroscopy (NIRS) probes consistently show saturations in the 40% range. ECG shows sinus tachycardia with a heart rate of 180 bpm. Arterial BP is 78/58 mm Hg. Chest x-ray shows no evidence of pulmonary congestion or significant infiltrates and lung fields are well expanded. The patient is on milrinone 0.4 mcg/kg/min and norepinephrine 1 mcg/kg/min. Urine output over the past 6 hours has averaged 1 cc/kg/hr. Limited bedside echo shows no significant pericardial effusion. The patient just received two 10 mL/kg boluses of normal saline. Which of the following interventions is most likely to benefit this patient?

A. IV furosemide

B. Decrease norepinephrine infusion rate

C. IV β-blocker therapy

D. Decrease milrinone infusion rate

E. Increasing the inspired FiO_2 concentration

15. A 10-month-old infant is treated for Kawasaki disease (KD) with intravenous immunoglobulin (IVIG) and aspirin. Which of the following statements regarding use of steroids in KD is most accurate?

A. A 24-hour single dose of IV steroid may be considered in addition to IVIG as primary therapy

B. Oral steroids may be used instead of aspirin if the patient remains afebrile but shows persistent elevation of acute inflammatory markers (ESR, CRP)

C. Steroids are contraindicated in Kawasaki patients

D. IV steroids may be used instead of IVIG in an uncomplicated patient

E. IV steroids may be considered if the patient has persistent or recrudescent fever after initial treatment with ASA and at least one dose of IVIG

16. A 7-year-old female whose parents recently emigrated from Mexico is diagnosed with acute rheumatic fever (RF). She complains of mild chest pain, but no shortness of breath. Cardiac examination reveals normal S_1 and S_2, with a soft holosystolic murmur at the apex. Neck veins do not appear to be distended. Abdominal examination shows no organomegaly. Echocardiogram shows small pericardial effusion, mild to moderate mitral valve regurgitation, mild aortic valve regurgitation, mildly dilated left ventricle with an ejection fraction of 60%. Which of the following treatment regimens should be initiated in the above patient?

A. IV steroids

B. Oral steroids

C. High-dose aspirin

D. β-Blocker therapy

E. IVIG + aspirin

17. Which of the following statements is true regarding immunosuppressive medications used in patients following heart transplantation?

A. Sirolimus is a calcineurin inhibitor

B. Tacrolimus is not available for intravenous use

C. Sirolimus acts by blocking gene transcription

D. Tacrolimus has been associated with improved survival over cyclosporine

E. Sirolimus is less nephrotoxic than cyclosporine

18. A 7-year-old female who was appropriately treated for her first episode of rheumatic fever (RF) with mild carditis is followed up at 3 months, 6 months, and then at 1 year. Serial follow-up echocardiograms show no residual pericardial effusion, trivial mitral valve regurgitation, no aortic valve regurgitation, normal left ventricular chamber size, and function. She is maintained on RF antibiotic prophylaxis and continues to remain asymptomatic without any recurrence of streptococcal sore throat. If there is no echocardiographic evidence of worsening ventricular or valvular function, which of the following is the best recommendation for ongoing secondary antibiotic prophylaxis?

A. Antibiotic prophylaxis should be continued for 5 years

B. Antibiotic prophylaxis should be continued for 10 years

C. Antibiotic prophylaxis should be continued until she is 21 years of age

D. Antibiotic prophylaxis should be continued until she is 40 years of age

E. She will need lifelong antibiotic prophylaxis

19. According to the 2007 AHA/ACC guidelines, infective endocarditis (IE) prophylaxis is recommended in which of the following clinical scenarios?

    A. A 7-year-old patient who has undergone cardiac transplantation 18 months ago with trivial tricuspid valve regurgitation prior to dental extraction

    B. An 8-year-old patient who has undergone device closure of ASD 4 months ago with residual shunt at the site of prosthetic device who is scheduled to undergo an upper gastrointestinal endoscopy

    C. A 9-year-old patient with TOF who underwent complete repair at 6 months of age and has an RV to PA conduit and is scheduled to have dental brace placement

    D. An 8-year-old patient with prosthetic mitral valve with previous history of IE who is scheduled for an outpatient cystoscopy

    E. A 12-year-old patient who has undergone percutaneous PDA closure 4 months ago who needs a root canal

20. A 14-year-old male is referred to your clinic for management of elevated LDL cholesterol. Six and seven months ago his LDL level was 196 mg/dL and 190 mg/dL, respectively, and he was advised appropriate dietary intervention and weight reduction regimen. At present his LDL level is 202 mg/dL, HDL is 38 mg/dL, and triglycerides are 120 mg/dL. His BMI is 31 kg/m^2 and his TSH level is normal. He has been compliant with his diet and exercise program and has lost 3 kg over the past year. He was adopted and therefore family history is not well known. Which of the following statements is most accurate?

    A. Continued dietary intervention alone will likely significantly reduce his LDL level over the next 6 months

    B. Oral statin therapy should be strongly considered

    C. Oral niacin therapy is the best first-line option due to its side effect profile

    D. Fibric acid derivatives should be considered

    E. If drug therapy is considered, bile acid–binding resins would be the first-line therapy given their favorable safety and side effect profile

21. A 16-year-old male recently diagnosed with hypertrophic cardiomyopathy (HCM) presents for evaluation. No other associated medical conditions are present. Medications include multivitamins. He is asymptomatic at rest but complains of shortness of breath with exertion. There is no history of syncope/presyncope or family history of HCM or sudden death. His resting HR is 80 bpm and BP is 130/80 mm Hg. His echocardiogram shows a septal thickness of 26 mm, ejection fraction = 70%, left ventricular outflow tract maximum instantaneous gradient 60 mm Hg. Cardiac MRI shows no late gadolinium enhancement. Recent Holter report showed frequent single PVCs, but no sustained tachycardia. On the basis of the above information, which of the following is the best initial treatment for this patient?

    A. ICD placement
    B. Digoxin
    C. Furosemide
    D. β-Blocker
    E. Nifedipine

22. Which of the following medications used in heart transplant recipients can inhibit smooth muscle proliferation and may have the advantage of inhibiting coronary allograft vasculopathy?

    A. Methylprednisolone
    B. Sirolimus
    C. Antithymocyte globulin (ATG)
    D. Cyclosporine
    E. Tacrolimus

23. A 19-year-old male with d-transposition of the great arteries who is status post arterial switch operation as an infant is known to have LV systolic dysfunction and is currently taking carvedilol, enalapril, and digoxin. You are seeing him in the ICU after he was admitted overnight for treatment of ventricular tachycardia. He is no longer having VT, but on examination, he has tremors and slurred speech. Which of the following is the most likely treatment he received for ventricular tachycardia?

    A. Esmolol
    B. Amiodarone
    C. Lidocaine
    D. Adenosine
    E. Digoxin

24. A 5-year-old female with idiopathic dilated cardiomyopathy undergoes induction with rabbit antithymocyte globulin (ATG) prior to orthotopic cardiac transplantation. Which of the following side effects of ATG is most common?

    A. Fever
    B. Rash
    C. Abdominal pain
    D. Hyperkalemia
    E. Myalgia

CHAPTER **14**

25. A 15-year-old male presents to the ER with fast heart rate (HR) and some shortness of breath. His ECG shows a regular narrow QRS tachycardia (HR 235 bpm) without discernible P waves. He was discharged 24 hours ago from the hospital following management of asthma exacerbation and received treatment in the intensive care unit. Vagal maneuvers have failed to bring down his HR. Which of the following statements regarding adenosine is true?

    A. Adenosine should be slowly pushed to avoid bronchospasm
    B. If bronchospasm results, it will only last several seconds, then resolve
    C. Patients who have undergone orthotopic heart transplant are less responsive to adenosine
    D. Transient hypertension may result from adenosine administration
    E. Flushing of the face is a common side effect

26. A 13-year-old female is newly diagnosed with idiopathic pulmonary arterial hypertension. She experiences shortness of breath at rest and has severe right ventricular enlargement with severe dysfunction. She is started on IV treprostinil, oral sildenafil, and ambrisentan. Which of the following is the correct statement among the following regarding her pharmacologic treatment?

    A. Ambrisentan is an endothelin A receptor agonist
    B. Treprostinil is a prostaglandin (PGE2) analogue
    C. Ambrisentan does not affect cytochrome P450 enzyme activity
    D. Sildenafil is a phosphodiesterase 3 inhibitor
    E. Epoprostenol would be favored over treprostinil due to its longer half-life

27. A 16-year-old male is evaluated by his cardiologist following a recent episode of unexplained syncope. His resting ECG and echocardiogram are normal, and the history is not typical for vasovagal syncope. His father is an immigrant from Southeast Asia and was diagnosed with Brugada syndrome 1 year ago. Which of the following tests would be helpful in making a definitive diagnosis in this patient?

    A. Epinephrine challenge test
    B. Cardiac MRI
    C. Isoproterenol provocative test
    D. Provocative testing with procainamide
    E. Exercise test

28. A 10-year-old female with known LQTS type 1 presents with status epilepticus to the emergency department. She is on oral nadolol therapy. Her ECG shows sinus rhythm (120 bpm) and her resting QT interval is 500 msec. The ER doctor prepares to administer IV phenytoin and consults the cardiologist regarding the safety of phenytoin use in the patient. Which of the following statements is accurate with regard to the current patient scenario?

    A. Phenytoin can prolong the QT interval and is therefore not safe in the patient
    B. Patient should be started on IV amiodarone before starting phenytoin
    C. Intravenous β-blocker can be administered concurrently with phenytoin drip
    D. Phenytoin has cardiac effects similar to mexiletine
    E. Phenytoin blocks cardiac potassium channels

29. An 18-year-old female patient with a history of repaired Ebstein anomaly is admitted to the ER with shortness of breath and tachycardia (HR of 150 bpm). She is found to be in atrial flutter with variable conduction on ECG evaluation. She is hemodynamically stable. An echocardiogram done 1 year ago showed normal left ventricular function with mild right ventricular dysfunction. Which of the following options is most appropriate in the immediate management of the patient?

    A. Flecainide
    B. Diltiazem
    C. Disopyramide
    D. Urgent electrical cardioversion
    E. Labetalol

30. You are caring for a 24-year-old female with tetralogy of Fallot status post repair using a valve-sparing technique. She is known to have renal dysfunction with a creatinine clearance of 50 mL/min, but she has never required dialysis. Which of the following medications requires dose adjustment for renal impairment?

    A. Adenosine
    B. Sotalol
    C. Amiodarone
    D. Warfarin
    E. Mexiletine

31. A newborn baby is noted to be bradycardic with an HR of 40 bpm. An ECG shows complete AV block. Infusion of which of the following medications would be most useful to increase the HR in this scenario?

    A. Milrinone
    B. Atropine
    C. Digoxin
    D. Isoproterenol
    E. Dobutamine

32. A 15-year-old female with Marfan syndrome is admitted to the intensive care unit with acute severe mitral valve regurgitation in the setting of a flail mitral valve leaflet. She is felt to be in a low cardiac output state with pulmonary edema. Heart rate is 120 bpm; blood pressure is 123/78 mm Hg. Her distal extremities are cool. Ejection fraction by echocardiogram is 70%. Which of the following medications would be most helpful in improving her cardiac output acutely prior to surgery?

    A. Nitroprusside infusion
    B. Intravenous Lasix
    C. Vasopressin infusion
    D. Intravenous digoxin
    E. Dopamine infusion

33. A 3-month-old child with unrepaired tetralogy of Fallot is referred to the ER by his pediatrician because his oxygen saturation during a well-child visit was only 62%. On examination, the patient is cyanotic but alert. His parents note that he has been less active for the past few days. His HR is 180 bpm, SpO$_2$ is 55% to 60%, respiratory rate is 40/min, and BP is 88/50 mm Hg. The lungs are clear on auscultation and a grade 3/6 harsh systolic ejection murmur is heard over the precordium. He is not on any medications. His lab work done at his pediatrician's office is available: Na 142, K 3.8, chloride 105, bicarbonate 26, BUN 15, creatinine 0.6, hematocrit 26, WBC 9,000, platelet count 350,000. Which of the following therapies can be expected to improve the patient's condition?

    A. Intravenous propranolol
    B. Phenylephrine infusion
    C. Packed red blood cell transfusion
    D. Morphine administration
    E. Intravenous furosemide

34. A 2-day-old child with hypoplastic left heart syndrome is started on prostaglandin E1 (PGE1). The parents have opted for a cardiac transplantation for the child and the cardiology team has decided to maintain him on PGE1 until a donor heart becomes available for transplantation. Which of the following statements is true with regard to the side effects of PGE1?

    A. Assisted ventilation may be necessary because of primary hypoxia
    B. Hypothermia is a potential side effect
    C. Patient needs to be monitored for hypertension
    D. Seizures are not associated with the administration of PGE1
    E. Cutaneous vasodilation and edema can develop as a side effect

35. Which of the following drugs used in the treatment of Marfan syndrome blocks TGF-β signaling?

    A. Losartan
    B. Propranolol
    C. Enalapril
    D. Verapamil
    E. Spironolactone

36. An 18-year-old man with dilated cardiomyopathy and LVEF of 30% comes for an outpatient evaluation to establish care. He has a chronically elevated potassium and is currently on no medications. Which of the following medications would be the best initial choice for CHF therapy?

    A. Eplerenone
    B. Spironolactone
    C. Captopril
    D. Carvedilol
    E. Enalapril

37. A 16-year-old patient who received a cardiac transplantation 10 years ago is managed as an outpatient. His LVEF has been in the 25% range for the past 1 year, and he is thought to have advanced coronary allograft vasculopathy. A 24-hour ECG monitor shows repeated episodes of atrial flutter. He is currently on the following oral medications: carvedilol, atenolol, spironolactone, digoxin, enalapril, warfarin, cyclosporine, oral steroids. The treating cardiologist elects to start him on amiodarone. Which of the following statements is correct with respect to drug interactions in the setting of amiodarone therapy?

    A. Digoxin dose does not need to be adjusted when adding amiodarone
    B. Enhanced AV nodal conduction can occur and can result in rapid ventricular response in the setting of atrial arrhythmias
    C. Cyclosporine levels may be elevated after beginning amiodarone
    D. INR should be checked periodically as it may become subtherapeutic
    E. Steroid dose should be decreased after adding amiodarone

38. Which of the following statements is true regarding the antiarrhythmic action of amiodarone?

    A. It shortens the QTc interval
    B. It produces some degree of calcium channel blockade
    C. It activates cardiac sodium channels
    D. It has vagolytic effects
    E. Presence of hypokalemia reduces its proarrhythmic potential

39. An 11-year-old female who received a heart transplant 10 years ago is maintained on tacrolimus, prednisone, and sirolimus. Which of the following statements is true with regard to associated side effects?

    A. The use of sirolimus is not associated with bone marrow suppression
    B. Lipid abnormalities typically do not develop until adolescence
    C. Tacrolimus is more commonly associated with the development of diabetes mellitus than cyclosporine
    D. Thiazides are the first-line antihypertensive agents in heart transplant recipients
    E. Sirolimus is more nephrotoxic than cyclosporine and tacrolimus

40. Which of the following drugs lowers pulmonary vascular resistance (PVR)?

    A. Nitrous oxide
    B. Ketamine
    C. Prostacyclin
    D. Dopamine
    E. Norepinephrine

41. A 4-year-old female who underwent a nonfenestrated Fontan procedure 6 days ago develops acute arterial thrombosis of her right great toe. An emergency echocardiogram shows normal systemic ventricular function without any thrombus and a patent Fontan pathway. She is receiving heparin 10 units/kg/hr through a central catheter in her internal jugular vein. She is currently on aspirin 81 mg/d, milrinone, and furosemide. She has been receiving frequent doses of fentanyl for severe pain. CBC today shows a hemoglobin of 12.8, white blood cell count of 12,000, and a platelet count of 60,000. Two days prior, her platelet count was 300,000. There is no evidence of any bleeding. The intensivist orders additional tests to clarify the diagnosis. Which of the following is most likely responsible for her drop in platelets?

    A. Milrinone
    B. Furosemide
    C. Aspirin
    D. Heparin
    E. Fentanyl

42. Which of the following medications is correctly listed with its teratogenic effect?

    A. Lithium: left-sided obstructive lesions
    B. Amiodarone: permanent fetal complete heart block
    C. Warfarin: defects in central nervous system
    D. ACE inhibitors: right-sided obstructive lesions
    E. High-dose folic acid: neural tube defects

43. An 18-year-old male patient with a history of TOF that was repaired 13 years ago presents to the emergency room with vomiting and complaints of visual disturbances (flashing lights and halos) and feeling dizzy. He has a history of underlying mild renal dysfunction. He was recently diagnosed with infectious mononucleosis. His oral intake has been reduced for the past few days, but he has been taking his digoxin, furosemide, and aspirin regularly. His HR is 40 bpm, respiratory rate is 18 breaths per minute, SpO_2 is 98%, and BP is 85/40 mm Hg. ECG shows underlying sinus rhythm, right bundle branch block with no evidence of peaked T waves, 3:1 AV block, ventricular bigeminy, and frequent three to four beat runs of premature ventricular contractions. Which of the following is the most likely to reveal the source of his symptoms?

    A. Serum potassium level
    B. Liver function tests
    C. B-type natriuretic peptide (BNP) level
    D. Aspirin level
    E. Digoxin level

44. A 6-year-old female is 2 days post repair of coarctation of aorta and subaortic membrane resection. She is intubated and appears comfortable on the ventilator (FiO_2 40%). She is noted to have persistently elevated BP (190 to 200/100 to 110 mm Hg) despite use of intravenous fentanyl and furosemide. Her HR is 100 bpm and SpO_2 is 90%. Chest x-ray shows some atelectasis in both lung fields. Her morning labs are as follows: hemoglobin 8.5, WBC 9,000, platelets 150,000, BUN 38, creatinine 1.9, ALT 250, AST 300. Her outpatient medications include the following: methylphenidate, albuterol prn, fluticasone/salmeterol twice daily, and montelukast daily. Which of the following treatment options would be best for this patient?

    A. Inhaled nitric oxide therapy
    B. Intravenous nicardipine
    C. Intravenous labetalol
    D. Sodium nitroprusside infusion
    E. Dexmedetomidine infusion

45. A 6-year-old male undergoes percutaneous pulmonary valvotomy for valvular pulmonary stenosis. His baseline SpO$_2$ is 98% on room air. His preprocedure echocardiogram had demonstrated a mean gradient of 55 mm Hg across the valve, right ventricular hypertrophy with normal systolic function, patent foramen ovale, normal branch pulmonary arteries, and normal left ventricular chamber size/systolic function. Following his procedure in the catheterization laboratory, his peak-to-peak gradient decreased from 80 to 30 mm Hg and SpO$_2$ was 95% (room air). Three hours later he is noted to be desaturating with SpO$_2$ in the 80s on room air and with poor peripheral perfusion. Which of the following treatment options would be most helpful in this patient?

    A. Inhaled nitric oxide therapy
    B. Milrinone therapy
    C. Phenylephrine therapy
    D. Intravenous β-blocker
    E. Intravenous furosemide

46. A 14-year-old patient on a statin to lower his cholesterol presents with fatigue, back pain, and soreness in the arms and legs. Which of the following lab values is most likely to reveal the etiology?

    A. Serum potassium level
    B. Creatine kinase level
    C. Serum creatinine
    D. Serum cholesterol level
    E. Complete blood count

47. A 1-week-old female infant is in the neonatal intensive care unit awaiting surgical palliation for tricuspid atresia with normally related great arteries and severe pulmonary stenosis. She is on prostaglandin to maintain ductal patency. Her oxygen saturations are 88% on room air and her lactate level is 0.6. The child is transported to the interventional radiology suite to have a peripherally inserted central catheter (PICC) line placed. Which of the following anesthetic induction regimens carries the highest risk of cardiopulmonary compromise in this patient?

    A. Inhalational anesthetic agent and ketamine
    B. Inhalational anesthetic agent and midazolam
    C. Ketamine and midazolam
    D. Midazolam and fentanyl
    E. Fentanyl and ketamine

48. A 3-year-old male presents to your office after receiving care in the ER for an episode of documented SVT the week prior. His baseline ECG demonstrates ventricular preexcitation. You decided to start him on β-blocker therapy to prevent further episodes of SVT. His parents have questions about a β-blocker potentially affecting his sleep and the possibility of worsening wheezing with occasional viral respiratory infections. Which of the following medications should have the least potential for CNS side effect and bronchoconstriction?

    A. Metoprolol
    B. Nadolol
    C. Propranolol
    D. Atenolol
    E. Sotalol

49. A 17-year-old male with a history of coarctation of the aorta status post repair at 12 years of age presents to the emergency department via ambulance after overdosing on his blood pressure medications at home. His heart rate is 35 bpm, blood pressure is 92/60 mm Hg. Blood glucose concentration is 65 mg/dL. Which of the following medications should be administered first?

    A. Glucagon
    B. Epinephrine
    C. Hydralazine
    D. Atropine
    E. Vasopressin

50. An 18-year-old woman with a history of mitral arcade and a remote history of atrial flutter has a tilting disc mechanical prosthesis. She is being treated with warfarin, and her INR level had been therapeutic (2.5 to 3.5) over the previous 2 years with minimal medication adjustment. More recently, she has required a 50% increase in her weekly warfarin dose to maintain similar INR levels. Initiation of which of the following would be most likely to produce this effect?

    A. Amiodarone
    B. Levothyroxine
    C. Propranolol
    D. Sertraline
    E. St. John's wort

51. Which of the following diuretics inhibits sodium and chloride transport in the distal convoluted tubule of the nephron?

    A. Furosemide
    B. Ethacrynic acid
    C. Spironolactone
    D. Bumetanide
    E. Chlorothiazide

52. A 3-year-old child underwent a Fontan procedure 5 days ago. Her postoperative course was complicated by bleeding and high venous pressures that warranted a return to the operating room on postop day 3 for fenestration and revision of her Fontan. She was intubated and sedated for 5 consecutive days beginning with the initial operation. After extubation, she is noticeably uncomfortable and agitated while taking shallow breaths. Which of the following would be the best approach to managing this patient's symptoms?

    A. Begin a dexmedetomidine infusion to manage her agitation and withdrawal
    B. Administer additional doses of midazolam and fentanyl to treat withdrawal
    C. Initiate fentanyl and midazolam infusions at a lower rate than that utilized while intubated
    D. Provide the patient with a hydromorphone patient-controlled analgesia (PCA) setup so that she can treat her own pain
    E. Emergent reintubation

53. An intubated 2-week-old infant post Norwood/Sano procedure for hypoplastic left heart syndrome has an aspiration event during suctioning of his endotracheal tube. His oxygen saturations precipitously decline from 85% to 40%, following which he becomes profoundly hypotensive. Which of the following medications would be immediately helpful in this situation?

    A. Vecuronium
    B. Midazolam
    C. Epinephrine 0.1 mcg/kg IV push
    D. Lidocaine 1 mg/kg
    E. Sevoflurane

54. A 5-year-old child presents with a pleural effusion 1 week after surgical intervention for Ebstein anomaly. He will require sedation for chest tube placement. Procedural sedation is planned with ketamine and midazolam. Which of the following agents is most important to have available during this procedural sedation?

    A. Propofol
    B. Fentanyl
    C. Muscle relaxant and glycopyrrolate
    D. Diazepam
    E. Epinephrine

55. A 15-year-old female with a history of moderately controlled asthma undergoes primary repair of coarctation of the aorta. On postoperative day 3, she remains hypertensive despite being on sodium nitroprusside at 8 mcg/kg/min. Her creatinine is 2.0 mg/dL and she is on a furosemide infusion to achieve adequate urine output in the setting of acute or chronic renal failure. Laboratory analysis reveals metabolic acidosis. The patient is becoming agitated and is no longer oriented to person or place. Which of the following is the most likely cause of her metabolic acidosis and altered mental status?

    A. Hypovolemia
    B. Narcotic-induced delirium
    C. Uremia
    D. Cyanide toxicity
    E. Ketoacidosis

56. A 5-day-old male infant is being treated as an inpatient for postnatal onset of AV reentrant tachycardia with propranolol. He has had a normal echocardiogram, a normal resting ECG, and is otherwise doing well. He continues to have frequent episodes of breakthrough supraventricular tachycardia and the decision is made to discontinue his propranolol and initiate flecainide therapy. Which of the following ECG changes are you most likely to observe on the day following the initiation of flecainide?

    A. ST depression
    B. QT prolongation
    C. PR shortening
    D. T-wave inversion
    E. QRS prolongation

57. An 18-year-old woman with a history of surgical repair of a secundum atrial septal defect at 3 years of age presents now with palpitations that began 3 days ago. Her BP is 112/78. On examination her rhythm is regular, she has no murmur or gallop, her lungs are clear, and she has no edema. Her ECG shows atrial flutter with 2:1 AV conduction at a ventricular rate of 150 bpm. She is then given a medication after which her ventricular rate suddenly increases to 220 bpm, and she feels lightheaded and fatigued. Which of the following medications was most likely given?

    A. Diltiazem
    B. Procainamide
    C. Lidocaine
    D. Esmolol
    E. Mexiletine

58. A 35-year-old man with d-transposition of the great arteries who underwent an atrial switch procedure as a child now presents with recurrent episodes of symptomatic intra-atrial reentrant tachycardia despite attempted catheter ablation and an adequate trial of sotalol therapy. His most recent labs include normal TSH and free T4, mildly elevated AST and ALT, BUN of 18 mg/dL, and creatinine of 0.9 mg/dL. On physical examination his rhythm is regular, there is no murmur. He has mild hepatomegaly and no peripheral edema. Echocardiogram demonstrates moderately decreased systemic right ventricular function, no significant valve dysfunction, and no evidence of baffle obstruction. Which of the following would be the best medical therapy for this patient at this time?

   A. Dofetilide
   B. Flecainide
   C. Amiodarone
   D. Metoprolol
   E. Dronedarone

59. You are considering starting dofetilide on a 25-year-old man with double-inlet left ventricle who continues to have recurrent intra-atrial reentrant tachycardia despite a surgical maze procedure and a Fontan revision. Which of the following is a contraindication to initiating dofetilide?

   A. Thyroid dysfunction
   B. Creatinine clearance of 45 mL/min
   C. Serum potassium level of 2.9 mmol/L
   D. QTc >440 msec in the presence of ventricular conduction delay
   E. Moderate systemic ventricular dysfunction

60. A 3-year-old female with ectopic atrial tachycardia has been treated with several antiarrhythmic medication combinations without sufficient control. She has been well controlled on amiodarone for the last 6 months and presents for follow-up. Which of the following adverse effects is most likely related to amiodarone therapy?

   A. Low parathyroid hormone level
   B. A rise in serum creatinine to twice normal
   C. Elevated TSH
   D. Elevated amylase and lipase
   E. Conjunctivitis

61. A 15-year-old female with a history of moderately controlled asthma undergoes primary repair of coarctation of the aorta. She has persistent hypertension after surgery. Which of the following antihypertensive agents would you avoid?

   A. Esmolol
   B. Nicardipine
   C. Clevidipine
   D. Hydralazine
   E. Lisinopril

62. A 12-year-old female with multifocal atrial tachycardia has been trialed on multiple combinations of antiarrhythmic medications in the past without good control. She has normal renal function, a normal baseline CBC, and normal liver function tests. You decide to trial her on propafenone, which works well to control her tachycardia. You obtain a CBC 1 month after starting propafenone to specifically assess for which of the following?

   A. A decreased platelet count
   B. An elevated white blood cell count
   C. A decreased red blood cell count
   D. An elevated platelet count
   E. A decreased white blood cell count

63. An 18-year-old male with a small membranous VSD that possesses a 4.1 m/sec left-to-right shunt without significant tricuspid or aortic regurgitation presents to the clinic for routine follow-up. He denies symptoms, and his echocardiogram does not reveal left heart enlargement. He inquires about the ability to participate in a drug trial to earn some extra cash. He states it is with a local drug testing company and it will be completed to assess the dosing and side effects of a medication on 50 participants. Which clinical phase trial is he describing?

   A. Phase 0
   B. Phase I
   C. Phase II
   D. Phase III
   E. Phase IV

64. A new antihypertensive medication is being developed. The preclinical testing has resulted in the data shown in **Figure 14.4** comparing five different medications, A to E.

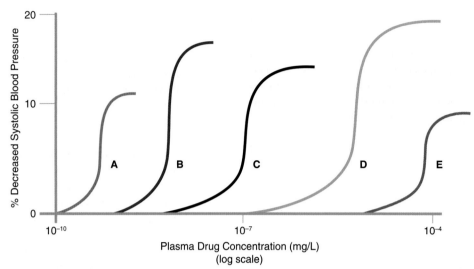

FIGURE 14.4

Which medication is the most efficacious at lowering systolic blood pressure?

A. Drug A
B. Drug B
C. Drug C
D. Drug D
E. Drug E

65. A new antihypertensive medication is being developed. The preclinical testing has resulted in the data shown in **Figure 14.5** comparing five different medications, A to E.

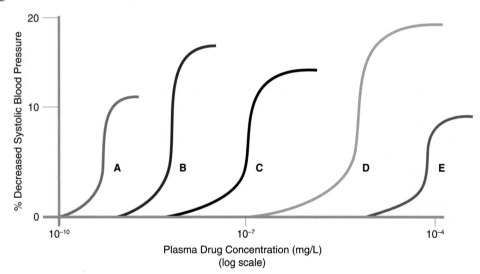

FIGURE 14.5

Which medication is the most potent?

A. Drug A
B. Drug B
C. Drug C
D. Drug D
E. Drug E

66. A 3-year-old female with a history of atrial tachycardia that is not responsive to propranolol is admitted to the hospital for initiation of flecainide. The medical student working with the team asks how long the patient will need to be in the hospital. The pediatric cardiology fellow states the patient will remain in the hospital until steady state of the medication is achieved and the medication is tolerated without reoccurrence of atrial tachycardia. How many half-lives are required for the patient to achieve steady state of flecainide?

    A. One
    B. Two
    C. Four
    D. Eight
    E. Ten

67. A 19-year-old male with a history of ASD status post device closure at the age of 5 presents for routine follow-up. He reports occasional palpitations and denies other symptoms. He is not on any medications. His echocardiogram reveals normal cardiac size and function with appropriate ASD device position and no obvious residual shunt. His ECG reveals normal sinus rhythm with normal intervals. He is just starting his second year of college and he states he has been participating in local drug trials. His last trial earned him $500, and he states it involved 1,500 participants. He reports the drug company was testing the drug "blindly" and he did not know if he got the "test drug" or the "gold standard drug." Which clinical phase trial did he participate in?

    A. Phase 0
    B. Phase I
    C. Phase II
    D. Phase III
    E. Phase IV

68. Which of the following is the mechanism of action of sildenafil?

    A. Blocks phosphodiesterase from degrading cyclic GMP in smooth muscle cells
    B. Blocks both endothelin A and B receptors
    C. Replaces the loss of endogenous prostaglandin I2
    D. Blocks calcium channels
    E. Suppresses production of prostaglandins and thromboxanes by irreversibly inactivating the cyclooxygenase enzyme

69. Which of the following best describes the mechanism of action of spironolactone?

    A. Inhibits Na–K–Cl cotransport in the thick ascending limb of the loop of Henle
    B. Inhibits carbonic anhydrase
    C. Inhibits sodium and chloride transport in the distal convoluted tubule
    D. Acts on the distal tubule to inhibit the effects of aldosterone
    E. Blocks L-type calcium channels in the heart

70. Which of the following is the mechanism of action of bosentan?

    A. Blocks phosphodiesterase from degrading cyclic GMP in smooth muscle cells
    B. Blocks both endothelin A and B receptors
    C. Replaces the loss of endogenous prostaglandin I2
    D. Blocks calcium channels
    E. Suppresses production of prostaglandins and thromboxanes by irreversibly inactivating the cyclooxygenase enzyme

71. A 19-year-old woman begins taking enalapril for mildly depressed left ventricular systolic function. Which of the following is true regarding this patient after starting this medication?

    A. Less angiotensin I will be converted to angiotensin II
    B. There will be increased production of aldosterone
    C. Heart rate will be increased
    D. There will be a reduction in circulating bradykinins
    E. The patient can be counseled that there are no concerns with pregnancy

CHAPTER 14

Answers

1. (B) Prolonged QT interval is noted on the given ECG. The patient likely has long QT syndrome (LQTS) in the clinical scenario.

Management with intravenous magnesium sulfate is reasonable for patients who present with LQTS and few episodes of torsades de pointes. Magnesium is unlikely to be effective in patients with a normal QT interval. The other agents in the scenario tend to prolong the QT interval and therefore are not recommended.

2. (E) The patient in this scenario likely has type 3 long QT syndrome (LQT3).

Class IIb recommendation: Intravenous lidocaine or oral mexiletine may be considered in patients who present with LQT3 and torsades de pointes. The other agents in the given scenario tend to prolong QT interval and therefore are not recommended.

3. (D) In the given scenario, the patient has a bileaflet mechanical aortic valve without any additional risk factors for thromboembolism (see below). The recommendation as per the ACC/AHA 2020 guidelines is to stop warfarin 3 to 4 days prior to the procedure without any need for heparin bridging. Class 1 recommendations for perioperative anticoagulation strategy as per ACC/AHA 2020 guidelines are quoted below.

Class 1 recommendation:

1. For patients with mechanical heart valves who are undergoing minor procedures (e.g., dental extractions or cataract removal) where bleeding is easily controlled, continuation of VKA anticoagulation with a therapeutic INR is recommended.
2. For patients with a bileaflet mechanical AVR and no other risk factors for thromboembolism who are undergoing invasive procedures, temporary interruption of VKA anticoagulation, without bridging agents while the INR is subtherapeutic, is recommended.

*Risk factors: atrial fibrillation, previous thromboembolism, LV systolic dysfunction, hypercoagulable conditions, older-generation thrombogenic valves (ball-cage or tilting disc), or more than one mechanical valve.

4. (B) Please refer to class 1 recommendations from ACC/AHA 2020 guidelines quoted below for postoperative anticoagulation management following mechanical valve placement and the class 2b recommendation on the concomitant use of aspirin therapy.

Class 1 recommendations:

1. In patients with a mechanical prosthetic valve, anticoagulation with a VKA is recommended.
2. For patients with a mechanical bileaflet or current-generation single–tilting disc AVR and no risk factors for thromboembolism, anticoagulation with a VKA to achieve an INR of 2.5 is recommended.
3. For patients with a mechanical AVR and additional risk factors for thromboembolism (e.g., AF, previous thromboembolism, LV dysfunction, hypercoagulable state) or

an older-generation prosthesis (e.g., ball-in-cage), anticoagulation with a VKA is indicated to achieve an INR of 3.0.

4. For patients with a mechanical mitral valve replacement, anticoagulation with a VKA is indicated to achieve an INR of 3.0.

Class 2b recommendation:

1. For patients with a mechanical surgical aortic valve replacement or mitral valve replacement who are managed with a VKA *and have an indication for antiplatelet therapy*, addition of aspirin 75 to 100 mg daily may be considered when the risk of bleeding is low.

5. (E) Anticoagulation with frequent monitoring needs to be continued through pregnancy in the setting of a mechanical valve and only stopped prior to delivery. The class 1 recommendations from the ACC/AHA 2020 guidelines are quoted below.

Class 1 recommendations:

1. Pregnant women with mechanical prostheses should receive therapeutic anticoagulation with frequent monitoring during pregnancy.
2. Women with mechanical heart valves who cannot maintain therapeutic anticoagulation with frequent monitoring should be counseled against pregnancy.
3. Women with mechanical heart valves and their providers should use shared decision-making to choose an anticoagulation strategy for pregnancy. Women should be informed that VKA during pregnancy is associated with the lowest likelihood of maternal complications but the highest likelihood of miscarriage, fetal death, and congenital abnormalities, particularly if taken during the first trimester and if the warfarin dose exceeds 5 mg/d.
4. Pregnant women with mechanical valve prostheses who are on warfarin should switch to twice-daily LMWH (with a target anti-Xa level of 0.8 to 1.2 U/mL at 4 to 6 hours after dose) or intravenous UFH (with an activated partial thromboplastin time [aPTT] 2 times control) at least 1 week before planned delivery.
5. Pregnant women with mechanical valve prostheses who are on LMWH should switch to UFH (with an aPTT 2 times control) at least 36 hours before planned delivery.
6. Pregnant women with valve prostheses should stop UFH at least 6 hours before planned vaginal delivery.
7. If labor begins or urgent delivery is required in a woman therapeutically anticoagulated with a VKA, cesarean section should be performed after reversal of anticoagulation.

6. (A) The patient was started on ACE inhibitor (captopril, enalapril, etc.). ACE converts angiotensin I to angiotensin II. It also inactivates or breaks down bradykinin. ACE inhibitors therefore increase bradykinin levels and decrease angiotensin II levels. Increased bradykinin levels are thought to be responsible for dry cough symptoms in patients taking

ACE inhibitors. Digoxin inhibits Na^+–K^+ ATPase pump. CCBs inhibit calcium entry into vascular smooth muscle cells. Angiotensin II receptor blockers (ARBs) inhibit the activation of angiotensin II receptors. Dry cough is not commonly recognized as a side effect of digoxin, CCBs, or ARBs.

7. (C) In the given scenario, atrial fibrillation with preexcitation is the diagnosis. This is the most likely rhythm with an irregularly irregular wide complex tachycardia in an otherwise healthy patient. In atrial fibrillation with preexcitation, antegrade conduction would be through both the AV node and accessory pathway, and some beats are likely to be fusion beats. Any AV nodal blocking agent (adenosine, digitalis, diltiazem, β-blocker) is likely to result in unopposed ventricular activation through accessory pathway and can result in ventricular fibrillation. Thus, AV nodal blocking agents are best avoided in this scenario. Direct current cardioversion is the treatment of choice. If this is not possible, amiodarone may be given in this situation as it can restore atrial fibrillation to sinus rhythm as well as decrease accessory pathway conduction. Amiodarone is a class III antiarrhythmic agent that slows cardiac conduction (including accessory pathway conduction).

8. (A) The ECG shows sinus rhythm with varying degrees of AV block (predominately 2:1 AV block with occasional Mobitz type 1 second-degree AV block (i.e., Wenckebach). Accelerated junctional rhythm is also seen in the first part of the tracing. Of the medications given above, digoxin is the most likely culprit to produce nausea/vomiting and high-grade AV block with activation of ectopic pacemakers (junctional, ventricular, etc.).

9. (C) In CPVT patients with VT/VF storm, intravenous β-blocker therapy is considered the first line of treatment. General anesthesia can be used as a last resort if β-blocker therapy is ineffective.

10. (C) Since he does not have hemodynamically significant ASD, patient is unlikely to benefit from RSV prophylaxis. He does not meet other criteria for prophylaxis based on the 2014 AAP guidelines for palivizumab prophylaxis. According to the more recent AAP guidelines, children who are 12 months of age or younger with hemodynamically significant cyanotic and acyanotic congenital heart disease may benefit from palivizumab prophylaxis.

Children younger than 12 months of age with congenital heart disease who are most likely to benefit from immunoprophylaxis include:

- infants with acyanotic heart disease who are being treated for congestive heart failure and who will require cardiac surgical procedures
- infants with moderate to severe pulmonary hypertension

The new guidelines do not provide specific recommendations for infants with palliated or unrepaired cyanotic heart disease. [*Pediatrics.* 2014;134(2):415-420]

11. (D) This patient is a candidate for RSV prophylaxis given the presence of acyanotic heart disease that requires therapy for congestive heart failure within the first year of life.

The primary benefit of immunoprophylaxis with palivizumab is a decrease in the rate of RSV-associated hospitalization. Results from double-blinded, randomized, placebo-controlled trials with palivizumab involving 2,789 infants and children with prematurity, chronic lung disease, or congenital heart disease demonstrated a reduction in RSV hospitalization rates of 39% to 78% in different groups. None of the clinical trials have demonstrated a significant decrease in the rate of mortality attributable to RSV infection in infants who receive prophylaxis. [*Pediatrics.* 2014;134(2):415-420]

12. (A) Furosemide inhibits Na^+–$2Cl^-$–K^+ cotransporter in the loop of Henle and is therefore termed a loop diuretic. Thiazide diuretics inhibit Na^+–Cl^- cotransporter. Digoxin inhibits Na^+–K^+ ATPase pump.

13. (D) The patient in the given scenario most likely has idiopathic/viral pericarditis. Ibuprofen and aspirin have been most commonly used and provide prompt relief of pain in most patients but they do not alter the natural history of the disease. High-dose aspirin (800 mg orally every 6 to 8 hours for 7 to 10 days followed by gradual tapering of the dose by 800 mg per week for three additional weeks) is usually recommended if aspirin is used. Although acute pericarditis appears to respond dramatically to corticosteroids, early use of corticosteroids has been associated with an increased risk of relapsing pericarditis in multiple studies.

Routine use of colchicine in the treatment of acute pericarditis has been supported by the Colchicine for Acute Pericarditis (COPE) trial that randomized patients into receiving aspirin alone versus aspirin + colchicine. A 4- to 6-week colchicine therapy may be considered in patients with acute pericarditis, especially in those who have not benefitted from NSAID therapy after 1 week. In this given scenario, ibuprofen is the best option given the side effect profile of colchicine, and it would also require a longer course than listed.

14. (B) NIRS saturation is a good surrogate for tissue level saturation/oxygenation. NIRS saturation can be substituted for a mixed venous saturation (MVO_2). The difference between SaO_2 and MVO_2 is a surrogate for cardiac output that is likely to be low given the difference of 40 (80 − 40) in this scenario, which would explain the pH of 7.2 (acidosis).

The pulmonary venous O_2 can be assumed to be close to 100% given the FiO_2 of 21% and clear lungs. The Q_p/Q_s in this scenario is 20.

Q_p/Q_s = (SaO_2 − MVO_2)/(pulmonary venous O_2 − SaO_2) = (80 − 40)/(100 − 80) = 40/20 = 2.

Thus, the patient has a low systemic cardiac output state and his lungs are getting at least two times the systemic blood flow. Norepinephrine is a potent vasoconstrictor. Weaning norepinephrine would lower systemic vascular resistance (SVR) and improve cardiac output, making the Q_p/Q_s more balanced. This should be the first line of management in addition to giving fluids that has already been tried in this patient. IV furosemide would decrease the intravascular volume and be detrimental for the patient. IV β-blocker therapy may decrease cardiac inotropy and worsen the low output state. Decreasing the milrinone would reduce the systemic cardiac output by increasing the SVR and by decreasing the cardiac inotropy. Increasing the FiO_2 would lower the PVR and lead to more pulmonary blood flow at the expense of systemic blood flow (increase in Q_p/Q_s).

15. (E) Initial therapy for KD during the acute phase is IVIG and high-dose aspirin. Single-dose pulse methylprednisolone should not be administered with IVIG as routine primary therapy for patients with KD. Administration of a longer course of corticosteroids (e.g., tapering over 2 to 3 weeks), together with IVIG 2 g/kg and ASA, may be considered for treatment of high-risk patients with acute KD, when such high risk can be identified in patients before initiation of treatment. In the case of persistence or recurrence of fever despite one dose of IVIG, it is reasonable to administer a second dose of IVIG (2 g/kg) to patients with persistent or recrudescent fever at least 36 hours after the end of the first IVIG infusion. Administration of high-dose pulse steroids (usually methylprednisolone 20 to 30 mg/kg intravenously for 3 days, with or without a subsequent course and taper of oral prednisone) may be considered as an alternative to a second infusion of IVIG or for retreatment of patients with KD who have had recurrent or recrudescent fever after additional IVIG. Administration of a longer (e.g., 2 to 3 weeks) tapering course of prednisolone or prednisone, together with IVIG 2 g/kg and ASA, may be considered in the retreatment of patients with KD who have had recurrent or recrudescent fever after initial IVIG treatment.

16. (C) The patient has mild to moderate carditis that needs therapy with high-dose aspirin (80 to 100 mg/kg/d in four divided doses in children). Oral prednisone is indicated for more severe carditis associated with a sicker patient in the setting of heart failure, severe valvular regurgitation, significant pericarditis/myocarditis, or reduced cardiac function. There is no recommendation for combining oral steroids with aspirin for treatment of acute RF. IVIG + aspirin is used in the treatment of KD. There is no indication for a β-blocker in pericarditis.

17. (C) Sirolimus acts at a more distal site in the lymphocyte activation cascade by blocking transcription of activation genes. Sirolimus (also known as rapamycin) is not a calcineurin inhibitor. Cyclosporine and tacrolimus are calcineurin inhibitors. Cyclosporine and tacrolimus are available for intravenous use. Tacrolimus offers no survival advantage over cyclosporine in heart transplant recipients. Sirolimus may be less nephrotoxic over the long term.

18. (C) The patient had mild carditis during RF but is free of residual heart disease now. Per guidelines, she will need RF antibiotic prophylaxis for at least 10 years or until 21 years of age, whichever is longer.

As per the current guidelines,

- RF patients with carditis and residual heart disease (persistent valvular disease) should receive treatment for a duration of 10 years or until 40 years of age (whichever is longer, sometimes lifelong) after the last attack of RF.
- RF patients with carditis but without residual heart disease (no valvular disease) should receive treatment for a duration of 10 years or until 21 years of age (whichever is longer) after the last attack of RF.

- RF patients without carditis should receive treatment for a duration of 5 years or until 21 years of age (whichever is longer) after the last attack of RF.

19. (E) Please refer to the guidelines as quoted below.
Class IIa recommendations:

Prophylaxis against IE is reasonable for the following patients at highest risk for adverse outcomes from IE who undergo dental procedures that involve manipulation of either gingival tissue or the periapical region of teeth or perforation of the oral mucosa:

- Patients with prosthetic cardiac valves or prosthetic material used for cardiac valve repair
- Patients with previous IE
- Patients with CHD
  - Unrepaired cyanotic CHD, including palliative shunts and conduits
  - Completely repaired CHD repaired with prosthetic material or device, whether placed by surgery or by catheter intervention, during the first 6 months after the procedure
  - Repaired CHD with residual defects at the site or adjacent to the site of a prosthetic patch or prosthetic device (both of which inhibit endothelialization)
- Cardiac transplant recipients with valve regurgitation due to a structurally abnormal valve

IE prophylaxis is not recommended for the following dental procedures: routine anesthetic injections through noninfected tissue, dental radiographs, placement/removal of orthodontic/prosthodontic appliances, shedding of deciduous teeth, and bleeding from trauma to lips/oral mucosa. IE prophylaxis is not recommended for the following respiratory procedures: bronchoscopy without biopsy, endotracheal intubation, or myringotomy with tube insertion. IE prophylaxis is not recommended for all gastrointestinal and genitourinary procedures including EGD and colonoscopy even with biopsy.

20. (B) The child is ≥10 years old and meets criteria for pharmacologic lipid-lowering therapy per the 2011 AAP guidelines since his LDL remained ≥190 mg/dL after a 6-month trial of diet and exercise modifications. Statin therapy is considered the first-line LDL lowering agent. A bile acid sequestrant or cholesterol absorption inhibitor may be added as a second agent if statin therapy alone is insufficient in lowering the LDL.

21. (D) The traditional therapeutic medication for HCM is β-blocker. If CCBs are used, then preferred medications would be diltiazem and verapamil. Dihydropyridine CCBs like nifedipine would cause peripheral vasodilation and reflex tachycardia that are both detrimental in an HCM patient with obstruction. Furosemide by reducing preload and therefore left ventricular filling (through its diuretic effect) could worsen the degree of obstruction in an HCM patient. ICD is not indicated at present as the patient has no clearly established sudden death risk factors (i.e., personal history of cardiac arrest or sustained VT, LV wall thickness of ≥30 mm, family history of sudden death in a first-degree relative, or unexplained syncope).

22. (B) Sirolimus can inhibit smooth muscle proliferation and may have the advantage of inhibiting coronary vasculopathy. Sirolimus is not a calcineurin inhibitor and may be used in combination with, or in lieu of, calcineurin inhibitors. Sirolimus may be less nephrotoxic over the long term.

23. (C) Lidocaine is considered a first-line agent in the acute treatment of ventricular tachycardia. It is a class Ib antiarrhythmic and is available IV. Lidocaine has a narrow therapeutic window and toxicity can occur at slightly higher levels. The most common side effects from lidocaine involve the central nervous system and include tremors, light-headedness, ataxia, dysarthria, mood/personality changes, hallucinations, and seizures. Lidocaine levels should be monitored, and dosing adjusted accordingly. Esmolol, verapamil, and amiodarone can be used in acute treatment of VT but generally do not have acute side effects of CNS toxicity. Adenosine effects on the AV node are short lived and except in very rare cases, adenosine has no role in the treatment of VT.

24. (A) All of the signs and symptoms listed can result from rabbit ATG infusion. The most common reported side effect is fever (over 60%). Other common side effects include rash (<25%), hyperkalemia (25% to 30%), abdominal pain (35% to 40%), myalgia (up to 40%), and shivering (55% to 60%).

25. (E) Both adenosine and β-blockers have the potential to exacerbate bronchospasm in this patient. Although the electrophysiologic effects of adenosine are temporary, the bronchospasm may persist for a long period of time. Heart transplant recipients are particularly sensitive to adenosine, and one-quarter to one-half the dose should be used initially as long periods of AV block may be noted with higher doses. Adenosine has a half-life of <2 seconds and is metabolized quickly in the blood. It therefore must be given as rapidly as possible in a large-bore IV as close to the heart as possible. Flushing and hypotension are common side effects. The bradycardia caused by adenosine may precipitate other arrhythmias including atrial fibrillation or ventricular tachycardia, so an external defibrillator should be readily available. The typical dose is 100 to 400 μg/kg in children.

26. (C) Combination therapy is increasingly used in children to treat severe pulmonary arterial hypertension despite the lack of published evidence. Ambrisentan is a selective endothelin A receptor antagonist. It does not induce or inhibit cytochrome P450 enzymes and is metabolized through glucuronidation. Therefore, it is much less hepatotoxic than bosentan. Treprostinil is a prostacyclin (PGI2) analogue and is not a prostaglandin (PGE2) analogue. It is favored over epoprostenol for long-term prostacyclin therapy due to its longer half-life. Sildenafil works through nitric oxide–cyclic GMP cascade, but it is a phosphodiesterase 5 inhibitor and not a phosphodiesterase 3 inhibitor. Milrinone is a phosphodiesterase 3 inhibitor.

27. (D) The ECG changes in Brugada syndrome can be dynamic and thus missed on a single ECG screening. Since the characteristic ECG hallmark may be concealed, drug challenge with sodium channel blockers (which may exacerbate the sodium channel dysfunction) to bring out the typical ECG changes has been proposed as a useful tool for the diagnosis of Brugada syndrome. Drugs employed for this purpose have included ajmaline, flecainide, procainamide, pilsicainide, disopyramide, and propafenone although the specific diagnostic value for all of them has not yet been systematically studied. Epinephrine challenge can be helpful in identifying concealed LQTS. Cardiac MRI may be used in the diagnosis of patients with arrhythmogenic right ventricular cardiomyopathy. Isoproterenol testing is commonly used in the EP lab to bring out arrhythmias. Exercise testing may be helpful in the diagnosis of CPVT.

28. (D) Phenytoin, lidocaine, and mexiletine are all class IB antiarrhythmic sodium channel blocking drugs characterized by rapid recovery of the blocked sodium channel. QT intervals may be slightly shortened by these drugs. There is no contraindication to phenytoin use in LQTS patients. There is at present no role for IV β-blocker or amiodarone in the absence of any significant ventricular ectopy. Class III agents like amiodarone, sotalol, and ibutilide block the potassium channels and prolong the QT interval.

29. (B) The patient is symptomatic with atrial flutter but is hemodynamically stable. Therefore, the priority of the physician is to treat her symptoms using medication(s). Electrical cardioversion is not the immediate first-line treatment for a stable patient. Of the medications given, IV diltiazem is the best option as it would slow down the rapid ventricular response and can produce symptomatic relief. IV β-blockers and sotalol are other options. Class IC antiarrhythmic agent flecainide can slow down the atrial conduction within the flutter circuit and therefore slow down flutter rate. Thus, it can convert fast flutter with AV block into slow flutter with 1:1 AV conduction if administered alone. Class I antiarrhythmic agent disopyramide has anticholinergic activity and may enhance AV node conduction and worsen the situation when administered alone. Therefore, flecainide and disopyramide are best administered in conjunction with an AV nodal blocking agent. IV labetalol is a nonselective β-blocker and is primarily used in hypertensive emergencies.

30. (B) Sotalol is excreted renally and the dosing needs to be adjusted if used in patients with significant renal dysfunction and is best avoided if possible in patients with severe renal dysfunction. In adults, sotalol is generally dosed every 12 hours, but in patients with a creatinine clearance below 60 mL/min, it should be dosed every 24 hours initially. If doses require escalation, then it should be done slowly with careful monitoring of the QTc. The other medications listed do not require renal dosing adjustments.

31. (D) Isoproterenol stimulates myocardial β1 receptors resulting in positive chronotropy and inotropy. It can result in the generation of a stable junctional/ventricular escape rhythm that is helpful in this setting allowing for additional time to pursue temporary pacemaker if necessary. Atropine is an anticholinergic/vagolytic agent and only works in reversing AV block to excessive vagal effect. It would not be helpful in this situation. Milrinone and dobutamine do not have the same effect as isoproterenol and therefore are not indicated. Digoxin may slow the junctional rate and thus is not indicated.

32. (A) The patient has low cardiac output despite an EF of 70% because a significant fraction of the left ventricular stroke volume can be expected to leak into the left atrium (LA) resulting in reduced forward systemic stroke volume. Elevated left atrial pressure can be expected and would result in pulmonary edema. She would benefit the most from a systemic vasodilator like nitroprusside that would increase her forward stroke volume and improve her cardiac output. IV furosemide would help by reducing pulmonary edema, but not primarily by improving forward stroke volume. Vasopressin is a vasoconstrictor and would be detrimental in this situation. Digoxin would not be helpful as the patient does not have myocardial dysfunction or reduced EF. Dopamine is not a systemic vasodilator and would not improve the patient's hemodynamics.

33. (C) The given clinical scenario does not suggest a TOF "Tet" spell. The RVOT murmur is still loud and the patient is alert, so there is unlikely to be an acute RVOT obstructive crisis. Given the patient's age, they are likely in their physiologic nadir for anemia of prematurity/infancy and their hematocrit is only 26, which is low for an unrepaired TOF patient. The low oxygen-carrying capacity in the setting of an underlying cyanotic heart disease could result in reduced activity levels.

Anemia could cause a drop in the SpO_2 in the following ways: Systemic vasodilation associated with anemia may shift blood flow from the lungs to the systemic circulation. Thus, there would be more right-to-left shunting as SVR drops causing a drop in SpO_2. Also, in the setting of low hemoglobin, tissue oxygen extraction would result in a much lower mixed venous saturation than compared to somebody with higher hemoglobin levels. In the absence of any right-to-left shunt, blood would be fully oxygenated in the lungs. But in the presence of a right-to-left shunt, a proportion of this blood (with lower mixed venous SpO_2) would mix with the oxygenated blood resulting in a much lower systemic SpO_2.

Since the patient is hypoxic, symptomatic treatment is indicated. Of the following options, blood transfusion would benefit the patient in the ER setting. It would increase his oxygen-carrying capacity and could also improve his SpO_2 for the above-mentioned reasons. Intravenous propranolol, phenylephrine infusion, and morphine administration are useful in patients who have a TOF spell that is not the case here. Furosemide therapy would not be helpful as pulmonary overcirculation is rare in TOF.

34. (E) Acute side effects of PGE1 include apnea (needing intubation), fever/hyperthermia, hypotension, and seizures. Cutaneous vasodilation and edema can develop. In patients who have been kept on long-term PGE1 therapy (beyond 2 weeks), various side effects including cortical hyperostosis has been described.

35. (A) Losartan is an angiotensin receptor 1 (AT1R) antagonist and has been shown to antagonize TGF-β signaling. The exact mechanism of action is uncertain, but activation of angiotensin type 1 receptors increases the expression of

TGF-β ligands and receptors and induces the activation of thrombospondin, a powerful TGF-β activator. Propranolol, enalapril, verapamil, or spironolactone does not have the above effect.

36. (D) Carvedilol is a nonselective β-blocker and α-blocker indicated for use in heart failure with reduced ejection fraction. While the remaining options may be used in heart failure with reduced ejection fraction, they all can potentially increase potassium levels. So in this patient with chronic hyperkalemia, the remaining options would not be ideal first choices. Eplerenone is a mineralocorticoid receptor (aldosterone receptor) antagonist with effects similar to spironolactone (including hyperkalemia). Enalapril and captopril are ACE inhibitors and both increase potassium levels as well.

37. (C) Amiodarone increases the levels of cyclosporine, digoxin, and warfarin (increased anticoagulant effect) by inhibiting the activity of cytochrome P450. In the setting of preexistent β-blocker therapy as in this patient, there is potential for heart block (not enhanced AV nodal conduction) due to the AV nodal blocking effect of amiodarone. There is no interaction requiring dose adjustment with steroids and amiodarone.

38. (B) Amiodarone (class III antiarrhythmic agent) is primarily a cardiac potassium channel blocker but it is also a broad-spectrum antiarrhythmic agent with multiple other effects on conduction. Because of potassium channel blocking, it prolongs repolarization and thus the QT interval. It also has some effect blocking cardiac sodium and calcium channels as well. It produces β-blockade, causes reduced AV nodal conduction, and is not a vagolytic agent. Hypokalemia exacerbates the proarrhythmic potential of amiodarone and can precipitate torsades de pointes.

39. (C) It is true that tacrolimus recipients (8%) more often develop diabetes mellitus than cyclosporine recipients (2%). Higher tacrolimus levels, HLA-DR mismatch, and older age at transplantation may predispose to posttransplant diabetes. Sirolimus use is associated with bone marrow suppression, especially when used in conjunction with tacrolimus. Lipid abnormalities are common even in younger children who are heart transplant recipients, and lipid-lowering therapy is often instituted in this subgroup. CCB and ACE inhibitors are typically used for managing hypertension in pediatric heart transplant recipients. Sirolimus is less nephrotoxic than cyclosporine or tacrolimus.

40. (C) Drugs that lower PVR include tolazoline (a nonselective competitive α-adrenergic receptor antagonist), nitric oxide (not nitrous oxide), dobutamine (not dopamine), milrinone, prostaglandins, prostacyclins, sodium nitroprusside, and sildenafil. Ketamine may increase PVR. Norepinephrine is a systemic vasoconstrictor and is not a pulmonary vasodilator.

41. (D) The patient in the given scenario is likely to have heparin-induced thrombocytopenia with thrombosis (HITT) that develops in a subset of patients with HIT. Heparin combines with platelet factor 4 (PF-4) complex and makes it immunogenic. The resulting antibodies to this complex may result in the formation of platelet aggregates (which can cause vaso-occlusion) and cause immune-mediated platelet destruction resulting in thrombocytopenia (usually a >50% drop in platelet count). Diagnosis is made using specific antibody assay. However, once a thrombotic complication is noted in the setting of suspected HIT, urgent medical therapy is indicated. The best course of action is to completely stop heparin and provide immediate alternative anticoagulation medications.

The degree of platelet drop in HIT patients is not enough to cause clinically significant bleeding, and therefore, platelet transfusion is not indicated. Low–molecular-weight heparins (enoxaparin) may not provoke HIT, may still cross-react with heparin antibodies, and are not used in HIT patients.

42. (C) Use of warfarin during pregnancy is associated with various teratogenic side effects including defects in calcification of the epiphyses (chondrodysplasia punctata), retarded intrauterine growth, psychomotor deficit, hypotonia, convulsions, nasal hypoplasia, ocular and CNS anomalies. Risk is higher during the first trimester (~10%), and the critical period is between the sixth and ninth weeks of gestation. The risk is estimated to be ~3% to 5% for administration during the second and third trimesters. Lithium has been associated with Ebstein anomaly and not left-sided obstructive lesions. Amiodarone can cause hypo- or hyperthyroidism, but complete heart block is not a typical finding and it is not permanent. ACE inhibitors can cause renal damage, cranial ossification defects, oligohydramnios, and delayed intrauterine growth, but right-sided obstructive lesions have not been described. They are contraindicated during pregnancy, especially in the second and third trimesters. High-dose folic acid therapy is known to be protective against neural tube defects.

43. (E) The patient has serious digoxin toxicity and is symptomatic (dizziness and mild hypotension) with high-grade AV block. He also has significant ventricular ectopy including nonsustained VT.

Intravenous atropine and temporary pacing are recommended in such patients with high-degree symptomatic AV block. Digoxin antibody Fab should be administered in patients showing serious signs of digoxin toxicity (symptomatic AV block, serious ventricular arrhythmias), and this patient would be a candidate.

Concomitant therapy with agents such as activated charcoal and cholestyramine has also been recommended in patients showing serious digoxin toxicity in an attempt to bind digoxin in the gut. Such agents facilitate gastrointestinal elimination as well as increase the systemic clearance of digoxin. Through both passive diffusion and enterohepatic recycling of digoxin, the intestine acts as a dialysis membrane, and the binding of the charcoal resin aids in the elimination of digoxin.

Digoxin is 50% to 70% eliminated through the kidneys unmetabolized without significant hepatic contribution, and therefore, liver dysfunction (due to recent infectious mononucleosis) is not the direct reason for elevated digoxin levels. In the setting of preexisting renal dysfunction, reduced oral intake following the viral illness could have contributed to exacerbated renal dysfunction (prerenal etiology) and associated hyperkalemia. This could result in

reduced renal excretion of digoxin and precipitate digoxin toxicity. Hyperkalemia exacerbates digoxin toxicity, and concurrent treatment of hyperkalemia would be beneficial, although the potassium level would not give the definitive cause of the AV block, and the QRS is not widened and the T waves are not peaked so the level is likely not severely elevated.

This patient needs the following management: IV fluids to improve renal perfusion and hypotension, treatment of hyperkalemia, IV atropine acutely (temporary pacing is also indicated), digoxin antibody therapy, and management of renal dysfunction. Intravenous lidocaine can be administered if the patient develops symptomatic ventricular arrhythmias before digoxin antibody becomes available.

44. (B) The patient has persistent postoperative hypertension that is significant, and in an intubated patient, it is not easy to evaluate symptoms. She should be treated for hypertension. She has a history of persistent asthma as judged by her medication list, and intravenous labetalol (β-blocker) can exacerbate bronchoconstriction and worsen her hypoxia. In the setting of concurrent renal and hepatic dysfunction, sodium nitroprusside is not safe due to potential buildup of cyanide. Nicardipine is a calcium channel blocker and can be used in situations where β-blocker and sodium nitroprusside are contraindicated. It does not have any adverse effects on the myocardium.

The patient's hypoxia is most likely due to atelectasis, and since there is no mention of pulmonary hypertension, there is no role for nitric oxide therapy. Dexmedetomidine is a highly selective α-2 receptor agonist and is used for sedation. It can produce dose-dependent decreases in BP and HR as a result of its α-2 agonist effect on the sympathetic ganglia with resulting sympatholytic effects. However, it is not indicated in the current scenario as the patient seems to be well sedated already.

45. (D) The clinical scenario is consistent with a "suicidal right ventricle" due to persistent dynamic infundibular/subpulmonary obstruction that can follow acute relief of a distal fixed pulmonary valve obstruction. The severe subvalvular obstruction in the absence of a distal fixed obstruction can result in complete/near-complete RVOT obstruction. This can lead to acute right ventricular failure with poor RV filling and right-to-left shunt through the patent foramen ovale. Intravenous β-blockers would be the drug of choice as they can relieve the dynamic RVOT obstruction and improve the hemodynamics. There is no role for pulmonary vasodilators like nitric oxide in this setting. Milrinone is an inotrope and can worsen the dynamic obstruction. Phenylephrine is a vasoconstrictor and is unlikely to produce any beneficial hemodynamic effects in this scenario. Intravenous diuretics like furosemide have no specific role in this situation. In fact, it may reduce right ventricular preload and worsen the condition.

46. (B) Very rarely, statins can cause life-threatening rhabdomyolysis. The most common symptom is muscle pain. Creatine kinase levels should be checked to rule out this condition. Rhabdomyolysis can cause severe muscle pain, liver damage, kidney failure, and death. Other side effects include diarrhea, liver damage, gastrointestinal problems such as diarrhea or nausea, rash and flushing, and neurologic side effects.

47. (B) Both the inhalational anesthetic agent and midazolam will cause a drop in systemic vascular resistance and unfavorably alter the Q_p:Q_s for this patient. Ketamine increases systemic vascular resistance and fentanyl has minimal hemodynamic effects. The combination of ketamine and an inhalational anesthetic or midazolam would be preferred to offset the vasodilatory effects of these agents.

Anesthetic induction requires an individual approach to each congenital heart disease patient. A careful presedation assessment is essential to determine the child's baseline cardiac reserve, cardiac physiology, and any noncardiac medical conditions that may impact sedation tolerance. Adequate sedation must be accomplished while simultaneously minimizing any anesthetic/sedation-related disruption in cardiopulmonary stability. Inhalational anesthetic agents have variable impact on the cardiopulmonary system. However, they all pose significant risk for hemodynamic compromise in the child with limited cardiac reserve. Decreases in systemic blood pressure due to vasodilation can occur with all inhalational anesthetics to some degree (halothane, isoflurane, and sevoflurane). Sevoflurane has the least impact on systemic blood pressure when compared with isoflurane and halothane.

48. (D) Atenolol and metoprolol are second-generation selective β-blockers primarily affecting β-1 adrenergic receptors. Although selectivity can be lost at higher concentrations, atenolol and metoprolol should have a reduced risk of bronchospasm since they do not affect β-2 adrenergic receptors. In addition, metoprolol is more lipid soluble than atenolol and therefore metoprolol can cross the blood–brain barrier more easily, which may result in greater CNS effects (such as sleep disturbances or depression) than atenolol. Propranolol, nadolol, and sotalol are nonselective β-blockers and would have more potential for bronchospasm than selective β-blockers.

49. (D) This patient has overdosed on β-blocker. β-Blocker toxicity manifests as bradycardia and hypotension and may involve hypoglycemia. Evidence of each of these signs are present, although the heart rate effect of β-blocker toxicity is most significant in this patient. Bradycardia can be counteracted by administering atropine, an anticholinergic. Hypotension may improve as the heart rate increases. Severe or recalcitrant hypotension, despite atropine, should be managed with IV fluids and vasoconstrictive agents (e.g., epinephrine, vasopressin, dopamine) if necessary. This patient's hypoglycemia is mild and does not require urgent treatment with glucagon. Hydralazine is a systemic vasodilator and is not indicated in the treatment of this patient.

50. (E) Amiodarone, levothyroxine, propranolol, and sertraline all have the potential to increase warfarin effect, leading to higher INR levels and a need to decrease warfarin dosage. St. John's wort, an herbal supplement that has been promoted to improve mood and treat depression, has been shown to decrease the efficacy of warfarin.

51. (E) Chlorothiazide is a thiazide diuretic that works by inhibiting sodium and chloride transport in the distal convoluted tubule. Furosemide, ethacrynic acid, and bumetanide are all loop diuretics that inhibit chloride–sodium–potassium cotransport in the thick ascending limb of the loop of Henle. Spironolactone competitively inhibits aldosterone in the distal tubule and is a relatively weak diuretic with potassium-sparing effects.

52. (A) A hydromorphone PCA would treat pain but not agitation. If the patient is having benzodiazepine withdrawal, the hydromorphone would not address this problem. Administration of fentanyl and versed intermittently or as an infusion would treat withdrawal but might worsen the situation if the patient is actually experiencing delirium. Withdrawal can occur following prolonged use of narcotics and benzodiazepines. Signs of withdrawal can include anxiety, insomnia, restlessness, yawning, stomach cramps, rhinorrhea, diaphoresis, mydriasis, vomiting, diarrhea, fever, muscle spasms, tremor, tachycardia, hypertension, and even seizures. Delirium on the other hand is a common complication observed in critically ill adults and children. Delirium can occur even after a short period of sedation. In adults, benzodiazepines appear to increase the risk for delirium. Some studies suggest that dexmedetomidine may reduce narcotic/benzodiazepine requirements and shorten the duration of mechanical ventilation for ICU patients. Dexmedetomidine infusions are also used to manage anxiety and alleviate withdrawal symptoms when narcotic/benzodiazepine weans are initiated. Dexmedetomidine is a centrally acting α-2-agonist. The drug has anxiolytic, sedative, and analgesic effects and does not interfere with respiratory drive. Dexmedetomidine can cause hypotension, hypertension, bradycardia, and atrial fibrillation but is generally well tolerated.

53. (A) This child is most likely having a pulmonary hypertensive crisis brought on by the aspiration event. Paralysis with vecuronium in combination with 100% oxygen can be administered immediately to try and reduce pulmonary vascular resistance (PVR) in the acute crisis. Sedation is an important component of treatment but midazolam does not have immediate onset of action. Vecuronium or the shorter-acting rocuronium will take effect within 120 seconds of administration. Epinephrine administration is not warranted in pulmonary hypertensive crisis because it will actually increase PVR at high doses. Lidocaine can be used prior to suctioning or intubation to prevent laryngospasm and also to treat ventricular arrhythmia but does not have a role in the acute management of pulmonary hypertension.

54. (C) Chest tube placement is painful and ketamine will provide both analgesia and sedation. Ketamine is also desirable because it will not interfere with this child's respiratory drive in case the pleural effusion is compromising the child's respiratory stability. Fentanyl and propofol will both cause respiratory depression, which increases the risk for further respiratory compromise. Fentanyl alone would provide good analgesia but inadequate sedation for this procedure. Diazepam is long acting and used to acutely treat seizures, which are unlikely during chest tube placement.

The correct answer is C because ketamine poses a risk for laryngospasm and bronchorrhea. Glycopyrrolate (or atropine) can be used to manage increased secretions and a muscle relaxant may be necessary if laryngospasm were to occur.

55. (D) This patient is demonstrating metabolic acidosis and alterations in her mental status. These are symptoms of cyanide toxicity. Sodium nitroprusside can cause cyanide toxicity and the risk is increased in patients with renal insufficiency. The US Boxed Warning for the drug states the following:

Except when used briefly or at low (<2 mcg/kg/min) infusion rates, nitroprusside gives rise to large cyanide quantities. Do not use the maximum dose for more than 10 minutes; if blood pressure is not controlled by the maximum rate (i.e., 10 mcg/kg/min) after 10 minutes, discontinue infusion. Monitor for cyanide toxicity via acid–base balance and venous oxygen concentration; however, clinicians should note that these indicators may not always reliably indicate cyanide toxicity. The following conditions increase the risk for cyanide toxicity when sodium nitroprusside is used: hepatic impairment, cardiopulmonary bypass, and therapeutic hypothermia. Sodium thiosulfate can be administered with nitroprusside to prevent cyanide toxicity, but thiocyanate toxicity remains a risk especially in patients with renal dysfunction. Avoidance of prolonged high doses and monitoring for metabolic acidosis, bradycardia, confusion, and convulsions are critical to prevent and detect cyanide toxicity during nitroprusside infusion. Elevated cyanide levels have been observed in children at doses of 1.8 mcg/kg/min. Monitoring of cyanide levels every 72 hours is recommended with prolonged use. Treatment includes supporting airway, breathing, and circulation, while administering the antidote hydroxocobalamin and sodium thiosulfate. [Sodium Nitroprusside: Pediatric Drug Information. Lexicomp, Inc.]

56. (E) Flecainide is a class IC antiarrhythmic. It is primarily a sodium channel blocker, and therefore, it prolongs phase 0 of the action potential in atrial myocardium, the His–Purkinje system, and the ventricular myocardium. This results primarily in an increase in the QRS duration. It can, however, also lengthen the PR interval. Generally, there is very little effect on the QT interval, the ST segments, or the T waves unless toxic levels are reached.

57. (B) Procainamide is a class IA antiarrhythmic and primarily blocks sodium channels and also potassium channels. This results in slower conduction through the atrial myocardium, the His–Purkinje system, and the ventricular myocardium with little to no effect on the sinus and AV node. The patient is in atrial flutter with 2:1 AV conduction. By giving procainamide, conduction through the atrial muscle can slow resulting in a slower atrial rate. The slower atrial rate can result in AV node conduction going from 2:1 to 1:1 thereby increasing the ventricular rate resulting in her change in clinical status. Diltiazem is a calcium channel blocker often used to slow AV node conduction during macroreentrant atrial arrhythmias. Lidocaine and mexiletine are class IB antiarrhythmics that affect ventricular muscle and

not AV node or atrial conduction. Esmolol is a β-blocker that would slow conduction through the AV node.

58. (A) According to the 2014 PACES/HRS expert consensus statement on the recognition and management of arrhythmias in adult congenital heart disease in patients with IART and complex congenital heart disease and concomitant ventricular dysfunction who have failed a catheter ablation attempt and have no treatable precipitating factors, the best choice of antiarrhythmic to maintain sinus rhythm is amiodarone or dofetilide. In this case, this patient has evidence of possible hepatic disease making amiodarone a less attractive choice as it can be hepatotoxic in addition to having several other potential long-term side effects. Dofetilide is excreted by the kidneys and dosing adjustments must be made in the face of renal dysfunction; however, this patient has a normal BUN and creatinine. Flecainide has been associated with an increased risk of mortality in those with depressed ventricular dysfunction and is generally avoided in patients with complex congenital heart disease and ventricular dysfunction. Dronedarone is not recommended in patients with a history of heart failure, moderate or severe systolic ventricular dysfunction, or moderate or complex congenital heart disease because of potential concerns over worsening heart failure and increased mortality. Metoprolol may be useful in this patient to prevent a rapid ventricular response in the setting of IART but is not likely to maintain long-term sinus rhythm.

59. (C) Dofetilide is a class III antiarrhythmic that selectively inhibits the rapid component of the delayed rectifier potassium current which can prolong the QT interval. Patients should be admitted and observed for QT prolongation and arrhythmia during initiation due to the risk of torsades de pointes. Dofetilide is excreted by the kidneys and the dose must be adjusted for impaired creatinine clearance. Dofetilide does not affect thyroid function. Contraindications to dofetilide treatment include creatinine clearance <20 mL/min, hypokalemia, QTc >440 msec or ≥500 msec in the presence of ventricular conduction delay.

60. (C) Amiodarone has many potential side effects. The most common side effects include the following: hypo- or hyperthyroidism; hepatitis resulting in a greater than twice normal AST and ALT level which can progress to hepatic failure in a small number; pulmonary toxicity commonly resulting in a cough, fever, dyspnea, opacities on chest x-ray, and a decreased DLCO on pulmonary function tests; dermatologic photosensitivity to UV light; rarely blue-gray skin discoloration; corneal microdeposits that are typically benign; and rarely optic neuropathy. Hypoparathyroid hormone, renal dysfunction, pancreatitis, and conjunctivitis are not known to be common side effects of amiodarone.

61. (A) This patient has moderately controlled asthma. Nonselective β-blockers can cause bronchospasm in asthmatics. Because esmolol is a selective β1-blocker, it will theoretically only act on the β1-receptors in the heart. However, caution is still warranted when considering its use in asthmatics. The other three antihypertensive agents (nicardipine, clevidipine, and hydralazine) would be better choices for establishing blood pressure control in this patient with moderately controlled asthma.

62. (E) Agranulocytosis has been reported with propafenone use and usually occurs within the first 2 months of initiation. If this is observed, the white blood cell count usually increases back to normal within 2 weeks of stopping propafenone. Propafenone use is not associated with changes in platelet count or red blood cell count.

63. (B) Clinic drug trials consist of preclinical, phase 0, I, II, III, and IV. This patient is looking to participate in a clinical drug trial that is assessing the dosing and side effects of a medication on 50 participants ("small group of subjects" <100 total). Therefore, he would be participating in a phase I drug trial. Preclinical trials include in vitro and in vivo nonhuman/laboratory studies establishing efficacy, toxicity, etc. Phase 0 trials are the first human trials of subtherapeutic doses on a very small amount of subjects (typically ≤10–15). Phase I consists of defining the appropriate dose as well as the safety profile/adverse effects of a medication in healthy volunteers (typically 20 to 100 subjects). Phase II begins to determine how well the drug works on a larger group of subjects (typically 100 to 300); of note, the medication does not yet have a presumed therapeutic effect. Phase III are large trials (300 to 3,000 subjects) that are often randomized against the already on the market standard of care drug ("the gold standard"). Phase IV trial occurs after FDA approval when the approved medication undergoes postmarketing surveillance of long-term adverse effects for a minimum of 2 years.

64. (D) The most efficacious medication will be the drug resulting in the largest desired response. Drug D reduces the systolic blood pressure the most, and thus, it would be the most efficacious medication listed. Efficacy (E_{max}) is the maximum effect a drug can be expected to achieve and higher doses will not increase the magnitude of the effect. Drug dose–effect relationships including dose-response curves are basic principles of pharmacodynamics—the drug's molecular, biochemical, and physiologic effects or actions.

65. (A) The most potent medication will be the drug producing a given level of response at the lowest dose. Drug potency is based upon the drug concentration at a steady state that produces 50% of its maximum effect (EC50). Of note, drug potency does not always equal maximal efficacy and it does not equal other important determinants of the drug-like duration of effect.

66. (C) A drug half-life is a basic principle of pharmacokinetics—the study of drug movement within the body; absorption, distribution, metabolism, and excretion. A drug's half-life is the time it takes for the ingested drug in the body to be reduced by half. Each drug has its unique half-life which can be affected (shortened or prolonged) by different states of well-being/disease (i.e., chronic liver or kidney disease, pregnancy, etc.). A drug's steady state is defined as the time during which the concentration of the drug within the body remains relatively stable if the medication is taken regularly no matter the dose size or interval. This typically equals

four to five drug half-lives. After one half-live, 50% of steady state will have been achieved; two = 75%, three = 87.5%, four = 93.75%, and five = 96.875%.

67. (D) Clinic drug trials consist of preclinical, phase 0, I, II, III, and IV. This patient is looking to participate in a clinical drug trial that is assessing the trial medication against the standard of care ("gold standard") medication in a randomized-blinded study including a very large subject population. Therefore, he would be participating in a phase III drug trial. Preclinical trials include in vitro and in vivo nonhuman/laboratory studies establishing efficacy, toxicity, etc. Phase 0 trials are the first human trials of subtherapeutic doses on a very small amount of subjects (typically ≤10–15). Phase I consists of defining the appropriate dose as well as the safety profile/adverse effects of a medication in healthy volunteers (typically 20 to 100 subjects). Phase II begins to determine how well the drug works on a larger group of subjects (typically 100 to 300); of note, the medication does not yet have a presumed therapeutic effect. Phase III are large trials (300 to 3,000 subjects) that are often randomized against the already on the market standard of care drug ("the gold standard"). Phase IV trial occurs after FDA approval when the approved medication undergoes postmarketing surveillance of long-term adverse effects for a minimum of 2 years.

68. (A) Sildenafil is a phosphodiesterase type 5 inhibitor, which blocks the degradation of cyclic GMP in smooth muscle cells and promotes vasodilation. Bosentan, ambrisentan, and macitentan are endothelin receptor antagonists (ERAs), which block endothelin receptors. Ambrisentan is a selective endothelin A receptor antagonist, while bosentan and macitentan are dual antagonists, blocking both A and B. Prostacyclin (also known as prostaglandin I2) was used classically in an intravenous fashion to restore the balance of endogenous thromboxanes and prostacyclins and induce vasodilation. Aspirin suppressed the production of prostaglandins and thromboxanes by irreversibly inactivating the cyclooxygenase enzyme.

69. (D) Spironolactone acts to inhibit aldosterone at the distal tubule, reducing potassium loss in the urine. The diuretic effect is relatively mild and is most commonly used concurrently with a loop or thiazide diuretics. Carbonic anhydrase inhibitors include acetazolamide and act in the proximal convoluted tubule. Thiazide diuretics act to inhibit sodium and chloride transport in the distal convoluted tubule. Loop diuretics such as furosemide act to inhibit Na–K–Cl cotransport in the thick ascending limb of the loop of Henle. Calcium channel blockers block L-type calcium channels in the heart.

70. (B) Bosentan, ambrisentan, and macitentan are endothelin receptor antagonists (ERAs), which block endothelin receptors. Ambrisentan is a selective endothelin A receptor antagonist, while bosentan and macitentan are dual antagonists, blocking both A and B. Sildenafil is a phosphodiesterase type 5 inhibitor, which blocks the degradation of cyclic GMP in smooth muscle cells and promotes vasodilation. Prostacyclin (also known as prostaglandin I2) was used classically in an intravenous fashion to restore the balance of endogenous thromboxanes and prostacyclins and induce vasodilation. Aspirin suppressed the production of prostaglandins and thromboxanes by irreversibly inactivating the cyclooxygenase enzyme.

71. (A) Enalapril, an angiotensin-converting enzyme (ACE) inhibitor, acts to decrease the amount of angiotensin I that is converted to angiotensin II. Angiotensin II is a potent vasoconstrictor, and as such, ACE inhibitors thus promote vasodilation by blocking the production of angiotensin II. ACE inhibitors also decrease the degradation of circulating bradykinins and reduce the production of aldosterone. Patients should be counseled to avoid pregnancy if on ACE-inhibitor medications, due to the high risk of major congenital malformations.

Surgical Palliation and Repair of Congenital Heart Disease

Nathaniel W. Taggart and Elizabeth H. Stephens

Questions

1. A 4-month-old child with a large membranous ventricular septal defect (VSD) and large secundum atrial septal defect (ASD) develops complete heart block shortly after surgical repair. A suture "bite" placed too deep in which of the following sites is most likely responsible for the heart block?

   A. Posterior-inferior rim of the VSD
   B. Anterior-superior rim of the VSD
   C. Anterior-superior rim of the ASD
   D. Posterior-superior rim of the ASD
   E. Posterior-inferior rim of the ASD

2. Which of the following surgical interventions carries the highest risk of pulmonary vascular obstructive disease among patients with tetralogy of Fallot and severe pulmonary stenosis?

   A. Central shunt
   B. Potts shunt
   C. Classic Blalock–Taussig (BT) shunt
   D. Modified BT shunt
   E. Late surgical repair

3. A 3-month-old female infant with Down syndrome undergoes successful repair of a balanced complete atrioventricular septal defect (AVSD). While discussing her long-term prognosis with her parents, you state that which of the following is the most common indication for reoperation after repair of AVSDs?

   A. Residual atrial shunt
   B. Residual ventricular septal defect
   C. Left ventricular outflow tract obstruction
   D. Right AV valve regurgitation
   E. Left AV valve regurgitation

4. Which of the following is the strongest predictor for developing left AV valve regurgitation after the repair of atrioventricular septal defects (AVSDs)?

   A. Presence of a preoperative mitral valve cleft
   B. Preoperative severe mitral regurgitation
   C. Postoperative left ventricular dysfunction
   D. Postoperative LV enlargement
   E. Postoperative LVOT obstruction

5. You perform a cardiac catheterization on a 12-month-old child with pulmonary atresia, VSD, and confluent pulmonary arteries status post placement of a 3.5-mm modified left-sided Blalock–Taussig (BT) shunt at 1 week of age. His systemic arterial saturation is 62% on room air. Body surface area is 0.5 m². The RPA diameter is 8 mm and the LPA diameter is 9 mm, just proximal to their first lobar branches. There is stenosis of the RPA proximal to the BT shunt insertion, measuring 6 mm in diameter. There are no significant aortopulmonary collateral arteries.

   Which of the following is the best intervention at this time?

   A. Revision of the BT shunt
   B. Placement of a right BT shunt
   C. RV-to-PA conduit; leave VSD open
   D. VSD closure, placement of an RV-to-PA conduit
   E. Takedown of BT shunt and placement of a bidirectional cavopulmonary anastomosis

6. A 3-year-old patient undergoes aortic valve replacement with a tissue bioprosthesis. Two days later, he develops complete heart block with no propagation of electrical activity through the AV node. Obstruction of which of the following would best explain this clinical scenario?

   A. Posterior descending coronary artery
   B. Right coronary artery
   C. Posterior descending coronary artery
   D. Left anterior descending coronary artery
   E. Left circumflex coronary artery

7. A 35-year-old female with a history of tricuspid atresia status post extracardiac, nonfenestrated Fontan at age 5 years presents with a 2-year history of dyspnea on exertion and cyanosis that is notably worse when in the standing position. What is the most likely cause of her symptoms?

   A. Hepatic arteriovenous malformation
   B. Fontan baffle leak
   C. Aortopulmonary collateral vessels
   D. Venovenous collateral vessels
   E. Pulmonary arteriovenous malformations

8. Which of the following operations carries the highest risk of postoperative sinus node dysfunction?

   A. Atrial switch (Mustard or Senning) procedure
   B. Secundum ASD patch repair
   C. Complete AV canal repair
   D. Tricuspid valve repair for Ebstein anomaly
   E. Mitral valve mechanical prosthesis replacement

9. A 6-month-old infant underwent repair of a perimembranous ventricular septal defect. Routine postoperative electrocardiogram is shown in **Figure 15.1**.

   Concomitant repair of which of the following lesions is mostly to have led to these findings?

   A. Mitral valve stenosis
   B. Subaortic membrane
   C. Tricuspid valve regurgitation
   D. Large secundum atrial septal defect
   E. Right ventricular outflow tract obstruction

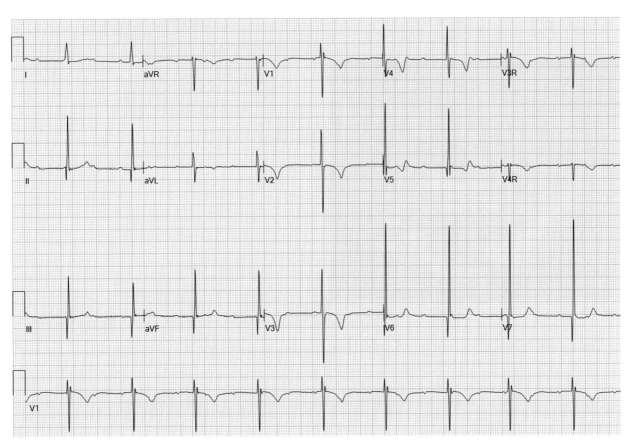

FIGURE 15.1

10. A 3-year-old patient is undergoing repair for tetralogy of Fallot and severe pulmonary stenosis. After initiation of cardiopulmonary bypass, using bicaval and aortic cannulation, the surgeon notes progressive left heart distention. This finding is most likely due to which of the following?

   A. Persistent left superior vena cava
   B. Ventricular septal defect
   C. Patent foramen ovale
   D. Aortic valve regurgitation
   E. Aortopulmonary collaterals

11. A 17-year-old male who had complete repair of a partial atrioventricular (AV) septal defect at 15 months of age presents with progressive shortness of breath. He has a 2/6 systolic crescendo–decrescendo murmur that is less prominent with Valsalva. Which of the following is most likely responsible for his symptoms?

   A. AV valve regurgitation
   B. Primary pulmonary hypertension
   C. Left ventricular outflow tract obstruction
   D. AV valve stenosis
   E. Residual atrial septal defect

12. A neonate presents with a murmur and is found to have the defect shown in **Figure 15.2** and **Video 15.1**.

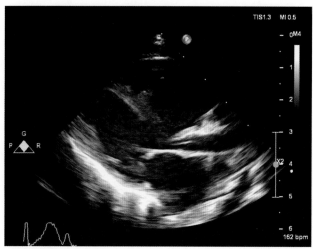

FIGURE 15.2

Which of the following will this patient most likely undergo as part of her surgical treatment?

A. Aortic arch repair
B. Aortic valvotomy
C. Mitral valve repair
D. Resection of intra-atrial membrane
E. Subaortic membrane resection

13. A 2-month-old infant presents with poor weight gain, tachypnea, and a murmur and is found to have the anomaly shown in **Figure 15.3**.

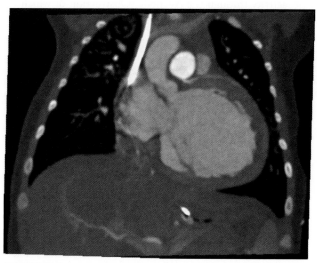

FIGURE 15.3

Which of the following preoperative findings is most closely associated with postoperative mortality and need for late reoperation in such a patient?

A. Mitral insufficiency
B. Tricuspid insufficiency
C. Left atrial dilation
D. Aortic valve insufficiency
E. Pulmonary valve insufficiency

14. Which of the following is the most common long-term complication after surgical repair of the defect shown in **Figure 15.4** and **VIDEO 15.2**?

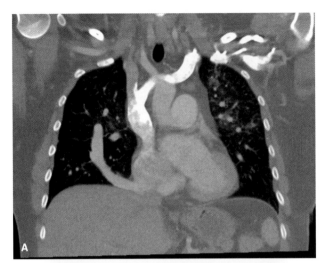

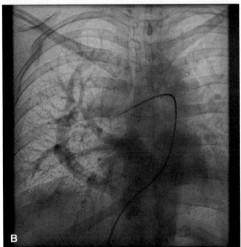

FIGURE 15.4

    A. Atrial arrhythmia
    B. Pulmonary vein obstruction
    C. Right ventricular enlargement
    D. IVC obstruction
    E. Pulmonary vascular disease

15. You are evaluating a 5-year-old child with a history of unbalanced AV canal, pulmonary atresia, bilateral superior venae cavae, and interrupted IVC. Initial palliation consisted of placement of bilateral bidirectional cavopulmonary anastomoses at 6 months of age, after which his oxygen saturation was 85% to 90%. Currently his saturation is 75% while sitting comfortably. Which of the following is most likely to have contributed to his progressive desaturation?

    A. Erythrocytosis
    B. Intrapulmonary shunting
    C. Development of coronary cameral fistulae
    D. Decreased chest wall compliance
    E. Increased pulmonary vascular resistance

16. You are asked to evaluate a 4-year-old child who recently moved to the United States from Russia. He has tricuspid atresia, normally related great arteries, pulmonary stenosis, and normal pulmonary and systemic venous connections. At 3 weeks of age, he had a modified Blalock–Taussig (BT) shunt. His height and weight are at the 15th percentile. The left ventricular impulse is slightly overactive. S_1 is normal, S_2 is single, and there is a 2/6 continuous murmur at the base of the heart. The liver is 1 cm below the right costal margin. The hemoglobin is 17 g/dL. The data in **Table 15.1** are obtained at the time of cardiac catheterization. An angiogram reveals normal size and distributed pulmonary arteries. An echocardiogram reveals an LV ejection fraction of 60%.

Table 15.1 Cardiac Catheterization Data

	Saturation	Pressure (mm Hg)
Right atrium	65%	Mean = 6
Left atrium	90%	Mean = 6
Pulmonary vein	99%	–
Left ventricle	82%	110/8
Aorta	82%	110/50
PA	82%	18/8, mean 11

PA, pulmonary artery.

Which of the following would you recommend?

    A. Delay any operative intervention until the hemoglobin reaches 19 g/dL
    B. Bidirectional cavopulmonary (Glenn) anastomosis and takedown of the BT shunt
    C. Kawashima operation and hepatic vein baffle to the pulmonary arteries
    D. Atriopulmonary connection and closure of the ASD and takedown of the BT shunt
    E. Extracardiac Fontan and takedown of the BT shunt

17. A 2-year-old female with a history of tetralogy of Fallot with pulmonary stenosis and an aortopulmonary collateral artery presents for routine follow-up 18 months after surgical repair. Surgery included transannular patch and ventricular septal defect closure. The collateral artery was not ligated. She was discharged from the hospital 5 days after surgery and is growing and developing appropriately. Her parents report no concerning symptoms.

On examination, she has a medium grade, to-and-fro murmur throughout the precordium. She is mildly tachypneic but comfortable with otherwise no increased work of breathing. Breath sounds are more pronounced over the left lung field. A chest x-ray is shown in **Figure 15.5**.

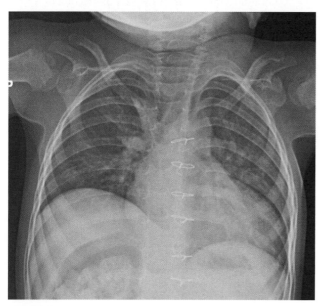

FIGURE 15.5

Which of the following is the best course of action for this patient?

A. No treatment needed at this time
B. Chest computed tomography
C. Chest tube insertion
D. Transcatheter occlusion of aortopulmonary collateral
E. Surgical diaphragm plication

18. A 1-day-old infant is found to be cyanotic. Oxygen saturation is 60% to 65% on room air. On examination, the child is breathing comfortably and is well perfused. Chest x-ray shows diminished pulmonary vascularity. Echocardiography demonstrates the findings shown in **Figure 15.6** and **VIDEO 15.3**.

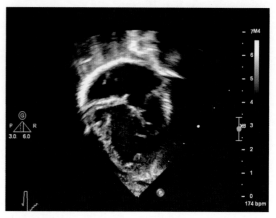

FIGURE 15.6

Which of the following procedures would be most likely to benefit this patient?

A. Balloon atrial septostomy
B. Enlargement of the bulboventricular foramen
C. Modified BT shunt placement
D. Pulmonary artery banding
E. Damus–Kaye–Stansel (DKS) anastomosis with modified BT shunt

19. A neonate presents with poor perfusion and a loud, harsh ejection-type murmur. Oxygen saturation is 95% on room air. Echocardiography demonstrates the findings shown in **Figure 15.7**.

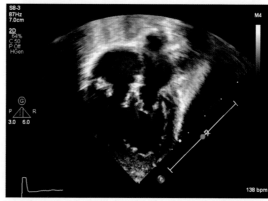

FIGURE 15.7

Which of the following is most likely to benefit this patient at this time?

A. Balloon atrial septostomy
B. Enlargement of the bulboventricular foramen
C. Coarctation repair and modified BT shunt placement
D. Pulmonary artery banding
E. Damus–Kaye–Stansel (DKS) anastomosis with modified BT shunt

20. A 2-year-old male undergoes successful surgical valvotomy for a stenotic dysplastic pulmonary valve resistant to balloon dilation. Postoperative echocardiography documents mild valvular regurgitation with a predicted gradient across the valve of 10 mm Hg. What is the likelihood that this child will need reintervention on his pulmonary valve within the next 10 years?

A. 50%
B. 40%
C. 30%
D. 20%
E. <10%

21. A 4-year-old child has pulmonary atresia and intact ventricular septum. She had placement of a modified Blalock–Taussig (BT) shunt as a neonate before being lost to follow-up. Her pulmonary artery trunk diameter is 10 mm. Pulmonary arteriolar resistance is 1.8 WU × m². Her hemoglobin is now 20 g/dL. Tricuspid valve Z-score is −3.5 and there is evidence of right ventricular sinusoids. Which of the following is the best next step in this patient's management?

A. Partial exchange transfusion with a goal hemoglobin of 15 g/dL
B. Ongoing follow-up until symptoms develop
C. Bidirectional cavopulmonary anastomosis with takedown of the BT shunt
D. ASD closure, tricuspid valve repair or replacement, and RV outflow tract reconstruction
E. Modified (extracardiac) Fontan and BT shunt takedown

22. A 3-month-old infant has pulmonary atresia with intact ventricular septum and a right modified Blalock–Taussig (BT) shunt. His oxygen saturation is 70% on room air. An angiogram documents confluent pulmonary arteries with membranous atresia of the pulmonary valve. The right ventricle (RV) is tripartite but diminutive. The tricuspid valve is well developed with moderate regurgitation and an annulus Z-score of −2.3. There is no evidence of right ventricle-dependent coronary circulation. Which of the following is the best treatment option for this patient?

A. BT shunt revision
B. Central shunt placement
C. RV outflow reconstruction
D. Unifocalization procedure with RV outflow reconstruction
E. Bidirectional cavopulmonary anastomosis with BT shunt takedown

23. The angiogram in **Figure 15.8** is performed in a 4-day-old term boy (3.8 kg) with pulmonary atresia with intact ventricular septum and a large patent ductus arteriosus (PDA).

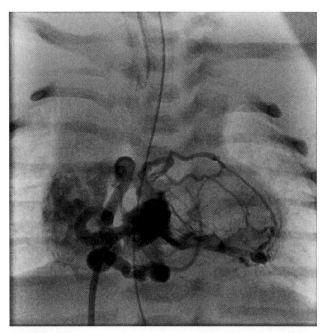

FIGURE 15.8

Which of the following treatments is best for this patient at this time?

A. Radiofrequency perforation and dilation of the RV outflow tract
B. PDA ligation, modified Blalock–Taussig shunt placement
C. PDA ligation, right ventricle-to-pulmonary artery conduit placement
D. PDA ligation, surgical pulmonary valvotomy
E. Continued prostaglandin infusion to allow for growth of the right ventricle

24. A 3-year-old child has pulmonary atresia with VSD. He has a history of hypoplastic central pulmonary arteries and multiple noncommunicating major aortopulmonary collateral arteries (MAPCAs), with multiple surgeries including a central shunt and bilateral unifocalization procedures. He undergoes reconstruction of the central confluence, placement of right ventricle-to-pulmonary artery (RV-PA) conduit, ligation of two MAPCAs, and VSD closure. When cardiopulmonary bypass is discontinued, his blood pressure is 84/60 mm Hg on multiple inotropic agents. Arterial blood oxygen saturation is 98% on 100% inhaled oxygen. Right ventricular systolic pressure is 69 mm Hg by direct measurement.

Transesophageal echo demonstrates patency of the conduit. Which of the following is the best next step?

A. Place on ECMO until hemodynamics improve
B. Fenestrate the VSD patch
C. Takedown the RV-to-PA conduit and place a central shunt
D. Replace of the RV-to-PA conduit with a larger conduit
E. Treat with inhaled nitric oxide

25. A term neonate (3.6 kg) presents with a murmur, mild hypoxia, and the echocardiographic findings shown in **Figure 15.9A,B** (**Video 15.4A,B**). Aortic arch is left sided and patent.

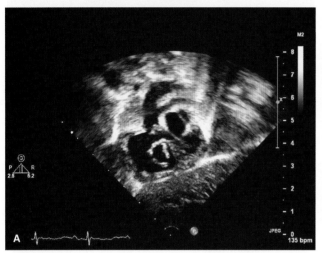
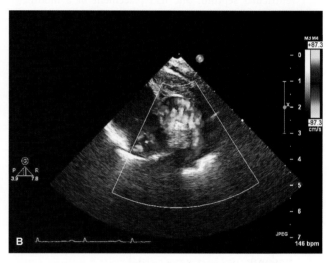

FIGURE 15.9

Which of the following is the best treatment plan for this infant?

A. Urgent balloon atrial septostomy
B. Prostaglandin E1 infusion
C. Modified BT shunt placement by 2 weeks of age
D. Complete repair within first month of life
E. Pulmonary artery banding by 4 months of age

26. After initial surgical intervention for the patient in Question 25, which of the following is the most likely indication for subsequent reoperation?

A. Valve regurgitation
B. Residual ventricular septal defect
C. Branch pulmonary artery stenosis
D. Conduit dysfunction
E. Progressive cyanosis

27. An asymptomatic 1-year-old female infant is referred for a murmur. Her blood pressure is 117/79 mm Hg (left arm) and 99/70 mm Hg (left leg). The echocardiogram confirms discrete coarctation of the aorta and bicuspid aortic valve with mild regurgitation. The mid-ascending aorta is mildly dilated. Left ventricular function is normal and wall thickness is at the upper limits of normal. Which of the following is the strongest reason to proceed with surgical intervention?

   A. Blood pressure
   B. Blood pressure gradient
   C. Left ventricular wall thickness
   D. Aortic valve dysfunction
   E. Ascending aorta dilatation

28. You are discussing the mortality risks to parents of a newborn with hypoplastic left heart syndrome. They ask about the risk of dying during the each of the stages of surgical palliation. You explain that current data suggest that the highest risk of mortality is during which of the following periods?

   A. Prior to stage 1 palliation
   B. Between stage 1 and stage 2 palliation
   C. During stage 2 palliation
   D. Between stage 2 and stage 3 palliation
   E. During stage 3 palliation

29. One day after bilateral pulmonary artery banding and PDA stent implantation ("hybrid" Norwood), a 7-day-old term neonate with aortic and mitral valve atresia develops progressive cyanosis and mild metabolic acidosis. His respiratory rate is 40 with an oxygen saturation of 65% on room air. His heart rate is 160 bpm, blood pressure is 65/42 mm Hg. His chest x-ray demonstrates increased pulmonary vascular markings. Which of the following best explains his worsening clinical status?

   A. Pulmonary hypertensive crisis
   B. Retrograde aortic arch obstruction
   C. Branch pulmonary artery obstruction
   D. Restrictive atrial septal shunt
   E. Hypovolemia

30. A neonate presents after delivery with respiratory distress and a loud murmur and is diagnosed with the defect shown in **Figure 15.10** and **VIDEO 15.5**.

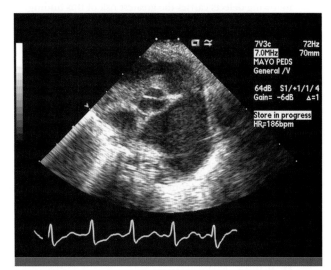

FIGURE 15.10

Oxygen saturation on room air is 75%. Which of the following procedures would most likely benefit this patient at this time?

   A. Patent ductus arteriosus stent implantation
   B. LeCompte maneuver with pulmonary artery plication
   C. Pulmonary balloon valvuloplasty
   D. Ventricular septal defect closure with transannular patch
   E. Pulmonary artery banding

31. Which of the following is the most common indication for reoperation after initial repair of the defect shown in **Figure 15.11** and **VIDEO 15.6A,B**?

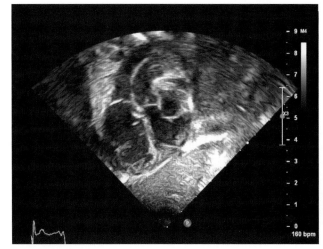

FIGURE 15.11

   A. Supravalvular pulmonary stenosis (PS)
   B. RV-PA conduit dysfunction
   C. Residual shunt
   D. AV valve regurgitation
   E. Coronary artery occlusion

32. A 3 month old is found to have a hoarse, weak cry after cardiac surgery. Laryngoscopy demonstrates immobility of the left vocal cord. Surgical intervention for which of the following defects carries the greatest risk of this finding?

    A. Complete atrioventricular canal

    B. Tetralogy of Fallot

    C. Bidirectional cavopulmonary anastomosis

    D. Coarctation of the aorta

    E. Total anomalous pulmonary venous return

33. A neonate is found to have d-transposition of the great arteries with a large ventricular septal defect (VSD), a large atrial septal defect, and severe left ventricular outflow tract (LVOT) obstruction. The patient's oxygen saturation is 68% on room air. Which of the following is the most appropriate initial intervention for this patient?

    A. Arterial switch operation

    B. Blalock–Hanlon septostomy

    C. Pulmonary balloon valvuloplasty

    D. Balloon atrial septostomy

    E. PDA stent implantation

34. A 2-year-old child with L-transposition of the great arteries, large membranous VSD with outlet extension, and history of critical pulmonary stenosis has been palliated with a modified BT shunt in the neonatal period and a bidirectional cavopulmonary anastomosis at 6 months of age. His oxygen saturation is 70%. He has good biventricular size and function, and no AV valve straddling. He is presenting for surgical intervention. Given this patient's anatomy, which of the following is the most reasonable surgical plan?

    A. Arterial switch and baffling of the IVC to the tricuspid valve

    B. Baffle LV flow across the VSD to the aortic valve (Rastelli-type repair) and placement of a pulmonary conduit

    C. Baffle the VSD to direct LV flow to the pulmonary valve and baffling IVC to the tricuspid valve

    D. Baffle LV flow across the VSD to the aortic valve, placement of a pulmonary conduit, and baffling of IVC to the tricuspid valve

    E. Extracardiac Fontan operation

35. You are performing an echocardiogram on a newborn infant in the neonatal ICU. You diagnose double outlet right ventricle with normally related great arteries and large, doubly-committed VSD, severe coarctation of the aorta, mild subaortic stenosis, and mitral valve which straddles the VSD. Both ventricles are normal in size. Which of the following is the best initial operation for this patient?

    A. Repair the coarctation and baffle the VSD to the aorta (Rastelli)

    B. Coarctation repair and mitral valve repair

    C. Coarctation repair only

    D. Norwood operation with placement of nonvalved RV-PA conduit

    E. Baffle VSD to aorta, repair coarctation, resect subaortic stenosis

36. A full-term infant (4 kg) is born with double outlet right ventricle, malposed great arteries, subpulmonary ventricular septal defect (VSD), and no left or right ventricular outflow obstruction. Oxygen saturation on room air is 80% to 85%. Which of the following initial operations should you recommend?

    A. Pulmonary artery banding

    B. Arterial switch with baffle closure of the VSD to the neo-aorta

    C. Systemic to pulmonary (BT) shunt

    D. Patch closure of the VSD

    E. Damus–Kaye–Stansel anastomosis and modified BT shunt

37. A term neonate with a harsh systolic murmur at birth is found to have double-inlet left ventricle with normally related great arteries, and a restrictive bulboventricular foramen. Prostaglandin E1 infusion is started. A subsequent echocardiogram documents a large ductus arteriosus. Which of the following is the most appropriate initial operation for this child?

    A. Modified Blalock–Taussig (BT) shunt

    B. Damus–Kaye–Stansel anastomosis with modified BT shunt

    C. Enlargement of the bulboventricular foramen

    D. Pulmonary artery banding

    E. Balloon atrial septostomy

38. A 3-year-old female is found to have a murmur during a routine physical examination. Echocardiogram reveals a secundum ASD with continuous left-to-right shunt. Which of the following factors would be the strongest indication for surgical repair rather than percutaneous closure of the ASD?

    A. Patient's age

    B. Deficient anterior-superior septal rim

    C. Severe tricuspid valve regurgitation

    D. Right ventricular dysfunction

    E. Estimated right ventricular systolic pressure = 40 mm Hg

39. A 2-month-old male with persistent stridor and tachypnea is found to have tracheomalacia and the defect shown in **Figure 15.12.**

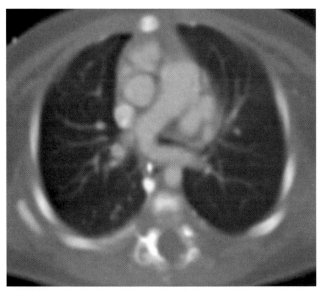

FIGURE 15.12

Which of the following will best help to alleviate the airway compression?

A. Reimplantation of the pulmonary artery anterior to the trachea
B. Pulmonary artery plication and LeCompte maneuver
C. Resection of the diverticulum of Kommerell
D. Division of the nondominant aortic arch
E. Division of the ductus arteriosus

40. A 31-year-old female with a history of coarctation of the aorta has a chest x-ray performed for chronic cough (see **Figure 15.13**).

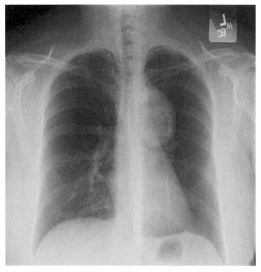

FIGURE 15.13

Which of the following treatments for coarctation of the aorta is most likely to have resulted in the finding in **Figure 15.13**?

A. Percutaneous balloon angioplasty
B. Transcatheter stent implantation
C. Subclavian flap repair
D. Synthetic patch repair
E. Surgical end-to-end anastomosis

41. A 37 year old presents with progressive exertional fatigue and weight gain over the past couple of years. He explains that he was born with a heart defect and had one operation when he was a baby but does not remember when he last saw a cardiologist.

Oxygen saturation is 97% on room air. On examination, he has a well-healed median sternotomy. S_2 is loud and single; no murmurs are present. Palpation of his abdomen reveals a fluid wave, and he has pitting edema to his knees. You document no jugular venous distension. Chest x-ray shows normal cardiac size and clear lung fields. Electrocardiogram is shown in **Figure 15.14**.

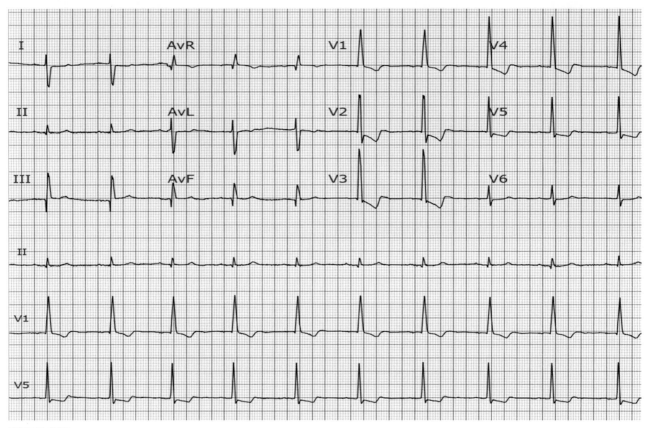

FIGURE 15.14

Which of the following defects did he most likely have?

A. Tetralogy of Fallot
B. Pulmonary atresia with intact ventricular septum
C. Transposition of the great arteries
D. Tricuspid atresia with malposed great arteries
E. Atrioventricular canal defect

42. A 13 year old presents with exertional desaturation and fatigue and is diagnosed with Ebstein anomaly. There is no history of syncope or palpitations. Electrophysiology testing does not provoke tachyarrhythmia. Which of the following procedures performed during surgical treatment of Ebstein anomaly has been shown to correlate most strongly with improvement in functional capacity after surgery?

A. Tricuspid valve repair
B. ASD or PFO closure
C. Right ventricular plication
D. MAZE procedure
E. Bidirectional cavopulmonary anastomosis

43. A 17-year-old young man (height 196 cm; weight 87 kg) is found to have ectopia lentis. Echocardiogram demonstrates a dilated aortic root (52 mm; Z-score 5.5), a bicuspid aortic valve with no stenosis and mild regurgitation, and bileaflet mitral valve prolapse with mild regurgitation. Which of the following is the best management option for this patient?

A. Initiate beta-blocker therapy and repeat echocardiogram in 6 months
B. Endoluminal ascending aorta graft
C. Composite graft aortic root replacement
D. Valve-sparing aortic root replacement
E. Mitral valve repair and aortic root replacement

44. A Warden procedure includes which of the following maneuvers?

A. Patch baffle from the base of the SVC across the atrial septum
B. Anastomosis of the vertical vein to the left atrial appendage
C. Transection of the SVC at its junction with the right atrium
D. Patch closure of the atrial septal defect
E. Reimplantation of the anomalous vessel(s)

45. A 15-year-old female present with dyspnea on exertion and difficulty swallowing. CT angiogram demonstrates the findings in **Figure 15.15**.

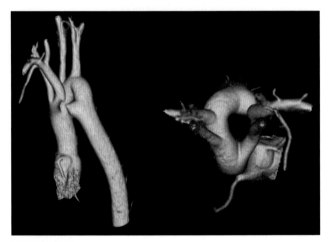

FIGURE 15.15

Which of the following is necessarily involved in the repair of this patient's defect?

A. Median sternotomy
B. Transection of the atretic aortic arch
C. Division of the ligamentum arteriosum
D. Resection of the diverticulum of Kommerell
E. Reimplantation of the anomalous brachiocephalic arteries

46. A neonate with critical aortic valve stenosis undergoes transcatheter aortic balloon valvuloplasty, resulting in moderate–severe regurgitation and a persistent peak systolic gradient of 45 mm Hg. A Ross procedure is recommended. The family asks about long-term outcomes after this procedure. Which of the following is the most likely indication for reoperation?

A. Arrhythmias
B. Subaortic stenosis
C. Neo-aortic valve failure
D. Coronary artery obstruction
E. Pulmonary homograft failure

47. Which of the following modifications to repair of Ebstein anomaly is most beneficial in patients with a history of supraventricular tachyarrhythmia?

A. MAZE procedure
B. Right reduction atrioplasty
C. Right ventricle plication
D. Pulmonary vein isolation
E. Bidirectional cavopulmonary anastomosis

48. An 8-day-old baby with d-transposition of the great arteries, intact ventricular septum, and atrial septal defect undergoes arterial switch operation with LeCompte maneuver and closure of the atrial septal defect. She is weaned from cardiopulmonary bypass, and the chest is closed before return to the ICU. Over the course of 2 hours in the ICU, she becomes progressively more hypotensive despite multiple fluid boluses and increasing infusions of epinephrine and vasopressin. Blood pressure is 63/47 mm Hg. Central venous pressure is 18 mm Hg. Lactate level is 5.0 mmol/L (normal = 0.6 to 3.2 mmol/L). Emergent bedside echocardiogram shows underfilled ventricles with normal systolic function and no pericardial fluid or thrombus. Which of the following is the best next step?

A. Emergent chest CT
B. Coronary angiography
C. Pericardial drain insertion
D. Reopen the sternotomy
E. Cannulation for ECMO support

49. Surgical treatment of which of the following constellation of defects might involve a Yasui procedure?

A. Pulmonary atresia with VSD and major aortopulmonary collateral arteries
B. Tricuspid atresia with malposed great arteries and aortic coarctation
C. D-transposition of the great arteries with VSD and left ventricular outflow obstruction
D. Posterior malaligned VSD with interrupted aortic arch
E. Truncus arteriosus with truncal valve dysfunction

50. A 14-year-old otherwise healthy male undergoes patch closure of a large secundum atrial septal defect. Three weeks after discharge from the hospital, he presents with low-grade fevers and chest pain that began about 4 days prior. His appearance is nontoxic with unlabored breathing. His heart rate is 89 bpm, blood pressure is 113/76 mm Hg. On examination, there is a pericardial friction rub, but heart sounds are clear. Chest x-ray shows clear lung fields with mildly enlarged cardiac silhouette (unchanged from the day of discharge). Echocardiogram shows a small circumferential effusion. Which of the following is the best next step?

A. Obtain blood cultures
B. Treat with high-dose aspirin
C. Treat with colchicine
D. Pericardiocentesis
E. Chest computed tomography

Answers

1. (A) A significant concern during the repair of membranous VSDs, particularly when performed on young infants, is damaging the AV node when suturing the patch in place. The AV node courses along the posterior-inferior rim of membranous VSDs. Damage to the node could result in high-grade AV block immediately or shortly after surgical repair. AV block is not a significant risk of secundum ASD repair.

2. (B) Many adults with congenital heart disease have had surgical creation of direct aorta to pulmonary artery communication, either via an ascending aorta to right pulmonary artery connection (Waterston shunt) or via a descending aorta to left pulmonary artery connection (Potts shunt). These techniques have since been abandoned, due to difficulty regulating the size of the shunt and a high rate of branch pulmonary stenosis. Inappropriately large surgical shunts carry a high risk of pulmonary hypertension and, ultimately, pulmonary vascular obstructive disease. Central shunts and modified BT shunts utilize synthetic shunts of specific size, allowing for more predictable shunt volume. Classic BT shunts (direct connection of the left or right subclavian artery to the ipsilateral branch pulmonary artery) were frequently complicated by shunt obstruction and are no longer performed. In the presence of severe pulmonary valve stenosis, the pulmonary vascular bed would be reasonably protected and not at risk of pulmonary vascular disease, even with late repair.

3. (E) Modern surgical repair of AVSDs has resulted in tremendous improvement in life expectancy and quality of life for children (and now adults) with Down syndrome. The need for late reoperation after complete AVSD repair is approximately 15% to 20%. While small residual atrial or ventricular shunts may persist after repair and right AV valve (tricuspid) regurgitation may be present, they are uncommon indications for reoperation. Unlike in partial AV septal defects, LVOT obstruction is an infrequent indication for reoperation among patients with complete AV canal defects. Left AV valve (mitral) regurgitation, on the other hand, is the most common reason for late reoperation.

4. (B) Intuitively, severe preoperative AV valve regurgitation predicts postoperative AV valve regurgitation. A cleft in the left AV valve is universal in AV canal defects and does not predict postoperative regurgitation. Left ventricular size and dysfunction may influence the degree of mitral regurgitation, but this association is not so strong.

5. (D) The Nakata index is commonly used to predict operability in patients with pulmonary atresia–VSD. Angiographic measurements of the central pulmonary arteries just proximal to the first lobar branches (and any MAPCAs that perfuse an entire pulmonary segment and can be unifocalized) are taken, and the cross-sectional area of each branch ($\pi \times$ radius^2) is calculated. The sum of these areas is divided by body surface area:

$$\text{Nakata index} = \frac{\text{LPA area (mm}^2) + \text{RPA area (mm}^2) + \text{MAPCA area (mm}^2)}{\text{BSA (m}^2)}$$

The calculation for this patient is as follows:

$$\text{Nakata index} = \frac{64 \text{ mm}^2 + 50 \text{ mm}^2}{0.5 \text{ m}^2} = 228$$

Patients with a Nakata index >200 are generally considered good candidates for complete repair (including unifocalization, if necessary). Patients with an index <200 may be candidates as well, but are at higher risk of pulmonary hypertension and right heart failure. They may be better off without surgical intervention or with limited surgical palliation. For the patient in the scenario, RPA patch angioplasty or stent placement would be indicated as part of the repair.

6. (B) Postoperative heart block, ST segment changes, or ventricular dysfunction with regional wall motion abnormalities should raise concern of compromised coronary artery perfusion. This may result from mechanical compression or obstruction by a prosthetic valve, transection of a coronary artery, or tension and kinking with coronary artery reimplantation. The child in this vignette presents a history typical of coronary artery obstruction after a procedure (aortic valve replacement) that presents risk of the same. While definitive identification of the compromised artery requires angiography, the AV node is supplied by a branch of the right coronary artery in 90% of humans, making disruption of the RCA the most likely cause of AV node dysfunction in this patient.

7. (E) Pulmonary arteriovenous malformations occur commonly in patients following Fontan procedures. Dyspnea on exertion and orthostatic or exertional cyanosis in Fontan patients can occur due to right-to-left shunting at a widely patent fenestration or due to right-to-left shunting from pulmonary arteriovenous malformations. These most commonly occur in the basal region of the lung.

8. (A) The sinus node is located in the posterior right atrium along the superiolateral aspect of the superior vena cava. As a result, surgical disruption of this area may result in damage to the sinus node. Of the choices available, only the atrial switch procedure affects the posterior aspect of the right atrium. In the Mustard/Senning atrial switch operations, systemic venous return is directed across the atrial septum to the left-sided, subpulmonary ventricle. This is done by suturing a patch baffle along the posterior (sinus venosus) wall of the right atrium, in close proximity to the sinus node.

9. (B) Figure 15.1 demonstrates complete heart block. Right bundle branch block is common after VSD repair, but complete heart block is rare after isolated VSD repair. The addition of surgical resection of a subaortic membrane or ridge introduces a risk of left bundle branch block, which along with the right bundle branch block from the VSD repair would result in complete heart block. The other lesions listed are not typically associated with a risk of left bundle branch block.

10. (E) The role of the cardiologist in the operating room includes providing accurate echocardiographic description of cardiac anatomy, particularly the presence of shunts that may complicate cardiopulmonary bypass. In this scenario, the patient develops left heart distention after being placed on bypass, which suggests ongoing pulmonary venous return to the left atrium. This results from persistent pulmonary blood flow that is not accounted for in the bypass circuit. The most likely cause in this situation is a systemic to pulmonary shunt, such as aortopulmonary collateral arteries. If the aorta is not cross-clamped, significant aortic valve regurgitation may result in left ventricular distension, but this is less likely to be the case for this patient. The other options are important findings to note prior to bypass, but would not cause left heart distension. A persistent left SVC typically drains to the coronary sinus and would result in blood return to the right atrium.

11. (C) While the most common cause of reoperation in patients with partial AV canal defects is mitral valve regurgitation, LVOT obstruction is a common cause and much more common than in the complete form of AVSD. Shortness of breath, cardiomegaly, and increased pulmonary vascularity may be caused by mitral valve regurgitation or LVOT obstruction. However, the ejection-type systolic murmur that diminishes with Valsalva presented in this patient clearly suggests outflow tract obstruction as the underlying problem.

Primary pulmonary hypertension is very rare in children, and one would expect to find diminished pulmonary vascularity on chest x-ray. Mitral stenosis may cause this patient's symptoms, but it is a less common late finding after partial AV canal defect repair and not suggested by the other findings in the vignette. A residual ASD could cause this patient's symptoms if it was large enough, but, again, LVOT obstruction is a more common postoperative complication.

12. (A) Figure 15.2 shows a parasternal long axis view of the left ventricular outflow tract. There is a posterior malalignment VSD, which narrows the LVOT. This type of VSD is commonly associated with aortic arch obstruction, either coarctation or interruption. Thus, surgical repair will likely involve aortic arch repair as well.

13. (A) Figure 15.3 demonstrates an anomalous left coronary artery originating from the pulmonary artery (ALCAPA). ALCAPA typically presents in the second or third month of life after pulmonary vascular resistance falls and the anomalous coronary artery loses perfusion pressure. Infants typically present with a dilated, poorly functioning left ventricle caused by myocardial ischemia. These children are at risk of ischemia and infarction of the mitral valve papillary muscles and resultant mitral valve regurgitation. The tricuspid valve papillary muscles are usually perfused by branches of the right coronary artery.

14. (B) Figure 15.4A,B shows a right lower pulmonary vein draining below the diaphragm to the right atrium–IVC junction. Scimitar syndrome is the eponym for this anomaly. Surgical repair typically depends on the proximity of the anomalous venous connection to the right atrium and the presence of an ASD. Typically, the anomalous connection is transected and the right veins are reimplanted, either into the right or into the left atrium. If implanted into the right atrium, the right pulmonary venous return is then directed across an ASD into the left atrium by a patch baffle. The most common complication of this type of repair is obstruction of pulmonary venous return.

15. (B) The development of pulmonary arteriovenous fistulae has been identified as a risk of the classic cavopulmonary anastomosis (Glenn). Subsequently, it has been found to relate to the absence of hepatic effluent blood in the pulmonary circulation. While this patient had bilateral modified (bidirectional) Glenn anastomoses, the absence of hepatic venous return within the pulmonary circulation (due to IVC interruption) results in a similar lack of the hepatic factor that would otherwise prevent the development of the pulmonary AV fistulae. When surgically feasible, incorporation of hepatic venous return into the pulmonary circulation often results in diminution of the fistulae.

16. (E) The questions being posed by this scenario are whether this patient is a candidate for a Fontan-type palliation and how should the operation be performed. This patient's cardiac hemodynamics are favorable for single-ventricle palliation, specifically the PA pressure is low (mean 11 mm Hg) with a reasonable transpulmonary gradient (5 mm Hg). This is not surprising in the context of pulmonary stenosis, which protects the pulmonary vascular bed from systemic pressure. Infants presenting with single-ventricle physiology typically are repaired in a staged fashion, consisting of a BT shunt shortly after birth, Glenn anastomosis by 6 to 9 months, and Fontan completion in young childhood. As this child is 3 years old, there is no obvious need to perform a Glenn anastomosis prior to Fontan completion. The modified Fontan, using an extracardiac conduit or a lateral tunnel approach, is favored over a direct RA-to-PA anastomosis (classic Fontan).

17. (A) The chest x-ray in **Figure 15.5** demonstrates an elevated right hemidiaphragm. The clinical scenario is consistent with paralysis of the right hemidiaphragm, likely a complication from her surgical repair. In the absence of respiratory distress or exercise limitation, treatment of this finding is not necessary. Her "comfortable" tachypnea should be well tolerated.

18. (C) The vignette above describes a neonate with single ventricle and inadequate pulmonary blood flow, as demonstrated by the child's oxygen saturation and paucity of pulmonary vascularity. This may result from valvular stenosis or obstruction at the VSD (bulboventricular foramen). The initial palliation, therefore, should be directed at increasing pulmonary blood flow. This is best accomplished by stenting the ductus arteriosus or placing a modified BT shunt from the subclavian artery to the branch pulmonary artery. Balloon atrial septostomy may be necessary if the ASD is restrictive, a rare occurrence in tricuspid atresia and not suggested by this patient's findings. Pulmonary artery banding would decrease pulmonary blood flow. A DKS anastomosis consists of a direct ascending aorta to MPA (end-to-side) anastomosis. This is used in single-ventricle situations where there is left ventricular outflow obstruction (subaortic stenosis, valvular stenosis/atresia, coarctation) and allows for retrograde perfusion of the coronary arteries via a reconstructed "neo-aortic" arch.

19. (E) A DKS anastomosis consists of a direct ascending aorta to MPA (end-to-side) anastomosis. This is used in single-ventricle situations where there is systemic outflow obstruction (subaortic stenosis, valvular stenosis/atresia, coarctation) and allows for retrograde perfusion of the coronary arteries via a reconstructed "neo-aortic" arch. After a DKS anastomosis, the native pulmonary valve functions as the "neo-aortic" valve. The neonate in the vignette has double-inlet left ventricle (as shown in **Figure 15.7**) and—based on the clinical presentation of poor perfusion but adequate oxygenation—malposed great arteries. As such, the pulmonary artery arises from the left ventricle, and the aorta arises from the diminutive right ventricle. Thus, systemic outflow is dependent on the size of the VSD (bulboventricular foramen). This patient presents with increased $Q_p:Q_s$, as evidenced by a systemic saturation of 95% and signs of poor systemic perfusion and a harsh ejection-type murmur. This may result from a restrictive VSD, subvalvular aortic stenosis, or aortic valve stenosis. In this situation, a DKS anastomosis allows for adequate systemic output and coronary artery perfusion. A BT shunt placed at the same time provides a stable source of pulmonary blood flow once the MPA

is separated from the PA branches. Surgical enlargement of the VSD risks damage to the cardiac conduction system causing rhythm disturbances and ventricular dysfunction. A BT shunt alone does not address the problem of systemic outflow obstruction. PA banding would not be indicated as the primary problem is inadequate systemic output, not excessive pulmonary blood flow.

20. (E) Pulmonary valve stenosis can be managed initially with percutaneous pulmonary balloon valvuloplasty or surgical valvotomy. Percutaneous valvuloplasty tends to produce better relief of stenosis, but patients are often left with a greater degree of regurgitation than the surgical approach. A good initial surgical outcome, as described in this patient, carries a low risk of need for future operation, probably not more than 5% over the next 10 years.

21. (E) The type of surgical intervention indicated depends on a patient's age, hemodynamics, and underlying cardiac anatomy. The vignette describes a child with pulmonary atresia and intact ventricular septum. These patients may qualify for a two-ventricle repair with placement of a conduit from the right ventricle to the pulmonary arteries (which may be confluent or surgically unifocalized). If the right ventricle is not usable as a functional pumping chamber, either because of hypoplasia or because of coronary to RV fistulae, then the patient is not a candidate for complete repair and requires some form of palliation. This patient has a very diminutive RV, demonstrated by a tricuspid valve Z-score of −3.5. It has been shown that when the tricuspid annulus Z-score is less than −3, the outcome is very poor after attempted complete repair. As a result, this patient should undergo palliation. Her low pulmonary vascular resistance suggests that she is a good candidate for a Fontan operation. At 4 years of age, a complete Fontan can be performed as a single operation, rather than first performing a staged bidirectional cavopulmonary anastomosis.

22. (C) Patients with pulmonary atresia and intact ventricular septum may qualify for a two-ventricle–type repair. If the right ventricle is not usable as a functional pumping chamber, either because of hypoplasia or because of coronary to RV fistulae, then the patient is not a candidate for complete repair and requires some form of palliation. It has been shown that when the tricuspid annulus Z-score is less than −3, the outcome is very poor after attempted complete repair. Infants with a Z-score of −2 to −2.5 and a functional tricuspid valve may undergo placement of an RV to PA conduit. This patient has a small but usable RV, demonstrated by a tricuspid valve Z-score of −2.3 and the absence of coronary cameral fistulae (RV-dependent coronary circulation). Low oxygen saturation suggests that he is outgrowing his BT shunt and should have the next stage operation, in his case a two-ventricle complete repair. Transcatheter perforation and balloon dilation of the atretic (membranous) valve or surgical valvotomy/RVOT reconstruction would be the preferred treatment options in this scenario.

23. (B) The angiogram demonstrates a very small RV chamber with multiple sinusoids and coronary cameral fistulae. These fistulae are common in pulmonary atresia with intact ventricular septum, where the RV is severely hypoplastic. Decompression of the RV by transcatheter or surgical means (e.g., pulmonary valvotomy or placement of a conduit) may decrease coronary perfusion pressure and cause diffuse myocardial ischemia. This patient should continue down a single-ventricle palliation pathway, with ductal stenting or placement of a modified BT shunt as the first stage.

24. (B) Successful outcome after complete repair of pulmonary atresia and VSD has been shown to correlate with the postoperative right ventricular systolic pressure. Poor systemic blood pressure and near-systemic RV systolic pressure suggest limited cardiac output due to increased pulmonary arterial resistance. Under these circumstances, the surgeon should reopen or fenestrate the VSD to allow the left ventricle to contribute to pulmonary blood flow. If pulmonary resistance cannot be improved by surgical or transcatheter means, these patients may require surgical palliation rather than complete repair. The patient described is at high risk of pulmonary hypertension given the history of hypoplastic pulmonary arteries.

25. (D) Figure 15.9 demonstrates a single great artery with branches originating posteriorly, just superior to the semilunar valve, consistent with truncus arteriosus. Complete repair of truncus arteriosus has become the favorable approach in US congenital cardiac surgery centers. This patient will need intervention early in life to prevent irreversible pulmonary vascular obstructive disease. Historically, these children underwent pulmonary artery banding procedures within the first month of life. Now, complete repair within the first month of life—with VSD closure, repair of the truncal (neo-aortic) valve if needed, and placement of a conduit from the RV to the pulmonary arteries—is the operation of choice in most centers. This child has nonrestrictive pulmonary blood flow and does not need a BT shunt. The pulmonary arteries arise directly from the common arterial trunk and there is no aortic arch interruption, so prostaglandin is not needed.

26. (D) All of the choices listed are potential indications for reoperation after repair of truncus arteriosus. Homograft or synthetic conduits tend to last 10 to 15 years but almost universally become stenotic and/or regurgitant and are less durable in the youngest patients. Truncal valve regurgitation is very common, but often can be managed without surgical intervention until it becomes moderate or severe. Residual VSDs and branch PA stenosis are infrequent reasons for reoperation. Cyanosis would not be expected in patients with truncus arteriosus after repair.

27. (A) Severity of coarctation of the aorta can be measured anatomically, via estimated Doppler gradient or by noninvasive blood pressure measurement. Whether to intervene and the timing of intervention depend primarily upon the blood pressure gradient. In the absence of systemic hypertension, LV dysfunction, or significant collateral arteries, a systolic blood pressure gradient of less than 20 mm Hg by itself is not an indication for surgical intervention. The patient has systemic hypertension in addition to a mild gradient and discrete coarctation, so surgical treatment is warranted.

28. (B) The classic Norwood procedure for hypoplastic left heart syndrome consists of three stages. Stage 1 consists of excision of any remaining atrial septal tissue, separation of the pulmonary arteries from the MPA trunk, placement of a BT shunt to the branch PAs, and construction of a neo-aortic arch using the MPA tissue. The right ventricle then serves as the systemic ventricle and the pulmonary valve functions as the systemic (neo-aortic) valve. This stage is usually performed within the first week of life in term neonates without comorbidities. Stage 2 consists of takedown of the BT shunt and placement of an SVC to PA anastomosis (bidirectional cavopulmonary anastomosis). This typically occurs around 6 to 9 months of age, depending on the patient growth and degree of cyanosis. The Norwood is completed in stage 3 with anastomosis of the IVC to the PAs via an extracardiac conduit or tunnel along the lateral wall of the right atrium (modified Fontan). This final stage may be performed as early as 2 years of age. As one would expect, the highest mortality occurs early during the Norwood stages. Specifically, it has been shown to be highest after stage 1 and prior to stage 2.

29. (D) This child is showing signs of poor perfusion and cyanosis. The presence of tachypnea and increased pulmonary vascularity suggest pulmonary congestion from pulmonary venous obstruction. In children with hypoplastic left heart syndrome, the only way for pulmonary venous return to reach the systemic circulation is through an ASD. A small, restrictive ASD would best explain the findings in this child. Pulmonary hypertensive crisis would present more acutely. Retrograde aortic arch obstruction from the PDA stent may manifest as coronary hypoperfusion and decreased ventricular function; desaturation would not be an initial sign. Obstruction of the branch PAs would result in decreased oxygenation, but lung fields would be clear on x-ray. Hypovolemia is unlikely to be the primary cause as evidenced by the pulmonary congestion on chest x-ray.

30. (B) The echocardiographic imaging in **Figure 15.10** shows a short axis view of the aortic valve. The branch pulmonary arteries are extremely large. Combined with the clinical findings, this likely represents tetralogy of Fallot with absent pulmonary valve (absent pulmonary valve syndrome). In this setting, the child's tracheobronchial tree is likely extrinsically compressed by the large pulmonary arteries, and relief of this obstruction is the highest priority. This is accomplished surgically by plication of the branch pulmonary arteries, often along with a LeCompte maneuver to move the pulmonary artery branches anterior to the trachea.

31. (A) The arterial switch procedure has replaced the atrial switch (Mustard/Senning) as the repair of choice for d-TGA. It provides a more anatomic repair, with the left ventricle serving as the systemic ventricle and the right ventricle as the pulmonary ventricle. Complications of the arterial switch are primarily related to the mobilization and relocation of the great arteries and coronary arteries. In d-TGA, the aorta is located anterior to the pulmonary artery. Relocation of the pulmonary artery anteriorly introduces the risk of supravalvar stenosis as the artery is stretched behind the ascending aorta. For this reason, the LeCompte maneuver is

CHAPTER 15

sometimes used. This is performed by transecting the main pulmonary artery and relocating the entire PA trunk and bifurcation anterior to the aorta. Distortion of the coronary arteries carries a higher risk of mortality than supravalvular PS but is less common overall.

32. (D) The clinical stem describes left vocal cord paralysis, likely due to an injury to the left recurrent laryngeal nerve. This branch of the vagus nerve course is underneath the aortic arch in the region of the left brachiocephalic arteries. It is at risk of injury during surgery in that region, such as with surgical repair of coarctation of the aorta.

33. (E) This patient's anatomy consists of a subpulmonary left ventricle with obstruction. This manifests clinically as severe hypoxemia due to inadequate pulmonary blood flow. The best intervention in this neonate to increase pulmonary blood flow is to stent the ductus arteriosus or place a modified BT shunt. This child is likely to not be a candidate for a traditional arterial switch operation due to the LVOT obstruction. The Blalock–Hanlon septostomy is an open surgical atrial septostomy that is no longer performed. Because LVOT obstruction is most often complex and not isolated to pulmonary valve stenosis, balloon valvuloplasty is unlikely to provide improvement in pulmonary blood flow. With a large ASD, the patient's cyanosis is not a result of inadequate atrial shunting/mixing, so septostomy is not likely to provide improvement in oxygenation.

34. (D) The patient in the vignette has complicated anatomy consisting of congenitally corrected TGA, pulmonary stenosis, and a large VSD. He has a bidirectional cavopulmonary anastomosis providing (presumably) the bulk of his pulmonary blood flow. His AV valve and the presence of two well-formed ventricles, however, are favorable for a two-ventricle, physiologic repair. This would be accomplished by directing the remainder of his systemic venous return across the atrial septum to the left-sided AV valve (tricuspid valve), baffle closure of the VSD to direct right ventricle output across the aortic valve, and placement of a pulmonary conduit from the morphologic left ventricle to the pulmonary arteries. Choice A would result in the stenotic pulmonary valve having to function as the neo-aortic valve. Choices B, C, and E would result in the IVC flow being directed to the systemic (subaortic) ventricle.

35. (D) The straddling of the mitral valve chordae precludes anatomic repair of this neonate's defect. As a result, the best option of the choices listed is a Norwood (aortopulmonary anastomosis with aortic arch repair) palliation with Sano (nonvalved RV-PA conduit). While the severe coarctation does not itself necessitate a single-ventricle repair, a Norwood-type aortic arch reconstruction is appropriate in this situation as the left AV valve morphology has already dictated a Fontan palliation. The Sano shunt is sometimes used as an alternative to a BT shunt to provide pulmonary blood flow from the right ventricle. Some advocate this approach rather than a BT shunt, as the pulsatile flow from a Sano shunt may promote better growth of the branch pulmonary arteries over time. Like the BT shunt, the Sano shunt is temporary and would be removed at the time of

bidirectional cavopulmonary anastomosis. In the presence of a functionally normal left AV valve (without straddling), repair of the VSD and coarctation and resection of the subaortic stenosis may be feasible.

36. (B) Taussig–Bing anomaly is a form of double outlet right ventricle where the VSD is located below the pulmonary valve. The physiology of this anomaly resembles that of complete transposition of the great arteries. The pulmonary artery receives primarily saturated blood from the left ventricle through the subpulmonic VSD. The aorta, which is remote from the VSD, receives desaturated systemic venous blood from the right ventricle. Given the arrangement of the great arteries relative to the VSD, the left ventricle cannot be baffled to the distant aortic valve. Instead, the great arteries are surgically switched, as they are for d-TGA, and the VSD is close to the pulmonic (neo-aortic) valve.

37. (D) This child's heart defect does not allow for complete (two-ventricle) repair. The pulmonary artery arises from a hypoplastic right ventricle which itself has no AV valve inflow. Thus, pulmonary blood flow is dependent on the size of the VSD and the size of the pulmonary valve. With a restrictive VSD (bulboventricular foramen) and severe subpulmonary stenosis, pulmonary blood flow is severely compromised and must be addressed. This is accomplished by placement of a BT shunt or stenting of the PDA. Later palliation would consist of a modified Glenn and, ultimately, a modified Fontan. A DKS anastomosis would be needed in the setting of malposed great arteries with systemic outflow obstruction. Enlargement of the VSD may improve outflow obstruction but is unlikely to provide adequate relief and risks injury to the conduction system. PA banding would further reduce pulmonary blood flow. Balloon atrial septostomy is not indicated in this situation.

38. (D) Most centrally located secundum ASDs can be closed safely and effectively in the cardiac catheterization laboratory. Indications for surgical repair of a secundum ASD include deficiency of the posterior-inferior septal rim and the presence of coexisting abnormalities that would benefit from surgical repair. Specific recommendations for surgical repair include moderate or severe tricuspid valve regurgitation, which would benefit from annuloplasty or repair of the valve.

39. (A) **Figure 15.12** shows an axial slice of a CT angiogram at the level of the pulmonary artery bifurcation. Notably, the left pulmonary artery branches late and courses behind the trachea. This is a left pulmonary artery sling. It may be associated with breathing difficulty and airway abnormalities, such as tracheomalacia or complete tracheal rings. Surgical repair involves transection of the LPA and reimplantation in the proximal pulmonary artery, anterior to the trachea.

40. (D) Of the interventions listed, synthetic patch repair of coarctation is known to carry a significant risk of pseudoaneurysm at the site of repair. In this patient, this is clearly seen as a large mass in the area of the previous coarctation repair.

41. (C) The clinical stem presents an adult with evidence of venous congestion involving the lower half of his body. In someone who has a history of congenital heart disease, this may be related to poor Fontan physiology, but the patient presented only had one operation as a baby. The electrocardiogram shown demonstrates sinus bradycardia with right ventricular hypertrophy. This would be consistent with a systemic right ventricle. Of the options listed, the most likely defect to explain all these findings is transposition of the great arteries after atrial switch operation. Atrial switch operation (Mustard/Senning) is performed by baffling SVC and IVC flow to the left-sided AV valve and into the subpulmonic ventricle. Obstruction of either baffle can occur and produces symptoms of central venous obstruction. SVC obstruction is more common and results in jugular venous distension and facial edema and may cause increased head size in infants with an open fontanelle. IVC obstruction, which is less common, may cause hepatomegaly, ascites, and lower extremity edema. SVC and IVC baffle obstruction is often amenable to stent placement in the interventional catheterization laboratory but may require surgical revision.

42. (B) Surgical treatment of Ebstein anomaly may involve any of the answer choices listed. In the current era, tricuspid valve repair typically involves a "cone" type repair with surgical delamination of the abnormal tricuspid valve leaflet tissue from the endocardial surface of the right ventricle and reconstruction of a valve at the level of the anatomic annulus. This approach increases the functional volume of the right ventricular cavity and may provide long-term benefits to right ventricular size and function. However, studies have not shown that tricuspid valve repair alone improves exercise capacity in patients with Ebstein anomaly. The only intervention that has correlated with such improvement is removal of a right-to-left shunt at the atrial level. Right ventricular plication is performed to facilitate right ventricular remodeling. A MAZE procedure may be performed to prevent or eliminate supraventricular arrhythmias. A bidirectional Glenn is sometimes used to offload a severely dysfunctional right ventricle. However, none of these interventions have been shown to improve patient exercise capacity.

43. (D) This patient has Marfan syndrome. The threshold for aortic root replacement in Marfan syndrome is an aortic root dimension of 50 mm or greater. Thus, he meets criteria for aortic root surgery. The question is whether he needs anything done for his aortic or mitral valve. In the absence of significant dysfunction of either valve (most commonly regurgitation), surgery is not indicated despite the presence of a bicuspid aortic valve and mitral valve prolapse.

44. (A) The Warden repair for sinus venosus ASD with anomalous right upper pulmonary veins involves transection of the SVC above the insertion of the pulmonary veins, baffling of the anomalous pulmonary vein/SVC stump to the ASD, and reimplantation of the upper SVC to the right atrial appendage.

45. (B) The symptoms described are consistent with a vascular ring. The CT images shown demonstrate a double aortic arch with atretic left arch. The "bird's beak" deformities

at the base of the left brachiocephalic artery and at the diverticulum of Kommerell on the descending aorta represent the ends of the fibrous ligament of the atretic arch. Note that this is *not* a ligamentum arteriosum from a prior ductus arteriosus, because it connects ascending aorta to descending aorta and not aorta to pulmonary artery. Resection of the diverticulum of Kommerell may be needed, but would be unlikely to cause significant airway or esophageal obstruction after transection of the atretic arch and, thus, may not necessarily be part of surgical repair.

46. (E) The Ross procedure involves autograft replacement of the stenotic native aortic valve with the native pulmonary valve. A homograft is then placed in the pulmonary position. While all of the choices are risks associated with the Ross procedure, the most common indication for reoperation is failure of the pulmonary homograft.

47. (A) The MAZE ablative procedure involves intraoperative cryoablation or radiofrequency ablation across several segments of the right atrium. This procedure is very effective in treating supraventricular tachyarrhythmias, including atrial fibrillation and atrial flutter. The remaining choices may be performed during repair of Ebstein anomaly but has not been shown to significantly reduce the risk of atrial arrhythmias. The Starnes procedure is typically performed in cases of neonatal Ebstein anomaly with severe right ventricle hypoplasia and significant tricuspid valve regurgitation. It involves patch occlusion of the tricuspid valve at the annulus, removal of the atrial septum, and placement of a systemic to pulmonary artery shunt (e.g., BT shunt). This procedure is performed in anticipation of a single-ventricle (Fontan) palliation.

48. (D) With poor perfusion (manifest by elevated lactate levels) in the face of elevated central venous pressure and normal systolic ventricular function, restriction to ventricular function is very likely. Underfilled ventricles suggest external restriction to filling. The absence of pericardial fluid effectively rules out tamponade due to pericardial effusion, thus pericardiocentesis is not indicated. Perioperative swelling can increase intrathoracic pressure and restrict diastolic filling, particularly in small babies. The treatment would be emergent opening of the sternotomy to relieve increased intrathoracic pressure. The available data support this intervention; additional imaging, such as a chest CT, is not indicated. Coronary artery obstruction can occur in patients with d-TGA after repair, but is unlikely given normal ventricular systolic function.

49. (D) The Yasui operation involves an ascending aorta to pulmonary artery (Damus–Kaye–Stansel) anastomosis, baffle closure of the VSD to the pulmonary artery (which now serves as part of the systemic outflow tract), and placement of a right ventricle to pulmonary artery conduit. Of the congenital heart lesions listed, a posterior malaligned VSD (with an adequate VSD size and LVOT obstruction) with interrupted aortic arch could be treated with a Yasui procedure as part of the repair. Surgical repair of the interrupted aortic arch is not implicit in a Yasui procedure but would need to be performed at the time of repair. Pulmonary

CHAPTER 15

atresia with VSD and MAPCAs may be treated with the unifocalization procedure with or without VSD closure and RV-PA conduit. Tricuspid atresia with malposed great arteries would be managed with a Norwood type of operation, without VSD closure. D-TGA with VSD and LVOT obstruction may be treated with a Rastelli, Nikaidoh, or REV operation, depending on anatomic considerations and institutional preferences. Truncus arteriosus with truncal valve dysfunction likely require truncal valve replacement in addition to the standard surgical repair.

50. (A) This patient's symptoms of fever and chest pain are most likely due to postpericardiotomy syndrome, which can occur following cardiac surgery, particularly repair of tetralogy of Fallot, atrial septal defects, and ventricular septal defects. While fever is often a presenting sign of postpericardiotomy syndrome, blood cultures should be drawn to evaluate for endocarditis. After appropriate workup, the initial treatment of postpericardiotomy syndrome is high-dose aspirin for 4 to 6 weeks. Steroids may benefit those who do not respond to aspirin alone. Colchicine is not used in the treatment of postpericardiotomy syndrome. Chest CT is not indicated as part of the initial workup. The presence of a friction rub indicates a pericardial effusion, but the patient's appearance and vital signs do not suggest a significant effusion or tamponade.

Adult Congenital Heart Disease

Frank Cetta, C. Charles Jain, Sabrina D. Phillips, and Bryan C. Cannon

Questions

1. A 37-year-old female saw her primary care provider who heard a murmur and ordered an echocardiogram. The echocardiogram showed a large secundum ASD and the pulmonary veins all entered the left atrium normally. The right atrium and ventricle were moderately enlarged, there was mild tricuspid regurgitation, and estimated right ventricular systolic pressure (RVSP) was 28 mm Hg. On questioning, you find out that she is an avid marathon runner. She has had no symptoms or any decline in functional status. According to the 2018 AHA/ACC guidelines, what do you tell her?

   A. There are insufficient data to guide what to do
   B. Closing the defect would be reasonable
   C. Since she is asymptomatic, there is a recommendation against closure
   D. She needs a cardiac catheterization to confirm hemodynamic significance

2. A 45-year-old male with tetralogy of Fallot presents to establish care. His last cardiology visit was many years ago. He underwent transannular patch repair as a child. He has felt well and has no symptoms. He enjoys biking, riding about 20 miles, 5 days per week. On examination, his jugular venous pressure is normal, he has an RV heave, S_1 is normal, S_2 is single, and there is a 1/6 early peaking systolic ejection murmur at the base followed by a 2/6 diastolic decrescendo murmur. The liver is not palpable and there is no edema. Echo revealed moderate–severe pulmonary regurgitation. The RV is severely enlarged and has moderately decreased function. There is moderate tricuspid regurgitation. The LV has normal size and function. MRI revealed an RV end-diastolic volume index of 189 mL/m^2 and RV ejection fraction of 36%. Exercise test showed exercise capacity at 107% age-predicted maximum. What is the most appropriate next step?

   A. Pulmonary valve replacement would be reasonable now
   B. Diagnostic catheterization to assess degree of pulmonary regurgitation
   C. Follow-up in 6 months with repeat echocardiogram, MRI, and exercise test
   D. Follow-up in 1 year with echocardiogram and MRI
   E. Follow-up in 2 years, echo in 2 years, MRI and exercise test in 3 years

3. A 54-year-old female with tetralogy of Fallot presents for annual evaluation. As a child she underwent repair with patch closure of the VSD, infundibular muscle resection, and pulmonary valvotomy. She has no other medical history. When you saw her last year, she described some slight decrease in energy. In the last 6 months, she noticed dyspnea even with climbing a single flight of stairs or doing chores around the house. On examination, her jugular venous pressure is moderately elevated, S_1 is normal, S_2 splits widely but varies with respiration, there is a 2/6 mid-peaking systolic ejection murmur at the base followed by a soft diastolic decrescendo murmur. The liver is palpable 3 cm below the costal margin and there is mild pitting edema in the lower legs. Echocardiogram reveals findings comparable to last year with a moderate to severely enlarged RV with mild systolic dysfunction, moderate pulmonary regurgitation with a pulmonary valve mean gradient of 22 mm Hg, severe tricuspid regurgitation, and a normal left ventricular size and function. What is the most appropriate next step?

A. Perform cardiac MRI for better assessment of RV size and function
B. Perform exercise testing
C. Follow-up in 6 months with repeat echocardiogram
D. Refer for percutaneous pulmonary valve replacement
E. Refer for surgery for pulmonary valve replacement and tricuspid valve repair

4. A 33-year-old male with tetralogy of Fallot is admitted with heart failure. His surgical history includes patch closure of the VSD and RVOT transannular patch augmentation at age 1, followed by pulmonary valve replacement at age 21, with subsequent pulmonary valve replacement and tricuspid valve repair at age 31. Prior to his last surgery, his right ventricle was severely enlarged and had severe systolic dysfunction. His ECG is shown in **Figure 16.1**.

Telemetry reveals brief runs of nonsustained ventricular tachycardia (VT). Echocardiogram shows unchanged appearance of the right ventricle, normal pulmonary prosthesis function, and moderate tricuspid regurgitation. But now the left ventricle is enlarged with an ejection fraction of 40% and moderate mitral regurgitation. Cardiac MRI shows severe RV enlargement and dysfunction along with extensive scarring. Regarding potential ICD implantation, which of the following is consistent with guideline recommendations?

A. Place an ICD at this time
B. EP study to assess for inducible VT prior to proceeding with ICD implantation
C. Undergo VT ablation rather than ICD implantation
D. ICD only recommended if he had prior cardiac arrest or cardiogenic syncope
E. ICD only recommended if the LV ejection fraction is <35%

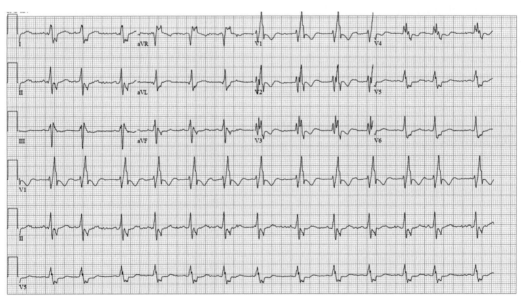

FIGURE 16.1

5. A 38-year-old male presents for progressive decline in exertional capacity over the past year. He has a history of tricuspid atresia, initially palliated with a left-sided subclavian artery to pulmonary artery (PA) shunt. At 8 years old he had a nonfenestrated atriopulmonary Fontan. Thereafter, numerous venovenous collaterals developed. He had ablation for atrial arrhythmias and no recent recurrence or need for chronic antiarrhythmic medication use. Systemic oxygen saturation was 91%. ECG shows sinus rhythm. Echocardiogram reveals normal left ventricular ejection fraction, mild mitral regurgitation, and a patent Fontan pathway without Doppler evidence of obstruction. Given his symptoms, he underwent cardiac catheterization. Mean right atrial pressure was 20 mm Hg, mean right and left pulmonary artery pressures were 19 mm Hg, and mean pulmonary capillary wedge pressure was 11 mm Hg. Angiography demonstrated no Fontan pathway obstruction or distal branch PA stenosis. What is the most appropriate next step?

   A. Refer for Fontan revision
   B. Refer for cardiac transplant
   C. Start epoprostenol therapy
   D. Start sildenafil therapy
   E. Start nocturnal oxygen therapy

6. A 67-year-old female is referred for a recently diagnosed small membranous VSD. She reports that she was told as a child that she had a "hole in her heart," but that it would likely close. She recently saw a new primary care doctor who heard a murmur and obtained an echocardiogram. The echo showed the small membranous VSD, normal biventricular size and function, trivial aortic regurgitation, mild tricuspid regurgitation, and an estimated right ventricular systolic pressure of 29 mm Hg. Your examination reveals normal S_1 and S_2 with normal P_2 component, a high-pitched 3/6 holosystolic murmur heard throughout the precordium and loudest at the left lower sternal border. She denies any symptoms and exercises regularly. What is the most appropriate next step?

   A. No further follow-up is necessary
   B. Cardiac MRI
   C. Follow-up in 1 year with repeat echocardiogram and cardiac MRI
   D. Follow-up in 3 years with repeat echocardiogram
   E. Refer for VSD closure

7. A 31-year-old male was referred for a bicuspid aortic valve. Prior echo and MRI evaluation have confirmed there was no coarctation of the aorta. He is in the military and the military physician is concerned that there is severe aortic valve regurgitation. The patient denies any symptoms. Current physical examination and echo are consistent with severe aortic regurgitation. As you review his echocardiogram, which of the following findings could warrant surgery at this time?

   A. LV end-diastolic dimension of 72 mm
   B. LV end-systolic dimension of 52 mm
   C. LV ejection fraction 56%
   D. Sinus of Valsalva of 46 mm
   E. Mid-ascending aorta of 51 mm

8. A 27-year-old female is admitted with new-onset atrial fibrillation with rapid ventricular response. She has a history of tricuspid atresia, status post bidirectional cavopulmonary anastomosis (Glenn), and lateral tunnel Fontan operations. Her ECG shows an atrial tachyarrhythmia with ventricular rate of 160 bpm, which has not improved despite IV diltiazem. You start her on anticoagulation, perform a transthoracic echo and a TEE that show no thrombus and patent Glenn and Fontan pathways. DC cardioversion successfully converts her to sinus rhythm. You elect to start sotalol therapy. Which of the following would be a significant risk factor for complications of sotalol?

   A. Concurrent use of warfarin
   B. Concurrent use of apixaban
   C. Concurrent use of dabigatran
   D. Hypokalemia
   E. Hyperkalemia

9. A 29-year-old male with a history of tetralogy of Fallot status post transannular patch repair in infancy presents for routine follow-up. He has recently noticed some abdominal swelling and has not been able to keep up with his father on family hikes. Examination reveals jugular venous distention to the mandible while upright with prominent x and y descents. There is a 1+ RV heave, S_1 is normal, S_2 is notable for a diminished P_2, 1/6 systolic ejection murmur, and a 2/6 very short early diastolic murmur at the base. There is also an early diastolic sound heard at the left lower sternal border. The liver is enlarged 4 cm below the costal margin. Echocardiogram reveals severe pulmonic regurgitation with a mildly dilated right ventricle with normal systolic function. Chest radiograph is shown in **Figure 16.2**. Which of the following is the most appropriate next step?

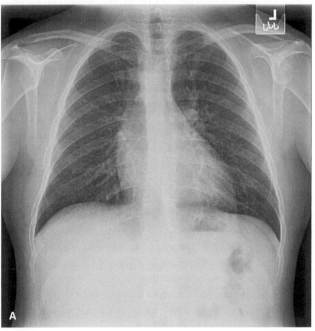
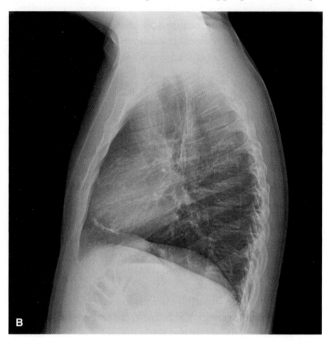

FIGURE 16.2

    A. Refer for percutaneous pulmonary valve replacement
    B. Recommend routine follow-up in 1 year
    C. Perform further evaluation for constrictive pericarditis
    D. Recommend regular exercise routine

10. A 36-year-old male with a history of bicuspid aortic valve was referred to you. He had a history of infective endocarditis with severe aortic regurgitation, which was treated with IV antibiotics and subsequent Ross procedure when he was 18 years old. He had subsequent degeneration of the pulmonary homograft with stenosis and underwent placement of a 27-mm homograft conduit. He now has progressive fatigue and dyspnea on exertion. Examination reveals normal jugular venous pressure, normal carotid impulses, a prominent RV heave and palpable P_2, normal S_1, S_2 notable for persistent splitting with a loud P_2, a harsh 3/6 systolic ejection murmur with a mid to late peak at the base, and no diastolic murmurs. Echocardiogram reveals normally functioning neo-aortic valve without root dilation, normal LV size and function, and moderately enlarged RV with reduced systolic function. The pulmonary conduit valve is difficult to visualize but there is a mean gradient of at 52 mm Hg and no clear regurgitation. The estimated right ventricular systolic pressure is 93 mm Hg. What do you recommend?

    A. TEE
    B. Cardiac CTA
    C. Exercise testing with measurement of VO_2
    D. Cardiac MR to assess indexed RVEDV

11. A 56-year-old female is referred with a newly diagnosed secundum ASD detected by echo during a work-up for palpitations. ECG demonstrates atrial fibrillation without rapid ventricular response. The shunt is exclusively left to right on echo, the right heart is severely dilated, and the TR velocity predicts an RVSP of 34 mm Hg. What is your plan of care and counsel to the patient?

A. Referral for device closure with expectation that her life expectancy is normal
B. Referral for surgical closure with expectation that her life expectancy is normal
C. Referral for surgical closure and Maze procedure with expectation that her life expectancy will be less than age-matched peers
D. Referral for cardiac cath to determine PVR

12. What is one of the earliest manifestations of cirrhosis from Fontan associated liver disease?

A. Thrombocytopenia
B. Elevation of alkaline phosphatase
C. Elevation of transaminases
D. Prolongation of INR
E. Elevated alpha-fetoprotein level

13. A 20 year old, new to your practice, with repaired tetralogy of Fallot had no cardiology follow-up for the last 10 years. He states that he is asymptomatic and able to do all activities of daily living without limitation. He does not exercise regularly and works as a toll booth operator. Echo demonstrated severe pulmonary valve insufficiency. Cardiac MRI demonstrates an RV end-diastolic volume index of 130 cc/m^2. What is the next best step in his care?

A. Return to clinic in 6 months with repeat echo
B. Refer for surgical or percutaneous pulmonary valve replacement
C. Exercise stress test for measurement of VO$_2$
D. Return to clinic in 12 months with repeat echo

14. Which of the following is an expected maternal cardiovascular adaptation to pregnancy?

A. Increase in systemic vascular resistance by 30%
B. Increase in colloid oncotic pressure by 20%
C. Little change in blood pressure during pregnancy
D. Decrease in heart rate during the second half of pregnancy
E. Increase in pulmonary vascular resistance by 20%

15. A 20-year-old female with a history of a celiac artery aneurysm is found to have a dilated aortic root measuring 48 mm, and the physical examination finding shown in **Figure 16.3**. BP is 120/50 mm Hg.

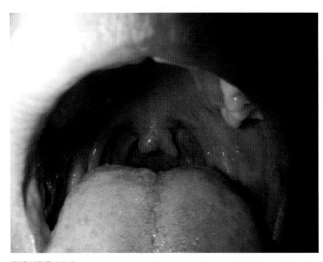

FIGURE 16.3

The next best step is:

A. Initiate beta-blocker therapy and repeat imaging in 6 months
B. Initiate ARB therapy and repeat imaging in 6 months
C. Initiate calcium channel blocker therapy and repeat imaging in 6 months
D. Perform TEE to quantitate the degree of aortic regurgitation
E. Refer for aortic root replacement

16. Which of the following is a major criterion for bacterial endocarditis?

A. Roth spots
B. Janeway lesions
C. New partial dehiscence of a prosthetic valve
D. Change in aortic regurgitation from mild to severe
E. One of two blood culture bottles positive for strep

17. Which patient should be screened with a hepatitis C antibody test?

A. 30 year old with a history of intranasal cocaine use, but no IV drug use
B. 18-year-old s/p Norwood, no history of drug use
C. 23-year-old female with small VSD, no prior surgery, no drug use, no transfusions
D. 30-year-old s/p surgical repair of a large membranous VSD in infancy

18. A 22-year-old female with a St. Jude mechanical mitral prosthesis is 17-week gestation. She is referred for a second opinion on anticoagulation management; currently using subcutaneous heparin (unfractionated). What is the most appropriate therapy for this patient?

    A. Continue subcutaneous heparin with aPTT monitoring
    B. Switch to IV heparin with aPTT monitoring
    C. Start warfarin with target INR 3.0
    D. Switch to LMWH injection daily with anti-Xa monitoring
    E. Start dabigatran

19. A 35-year-old male with prior St. Jude aortic valve replacement and normal LV function presents for management of anticoagulation prior to vasectomy. What is the most appropriate recommendation?

    A. Stop warfarin 3 to 5 days prior to vasectomy, resume warfarin on the evening of procedure
    B. Stop warfarin 5 days prior to vasectomy, start lovenox 1 mg/kg twice daily 3 days prior to surgery with last dose 12 hours prior, resume lovenox and warfarin on the evening of procedure, continue lovenox until INR >2
    C. Stop warfarin 5 days prior to vasectomy, start lovenox 1 mg/kg twice daily 3 days prior to surgery with last dose 24 hours prior, resume lovenox and warfarin on the evening of procedure, continue lovenox until INR >2
    D. Stop warfarin 5 days prior to vasectomy, start lovenox 1 mg/kg twice daily 3 days prior to surgery with last dose 24 hours prior, resume warfarin on the evening of procedure

20. A 23-year-old female presents at 12-week gestation for cardiology consultation. She reports a history of "heart surgery" in childhood. She has not seen a cardiologist for 8 years. Which patient characteristic is the most predictive of increased risk of maternal and fetal complications?

    A. NYHA class II heart failure symptoms
    B. Prepregnancy peak VO_2 75% of predicted
    C. Room air oxygen saturation of 89%
    D. Bioprosthetic aortic valve with normal function

21. A 35 year old with Eisenmenger syndrome and chronic secondary erythrocytosis has been undergoing phlebotomy every 3 months by another physician. Baseline oxygen saturation is 75% in room air. Echo demonstrates a large VSD with right-to-left shunting but good biventricular function. What is this patient's greatest risk for stroke?

    A. Iron deficiency
    B. Dehydration
    C. Hgb = 20 g/dL
    D. Thrombocytopenia
    E. Leukopenia

22. In which of the following patients is pregnancy absolutely contraindicated?

    A. 20 year old with bicuspid aortic valve and mean gradient of 30 mm Hg
    B. 20 year old with Marfan syndrome and ascending aorta diameter of 32 mm
    C. 20 year old with Ebstein anomaly, severe RV enlargement, and tricuspid regurgitation
    D. 20-year-old female with an unrepaired VSD and PA systolic pressure of 80 mm Hg

23. A 25-year-old female with d-TGA underwent arterial switch operation in infancy. Twice while shoveling snow, she developed a dull ache between her scapulae. Symptoms abated with rest. She walks up to 3 miles per day without symptoms. In addition to routine echocardiography, you would recommend which of the following?

    A. Coronary angiography
    B. Transesophageal echocardiogram
    C. Fasting lipid panel
    D. Cardiac MRI with gadolinium
    E. No additional evaluation

24. A 40-year-old female with d-TGA had a Mustard procedure. On examination, her heart rate is 40 bpm and regular. Resting oxygen saturation is 92%. Jugular venous pressure is elevated 10 cm above the angle of the sternum. ECG shows junctional rhythm. During exercise testing, she has sinus rhythm with a peak heart rate of 65 bpm and with poor exercise capacity. Prior to transvenous pacemaker placement, evaluation should include which of the following?

    A. Thrombophilia laboratory assessment
    B. Coronary artery CTA
    C. Electrophysiology study to evaluate for inducible ventricular tachycardia
    D. Cardiac catheterization to evaluate for SVC obstruction and baffle leak
    E. Cardiac catheterization to evaluate for proximal coronary obstruction

25. A 20 year old presents for his first ACHD visit. He has not seen a cardiologist for the last 10 years. His medical record describes a grade II/VI high-pitched holosystolic murmur consistent with known small membranous VSD. On current examination, a right ventricular heave is present, and a prominent thrill is palpable at the left upper sternal margin. Which of the following is the most likely diagnosis?

    A. Supravalvular pulmonary stenosis
    B. Double-chambered right ventricle
    C. Increase in left ventricular pressure
    D. Decrease in VSD size
    E. Increase in VSD size

26. A 48-year-old male with d-TGA, status post Mustard operation in infancy presents with progressive dyspnea. Heart rate is 90 bpm and blood pressure 122/78 mm Hg. Examination reveals mildly elevated jugular venous pressure, a prominent RV heave, normal S_1 and S_2, and 2/6 holosystolic murmur at the left lower sternal border with an early diastolic filling sound. The liver cannot be palpated. Echocardiogram reveals severe systemic right ventricle dilation. Estimated ejection fraction 15%, moderate systemic AV valve regurgitation, and estimated pulmonary artery systolic pressure of 60 mm Hg. A CT shows patent coronary arteries and systemic venous baffles. What do you tell him regarding management options?

   A. He should begin pulmonary vasodilators
   B. There are insufficient data to recommend medical therapy to improve function
   C. He should be started on warfarin therapy
   D. He should undergo replacement of the systemic AV valve

27. A 65-year-old female presents for preoperative assessment prior to knee surgery. She has a history of coarctation of the aorta which was repaired surgically in infancy and also bicuspid aortic valve for which she underwent replacement with a 25-mm bileaflet mechanical valve last year. She has no other significant past medical history besides hypertension. Her medications include warfarin (INR goal 2.5), aspirin 81 mg daily, and losartan 50 mg daily. Echocardiogram reveals a normally functioning aortic prosthesis with mean gradient of 7 mm Hg and trivial prosthetic regurgitation. Peak gradient across the coarctation is 6 mm Hg and cross-sectional imaging performed prior to cardiac surgery last year showed no significant recoarctation. What is the appropriate anticoagulation regimen prior to surgery?

   A. Continue warfarin and aspirin until the day of surgery
   B. Stop warfarin and aspirin 5 days prior to surgery, initiate IV heparin 2 days prior to surgery
   C. Stop warfarin 5 days prior to surgery, continue aspirin, initiate enoxaparin 3 days prior to surgery
   D. Stop warfarin 5 days prior to surgery, continue aspirin, no bridging needed
   E. Stop warfarin and aspirin 5 days prior to surgery, no bridging needed

28. A 24-year-old female presents to the ACHD clinic at 12-week gestation of her first pregnancy. She was recently diagnosed with a bicuspid aortic valve. She has never had an intervention. Her echocardiogram was performed 6 months ago. It demonstrated mild eccentric aortic valve regurgitation, a bicuspid aortic valve with fusion between the right and left cusps. Mean gradient was 14 mm Hg. Left ventricular wall thickness, chamber dimensions, and ejection fraction were all within the normal range. Her ascending aorta measured 32 mm at the sinus, 37 mm at the mid-ascending level. What would you recommend?

   A. Proceed with pregnancy, expect vaginal delivery
   B. Proceed with pregnancy, expect cesarean section for delivery
   C. Obtain an MRI of the thoracic aorta before giving an opinion
   D. Start an angiotensin receptor blocker
   E. Recommend immediate termination

29. A 24-year-old female presents at 6-week gestation of her first pregnancy. She was born with a bicuspid aortic valve and eventually required aortic valve replacement with mechanical prosthesis. She tells you that she usually runs her INR "a bit high" at 3.0 to 3.5. Her average daily dose of Warfarin is 4 mg daily. How would you manage her anticoagulation during this pregnancy?

   A. Discontinue Warfarin immediately and begin low–molecular-weight heparin
   B. Continue Warfarin at the present dose, discontinue at 36-week gestation and switch to low–molecular-weight heparin
   C. Continue Warfarin and aspirin throughout pregnancy
   D. Discontinue Warfarin immediately and start low–molecular-weight heparin, resume warfarin therapy at 12-week gestation
   E. Terminate pregnancy

30. A 20-year-old female with a history of surgical repair of a secundum ASD and short arms with the thumbs that are displaced proximally along the length of the arm comes to clinic in anticipation of pregnancy. She asks about the risk of her baby inheriting her genetic syndrome. Assuming complete penetrance, what percent would you quote to her?

   A. 100%
   B. 75%
   C. 50%
   D. 25%
   E. 10%

31. She further asks, if her baby has the same syndrome, what is the chance the infant will have any form of congenital heart disease (CHD)?

    A. 100%
    B. 75%
    C. 50%
    D. 35%
    E. 3% to 5%

32. A 30-year-old female presents to the ACHD clinic complaining of shortness of breath, intermittent palpitations, and dyspnea with exertion. She notes that she was able to run ten miles per day fairly briskly when she was 20 years old. Now she is barely able to cover a mile without feeling exhausted. A 12-lead electrocardiogram was performed and demonstrated sinus rhythm and an rSR' pattern in lead V1. Physical examination demonstrates a right ventricular lift, a normal first sound, and widely fixed and split second sound; the intensity of the pulmonary component of the second heart sound was normal. There is a 2/6 systolic ejection murmur at the left upper sternal border and 2/4 low-pitched diastolic rumble at the lower sternal border. No third or fourth heart sounds. No rubs. The abdomen is soft and nontender. There is no hepatosplenomegaly. Jugular venous pulsations are normal. Transthoracic echocardiography demonstrated a centrally located secundum ASD with adequate rims. Pulmonary venous connections were normal and there was only mild tricuspid valve regurgitation. Based on this clinical scenario and imaging, what is the next most appropriate step?

    A. Cardiac catheterization to measure Q_p/Q_s and pulmonary vascular resistance
    B. Transesophageal echocardiography
    C. Cardiac MRI
    D. Either surgical closure or device closure based on patient preference
    E. No intervention, patient has irreversible pulmonary hypertension

33. In the patient from the previous question, the source of the diastolic murmur is?

    A. Flow through an ASD
    B. Flow across the pulmonary valve
    C. Flow across the tricuspid valve
    D. Flow across the mitral valve
    E. It is a normal murmur in children

34. A 48-year-old male with a history of d-TGA, status post Senning operation, is being evaluated in the ACHD clinic. It is noted that total cholesterol is 260, LDL 190, and HDL 45. His pooled cohort risk assessment score is 12.5%. Which of the following medications would you recommend?

    A. Niacin
    B. Gemfibrozil
    C. Simvastatin
    D. Aspirin
    E. Losartan

35. A 25 year old with a history of tricuspid valve atresia who had an atrial–pulmonary Fontan connection performed at age 8 was seen for a routine follow-up visit. He recently started feeling palpitations. A Holter monitor was performed. It demonstrated sinus bradycardia and brief (10 beat) runs of nonsustained supraventricular tachycardia. An echocardiogram demonstrated a left ventricular ejection fraction of 45%. There is trivial mitral valve regurgitation. The right atrium is dilated. There is spontaneous echo contract demonstrated in the inferior vena cava as it enters the right atrium. There is a patent fenestration. The mean gradient through the fenestration is 7 mm Hg.

    Which of the following is the best anticoagulation strategy in this patient?

    A. No anticoagulation
    B. Aspirin
    C. Warfarin
    D. Aspirin and warfarin
    E. Aspirin and clopidogrel

36. In the patient described in the previous question, the Fontan fenestration gradient correlates best with which of the following?

    A. Right atrial mean pressure
    B. Left atrial mean pressure
    C. Left ventricular end-diastolic pressure
    D. Pulmonary capillary wedge pressure
    E. Transpulmonary gradient

37. A 25 year old is referred for evaluation of a murmur that was recently heard during a general physical. On examination, there is a regular rate and rhythm. No lift or thrill. First heart sound is normal in intensity. Second heart sound is hard to distinguish. There is a 3/6 continuous murmur, heard best at the left sternal border. It peaks around the second heart sound. No third or fourth heart sounds. No rubs. Right radial, right carotid, and femoral pulses are all easily palpable. Blood pressure is 120/40 mm Hg in both the right and left arms. Which test is most likely to define the source of the murmur?

   A. ECG
   B. Transesophageal echocardiogram
   C. Transthoracic echocardiogram
   D. Exercise ECG
   E. Dobutamine stress echocardiogram

38. An 18 year old with unrepaired pulmonary valve atresia/VSD (PA/VSD) comes to clinic for an annual evaluation. On examination, the patient has upper and lower extremity clubbing. There is a regular rate and rhythm. A parasternal lift is present but no thrill. First heart sound is normal. Second heart sound is single. There is a 3/6 continuous murmur which is heard best at the right scapula. No third or fourth heart sounds. Blood pressure is 120/40 mm Hg in both the right and left arms. The origin of the murmur is most likely:

   A. Right coronary artery fistula
   B. Aortic valve regurgitation
   C. Mitral valve stenosis
   D. Patent ductus arteriosus
   E. Pulmonary valve regurgitation

39. A 25 year old presents to clinic with a 3-month history of exercise intolerance. She also recently had palpitations. Holter monitor demonstrated sinus rhythm. She was wearing the Holter monitor when she had three episodes of palpitations. Echocardiogram demonstrated a 20-mm secundum atrial septal defect with adequate anterior/superior and posterior/inferior rims. Echocardiogram also demonstrated RA and RV dilation with preserved function, trivial pulmonary regurgitation, severe tricuspid regurgitation, and RV systolic pressure was 35 mm Hg.

   What is the next best step in this patient's management?

   A. Diagnostic cardiac catheterization to determine pulmonary vascular resistance
   B. Transcatheter closure of the ASD
   C. Annual follow-up
   D. Electrophysiology study
   E. Surgical repair of ASD with tricuspid valve repair

40. A 20 year old with a history of tricuspid valve atresia, status post a classic Glenn to the right pulmonary artery and subsequent lateral tunnel Fontan to the left pulmonary artery presents with a history of progressive cyanosis and exercise intolerance. He undergoes cardiac catheterization, superior vena cava saturation is 75%, right pulmonary artery 75%, left pulmonary artery 78%, descending aorta 88%. Right upper pulmonary vein 88%, left upper pulmonary vein 98%.

   The ratio of pulmonary blood flow (QP) to systemic blood flow (QS) is:

   A. 1.3 to 1
   B. 1.5 to 1
   C. 1.8 to 1
   D. 2 to 1
   E. Cannot be calculated

41. A 31 year old with a history of tricuspid valve atresia and an atrial–pulmonary Fontan connection performed in 1989 presents to the ACHD Clinic. The patient has progressive dyspnea on exertion. Physical examination is remarkable for oxygen saturation of 94%, elevated jugular veins, single first and second heart sounds, and no murmurs. Liver edge is palpable 8 cm below the costal margin. No ascites, no edema. Liver function including transaminases, total bilirubin, and alkaline phosphatase are all normal. Hepatitis C screening is ordered. Which of the following is a true statement regarding hepatitis C?

   A. A positive antibody test indicates active hepatitis C infection
   B. 20% of patients who had cardiac surgery prior to 2000 have hepatitis C infection
   C. Hepatitis C virus polymerase chain reaction testing confirms presence of infection
   D. Hepatitis C cannot be transmitted from an infected mother to her neonate
   E. Normal liver function testing makes a diagnosis of hepatitis C unlikely

42. BNP levels have been reported to have prognostic value in which subset of patients with congenital heart disease?

   A. Eisenmenger syndrome
   B. Tetralogy of Fallot
   C. Ebstein anomaly
   D. Congenitally corrected TGA
   E. Shone syndrome

43. A 22-year-old female presents for evaluation of a murmur. She has been asymptomatic. An echocardiogram shows a primum ASD. There is moderate right atrial and right ventricular enlargement. Her tricuspid valve is normal with no tricuspid regurgitation. ECG shows right atrial enlargement and left axis deviation. Left ventricular size and function are normal. No shunt is evident at ventricular level.

The next most appropriate step in the care of this patient would be?

A. Referral for surgical ASD closure

B. Referral for ASD device closure in the cardiac cath lab

C. Initiation of ACE inhibition

D. Cardiac cath with coronary angiography

E. Observation with follow-up in 2 years

44. A 26 year old with tetralogy of Fallot had an episode of syncope while playing basketball. He had no pulse and an AED was placed within 2 minutes of the episode of syncope. Tracings from the AED show ventricular tachycardia at a rate of 260 bpm and an AED shock was delivered with conversion to sinus rhythm. An echocardiogram showed free pulmonary regurgitation, moderate right ventricular enlargement, and normal right ventricular systolic function.

Which of the following statements is true about implantable cardioverter-defibrillator placement in this patient?

A. Catheter-based VT ablation is an alternative to ICD placement

B. Incidence of ICD-related complications is the same as the adult postmyocardial infarction population

C. Inappropriate ICD shocks occur in <10% of patients with tetralogy of Fallot

D. Amiodarone can be offered as an alternative to ICD placement

E. Transvenous ICD can be placed despite severe pulmonary regurgitation

45. You are seeing a 24-year-old female with a history of a dysmorphic right thumb. She was recently diagnosed with a secundum atrial septal defect. Which of the following genetic mutations is most likely in this patient?

A. TGFBR2

B. FBN1

C. Trisomy 21

D. TBX5

E. NKX 2.5

46. A 16 year old is being evaluated for a systolic murmur that was heard during a preparticipation sports examination. She tells you that two of her family members had surgical repair of an ASD. Her ECG demonstrated second-degree Type II AV block. Which gene mutation is most likely in this patient?

A. NKX 2.5

B. TBX5

C. GATA IV

D. NOTCH I

47. Which structure is associated with the septum primum?

A. Valve of the fossa ovalis

B. Superior limbus of the atrial septum

C. Inferior limbus of the atrial septum

D. Right atrial appendage

E. Endocardial cushion

48. Which of the following patients has the highest risk of cardiac complication during pregnancy?

A. 32-year-old G2P1 with a large (15-mm) secundum atrial septal defect (ASD) with estimated RV pressure of 30 mm Hg, moderate right ventricular enlargement with normal right ventricular systolic function

B. 20-year-old G1P0 with tricuspid atresia status post extracardiac Fontan, no history of arrhythmia or thromboembolic event, NYHA functional class I, systemic ventricular ejection fraction 55%

C. 25-year-old G1P0 with repaired tetralogy of Fallot. One prior episode of atrial fibrillation treated with sotalol, severe pulmonary valve regurgitation with moderate right heart dysfunction on echocardiogram. Peak VO$_2$ 58% of predicted

D. 30-year-old G2P1 with bicuspid aortic valve with a mean systolic gradient across the aortic valve of 30 mm Hg. No history of syncope, chest pain, CHF, or arrhythmia. Peak VO$_2$ 95% of predicted

49. A 22-year-old female with a history of partial AV septal defect and cleft mitral valve presents for evaluation at 6-week gestation. Her partial AV canal defect was repaired at age 2 with no residual defect. She had severe mitral valve regurgitation from her cleft mitral valve repaired 3 years ago. Her left ventricular ejection fraction was reduced to 40% postoperatively, and she has been on a medical regimen of lisinopril, carvedilol, digoxin, and aspirin since surgery. Her ejection fraction was noted to be 60% on her last echocardiogram 9 months ago. Which of the following statements is true regarding her medical therapy?

    A. Lisinopril should be continued until 24-week gestation. It should be discontinued then as fetal renal dysfunction can develop in the third trimester
    B. Lisinopril should be discontinued and an angiotensin receptor blocker should be initiated
    C. Lisinopril should be discontinued now and hydralazine plus a nitrate should be initiated
    D. Lisinopril should be continued throughout pregnancy since it has already been used during a period of critical embryogenesis

50. An asymptomatic, sedentary 62-year-old male with hypertension and hyperlipidemia underwent stress echocardiography for preoperative clearance before knee replacement surgery. The baseline echocardiogram demonstrated a coronary fistula to the right atrium. The cardiac chamber sizes were within normal limits. There was no evidence of ischemia during the test by ECG or imaging criteria. Cardiac examination reveals normal S_1 and S_2, no murmur, and no S_3. You should recommend:

    A. Cardiac catheterization for further delineation of the fistula
    B. Cardiac CT for further delineation of the fistula
    C. No further testing or intervention
    D. Surgery for closure of the fistula

51. A 23-year-old female with a history of bicuspid aortic valve presents to your office at 6-week gestation. She has previously undergone aortic valve replacement with a 21-mm St. Jude mechanical valve. She is currently taking warfarin for anticoagulation with a target INR of 2.5 with an average daily dose of 7 mg. What is the best recommendation for further management?

    A. Continue warfarin but decrease daily dose to 5 mg daily
    B. Continue warfarin until 34-week gestation then discontinue warfarin and start unfractionated heparin until delivery
    C. Discontinue warfarin now, start Lovenox injection daily, continue at dose of 1 mg/kg daily
    D. Discontinue warfarin now, start Lovenox injection and continue at dose to achieve therapeutic anti-Xa levels

52. A 19-year-old patient with tricuspid atresia who is status post RA-PA Fontan connection requests reversible contraception. She had a thrombus in her right atrium 2 years ago, and is taking warfarin anticoagulation. She is unmarried and has had 2 partners. Which of the following should you recommend?

    A. Essure fallopian tubal implant
    B. Mirena intrauterine device
    C. Diaphragm
    D. Low-dose estrogen cyclical oral contraception
    E. Depo-Provera intramuscular injection

53. A 19 year old presents for evaluation. His family history is notable for an aortic dissection in his mother (at an unknown aortic dimension). Physical examination is normal except for mild hypertelorism and a bifid uvula. He does not have ectopia lentis. Blood pressure 110/50 mm Hg. Echocardiogram demonstrates a sinus of Valsalva dimension of 32 mm. Which of the following is most appropriate?

    A. Initiation of beta blocker and repeat imaging in 6 months
    B. Initiation of ARB and repeat imaging in 6 months
    C. No therapy and repeat imaging in 6 months
    D. Surgical referral for valve sparing aortic root replacement
    E. Initiation of calcium channel blocker and repeat imaging in 6 months

54. A 42-year-old male with trisomy 21 and an unrepaired AV septal defect presents to the office to establish care. His caregivers have noted that he is more short of breath during daily activities over the last year. His room air oxygen saturation is 80% and his hemoglobin is 17 g/dL, MCV 70. Which of the following is most appropriate?

    A. One unit phlebotomy with 500 cc saline replacement
    B. One unit phlebotomy without saline replacement
    C. Initiate oral iron therapy and recheck hemoglobin in 1 month
    D. Initiate IV iron therapy and recheck hemoglobin in 2 weeks
    E. Refer for hematology consultation

55. A 28-year-old female presents at 24-week gestation with dyspnea on exertion, orthopnea, and paroxysmal nocturnal dyspnea. Physical examination is notable for a 4/6 late peaking systolic murmur heard at the upper sternal margins with radiation to the carotids. Echocardiogram demonstrates a heavily calcified bicuspid aortic valve with severe stenosis, systolic mean Doppler gradient: 80 mm Hg. What is the most appropriate management strategy?

    A. Advise bed rest and see the patient back in 4 weeks
    B. Balloon valvotomy
    C. Delivery of the fetus now with immediate replacement of the aortic valve
    D. Percutaneous aortic valve implantation
    E. Surgical replacement of the aortic valve and continuation of the pregnancy

56. A 32-year-old male with a history of coarctation of the aorta repaired at age 9 (end-to-end) presents for follow-up. Echocardiogram demonstrates a coarctation gradient of 7 mm Hg with a normal abdominal aorta Doppler signal. Blood pressure in the office is 160/92. Laboratory data reveal a total cholesterol of 354, LDL cholesterol of 200, HDL of 34, triglycerides of 130. What is the best therapy for his dyslipidemia?

    A. Low-fat, low-cholesterol diet alone
    B. Diet plus Niaspan 500 mg daily
    C. Diet plus fish oil 3 g daily
    D. Diet plus simvastatin 40 mg daily
    E. Diet plus gemfibrozil

57. A 32-year-old male with a history of coarctation of the aorta repaired at age 9 (end-to-end) presents for follow-up. Echocardiogram demonstrates a coarctation gradient of 7 mm Hg with a normal abdominal aorta Doppler signal. Blood pressure in the right arm is 160/92, right leg 162/94 mm Hg, heart rate 50 bpm. Laboratory data reveal total cholesterol of 354, LDL cholesterol of 200, HDL of 34, and triglycerides of 130. What is the best therapy for his hypertension?

    A. Stent implantation to relieve the coarctation gradient
    B. Metoprolol 25 mg twice daily
    C. Diltiazem 120 mg daily
    D. Losartan 25 mg daily
    E. Lasix 20 mg daily

58. A 45-year-old male underwent stress echocardiography to evaluate chest pain. He has no other medical history. The stress echocardiogram was negative for ischemia, but views of the atrial septum demonstrated a patent foramen ovale (PFO) with tiny bidirectional shunt by color Doppler imaging. Agitated saline injection was positive for small right-to-left shunt. The echocardiogram was otherwise normal. What should you recommend?

    A. No further testing
    B. Coumadin therapy with a target INR of 2 to 3
    C. Device closure of the patent foramen ovale
    D. Surgical closure of the patent foramen ovale
    E. Cardiac MRI to evaluate right ventricular volumes

59. A 75-year-old female presented to her primary care physician with complaints of exercise intolerance, worsening over the past year. She has extreme dyspnea on exertion and lightheadedness. This has progressed to the point that she is only comfortable while lying supine. She has no lower extremity edema and she denies chest pain. Transthoracic echocardiogram demonstrates normal chamber sizes and normal valvular function. There is a sigmoid ventricular septum of normal thickness. Exercise testing demonstrates poor exercise capacity with a low oxygen saturation of 90% at the start of the test and 82% at 2 min of exercise. What is the next best step for evaluation?

    A. Pulmonary function tests with methacholine challenge
    B. V/Q scan
    C. Cardiac catheterization
    D. Adenosine sestamibi cardiac perfusion scan
    E. Measurement of oxygen saturation while supine

60. A 60-year-old female presents for evaluation of a secundum ASD. Her past medical history is notable for systemic hypertension, now treated with three drugs. An echocardiogram was performed to evaluate a complaint of dyspnea on exertion. The transthoracic echocardiogram demonstrated a 7-mm secundum ASD with left-to-right shunt, normal left ventricular systolic function, mildly increased left ventricular wall thickness without regional wall motion abnormalities, and moderate right ventricular enlargement with normal systolic function. There was no valvular dysfunction. What do you recommend?

    A. Observation, return to clinic in 3 years
    B. Surgical closure of the ASD
    C. Left and right heart catheterization
    D. Aspirin therapy and return to clinic in 1 year
    E. Start sildenafil therapy and return for cardiac catheterization in 1 year

61. A 22-year-old female with a history of bicuspid aortic valve presents to your office at 12 weeks of pregnancy. She is physically active with no symptoms. Her echocardiogram demonstrates a bicuspid aortic valve with a systolic peak Doppler gradient of 44 mm Hg. The left ventricular chamber size and function are normal. The aortic dimension is normal. There is no evidence for coarctation. What would you estimate is her risk of cardiac complication during the pregnancy?

    A. 1%
    B. 5%
    C. 10%
    D. 25%
    E. 50%

62. A 29-year-old male with a history of coarctation of the aorta status post surgical repair at age 3 years presents for routine follow-up. A cardiologist has not seen him in 12 years. He has no complaints. On physical examination, blood pressure is 120/80 in the right arm and unobtainable in the left arm. There is no radial–femoral delay. Cardiac examination reveals a normal S$_1$ followed by a systolic ejection click and a 2/6 mid-peaking systolic murmur. What imaging studies would you recommend?

    A. Transthoracic echocardiogram
    B. Transthoracic echocardiogram and CT scan of the aorta
    C. Transthoracic echocardiogram and MRI scan of the aorta
    D. Cardiac MRI
    E. Transthoracic echocardiogram, MRI scan of the aorta, and MRA scan of the brain

63. A 27-year-old female with Marfan syndrome presents for routine follow-up. Her echocardiogram demonstrates a sinus of Valsalva dimension of 42 mm with a mid-ascending aorta dimension of 39 mm, mitral valve prolapse, and trivial mitral regurgitation. Her only complaint is of fatigue, which by description is daytime hypersomnolence rather than decline in stamina. She is currently taking metoprolol succinate 25 mg daily and losartan 25 mg daily. On examination, her blood pressure is 100/60, HR 60 bpm. What would you recommend?

    A. Overnight oximetry
    B. Discontinue metoprolol and increase losartan
    C. Continue current medical regimen and return in 1 year
    D. Discontinue losartan and increase metoprolol
    E. Discontinue both losartan and metoprolol and initiate amlodipine

64. A 36-year-old male with a history of repaired tetralogy of Fallot is seeing a local psychiatrist for moderate depression. The psychiatrist would like to know which of the following medications would be safest for the patient given his cardiac history.

    A. Sertraline
    B. Citalopram
    C. Venlafaxine
    D. Bupropion
    E. Amitriptyline

65. Dabigatran therapy would be most appropriate for which patient?

    A. 23 year old with Ebstein anomaly with persistent atrial fibrillation
    B. 23-year-old male with bicuspid aortic valve status post mechanical aortic valve replacement who has difficulty checking his INR regularly
    C. 10-week pregnant, 23-year-old female who has a mechanical mitral valve prosthesis
    D. 23 year old with atrial fibrillation who needs bridging anticoagulation for noncardiac surgery
    E. 23-year-old male with atrial fibrillation who has had recent GI bleeding while taking warfarin

66. Simvastatin has an important drug–drug interaction with which antihypertensive agent?

    A. Metoprolol
    B. Lisinopril
    C. Amlodipine
    D. Hydrochlorothiazide
    E. Losartan

67. Which drug has a Class D pregnancy classification?

    A. Metoprolol
    B. Atenolol
    C. Amlodipine
    D. Verapamil
    E. Diltiazem

68. A 38-year-old female with a mechanical mitral valve and chronic atrial fibrillation presents with a complaint of menometrorrhagia. She is not interested in any future pregnancies. Which choice below prevents future pregnancy and requires the least manipulation of her anticoagulation management?

    A. Ortho Tri-Cyclen
    B. Depo-Provera
    C. Essure implantation
    D. Endometrial ablation
    E. Hysterectomy

69. A 29 year old with repaired tetralogy of Fallot and moderate residual pulmonary valve regurgitation is started on Flecainide for atrial fibrillation. How should the drug be initiated?

A. Outpatient initiation at full dose with ECG daily for 3 days to check QT interval

B. Outpatient initiation at full dose with ECG daily for 3 days to check QRS duration

C. Outpatient initiation at half dose for 1 day, increasing to full dose if no side effects

D. Inpatient initiation at full dose for five doses with daily ECG to check QT interval

E. Inpatient initiation at full dose for five doses with daily ECG to check QRS duration

70. A 30-year-old male with a history of repaired tetralogy of Fallot is treated with amiodarone for atrial fibrillation. What testing should you obtain at least annually?

A. TSH, AST, bilirubin, alkaline phosphatase, pulmonary function tests

B. TSH, BUN, creatinine, pulmonary function tests

C. Pulmonary function tests, AST, bilirubin, alkaline phosphatase, creatinine

D. AST, bilirubin, alkaline phosphatase, BUN, creatinine, lipid panel

E. TSH, pulmonary function tests, CPK

71. Which pulmonary vasodilator has the highest incidence of lower extremity edema?

A. Bosentan

B. Sildenafil

C. Tadalafil

D. Iloprost

E. Atenolol

72. Patients prescribed the "mini pill" progesterone only oral contraceptive should be counseled to do which of the following?

A. Use barrier contraception for the first 60 days after initiation

B. Avoid prolonged sun exposure

C. Expect cessation of all menstrual flow

D. Stop using SBE prophylaxis

E. Take the dose at the same time daily

73. A 45-year-old female is evaluated for exertional dyspnea and decreased exercise tolerance. On examination, a 2 to 3/6 systolic ejection murmur is appreciated at the left upper sternal border and the second heart sound is widely split and fixed. An ECG demonstrates right atrial enlargement and right ventricular hypertrophy. Echocardiography is shown in **Figure 16.4**.

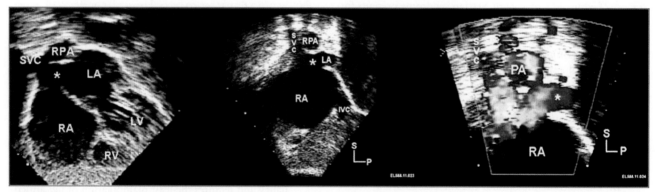

FIGURE 16.4

Which of the following is the best course of action?

A. Observe the patient without intervention

B. Perform cardiopulmonary exercise testing to determine need for intervention

C. Recommend surgical ASD closure only

D. Recommend surgical ASD closure with pulmonary venous baffle

E. Recommend device closure of the ASD

74. A 52-year-old female falls while snow skiing and injures her wrist. On seeking medical care, a systolic murmur is identified, and she is referred for cardiac evaluation. She is normotensive. Her physical examination demonstrates a holosystolic murmur heard best at the left sternal border. An ECG is normal. A transthoracic echocardiogram demonstrates a muscular ventricular septal defect (VSD) in the midseptum with a peak systolic velocity of 5 m/s. There is no chamber enlargement. The right ventricular systolic pressure is estimated to be normal by tricuspid regurgitant velocity. Which of the following is the best initial management of this lesion?

A. No intervention
B. Surgical closure of the VSD
C. Cardiac catheterization to quantify ventricular level shunting
D. Restriction of vigorous physical activity with no immediate intervention
E. Device closure of the VSD

75. A 28-year-old male is found to have cardiomegaly on chest x-ray. An echocardiogram demonstrates flow acceleration at the level of the pulmonary valve (peak velocity 2.1 m/s) and moderate dilation of the right-sided chambers. Which of the following is the best next step?

A. Additional echocardiographic imaging to demonstrate PDA
B. Additional echocardiographic imaging to demonstrate ASD
C. Cardiac catheterization with pulmonary balloon valvuloplasty
D. Serial annual evaluation to assess for ventricular dysfunction
E. Cardiopulmonary exercise testing

76. An 18-year-old female had neonatal arterial switch operation for d-TGA. She presents to a cardiology clinic after 4 years without medical care. She has slowly developed exertional dyspnea and now can only climb one flight of stairs without resting. Her physical examination reveals normal jugular venous pressure and pulsation. A grade 3/6 ejection systolic murmur is audible at the upper left sternal border with no diastolic murmur. Which of the following is the most likely explanation of the symptoms?

A. Supravalvar pulmonary stenosis
B. Atrial fibrillation
C. Pulmonary valve regurgitation
D. Aortopulmonary window
E. Subacute bacterial endocarditis

77. A 40-year-old female with a membranous VSD underwent prosthetic patch repair as a child. Subsequently, at age 18 years, she was successfully treated for *Streptococcal viridans* endocarditis involving her mitral valve. Regarding future endocarditis prevention at the time of dental work, which of the following includes the most appropriate counseling?

A. *S. viridans* is an unusual pathogen for endocarditis
B. Prophylactic antibiotics are not indicated in the absence of a residual shunt
C. Prophylactic antibiotics are indicated due to the history of bacterial endocarditis
D. Prophylactic antibiotics are indicated daily due to her history of VSD repair
E. No prophylactic antibiotics are indicated

78. A 43-year-old male with d-TGA underwent a Mustard procedure in early childhood. His pulse oximetry reveals an oxygen saturation of 96% at rest. His family history includes colon cancer in his father at the age of 40, and the patient is scheduled for elective colonoscopy. Regarding endocarditis prevention at the time of colonoscopy, which of the following includes the most appropriate counseling?

A. Routine antibiotic prophylaxis should be administered
B. Broad-spectrum antibiotic prophylaxis with anaerobic coverage should be administered
C. No antibiotic prophylaxis is indicated
D. Full colonoscopy should be delayed due to endocarditis risk
E. Limited sigmoidoscopy should be performed

79. A 25-year-old male with Ebstein anomaly had a witnessed, transient loss of consciousness while walking down his apartment stairs immediately after eating dinner. He had brief upper extremity twitching as he regained consciousness. Evaluation in the emergency room reveals normal blood pressure and perfusion. The patient had no prodrome. His ECG demonstrates sinus rhythm, right atrial enlargement with prominent peaked P waves, first-degree atrioventricular block, and right bundle branch block. Which of the following is the most concerning explanation for this patient's symptoms?

A. Neurocardiogenic (vasovagal) syncope
B. Seizure disorder
C. Ventricular tachycardia
D. Atrioventricular reentrant (accessory pathway) tachycardia
E. Complete heart block

80. A 32-year-old female with tricuspid atresia had a lateral tunnel Fontan palliation as a teenager. She has been followed since that intervention with minimal functional limitation. In the past 2 weeks, she has noted increasing abdominal girth and decreasing exercise tolerance. On examination, she is bradycardic and her liver edge is palpable 4 cm below the costal margin. Her ECG demonstrates junctional rhythm at 42 bpm. Which of the following is the most appropriate intervention at this time?

A. Increased diuresis
B. Pacemaker placement
C. Fontan revision surgery
D. Cardiopulmonary rehabilitation
E. Digoxin therapy

81. A 50-year-old male is undergoing right-sided diagnostic heart catheterization in the setting of biventricular systolic dysfunction. He acutely develops third-degree atrioventricular block and subsequent hypotension. A pacing catheter is placed emergently. An echocardiogram is performed in the catheterization suite, and chordal attachments are noted from the left-sided atrioventricular valve to the interventricular septum. Which of the following is the underlying congenital lesion that explains these events?

A. Partial atrioventricular septal defect
B. Congenital pulmonary stenosis
C. Congenitally corrected transposition
D. Double-chambered right ventricle
E. Parachute mitral valve

82. A 41-year-old male is new to your practice after living in remote Africa for the past 5 years. He was born with pulmonary atresia with an intact ventricular septum, and palliation was performed in early childhood with placement of a central shunt. He has routinely had therapeutic 300 mL phlebotomy. He denies symptoms including headaches, visual changes, or other neurologic symptoms before or after phlebotomy. He is euvolemic on examination. His initial laboratory results include hemoglobin 21 g/dL and hematocrit 70%. Which of the following is the next best step?

A. Administer IV 500 mL isotonic crystalloid
B. Initiate therapeutic heparinization
C. Initiate iron chelation
D. Therapeutic phlebotomy with crystalloid volume replacement
E. Order serum iron studies

83. A 38-year-old female with tetralogy of Fallot had a right ventricle to pulmonary artery homograft connection. She requires pulmonary valve replacement. She is an active smoker and has a family history of premature coronary artery disease. Fasting cholesterol panel is normal. Prior to surgical intervention that is scheduled in 1 week, which of the following is most urgent?

A. Tobacco cessation
B. Routine preoperative laboratory evaluation only
C. Coronary angiography
D. Prophylactic statin therapy
E. Surveillance blood cultures

84. An 18-year-old male is referred to you after his primary provider hears an early systolic click at the apex. Echocardiogram confirms a bicuspid aortic valve with normal function. There is no family history of heart disease. He has two healthy siblings, and his parents accompany him. Your recommendations for the patient's first-degree relatives should include which of the following?

A. Physical examination of first-degree relatives to assess for aortic valve click
B. Echocardiographic screening of all first-degree relatives
C. Cardiac MRI of any first-degree relatives with abnormal physical examination findings
D. Cardiac MRI of the patient to determine need for family screening
E. No evaluation of first-degree family members is needed

85. A 20-year-old female returns for routine follow-up after repair of coarctation of the aorta in early childhood. Physical examination demonstrates normal femoral pulses and no brachiofemoral delay. Her right upper extremity and lower extremity blood pressures are equivalent. She has had serial echocardiograms demonstrating no recoarctation of the aorta. At this time, ongoing evaluation should include which of the following?

A. Coronary angiography
B. Neurocognitive testing
C. MRI/MRA of the head and CT or MRI of the thoracic aorta
D. TEE
E. 24-hour Holter monitor

86. A 35-year-old patient with trisomy 21 and repaired partial AVSD is admitted for new onset atrial fibrillation with rapid ventricular conduction. The ventricular rate decreases appropriately with medical therapy and perfusion is normal. On physical examination, there is a prominent apical impulse, and a grade III/VI harsh systolic ejection murmur is heard at the upper sternal border. Echo reveals a mean left ventricular outflow tract (LVOT) gradient of 55 mm Hg at rest. Which of the following is the best choice for therapeutic intervention?

   A. Chronic beta-blockade therapy
   B. Chronic amiodarone therapy
   C. Chronic ACE inhibition
   D. Aortic balloon valvuloplasty
   E. Surgical outflow tract repair

87. A 35-year-old patient with trisomy 21 and repaired complete AVSD has routine follow-up evaluation. She is noncompliant with CPAP therapy for obstructive sleep apnea. She is known to have a residual shunt. Her echocardiogram reports mild tricuspid regurgitation with a velocity of 5 m/s. Cardiac catheterization is performed under general anesthesia to evaluate right ventricular hypertension. The right ventricle and pulmonary artery pressures are found to be normal. Which of the following is the most likely explanation for the discrepancy in echo and catheterization data?

   A. Improved right ventricular pressure with adequate ventilation
   B. Left ventricle to right atrial shunting contaminating the TR jet
   C. Doppler contamination with right ventricular outflow signal
   D. Transient pulmonary vasospasm
   E. No discrepancy is present

88. A 52-year-old tow truck driver had repair of tetralogy of Fallot at 4 years of age. He presents to the emergency department due to syncope while loading a car onto his truck. He had no prodromal symptoms. He had only one surgery in childhood. He had last sought cardiac care in 1970. His ECG shows sinus rhythm at 80 bpm, PR interval 100 ms. There is right bundle branch block and the QRS duration is 199 ms. An electrophysiology study is most appropriate to evaluate for which of the following?

   A. Inducible ventricular arrhythmia
   B. Inducible atrial arrhythmia
   C. Sinus node dysfunction
   D. Atrioventricular node dysfunction
   E. Accessory pathway characteristics

89. A 35-year-old male with congenitally corrected L-TGA and no previous surgery was found to have periods of complete heart block. Therefore, a dual chamber transvenous pacemaker was placed. The echo immediately after the intervention demonstrated stable findings including mildly reduced systolic function of the systemic ventricle and minimal systemic atrioventricular valve regurgitation. Six months later, the patient returns with new onset of paroxysmal nocturnal dyspnea and decreased exercise tolerance. Pacemaker interrogation is unremarkable. Repeat echo demonstrates moderate systemic ventricular systolic dysfunction and moderate mitral valve regurgitation. Which of the following is the most likely explanation for these changes?

   A. Myocardial ischemia
   B. Pacemaker-induced dysfunction
   C. Paradoxical supraventricular tachycardia
   D. Obstructive sleep apnea
   E. Subacute bacterial endocarditis

90. A 32-year-old female with lateral tunnel Fontan palliation of tricuspid atresia presents to an emergency department with sinus tachycardia and tachypnea after a presyncopal event. There was concern for pulmonary embolism and after placing a right upper extremity IV, a ventilation perfusion scan (VQ scan) demonstrated no perfusion of the left lung with normal perfusion of the right lung. Prior to initiation of treatment for pulmonary embolus occluding the left pulmonary artery, what would you recommend that the treating team perform next?

   A. Repeat the study with a lower extremity IV
   B. Perform a transesophageal echocardiogram
   C. Place a central venous line
   D. Perform invasive pulmonary angiography
   E. Draw blood for thrombophilia assays

91. A 48-year-old male undergoes computed tomography angiogram in the setting of exertional chest discomfort. His right coronary artery arises from the left coronary cusp of the aorta with a proximal intramural course, subsequently passing between the pulmonary artery and the aorta that are normally positioned. Which of the following is the best intervention?

   A. Saphenous vein graft to the distal left main coronary artery
   B. Internal mammary artery anastomosis to the distal left main coronary artery
   C. Unroofing of intramural right coronary artery
   D. Coronary button translocation to the left coronary cusp
   E. No intervention is indicated

92. A 40-year-old male with congenital heart disease operated in infancy undergoes right-and left-sided cardiac catheterization with this anterior–posterior image of catheter position (**Figure 16.5**). The course of the catheter (not the wire) is best described as which of the following?

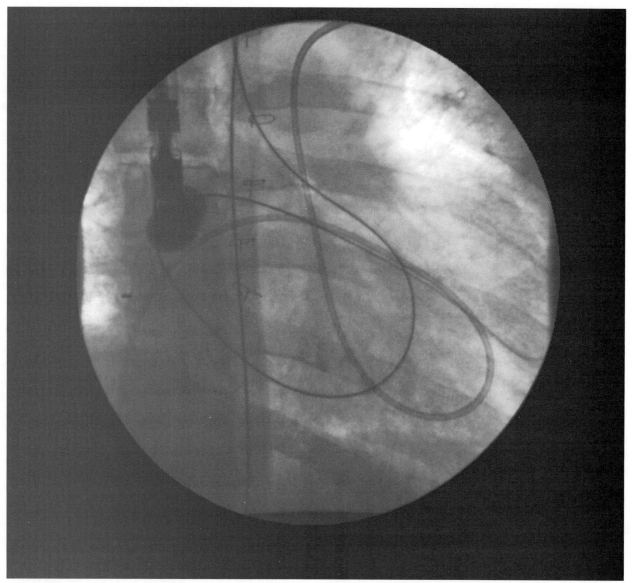

FIGURE 16.5

A. IVC, systemic venous baffle, mitral valve, morphologic left ventricle, aorta

B. IVC, systemic venous baffle, tricuspid valve, morphologic right ventricle, pulmonary artery

C. IVC, systemic venous baffle, mitral valve, morphologic left ventricle, pulmonary artery

D. IVC, systemic venous baffle, tricuspid valve, morphologic left ventricle, pulmonary artery

E. IVC, pulmonary venous baffle, tricuspid valve, morphologic right ventricle, pulmonary artery

93. A 55-year-old female presents to establish care. She has not been seen for many years. She has a history Shone complex with prior coarctation repair and resection of subaortic membrane, as well as a parachute mitral valve without significant disease. She is feeling well and has no complaints. Her blood pressure is 138/88 mm Hg with heart rate 72 bpm. Examination and echocardiography have no concerning findings. Laboratory evaluation (fasting) is notable for a hemoglobin A1c of 7.3%, total cholesterol 239 mg/dL, HDL 45 mg/dL, LDL 167 mg/dL, and triglycerides 157 mg/dL. She is a prior smoker and has a family history of premature coronary disease. What is the most appropriate next step?

   A. Calculate an ASCVD risk score
   B. Initiate shared decision making about possible initiation of a low-intensity statin
   C. Start high-intensity statin
   D. Perform CT coronary calcium scan
   E. Perform cardiac CT

94. **Figure 16.6** shows a chest radiograph of a patient who most likely has which of the following?

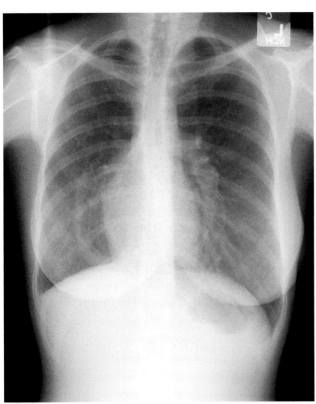

FIGURE 16.6

   A. VSD
   B. ASD
   C. Intact atrial septum
   D. Left SVC
   E. Anomalous coronary artery

95. An unoperated 40 year old has an echocardiogram that shows congenitally corrected TGA. The ECG of this patient would most likely show which of the following?

   A. Q waves in leads I and AVL
   B. Northwest QRS axis
   C. Left axis deviation
   D. Complete heart block
   E. Right bundle branch block

96. A teenager presents with progressive symptoms of stridor during exercise. In retrospect, he recalls having these symptoms for most of his life. His mother told him that periodically he was cyanotic as a baby. In the office, his oxygen saturation in room air is 99%. The CT scan shown in **Figure 16.7** was performed.

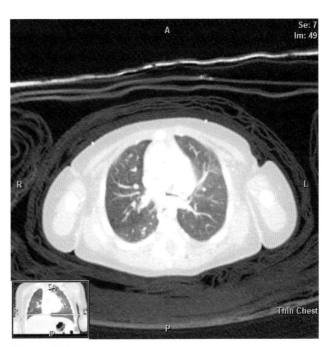

FIGURE 16.7

Which of the following would be most likely?

   A. Anterior indentation of the esophagus on barium esophogram
   B. Large VSD seen on echo
   C. Left SVC seen on CT
   D. Partial anomalous pulmonary venous connections
   E. Short stature and webbed neck

97. A 19 year old with congenital complete AV block presents for a routine follow-up evaluation. She has been doing well with no symptoms. Her baseline ECG and 24-hour Holter both show complex ventricular ectopy with frequent multiform premature ventricular contractions (PVCs). There is no evidence of AV conduction with an average ventricular rate of 64 bpm. Her echocardiogram shows mild ventricular dysfunction with an ejection fraction of 45%.

The next most appropriate step in the care of this patient would be:

A. Pacemaker implantation
B. Close follow-up for development of symptoms
C. Initiation of amiodarone therapy
D. Electrophysiology study
E. Initiation of ACE inhibitor therapy

98. A 24 year old with a large unrepaired VSD and pulmonary hypertension presents after an episode of syncope preceded by palpitations. A 24-hour Holter shows a 10 minute episode of monomorphic ventricular tachycardia at a rate of 180 bpm during which the patient reports symptoms of dizziness. His echocardiogram shows normal left ventricular function with an ejection fraction of 58%. There is a large VSD with bidirectional shunting. An electrophysiology study reveals inducible ventricular tachycardia at a rate of 210 bpm with a blood pressure drop to 50/30 which spontaneously converts to sinus rhythm after 1 minute. The patient is cyanotic with a resting saturation of 84% but otherwise doing well with minimal symptoms. The next most appropriate step in the care of this patient would be:

A. Implantation of a transvenous implantable cardioverter-defibrillator (ICD)
B. Implantation of an epicardial ICD
C. Initiation of amiodarone therapy
D. Surgical closure of the ventricular septal defect
E. Initiation of bosentan and a beta blocker and repeat EP study

99. A 24 year old with tricuspid atresia who has undergone an atriopulmonary Fontan procedure presents complaining of fatigue. Echo shows good left ventricular function. The ECG shown in **Figure 16.8** is obtained.

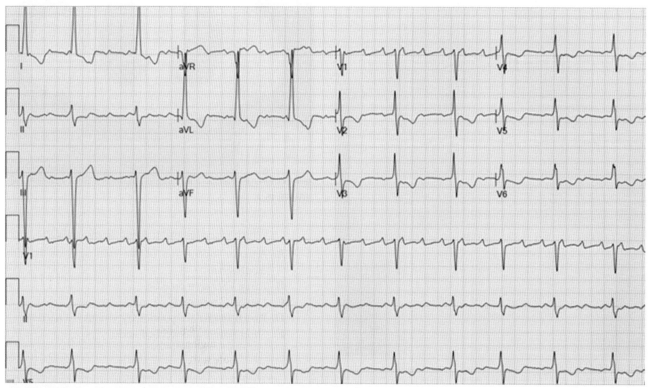

FIGURE 16.8

A. Ventricular tachycardia requiring lidocaine
B. Incisional atrial flutter requiring cardioversion
C. Normal sinus rhythm requiring evaluation for other sources of fatigue
D. Ventricular dyssynchrony requiring a biventricular pacemaker
E. Sinus node dysfunction requiring a pacemaker

100. A 20-year-old obese female presents to the clinic complaining of shortness of breath with exertion for 9 months. She denies any other symptoms. She has no significant past medical or surgical history. On physical examination, she has a normal S_1 and a fixed split S_2 with a I/VI systolic ejection murmur at the upper left sternal border. The rest of her examination is unremarkable. The echocardiogram has very poor acoustic windows, but shows normal left ventricular function and a mildly dilated right ventricle. An ECG is obtained and shown in **Figure 16.9**.

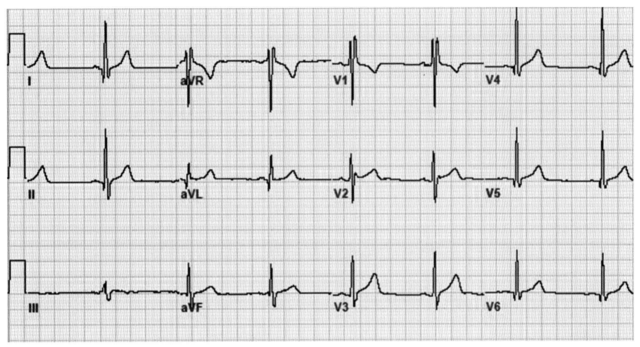

FIGURE 16.9

The additional test most likely to reveal the diagnosis in this patient is:

A. Coronary angiography
B. Thyroid function tests
C. Agitated saline contrast echocardiogram
D. Pulmonary function testing
E. Exercise treadmill test

101. A 20-year-old male with d-TGA, status post arterial switch presents to establish care in the ACHD clinic. He was last seen 5 years ago, but stopped seeing his cardiologist since he felt well and was "too busy" to make an appointment. He denies any symptoms, but has no established exercise program. What testing should be recommended at this time?

A. Pulmonary function tests to evaluate for restrictive lung disease
B. Stress echocardiogram
C. Coronary angiography
D. Six-minute walk

102. A 26 year old with d-transposition of the great arteries had a Mustard operation at 3 years of age. He has been doing well with no symptoms and works full time as an accountant. On examination, his blood pressure is 110/65 and has no murmurs or gallops. An echocardiogram shows a dilated right ventricle with moderately depressed right (systemic) ventricular function and moderate tricuspid regurgitation. An ECG is obtained and is shown in **Figure 16.10**.

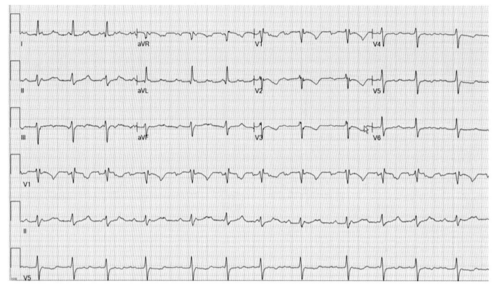

FIGURE 16.10

Which of the following medications is indicated for his clinical situation?

A. Digoxin

B. Lisinopril

C. Amiodarone

D. Carvedilol

E. Rivaroxaban

103. A 27 year old with a history of a large primum atrial septal defect underwent repair at age 14 years. She has been doing well with normal biventricular function and no symptoms. Three days prior to her visit with you, she began feeling fatigued and short of breath. She presents to the ER after an episode of syncope while running to catch a bus. Her blood pressure is 94/62 and she is alert. An echocardiogram shows a small residual atrial septal defect and a decrease in her left ventricular ejection fraction from 55% 2 months ago to 45% now. Her ECG is shown in **Figure 16.11**.

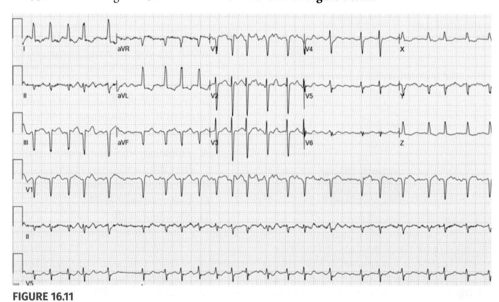

FIGURE 16.11

Which of the following is indicated for her clinical situation?

A. Coumadin for 3 weeks, then DC cardioversion

B. Emergent cardioversion in the emergency room

C. IV amiodarone bolus

D. Transesophageal echocardiogram and DC cardioversion

E. Device closure of the residual ASD

104. Which of the following patients should be transferred to a regional center specializing in care for adults with congenital heart disease for cholecystectomy?

    A. 42-year-old female with a bicuspid aortic valve and severe aortic valve regurgitation; echocardiogram demonstrates left ventricular end-diastolic dimension of 60 mm with ejection fraction of 62%

    B. 36-year-old male with tricuspid atresia status post lateral tunnel Fontan. No history of heart failure or arrhythmia

    C. 50-year-old female with atrial septal defect and pulmonary valve stenosis. Echocardiogram demonstrates right ventricular systolic pressure of 50 mm Hg and peak velocity across the pulmonary valve of 3 m/s

    D. 52-year-old female with unrepaired membranous ventricular septal defect; echocardiogram demonstrates peak velocity across the defect of 5 m/s, left ventricular end-diastolic dimension of 50-mm, end-diastolic pulmonary valve regurgitation velocity of 1.4 m/s

105. A 37-year-old female with a history of subaortic membrane that was resected at 8 years old presents with progressive dyspnea on exertion over the past couple of years and recent exertional presyncopal episodes without palpitations. On examination, LV impulse is normal, she has a normal S_1, A_2 is preserved but S_2 has paradoxical splitting, there is a 3/6 systolic ejection murmur, and diastole is quiet. Carotids are not palpable. Echocardiogram reveals normal left ventricular ejection fraction, mild left ventricular hypertrophy with abnormal diastolic function. There is a subaortic membrane and a bicuspid aortic valve which is thin and mobile with trivial regurgitation. Continuous wave Doppler shows a maximum gradient of 36 mm Hg and a mean gradient of 22 mm Hg. Which of the following is the most appropriate next step?

    A. Refer for surgical resection of the subaortic membrane

    B. No intervention needed, follow-up in 1 year

    C. No intervention needed, follow-up in 3 years

    D. Cardiac MRI for further assessment

106. A 24-year-old female presents for evaluation of supravalvar aortic stenosis. She has a known elastin mutation. She has never had intervention. Echocardiography demonstrates discrete narrowing of the proximal ascending aorta with a mean Doppler gradient of 40 mm Hg. Left ventricular size, ejection fraction, and wall thickness are within normal limits. The patient is asymptomatic with activities of daily living. She is contemplating a pregnancy in the near future. You recommend:

    A. Surgical intervention to relieve the obstruction

    B. Permanent contraception given the elastin mutation and risk of fetal transmission

    C. Proceed with pregnancy without further testing

    D. Initiate beta blockade

107. A 22 year old is referred for evaluation of valvular pulmonary stenosis. Echocardiography demonstrates a maximal instantaneous velocity across of the pulmonary valve of 3.2 m/s. The patient is asymptomatic. What should be recommended?

    A. Cardiac catheterization to confirm the degree of obstruction

    B. Referral for percutaneous valve implantation

    C. Cardiac MRI to calculate indexed RV end-diastolic volume

    D. Repeat echocardiogram in 3 years

Answers

1. (B) For asymptomatic patients with secundum ASDs, right heart enlargement, and no pulmonary hypertension, there is a 2A recommendation to proceed with ASD closure (compared to a grade 1 recommendation for those who are symptomatic). Her right heart is moderately enlarged and RVSP is normal. Therefore, there is no need for invasive Q_p/Q_s measurement as there is no concern for pulmonary hypertension.

2. (A) The 2018 AHA/ACC ACHD guidelines varied from the original 2008 statement. The 2008 guidelines stated that pulmonary valve replacement for repaired tetralogy of Fallot was only recommended if the pulmonary regurgitation was severe and had any of the following symptoms: ≥moderate RV enlargement or dysfunction, ≥moderate tricuspid regurgitation, or symptomatic arrhythmias. *The 2018 guidelines state that in asymptomatic individuals (Physiological Stage A)* *with ≥moderate pulmonary regurgitation, pulmonary valve replacement is reasonable if there are any two of the following: mild or moderate RV or LV systolic dysfunction, severe RV dilation (RVEDVI ≥160 mL/m², RVESVI ≥80 mL/m², or RVEDV/LVEDV >2.0), RVSP ≥2/3 systemic pressure, or progressive reduction in exercise tolerance.* As this patient has moderate–severe pulmonary regurgitation and a severely enlarged RV with moderate systolic dysfunction, pulmonary valve replacement would be reasonable at this time.

3. (E) This patient with repaired tetralogy of Fallot and moderate pulmonary regurgitation has progression of symptoms and is now NYHA Class III. The 2018 AHA/ACC guidelines recommend that for symptomatic patients with ≥moderate pulmonary regurgitation, pulmonary valve replacement is reasonable. Results of MRI, exercise testing, or repeat echocardiogram would not outweigh her symptoms and heart failure. Although tricuspid regurgitation may improve after percutaneous pulmonary valve implantation, given the severity of the TR and the tricuspid valve dilation, surgery may be more effective for this patient. However, when answering a question similar to this on the boards realize that guideline recommendations (hence the correct answer on the test) and clinical practice for the individual patient may differ regarding choice of catheter versus surgical intervention.

4. (A) According to the 2018 AHA/ACC guidelines, ICD implantation would be reasonable for primary prophylaxis in a patient with tetralogy of Fallot given numerous risk factors (LV dysfunction, nonsustained VT, QRS duration ≥180 ms, and extensive RV scarring). While proceeding with electrophysiology study and potential ablation is reasonable, these are not necessary prior to ICD implantation.

5. (D) According to the AHA/ACC 2018 guidelines, pulmonary vasoactive medications are reasonable to use in patients with Fontan physiology for improvement in exercise tolerance. He has a borderline increased transpulmonary gradient of 8 mm Hg, suggestive of pulmonary vascular disease in a patient after Fontan. PDE5 inhibitors such as sildenafil and endothelin antagonists have been utilized in this patient population. There are limited data regarding prostacyclin analogues (e.g., epoprostenol); and furthermore, this medication requires continuous intravenous infusion, thus it would not be preferred over oral sildenafil therapy. Oxygen therapy is unlikely to improve his saturation significantly given his known venovenous collaterals. Fontan revision is mostly recommended when there are refractory atrial tachyarrhythmias. While transplant referral may be reasonable, medical therapy is a more appropriate next step

6. (D) According to the 2018 AHA/ACC guidelines, this patient is IA with a simple congenital abnormality and is Physiological Stage A with no symptoms. Physical examination and echocardiogram are reassuring that this is a small, restrictive VSD with no left heart enlargement or pulmonary hypertension. There is no significant associated valve disease. Thus, she likely will never need closure of this VSD due to the shunt. But routine follow-up is recommended to assess progression of aortic valve regurgitation. Aortic valve

cusp prolapse may occur in patients with membranous VSDs. The guidelines do not have recommendations for use of cardiac MRI in long-term follow-up of VSDs in adults.

7. (B) According to the AHA/ACC Valve guidelines, surgery is indicated for asymptomatic individuals with severe aortic regurgitation if there is significant LV enlargement (LVESV >50 mm, LVESVi >25 mm/m²) or dysfunction (LV ejection fraction <55%). In addition, in patients with bicuspid aortic valves, aortic dilation >55 mm in those without risk factors (family history, rapid growth, or coarctation) or >50 mm in those with risk factors, is an indication for ascending aorta and valve replacement.

8. (D) Sotalol is a Class III antiarrhythmic, blocking the IK$_r$ channel, thus it delays ventricular repolarization and can prolong the QT interval. Excessive prolongation of the QT interval can lead to polymorphic VT (torsades de pointes). This is more likely to occur with hypokalemia, hypomagnesemia, and bradycardia. The type of anticoagulant does not make torsades more likely. The 2018 AHA/ACC guidelines recommend anticoagulation with a vitamin K antagonist (i.e., warfarin) in all patients after Fontan with atrial arrhythmias and no contraindications to anticoagulation. However, novel agents are currently under investigation for this purpose also.

9. (C) This patient with prior surgical repair of tetralogy of Fallot has now developed right-sided heart failure from constrictive pericarditis and severe pulmonary regurgitation. This is suggested by his elevated jugular venous pressure and the contour with prominent descents classic for constrictive physiology. In addition, he has a pericardial knock. The lateral film shows calcification of the diaphragmatic pericardium. Further evaluations with echocardiography, MRI, and/or catheterization are important prior to surgical referral. Percutaneous pulmonary valve replacement would not address the pericardial disease. He has newly diagnosed heart failure, so recommending routine follow-up or exercise without further assessment is not appropriate.

10. (B) There are multiple complications of the Ross procedure including pulmonary homograft degeneration, neo-aortic valve degeneration, aortic root dilation, and coronary ostial narrowing/occlusion. This patient had degeneration of his pulmonary homograft requiring placement of a conduit and this has now degenerated. He has symptomatic RV-PA conduit obstruction and warrants intervention. Given the loud and palpable P$_2$, this is unlikely to purely be valvular stenosis and rather there is sub- or supravalvular stenosis as well. Given the multilevel obstruction, he will need either surgical replacement of the entire conduit or percutaneous valve replacement with stenting of the conduit. CT imaging specifically to evaluate the extra-anatomic conduit and the course of the coronary arteries relative to the conduit will be essential for either percutaneous or surgical planning. In this situation, CT imaging is superior to MR.

11. (C) The shunt is exclusively left to right and there is RV enlargement. Therefore, the shunt is large. In this scenario, PVR is likely low enough that it can be argued that calculation of pulmonary pressures and resistance at cardiac cath are not essential. She will require some form of coronary artery imaging given her age >40 to 45 years. Life expectancy with a large ASD is reduced in adults >40 years, with arrhythmia and elevated PA pressures. Treating her solely with device closure will not be sufficient to address the Afib. Surgical closure with Maze is likely the best course. This would also be true if there was severe TR associated with the ASD. Tricuspid valve repair could be addressed at time of surgical ASD closure.

12. (A) One of the earliest signs of cirrhotic liver disease from any etiology is thrombocytopenia. It is present in at least 70% of patients with cirrhosis. The pathophysiology is due to splenic sequestration, decreased production of thrombopoietin (TPO), and decreased bone marrow production. A platelet count <100,000 is a marker for advanced liver disease and increased mortality. Elevation of biomarkers that detect synthetic dysfunction appear late in FALD. Elevation of the INR, in a patient not receiving a vitamin K antagonist, may be an earlier manifestation of synthetic liver dysfunction. Alpha fetoprotein is a marker for hepatocellular carcinoma.

13. (C) Objectively assessing functional capacity and VO$_2$ can be very helpful during the assessment of adults with CHD. Arrhythmias that may prompt earlier intervention may be provoked with exercise. In an adult with ToF and severe residual PR, most would recommend PVR if there are overt symptoms, new arrhythmia, RVEDVi >150 mL/m^2, RV/LV >2:1, > mild TR, > mild RV systolic dysfunction, *or* any LV dysfunction.

14. (C) During a normal pregnancy, the following physiologic changes occur: blood volume increases by 40%, systemic and pulmonary vascular resistance decrease, and heart rate increases. This all leads to a 30% increase in cardiac output. Blood pressure is the least affected by pregnancy.

15. (E) The image shows a bifid uvula. The patient has peripheral aneurysms. She likely has Loeys–Dietz. These patients have increased risk of aortic dissection when the aortic root is >40 mm. Surgical intervention is recommended in Loeys–Dietz patients at 40 mm. In this patient, valve-sparing root replacement may not be possible if there already is significant aortic valve regurgitation. Prior to reaching 40 mm, aggressive medical management with ARBs is indicated for all patients with Loeys–Dietz.

16. (C) Review the modified Duke criteria (see below). A and B are minor criteria, D (changing degree of regurgitation) does not satisfy a major criterion, E—*both* culture bottles should be positive to satisfy a major criterion.

Major criteria:

- Blood culture positive for IE
- Typical microorganism consistent with IE from two separate blood cultures: *Viridans streptococci*, *Streptococcus bovis*, HACEK group, *Staphylococcus aureus*, or community-acquired enterococci in the absence of a primary focus…or…Microorganisms consistent with IE from

persistently positive blood cultures defined as follows: At least two positive cultures of blood samples drawn >12 hours apart; or all of three or a majority of ≥four separate cultures of blood (with first and last sample drawn at least 1 hour apart)

- Single positive blood culture for *Coxiella burnetii* or anti-phase 1 IgG antibody titer >1:800. Evidence of endocardial involvement
- Echocardiogram positive for IE (TEE recommended for patients with prosthetic valves, rated at least "possible IE" by clinical criteria or complicated IE [paravalvular abscess]; TTE as first test in other patients) defined as follows:
  - Oscillating intracardiac mass on valve or supporting structures, in the path of regurgitant jets, or on implanted material in the absence of an alternative anatomic explanation; or
  - Abscess; or
  - New partial dehiscence of prosthetic valve; or
  - New valvular regurgitation (worsening, changing or preexisting murmur are *not* sufficient)

17. (A) Intranasal cocaine use is a risk for HCV infection. The patients described in (**B**) and (**D**) had blood transfusions, but after 1992 and neither were born before 1965. The patient described in C has no risk factors.

The following need screening for hepatitis C infection:

- Born between 1945 and 1965
- Injection drug use or intranasal illicit drug use
- Hemodialysis
- Needle stick/heath care exposures
- Children of HCV infected mothers
- Transfusion or organ transplant before 1992
- Unexplained liver disease

18. (C) She needs to start warfarin therapy to avoid valve thrombosis. Subcutaneous heparin is an inferior choice for therapeutic anticoagulation long term and IV heparin long term is not practical. LMWH can be used, but needs *weekly* anti-Xa monitoring, not daily. NOAC/DOACs have not been approved for use in pregnancy.

19. (A) Patients with bileaflet mechanical *aortic* valve replacements and no other risk factors for thrombosis do not need bridging.

20. (C) Cyanosis is an important risk factor for maternal and fetal complications. While baseline exercise intolerance and NYHA class II symptoms are important to note, cyanosis is a more important risk factor. Bioprosthetic valves with normal function confer less risk than mechanical valves.

21. (A) Microcytosis caused by iron deficiency in patients with secondary erythrocytosis creates the greatest risk for thromboembolic events. Phlebotomy for these patients is rarely performed in the current era. It is reserved for patients with neurologic symptoms or prior to surgery. Hydration is also a successful therapy for these patients. Thrombocytopenia and mild leukopenia are characteristic of patients with unrepaired cyanotic CHD.

22. (D) Women with Eisenmenger syndrome are at exceptionally high risk of complication and death during pregnancy and the peripartum period. Pregnancy should be avoided in these patients. The patient described in answer A has one predictor of cardiac complications (predicted risk 25%) but has a low risk of death. Patients with Marfan syndrome can have dissection during pregnancy, but pregnancy is not absolutely contraindicated unless the aorta is >40 mm. The patient described in answer C has a risk of cardiac complications, but no absolute contraindication.

23. (A) The arterial switch operation for d-TGA requires reimplantation of coronary artery buttons. There is risk of both early and late coronary obstruction. There is evidence that the risk may be greater with single coronary artery anatomy. Symptoms of coronary ischemia may present in atypical fashion. The history of exertional chest pain that resolved with rest warrants evaluation. Coronary angiography is the gold standard for coronary assessment, although computed tomography angiography may be appropriate.

24. (D) Mustard and Senning atrial switch procedures are associated with sinus node dysfunction and atrial arrhythmias. Other complications are baffle leaks and baffle obstruction. Placement of transvenous, intracardiac pacemaker leads may worsen baffle stenosis, and paradoxical embolus may occur across a baffle leak. Incorrect positioning of ventricular leads across the baffles is occasionally observed. Pacemaker placement in this patient should be performed at a center with experience in adult congenital cardiac care. There is no history given for thrombophilia. While sudden death does occur in patients with repaired d-TGA, there is no history of atrial or ventricular tachycardia in this patient even with exercise.

25. (B) Isolated membranous VSD is associated with the development of DCRV that may occur in adulthood. DCRV is defined by a proximal portion of the RV that is at high pressure, separated by abnormal muscular hypertrophy from a distal low-pressure zone. The pulmonary arterial pressure is distal to the obstruction and should be normal. The development of DCRV is often heralded by an increase in murmur intensity, onset of a thrill, and findings of RV pressure loading including an increased right ventricular impulse and RVH by ECG. Surgical resection of the muscle bundle is needed.

26. (B) The 2018 ACHD guidelines concluded that at this time there is insufficient evidence to recommend medications, such as ACE inhibitors or beta blockers, for patients with failing systemic right ventricles. His pulmonary hypertension is likely postcapillary in nature and pulmonary vasodilators would worsen his symptoms. His AV valve regurgitation is only moderate and likely due to ventricular dilation; furthermore, his ventricle may not tolerate AV valve replacement. There is no evidence to suggest obstruction of the systemic venous baffles given only mild jugular venous distention, no hepatomegaly, and patent baffles demonstrated on echocardiogram.

27. (D) The patient has a bileaflet mechanical aortic valve which functions normally. There is a relatively low likelihood of thrombosis with a brief period of holding anticoagulation. She has no additional risk factors for thrombosis (e.g., prior venous thromboembolism, atrial fibrillation, or solid organ malignancy), it is appropriate to hold warfarin 5 days prior to surgery, continue aspirin, and no bridging is needed. Alternatively, if she had risk factors for thrombosis, malfunctioning aortic prosthesis, or if the mechanical prosthesis was in another position, then bridging with a heparin product would be recommended.

28. (C) This young woman has never had alternative imaging of her aorta. Since she has dilation of the ascending aorta, it would be appropriate to perform more extensive imaging at least once early in adulthood and prior to pregnancy. She has mild aortic valve stenosis and regurgitation and likely would tolerate pregnancy well. Unless obstetrical complications occur, one would expect a normal spontaneous vaginal delivery. ACE inhibitors and angiotensin receptor blockers are contraindicated during pregnancy.

29. (B) It is considered safe to continue Warfarin at a dose of 5 mg or less daily if an INR of 3.0 can be obtained during pregnancy. The risk of warfarin embryopathy at a dose of less than 5 mg daily is felt to be low enough that one could continue Warfarin during pregnancy. Alternatively, if one cannot maintain an INR of 3.0 on this dose and need a higher dose, then Warfarin should be discontinued by the 6th week of gestation and resumed after the 12th week of gestation. Low–molecular-weight heparin 1 mg/kg twice daily should be administered. The patient should have her Anti-Xa level checked weekly or twice weekly depending on the clinical situation. Anti-Xa levels of 0.7 to 1.3 should be obtained. If this is a mechanical AV valve, one would want to have a higher Anti-Xa level. Warfarin should be discontinued at 36-week gestation in anticipation of delivery. Patients should be switched to low–molecular-weight heparin at this time. The last dose of low–molecular-weight heparin should be 12 hours prior to planned delivery. Postpartum if there is no unexpected bleeding, warfarin therapy can be reinstituted while bridging with low–molecular-weight heparin until the INR is at least 2.0. Pregnancy is considered a hypercoagulable state due to the elevated estrogen levels. Patients remain in this state of hypercoagulability in the first several weeks postpartum.

30. (C) The woman likely has Holt–Oram syndrome (radial hypoplasia associated with secundum atrial septal defect). It is inherited on an autosomal dominant fashion; therefore 50% of her offspring would be expected to inherit this syndrome assuming complete penetrance.

31. (B) See Answer 30. In patients with Holt–Oram syndrome, 75% have CHD.

32. (D) This case scenario demonstrates a typical presentation of a young adult with a previously undiagnosed ASD. Transthoracic imaging prior to intervention demonstrates a centrally located defect that is amenable to device closure. This defect can also be closed surgically. If the pulmonary veins were adequately visualized entering the left atrium, then no further imaging is required. Her clinical examination is consistent with a large left-to-right shunt from an atrial level defect (presence of diastolic rumble). There is no evidence on echocardiography or clinical examination for pulmonary hypertension, therefore cardiac catheterization would not be needed.

33. (C) The diastolic flow rumble in a patient with an ASD is due to excess flow across a normal tricuspid valve. Presence of this sound is associated with a Q_p/Q_s >1.5 to 2.0. The systolic murmur, similarly, is due to excess flow across an otherwise normal pulmonary valve. Flow across the ASD is of low velocity and inaudible. Young children with large VSDs will have a diastolic flow murmur due to flow across the mitral valve. Diastolic murmurs are not "normal."

34. (C) The 2013 ACC/AHA guidelines recommend either high intensity or moderate intensity statin regimen for patients with an ASCVD risk score that is ≥7.5%. Gemfibrozil and Niacin are not statins. Aspirin therapy is not contraindicated but would not address this issue directly. Losartan does not treat hyperlipidemia

35. (C) The patient has a residual right-to-left shunt and atrial arrhythmia with spontaneous echo contrast in the right atrium. Risk of paradoxical embolus is important. Based on the ACHD guidelines, warfarin therapy is indicated.

36. (E) The fenestration gradient is equal to the transpulmonary gradient (RA or Fontan pressure minus LA pressure). Values of 5 to 8 mm Hg usually are expected. An increased gradient correlates with obstruction in the Fontan circuit, lungs or pulmonary veins. It is primarily dependent on total pulmonary vascular resistance. Elevated LA or ventricular end-diastolic pressures do not change the transpulmonary gradient. A low fenestration gradient is associated with hypovolemia.

37. (C) The murmur described in the examination is continuous and it peaks around the second heart sound—typical of a PDA. An audible PDA usually can be visualized with transthoracic echocardiography. If that imaging is suboptimal, CT or MRI of the chest may be helpful. If the PDA is audible, especially in a patient with a wide pulse pressure, one would expect left ventricular and left atrial enlargement. This patient should undergo closure of the PDA, usually via a transcatheter procedure.

38. (D) The continuous murmur is typical of a PDA or systemic arterial to pulmonary artery collateral vessels (common in patients with pulmonary atresia). Patients with PA/VSD frequently have a right-sided aortic arch and the PDA may be best heard over the right back. A right coronary fistula may produce a continuous murmur but is unlikely to be heard best in the back. The other choices do not generate continuous murmurs.

39. (E) The patient has an ASD that technically would be amenable to device closure. But, other issues need to be addressed such as intervention for the tricuspid

valve—dictating that the patient is best served with surgical management. Patients who may need additional cardiac surgery for coronary revascularization, valve repair, or arrhythmia surgery should be treated with surgery rather than sole transcatheter device closure of the ASD.

40. (E) The patient has two sources of pulmonary blood flow, the SVC exclusively supplies the RPA, the IVC flow via the Fontan conduit supplies the LPA exclusively. In addition, the patient has substrate for right lung fistula due to the classic Glenn procedure. Pulmonary blood flow cannot be accurately quantitated nor can pulmonary vascular resistance be assessed.

41. (C) Polymerase chain reaction is needed to confirm presence of active infection. Antibody positivity indicates immunization or prior infection. Prior to 1992, no formal testing was available for what was formerly called "non A-non B hepatitis." It is estimated that 5% of patients with congenital heart disease who had cardiac surgery prior to 1992 are infected with hepatitis C.

42. (A) Serum BNP levels >140 pg/mL correlated with poor long-term outcome in patients with Eisenmenger syndrome (*Reardon LC, et al. Am J Cardiol 2012; 110:1523-6*). Elevated BNP correlates with ventricular dilation, dysfunction, and heart failure symptoms but has not been studied specifically in the other lesions listed. Although based on data from just one study, this question has appeared on several board examinations.

43. (A) The patient in this scenario has a primum ASD. A primum ASD is located in the most anterior and inferior aspect of the atrial septum at the level of the mitral and tricuspid valves. It is associated with a cleft mitral valve. Any ASD with moderate right ventricular volume overload should be closed. There is decreased mortality after surgical closure (compared to medical treatment), although nonfatal cardiovascular complications are similar. Unlike secundum ASDs, primum ASDs should not be closed using a device in the cath lab. Although there is right atrial enlargement, the patient is not hypertensive and there is no definitive role for ACE inhibition in shunt lesions. Patients with primum ASDs will frequently have left axis deviation on ECG that is related to the lesion rather than any coronary artery disease. There is no indication for a cardiac cath (unless there is concern for pulmonary hypertension).

44. (E) Any patient who survived a cardiac arrest due to nonreversible causes should have an ICD placed. There is no evidence of a reversible cause in this patient. Ablation may be offered as an alternative in a patient with a slow, stable, monomorphic ventricular tachycardia, but not the fast ventricular tachycardia resulting in cardiac arrest seen in this patient. The incidence of ICD complications was reported to be 30% in one study of patients with tetralogy of Fallot, compared to about 10% in the postmyocardial infarction population. The incidence of inappropriate shocks in tetralogy of Fallot is about 25%, which is similar to that seen in other congenital heart lesions. Antiarrhythmic medications are not as effective as an ICD in preventing recurrent arrhythmias. Beta blockers, amiodarone, and sotalol do not decrease the risk of appropriate ICD shocks in patients with tetralogy of Fallot. A transvenous system can be performed in a patient with free pulmonary regurgitation. Patients with residual intracardiac shunts should not have transvenous pacing/ICD leads.

45. (D) TBX5 mutation is associated with Holt–Oram syndrome. It is inherited in an autosomal dominant fashion. TGFBR 1 & 2 with Loeys–Dietz; FBN1 with Marfan syndrome; Trisomy 21 is Down syndrome; NKX 2.5 with ASD + heart block.

46. (A) NKX 2.5 mutation is associated with familial occurrence of ASDs and progressive AV block. The GATA IV mutation is associated with ASDs *without* AV block. TBX5 is associated with Holt–Oram syndrome, NOTCH mutations are associated with AVSD.

47. (A) The embryologic origin of the valve of the fossa ovalis is derived from septum primum. The superior limbus and inferior limbus originate from the septum secundum. Atrial appendage morphology is not related to development of the atrial septum. The endocardial cushions are important in septation of the atrioventricular septum and delamination of the atrioventricular valves.

48. (C) The cardiac disease in pregnancy (CARPREG) investigators demonstrated in a prospective multicenter study that maternal cardiac risk could be predicted with the use of a risk index. Cardiac events were defined as pulmonary edema, arrhythmia, stroke, or cardiac death. The four predictors of primary cardiac events were (1) prior cardiac event, (2) baseline NYHA class >II or cyanosis, (3) left heart obstruction (mitral valve area <2 cm^2, aortic valve area <1.5 cm^2, or *peak* LVOT gradient >30 mm Hg by echocardiography), and (4) reduced systemic ventricular systolic function (EF <40%). The risk of maternal cardiac complication with zero predictors was 5%, with one predictor it was 25%, and with greater than one predictor the risk was 75%. The risk score was further refined by the Boston Adult Congenital Heart Disease Group in a study that demonstrated that including decreased subpulmonary ventricular function and/or severe pulmonary regurgitation as a predictor in the risk index improved the accuracy of the assessment. Of the answers listed, the patient described in (**C**) has the highest predicted risk with a prior cardiac event (history of atrial fibrillation) and severe pulmonary valve regurgitation. Her poor peak VO$_2$ may be a further indication of poor outcome, even if she has no complaints clinically. The 32-year-old patient has no predictors. The 30-year-old patient has one predictor. The 20-year-old patient could be considered to have one predictor—poor subpulmonary ventricular function.

49. (C) ACE inhibitors can cause fetal renal dysfunction in the third trimester, but have also been demonstrated to be a teratogen. Therefore, ACE inhibitors should be avoided throughout pregnancy. ARBs should be considered to have the same risk profile and should be avoided. Hydralazine and nitrates are safe in pregnancy and together provide similar physiologic response to ACE inhibition.

50. (C) Small coronary fistulae with no symptoms, no murmur, and no evidence of hemodynamic compromise do not need further evaluation or treatment.

51. (D) Patients with mechanical valve prostheses pose significant difficulties for anticoagulation management. Warfarin probably provides the optimum anticoagulation, but it is a teratogen and should be avoided if possible during the first trimester of pregnancy. Also, warfarin crosses the placenta, and a fetus of a mother anticoagulated with warfarin should not be delivered vaginally secondary to the risk of fetal intracranial bleeding. However, studies have shown that if *therapeutic* anticoagulation can be achieved with a daily dose of <5 mg daily, the risk of warfarin embryopathy is quite low. A currently accepted management strategy is to provide alternative anticoagulation during at least the first trimester. Low–molecular-weight heparin is an attractive alternative to warfarin as it does not cross the placenta. However, weight-based dosing alone is not effective anticoagulation during pregnancy secondary to altered volume of distribution and drug metabolism. If low–molecular-weight heparins are used, anti-Xa levels must be followed closely (at least weekly) to ensure adequate anticoagulation.

52. (E) Depo-Provera injection provides the best option for this patient, though there is some risk of hematoma at the injection site. Essure tubal implants were an irreversible form of contraception and implanted in >500,000 women worldwide, but subsequently have been withdrawn from the market. Mirena IUD is reversible and safe to implant, but is not the best option in patients who are not monogamous as the incidence of pelvic inflammatory disease may be increased. Barrier contraception such as a diaphragm does not have the same efficacy as Depo-Provera, but the patient should be encouraged to use condoms with a new partner to prevent sexually transmitted disease. Estrogen containing oral contraception would not be a good choice in a patient at risk for thrombus.

53. (B) This patient likely has Loeys–Dietz syndrome, a mutation of TGF-β receptor that results in arterial fragility. ARBs have been shown to reduce TGF-β signaling and reduce the risk of arterial complications in animal models. ARBs are the drug of choice in this situation. While patients with Loeys–Dietz can have aortic complication at this degree of dilatation, it is acceptable to follow closely with routine imaging.

54. (C) This patient had appropriate secondary erythrocytosis related to his cyanosis. This increase in hemoglobin is necessary to provide appropriate oxygen delivery and is not associated with stroke or other small vessel occlusion unless the patient is microcytic. Microcytotic red cells are less deformable as they traverse small capillary beds. This patient likely feels unwell because he has poor oxygen delivery. He should be treated with iron therapy for 1 month with a goal of normalizing the MCV and ferritin.

55. (E) This patient has symptomatic aortic stenosis. Bed rest may be advisable, but 4 weeks is too long for a follow-up interval. Balloon valvotomy is not a good choice since the valve is calcified. Delivery of the fetus now is not optimal since this degree of prematurity would provide a high risk of neonatal complication and death. Percutaneous valve implantation is currently not an option in this situation and would likely carry some risk to mother and fetus. Surgical replacement of the aortic valve can be done with low risk to mother and relatively low risk to the fetus and is the best option in this scenario.

56. (D) This patient is at higher risk of coronary artery disease given his history of coarctation. His LDL cholesterol goal should be 70 mg/dL or less. Diet can be helpful, but the patient will benefit from a statin drug to lower LDL. Niaspan, fish oil, and gemfibrozil do not have significant LDL lowering effects.

57. (D) This patient does need treatment for hypertension. While a recurrent coarctation can cause residual hypertension, there is no evidence from the echocardiogram that the patient has any significant residual obstruction; hence, stent implantation is unlikely to provide much benefit. This patient likely has hypertension related to stiff arterial vasculature and a relatively late coarctation repair. All the drugs listed can treat hypertension, but Metoprolol and Diltiazem would not be favored given the low resting heart rate. Lasix will probably not be effective in controlling the hypertension and would not be a first-line choice. Losartan has the most advantages with a low side effect profile, no heart rate changes, and possible protection against aortic dilatation (for which this patient is at risk).

58. (A) PFO is present in 25% to 30% of the adult population. Currently there are no data that treatment with medication or closure to prevent paradoxical emboli is indicated in an asymptomatic patient. PFO should not cause right ventricular volume overload; hence, MRI would not provide clinically useful information.

59. (E) The patient has symptoms of platypnea–orthodeoxia syndrome, related to positional right-to-left shunting across a PFO. Elderly patients with a PFO are more prone to right-to-left shunting as the cardiac geometry changes with age. A normal supine saturation would make this diagnosis more likely combined echocardiographic confirmation. Treatment would be closure of the PFO. Pulmonary function test with methacholine challenge would be helpful for diagnosing asthma, but asthma would not explain the patient's decline in saturation. V/Q scan would be helpful to determine whether there had been pulmonary emboli, but the patient would potentially have right heart changes on echocardiography if emboli were so extensive to cause this degree of desaturation. Diastolic dysfunction or coronary artery disease can lead to dyspnea on exertion, but this degree of desaturation would be unlikely.

60. (C) ASDs can cause right heart enlargement secondary to left-to-right shunting, but at this age and with the history of hypertension, it is possible that the left-to-right shunt volume is increased secondary to left ventricular diastolic dysfunction. If the left ventricular filling pressures are extremely high, the patient may become more dyspneic with closure of the ASD since the left atrial pressure will increase after ASD closure. Therefore, the best initial step in this patient's evaluation is to perform left and right heart catheterization to determine filling pressures. If the pressures are elevated, balloon occlusion of the ASD can be performed to ensure that left atrial pressures do not become excessively increased with ASD closure.

61. (D) This patient has one risk factor—left heart obstruction (mitral valve area <2 cm^2, aortic valve area <1.5 cm^2, or *peak* LVOT gradient >30 mm Hg by echocardiography). In the CARPREG model, one risk factor predicts a 25% risk of cardiac complication during pregnancy.

62. (E) This patient is best served by transthoracic echocardiogram to evaluate the function of the left ventricle and the bicuspid aortic valve, MRI scan of the aorta to evaluate for thoracic aorta dilation and complications at the coarctation repair site, as well as MRA scan of the brain to evaluate for intracranial aneurysms since patients with a history of coarctation have an increased risk of intracranial aneurysm. The other choices listed could evaluate the heart and the thoracic aorta, but would not evaluate the intracranial vasculature.

63. (A) Blood pressure medications can cause fatigue as a side effect, but this patient is complaining of hypersomnolence. Patients with Marfan syndrome should be screened for obstructive sleep apnea as they are at high risk for this condition, which can result in daytime hypersomnolence, hypertension, and aortic dilatation. Overnight oximetry is a simple, but effective, screening tool to evaluate possible obstructive sleep apnea.

64. (A) Sertraline has a low risk of cardiac complications. Citalopram and amitriptyline can cause prolonged QT that could be a problem in a patient with tetralogy of Fallot. Venlafaxine and bupropion both inhibit the neuronal uptake of norepinephrine and can cause hypertension and tachycardia.

65. (A) Dabigatran is an oral direct thrombin inhibitor. Unlike warfarin, dabigatran therapy does not need to be monitored to ensure achievement of therapeutic anticoagulation. It is currently approved for use in patients with atrial fibrillation, but not for use with mechanical valves. There are no data currently regarding the use of this agent during pregnancy. Dabigatran is not useful for bridging anticoagulation as it is recommended that dabigatran should be discontinued 1 to 2 days prior to surgery (with abnormal creatine clearance, this recommendation increases to 3 to 5 days). Dabigatran should not be used in patients with significant bleeding issues as there is no direct reversal agent available.

66. (C) Concomitant use of amlodipine and simvastatin increases the risk of myopathy and rhabdomyolysis. If it is necessary to use both drugs, it is recommended that the dose of simvastatin not exceed 20 mg/day.

67. (B) Atenolol has an FDA pregnancy classification of class D—*There is positive evidence of human fetal risk, but the benefits from use in pregnant women may be acceptable* *despite the risk (e.g., if the drug is needed in a life-threatening situation or for a serious disease for which safer drugs cannot be used or are ineffective)*—because a study in hypertensive women taking atenolol demonstrated lower birth weight infants. The other drugs are labeled class C—*Either studies in animals have revealed adverse effects on the fetus (teratogenic or embryocidal or other) and there are no controlled studies in women or studies in women and animals are not available. Drugs should be given only if the potential benefit justifies the potential risk to the fetus.*

68. (D) Endometrial ablation is a safe, minimally invasive procedure that can reduce menstrual bleeding significantly (especially in women >35 years of age) and can be performed without interruption of anticoagulation. Endometrial ablation should not be performed if interested in future pregnancies. Hysterectomy can provide the same relief of symptoms, but for this patient to have hysterectomy, she would have to interrupt her warfarin anticoagulation and undergo a surgical procedure. Oral estrogen containing contraception can be a good choice to treat menometrorrhagia in some patients, but is not favorable in this patient secondary to the increased risk of thrombosis. Depo-Provera can improve menometrorrhagia, but is not as effective as endometrial ablation. Essure tubal ligation prevented pregnancy, but did not treat menometrorrhagia. Its use was discontinued at the end of 2018 when the manufacturer suspended sales. Worldwide, 750,000 women reportedly had it implanted. Multiple side effects were reported to the FDA.

69. (E) Flecainide is a class IC antiarrhythmic agent. It can cause pro-arrhythmia and QRS prolongation, so is best initiated in hospital with continuous monitoring for five doses with a daily ECG to check the QRS duration.

70. (A) Amiodarone can cause liver, pulmonary, and thyroid toxicity. Therefore, TSH, liver function tests, and pulmonary function tests should be monitored routinely. Liver function tests ideally should be reviewed twice yearly and thyroid function tests every 3 to 6 months.

71. (A) One of the most common side effects of Bosentan is lower extremity edema. This side effect is not significant in the other drugs listed. Beta blockers are not considered pulmonary vasodilators.

72. (E) It is very important that the drug be taken at the same time daily for optimum effectiveness. It does not take 60 days for the pill to become effective. Rash can occur, but not sun sensitivity. Amenorrhea can occur, but is not the norm. Antibiotics may reduce the effectiveness of contraception, but patients who need SBE prophylaxis should continue using antibiotics when appropriate and be counseled to use alternative contraception for that cycle.

73. (D) The physical examination and ECG are consistent with the echocardiographic image demonstrating a sinus venosus defect with partial anomalous pulmonary venous return with the right superior pulmonary vein draining to the superior vena cava—right atrial junction. Given the cardiac chamber dilation with respiratory and exercise symptoms, it is appropriate to proceed with surgical intervention. ASD closure alone will allow persistent left-to-right shunting through the right superior pulmonary vein. To eliminate this shunt and volume load of the right heart, ASD closure and surgical pulmonary venous redirection to the left atrium are indicated. Device closure is reserved for secundum ASDs only. But in recent years, case series of transcatheter therapy for sinus venosus defects have been reported. Midterm follow-up data for these techniques are not yet available.

74. (A) Small VSDs may be detected at any age, particularly in patients who have avoided medical care. Management of this patient is based on the hemodynamic effects of the lesion. Evidence that the ventricular level shunt is small and of no hemodynamic consequence includes the absence of LA and LV enlargement, normal RV systolic pressure, and a very high flow velocity across the VSD, although the latter may be the least trustworthy of these findings. No intervention or additional evaluation is required. The patient should be reassured about the benign nature of this lesion. There is no need for SBE prophylaxis.

75. (B) The flow acceleration demonstrated by echocardiogram is mildly elevated. Mild pulmonary valve stenosis should not result in RA and RV enlargement. Additional evaluation is needed to explain the chamber dilation. PDA with normal pulmonary vascular resistance would result in increased pulmonary venous return and enlarged left-sided chambers. Hemodynamically significant ASD would result in left-to-right shunting with RA and RV dilation.

76. (A) Arterial switch operation for d-TGA has been the preferred surgical procedure since the early 1980s. The most common late postoperative complication after the arterial switch operation is supravalvar pulmonary stenosis. This may be amenable to stent implantation with care taken to avoid the pulmonary valve. Balloon valvuloplasty without stenting has a low success rate. Stenosis of the aorta is less common. Coronary ostial stenosis is a known complication but is not consistent with the physical examination. Atrial arrhythmias late after arterial switch operation are rare.

77. (C) The 2007 ACC/AHA guidelines continue to recommend prophylactic antibiotics prior to dental work for anyone with a prior history of bacterial endocarditis. For nonvalvular prosthetic patch material, antibiotic prophylaxis is recommended for only the first 6 months following surgery in the absence of a residual peripatch shunt. There is no indication for daily antibiotics. *S. viridans* remains a common pathogen for infective endocarditis.

78. (C) Antibiotic prophylaxis is not indicated for patients undergoing nondental interventions (colonoscopy or upper endoscopy) in the absence of active systemic infection. Comprehensive care of patients with congenital heart disease includes preventative screening procedures at recommended ages.

79. (C) While there is a clear association between Ebstein anomaly and atrioventricular reentrant accessory pathway tachycardia, patients with Ebstein anomaly are also at risk for life-threatening ventricular arrhythmias. This is particularly true for patients with deterioration in hemodynamic status. Atrioventricular reentrant accessory pathway tachycardia is less likely to cause a sudden loss of consciousness. The absence of prodromal symptoms also makes a ventricular tachycardia more likely. Myoclonus is common in any loss of consciousness. This patient requires additional arrhythmia monitoring and evaluation of hemodynamic status and cardiac function.

80. (B) The symptoms and physical examination findings are consistent with elevated IVC and central venous pressures in this Fontan circulation. While these symptoms could be consistent with obstruction in the Fontan connection, the ECG demonstrates junctional bradycardia. This is a common and often delayed finding in multiple forms of congenital heart disease after Mustard, Senning, and Fontan procedures. The onset of junctional rhythm may cause significant hemodynamic impact. This is a class I indication for atrial or dual chamber pacemaker placement.

81. (C) In congenitally corrected TGA, the conduction system is abnormal in location and structure, making it vulnerable to physical trauma during catheterization in addition to spontaneous heart block associated with increasing age. The diagnosis of this congenital cardiac abnormality may be delayed into adulthood in individuals with adequate systemic ventricular function and no obvious murmur from a VSD or pulmonary/subpulmonary stenosis.

82. (E) Routine phlebotomy for erythrocytosis in cyanotic patients is not recommended in the absence of symptoms and often leads to iron deficiency anemia with resulting microcytosis. Microcytosis independently increases viscosity, perpetuating a cycle of phlebotomy and worsening microcytosis leading to symptoms. For euvolemic patients with hemoglobin >20 g/dL and hematocrit >65% with symptoms of hyperviscosity, therapeutic phlebotomy with equal volume crystalloid replacement is indicated.

83. (C) The 2008 ACC/AHA valvular heart disease updated guidelines recommend cardiac catheterization with coronary angiography for "men aged 35 years or older, premenopausal women aged 35 years or older who have coronary risk factors, and postmenopausal women" (Class I, Level of evidence: C) Tobacco cessation 1 week prior to surgery may increase respiratory secretions in the perioperative period. There is no indication for statin therapy at this time.

84. (B) Both bicuspid aortic valve anatomy and isolated ascending aortic dilation have been identified in first-degree family members of patients with bicuspid aortic valve. The abnormalities resulting in bicuspid aortic valves have clear association with abnormal aortic dilation and are not a process isolated to the aortic valve alone. For patients with bicuspid aortic valve, all first-degree relatives should be screened with transthoracic echocardiograms. Cardiac MRI is not recommended as first-line screening. Screening is recommended regardless of physical examination findings

since ascending aortic dilation may be present in the setting of a normal physical examination.

85. (C) Patients with repaired coarctation of the aorta have associated risk for cerebral aneurysms and for pseudoaneurysm formation at the site of prior surgical repair. While there is no evidence of aortic recoarctation by physical examination or by echocardiographic evaluation of the aortic lumen and blood flow, this does not exclude pseudoaneurysm formation. CT or MRI imaging of the thoracic aorta should be performed. Cardiac catheterization is not required. Head MRI with MR angiography may be utilized for cerebral aneurysm screening. Neurocognitive testing may be appropriate for an individualized patient.

86. (E) Late postoperative complications following AVSD repair include LVOT obstruction, heart block, and left atrioventricular valve regurgitation. New onset of atrial arrhythmias should prompt a thorough anatomic and hemodynamic evaluation for postoperative complications resulting in atrial fibrillation. Treating the arrhythmia with medical therapy without additional evaluation is insufficient. Isolated LVOT obstruction with a mean gradient >50 mm Hg or a maximum instantaneous gradient >70 mm Hg is an indication for surgical intervention. Afterload reduction with ACE inhibition is relatively contraindicated in the presence of fixed LVOT obstruction and may result in hypotension and coronary hypoperfusion.

87. (B) Left ventricle to right atrial shunting in the setting of normal right-sided pressures results in a high-velocity left-to-right shunt. This Doppler signal may contaminate the tricuspid regurgitation signal. Initiation of pulmonary vasodilator therapy without additional investigation would be inappropriate. Patients with trisomy 21 are at increased risk of obstructive sleep apnea and pulmonary hypertension.

88. (A) Risk factors for sudden death after repair of tetralogy of Fallot are QRS duration >180 ms, poor right ventricular hemodynamics, older age at repair, and prolonged palliative shunts. Invasive electrophysiology study is appropriate to provide additional risk stratification, but some would argue for internal defibrillator placement regardless of the outcome. Atrial arrhythmia and atrioventricular node dysfunction are both known complications following surgical repair, but are not the primary indication for additional electrophysiology study at this time.

89. (B) Progressive systemic ventricular dysfunction may occur following initiation of ventricular pacing. The ventricular lead crosses the right-sided mitral valve (in L-TGA) and may cause mitral regurgitation. Following pacemaker placement, surveillance of the patient should be increased to detect these changes. Biventricular pacing may reverse these effects in some patients. Supraventricular tachycardia should be detected by pacemaker interrogation.

90. (A) Patients with Fontan palliation are at increased risk for systemic venous thromboembolic events. Pulmonary embolism may present with variable symptoms. This patient's presentation is consistent with a pulmonary embolism but is not specific for this diagnosis. Streaming of blood flow in the Fontan circulation may result in superior vena cava blood flowing preferentially to one lung with inferior vena cava flow to the other lung. Contrast or isotope may need to be injected into upper and lower extremities to accurately demonstrate bilateral pulmonary perfusion. Invasive pulmonary angiography remains the gold standard, but may not be required in this scenario.

91. (C) Anomalous coronary arteries are detected as incidental findings in the current era of advanced imaging. The intramural course of the anomalous artery in a long segment through the wall of the aorta is a risk factor for cardiac ischemia and death. The preferred intervention is an unroofing of this segment, opening the internal portion of the aortic wall to the aortic lumen. Bypass grafting a vessel that is not stenotic at baseline will typically result in a failed graft. Coronary button translocation is not required if unroofing is successful. Unroofing may be unsuccessful if the intramural course is very short.

92. (C) The anatomy demonstrated is d-TGA after a Mustard procedure. The wire and small balloon catheter can be traced retrograde from the aorta to the right-sided, morphologic right ventricle, tricuspid valve, and pulmonary venous baffle with a balloon inflated in the pulmonary venous baffle adjacent to the TEE probe tip. The wire extends beyond the heart border in a left-sided pulmonary vein. The larger catheter can be followed antegrade through the inferior vena cava, systemic venous baffle, mitral valve, morphologic left ventricle, and proximal pulmonary artery. The pulmonary artery runs parallel to the aorta.

93. (C) Laboratory evaluation reveals a hemoglobin A1c >6.5% which is consistent with diabetes, and she also has hyperlipidemia with LDL >130. In adults 40 to 75 years old with diabetes, especially those with risk factors for atherosclerosis (e.g., hyperlipidemia, prior smoking, positive family history, hypertension, coarctation) or >50 years old, it is reasonable to initiate high-intensity statin therapy. Shared decision making is appropriate, but the statin should not be low-intensity given her increased risk. In patients with diabetes, you do not need to calculate ASCVD risk score or perform CT coronary calcium scan. Cardiac CTA could be an appropriate screen for coronary artery disease if she had angina, which she does not.

94. (C) This is a classic chest radiograph (CXR) (**Figure 16.4**) of a patient with Scimitar syndrome. There is anomalous connection of right lower pulmonary vein to the IVC. This is evident on the CXR. Sometimes the right upper and middle pulmonary veins also connect to the IVC. In 25% of cases, there is associated intracardiac congenital heart disease (usually an ASD). But in the majority of cases, the atrial septum is intact. Scimitar patients also have right lower lobe hypoplasia, sequestration, and arterial supply from a vessel originating from the descending aorta. Due to right lung hypoplasia, the cardiac silhouette is shifted rightward.

95. (D) In an unoperated 40-year-old patient who has congenitally corrected TGA, complete heart block and need for pacemaker insertion are very common. Q waves in leads I and AVL are seen in anomalous left coronary artery from the pulmonary artery (ALCAPA). Northwest (superior) and left QRS axes are seen in AVSD. RBBB is associated with Ebstein anomaly and patients after surgery for VSD and ToF repair.

96. (A) The CT (**Figure 16.5**) demonstrates a patient with an LPA sling. There is origin of the LPA from the RPA, not at the level of the true PA bifurcation. The LPA crosses between the bronchus and the esophagus. On barium esophogram, an anterior indentation occurs.

97. (A) Congenital complete AV block occurs in 1 per 14,000 to 20,000 live births and is thought to be the result of transplacental passage of autoantibodies against Ro and La intracellular ribonuclear proteins from the mother who may have a clinical autoimmune disease such as systemic lupus erythematosus or Sjögren syndrome. These patients may be completely asymptomatic throughout childhood and adolescence and require no active cardiology intervention, but there are certain findings that require intervention regardless of symptoms. According to the ACC/AHA/HRS 2008 guidelines for device-based therapy of cardiac rhythm abnormalities, permanent pacemaker implantation is indicated for congenital third-degree AV block with a wide QRS escape rhythm, complex ventricular ectopy, ventricular dysfunction (Class I indication, Level of evidence: B). This is independent of the presence of symptoms as a wide complex escape rhythm may be unreliable and result in abrupt pauses that may result in cardiac arrest. Ventricular dysfunction is not common and when present is best treated with pacemaker implantation, although ACE inhibition may be used in combination with device therapy. There is no indication for an electrophysiologic study in patients with congenital complete AV block. There is no role for amiodarone, especially since it may slow the underlying junctional escape rhythm.

98. (B) An epicardial ICD system is the most appropriate step in this patient who is at risk for an arrhythmic sudden death. According to the ACC/AHA/HRS 2008 guidelines for device-based therapy of cardiac rhythm abnormalities, in patients with congenital heart disease, spontaneous sustained VT or unexplained syncope with inducible sustained hypotensive VT are considered Class I ICD indications when other remediable causes (hemodynamic or arrhythmic) have been excluded. The ACC/AHA 2008 guidelines for ACHD state that epicardial pacemaker and device lead placement should be performed in all cyanotic patients with intracardiac shunts who require devices (Class I indication). In a study by Khairy et al., transvenous leads incurred a >2-fold increased risk of systemic thromboemboli in patients with any intracardiac shunt independent of the administration of Coumadin or aspirin, so consideration for epicardial lead placement should be given to all patients with intracardiac shunts. An ICD is superior to amiodarone in the prevention of sudden cardiac death. As the patient has pulmonary hypertension, surgical repair would likely result in right ventricular failure and therefore would not be a viable option. Although bosentan is likely indicated with her pulmonary hypertension, she has a class I indication for an ICD. There is no reason to repeat her EP study

99. (B) This patient is having an atrial arrhythmia called incisional atrial flutter or intra-atrial reentrant tachycardia (IART). This arrhythmia is a unique type of atrial flutter seen in patients who have had previous cardiac surgeries on their atria or have extensive scarring of the atria for other reasons. It is present in about 7% of patients following the Fontan operation. IART tends to have slower rates than atrial flutter. The ECG is different in that there frequently is an isoelectric baseline in between two consecutive P waves, unlike atrial flutter where there is typically constant activity creating the "saw-tooth" pattern (see **Figure 16.12** with *arrows* pointing to the IART P waves). Patients who have baseline bradycardia and present with faster heart rates or have no variation in their heart rate should have an ECG to evaluate for IART. The T wave must be closely examined for the presence of P waves and a P wave will often be obscured by the QRS complexes. This arrhythmia typically requires cardioversion, although evaluation for the presence of a thrombus and/or anticoagulation therapy is indicated prior to cardioversion to help prevent embolization of a thrombus which may have formed due to stasis in the atria from the arrhythmia. As the function on echocardiogram was normal, dyssynchrony is an unlikely cause of the patient's symptoms and a biventricular pacemaker would not likely be beneficial. The ventricular rate in this ECG is too slow for ventricular tachycardia. Although the P wave axis is relatively normal (between 0 and 90 degrees), this patient is not in sinus rhythm. The patient may have underlying sinus dysfunction, but there is no evidence based on this ECG.

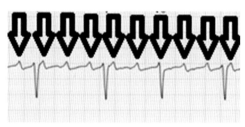

FIGURE 16.12

100. (C) The patient in the scenario most likely has an ASD. The most common presentation of a small to moderate defect is exercise intolerance typically in the second decade of life. The fixed split second heart sound and pulmonary flow murmur from left-to-right shunting at the atrial level are classic findings. The ECG will frequently show an incomplete right bundle branch block with an rSR' in lead V1 and may show right atrial enlargement. Imaging ASDs may be challenging in adults, particularly in obese individuals. An

agitated saline contrast echocardiogram (agitated saline is injected into a peripheral vein while imaging the right and left atrium) may show contrast in the left atrium, indicating a shunt at the atrial level. Alternatively, transesophageal imaging or cardiac magnetic resonance imaging may be performed to make the diagnosis. An exercise treadmill test is nonspecific and is unlikely to yield a diagnosis. Although she may have hypothyroidism, the murmur is not consistent with a thyroid problem and she is not bradycardic. She has no direct indication of pulmonary disease, so pulmonary function testing is unlikely to be helpful. Despite her obesity, coronary artery disease in an 18 year old would be very rare and does not explain the ECG or examination findings.

101. (B) Noninvasive testing for ischemia provocation is recommended every 3 to 5 years for patients after arterial switch procedures. Six-minute walk is not indicated for ischemia provocation. The patient has no pulmonary symptoms, so PFTs are not needed.

102. (E) The ECG tracing shows intra-atrial reentrant tachycardia (IART) with variable conduction. (See also **Figure 16.13**.)
    Clues to the IART are:

- Heart rate above normal in a patient with sinus node dysfunction
- Marked variability of ventricular rate or no heart rate variability (i.e., heart rate always 90 bpm)
- Abnormal P wave axis
- Prolongation of PR interval
- Variability of PR interval throughout the tracing

The ACCP evidence-based clinical practice guidelines recommend that antithrombotic therapy be initiated for both atrial fibrillation and atrial flutter. As he is clinically stable, there is no indication for cardioversion and as long as he does not have a rapid ventricular response to his arrhythmia, he should be anticoagulated for 3 weeks and then undergo a cardioversion. Both warfarin and rivaroxaban are reasonable medications for anticoagulation. Rivaroxaban is a novel anticoagulation agent that has a similar efficacy and safety profile to warfarin, but has the advantage of not needing to check INR to adjust the dosage. Although digoxin and beta blockers may slow conduction in the AV node preventing rapid conduction of an atrial arrhythmia, there is no evidence of rapid conduction of the arrhythmia in this patient. Although it would be reasonable to start digoxin or beta blockers, anticoagulation is more important. ACE inhibition may be beneficial in patients with a systemic right ventricle, but would not have any effect on this acute arrhythmia. There is no indication to start amiodarone immediately. Amiodarone may have significant side effects, it is typically not the first choice for long-term therapy in young, otherwise healthy patients.

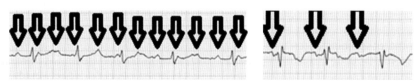

FIGURE 16.13 IART with arrows showing P waves marching with variable PR intervals intervals.

103. (D) The tracing shows an irregularly irregular rhythm characteristic of atrial fibrillation. There is chaotic atrial activity with no definitive P waves. The ventricular response is relatively fast with an average rate of 136 bpm, but a stretch in the middle of the tracing with a heart rate over 150 bpm. The episode of syncope that she had is likely due to a rapid ventricular response caused by a catecholamine surge when running for the bus. Her decreased function is also likely due to the arrhythmia. Although it would be ideal to anticoagulate for 3 weeks and then cardiovert, the acute nature of her syncope and depressed function as well as symptoms necessitate cardioversion. Although the ventricular response is relatively rapid, her vital signs are stable and there is no indication for emergent cardioversion. Performing a transesophageal echocardiogram to rule out a large thrombus that might be dislodged by the cardioversion is indicated in this situation. If a large thrombus is present, it is reasonable to anticoagulate for a period of time prior to performing the cardioversion. If there is no thrombus, a cardioversion can be performed immediately, although there is some risk of a small thrombus that cannot be seen on echocardiogram dislodging and causing a stroke. DC cardioversion is likely to be more effective and quicker than IV amiodarone at converting the atrial fibrillation. There is no indication for urgent device closure of the residual ASD and this will not acutely correct the current problem of atrial fibrillation.

104. (B) ACC guidelines suggest that patients with prior Fontan procedure, severe pulmonary arterial hypertension, cyanotic CHD, complex CHD, or patients with malignant arrhythmia be referred to regional ACHD centers for noncardiac surgery. (A) is not correct as the patient does not have complex CHD without evidence of heart failure; the patient described in (C) does not have pulmonary artery hypertension, but right ventricular hypertension; and the patient in (D) has no evidence of significant VSD.

105. (A) The 2018 AHA/ACC ACHD guidelines give a class I recommendation for surgical intervention in patients with subaortic stenosis with maximum instantaneous gradient (MIG) > 50 mm Hg or symptoms attributable to the subaortic stenosis, heart failure, ischemic symptoms, or systolic dysfunction. This is in contrast to the 2008 guidelines which gave a class I recommendation for surgical intervention if MIG >50 mm Hg or mean >30 mm Hg regardless of symptoms or for those with moderate subaortic stenosis (MIG <50 mm Hg or mean <30 mm Hg) who have LV systolic dysfunction or progressive aortic regurgitation and LV dilation. It is important to also consider the examination as this supports severe obstruction and also to consider the dynamic nature of subaortic obstruction. This patient also had an exercise echocardiogram during which MIG was 92 mm Hg and mean gradient was 59 mm Hg. Thus surgical intervention is warranted now. The guidelines do not comment on the use of cardiac MRI for subaortic stenosis.

106. (A) Class I indications for surgical intervention of supravalvar AS include a mean gradient of 50 mm Hg or greater in asymptomatic patients. Patients with lesser degrees of obstruction should be considered for surgical intervention if they are symptomatic, have LVH, or are planning a pregnancy.

107. (D) Asymptomatic patients with maximum instantaneous pulmonary valve gradient >30 mm Hg should have follow-up echocardiograms every 2 to 5 years. There is no indication for cardiac catheterization or intervention in this patient.

SUGGESTED READINGS

AASLD/IDSA HCV Guidance Panel. Hepatitis C guidance: AASLD-IDSA recommendations for testing, managing, and treating adults infected with hepatitis C virus. *Hepatology*. 2015;62(3):932–954.

ACC/AHA/HRS 2008 guidelines for device-based therapy of cardiac rhythm abnormalities: Executive summary. *Circulation*. 2008;117:2820–2840.

AHA Scientific Statement. Diagnostic criteria for infective endocarditis. *Circulation*. 2005;111:e394–e434.

Ammash N, Warnes CA. Cerebrovascular events in adult patients with cyanotic congenital heart disease. *J Am Coll Cardiol*. 1996;28(3):768–772.

Bonow RO, Carabello BA, Chatterjee K, et al. 2008 focused update incorporated into the ACC/AHA 2006 guidelines for the management of patients with valvular heart disease: A report of the American College of Cardiology/American Heart Association Task Force on Practice Guidelines. *Circulation*. 2008;118(15):e523–e661.

Connolly SJ, Gent M, Roberts RS, et al. Canadian implantable defibrillator study (CIDS): A randomized trial of the implantable cardioverter defibrillator against amiodarone. *Circulation*. 2000;101:1297–302.

Epstein AE, Dimarco JP, Ellenbogen KA, et al. ACC/AHA/HRS 2008 guidelines for device-based therapy of cardiac rhythm abnormalities: Executive summary. *Circulation*. 2008;117:2820–2840.

Haberer K, Silversides CK, Siu SC. Pregnancy in young women with congenital heart disease. In: Shaddy RE, Penny DJ, Feltes TF, Cetta F, Mital S, eds. *Moss and Adams' Heart Disease in Infants, Children and Adolescents*. 10th ed. Wolters Kluwer; 2022:1582–1595.

Hiratzka LF, Bakris GL, Beckman JA, et al. 2010 ACCF/AHA/AATS/ACR/ASA/SCA/SCAI /SIR/STS/SVM guidelines for the diagnosis and management of patients with thoracic aortic disease. *Circulation*. 2010;121:e266–e369.

John AS, Gurley F, Schaff HV, et al. Cardiopulmonary bypass during pregnancy. *Ann Thorac Surg*. 2011;91(4):1191–1196.

Khairy P, Harris L, Landzberg MJ, et al. Implantable cardioverter-defibrillators in tetralogy of Fallot. *Circulation*. 2008;117(3):363–370.

Khairy P, Landzberg MJ, Gatzoulis MA, et al. Transvenous pacing leads and systemic thromboemboli in patients with intracardiac shunts: A multicenter study. *Circulation*. 2006;113(20):2391–2397.

Khairy P, Ouyang D, Fernandes SM, et al. Pregnancy outcomes in women with congenital heart disease. *Circulation.* 2006; 113(4):517–524.

Konstantinides S, Geibel A, Olschewski M, et al. A comparison of surgical and medical therapy for atrial septal defect in adults. *N Engl J Med.* 1995;333(8):469–473.

MacCarrick G, Black JH, Bowdin S, et al. Loeys-Dietz syndrome: A primer for diagnosis and management. *Genet Med.* 2014; 16:576–587.

Michaelsson M, Jonzon A, Riesenfeld T. Isolated congenital complete atrioventricular block in adult life. A prospective study. *Circulation.* 1995;92:442–449.

Nishimura RA, Otto CM, Bonow RO, et al. 2017 AHA/ACC guideline for the management of patients with valvular heart disease. *J Am Coll Cardiol.* 2017;70:252–289.

Nishimura RA, Warnes CA. Anticoagulation during pregnancy in women with prosthetic valves; evidence, guidelines and unanswered questions. *Heart.* 2015;101:430–435.

Phillips SD, O'Leary PW. Echocardiographic evaluation of the functionally univentricular heart after Fontan operation. In: Eidem BW, Johnson J, Lopez L, Cetta F, eds. *Echocardiography in Pediatric and Adult Congenital Heart Disease.* 3rd ed. Wolters Kluwer; 2021:756–776.

Rigatelli G, Cardaioli P, Hijazi ZM. Contemporary clinical management of atrial septal defects in the adult. *Expert Rev Cardiovasc Ther.* 2007;5(6):1135–1146.

Sanikommu V, Lasorda D, Poornima I. Anatomical factors triggering platypnea-orthodeoxia in adults. *Clin Cardiol.* 2009;32(11):e55–e57.

Singer DE, Albers GW, Dalen JE, et al. Antithrombotic therapy in atrial fibrillation: American College of Chest Physicians Evidence-Based Clinical Practice Guidelines (8th Edition). *Chest.* 2008;133(6 Suppl):546S–592S.

Siu SC, Sermer M, Colman JM, et al. Prospective multicenter study of pregnancy outcomes in women with heart disease. *Circulation.* 2001;104(5):515–521.

Soliman OI, Geleijnse ML, Meijboom FJ, et al. The use of contrast echocardiography for the detection of cardiac shunts. *Eur J Echocardiogr.* 2007;8(3):S2–S12.

Stephenson EA, Lu M, Berul CI, et al. Arrhythmias in a contemporary Fontan cohort: Prevalence and clinical associations in a multicenter cross-sectional study. *J Am Coll Cardiol.* 2010;56(11):890–896.

Stout KK, Daniels CJ, Aboulhosn JA, et al. 2018 AHA/ACC guideline for the management of adults with congenital heart disease. A report of the American College of Cardiology/American Heart Association Task Force on Clinical Practice Guidelines. *J Am Coll Cardiol.* 2019;73(12):e81–e192.

Walsh EP. Arrhythmias in patients with congenital heart disease. *Card Electrophysiol Rev.* 2002;6(4):422–430.

Yap SC, Roos-Hesselink JW, Hoendermis ES, et al. Outcome of implantable cardioverter defibrillators in adults with congenital heart disease: A multi-centre study. *Eur Heart J.* 2007;28(15): 1854–1861.

Statistics and Research Design

John Detterich and Justin M. Horner

Questions

1. Of the following types of data-descriptive term pairs, which is the pair that incorrectly matches the data with the type of data?

   A. Blood groups—nominal data
   B. American Heart Association (AHA) class—ordinal data
   C. Number of surgical procedures—discrete data
   D. Pulmonary vascular resistance—categorical data
   E. Index—continuous data

2. A pediatric cardiology fellow is interested in studying the potential relationship between exposure to lithium and Ebstein anomaly with an observational study. He decided to use a case-control methodology for his study. Of the following observations of studies, which is a disadvantage for this case-control study?

   A. Information on exposure and past history is primarily based on interview and may be subject to recall bias
   B. Exposure patterns, for example, the composition of oral contraceptives, may change during the course of the study and make the results irrelevant
   C. Not suited for the study of rare diseases because a large number of subjects are required
   D. Expensive to carry out because a large number of subjects are usually required
   E. Baseline data may be sparse because the large number of subjects do not allow for long interviews

3. A new drug is available for the treatment of heart failure and is undergoing phase III trials in adults with heart failure. Of the following statements, which most closely describes a phase III trial for a medication?

   A. A small group (20 to 80 subjects) of volunteers to assess the safety and pharmacokinetic profile of the medication
   B. Randomized controlled, multicenter trial on a relatively large group (300 to 3,000 or more subjects) depending on the medical condition in order to assess the drug's effectiveness and to compare it with an accepted therapy
   C. A large group (20 to 300 subjects) to assess safety in a larger group of patients as well as effectiveness of the drug
   D. Administration of a single subtherapeutic dose of the drug to a small group (10 to 15 subjects) to gather preliminary data on pharmacokinetics and pharmacodynamics
   E. Involves safety surveillance and ongoing technical support of a drug after permission for it to be distributed

4. A pediatric cardiologist would like to compare atrioventricular (AV) valve regurgitation severity data from two unpaired groups of children that are relatively small in number (<5). Of the following statistical methods, which should he select?

   A. Chi-squared (χ^2) test
   B. Fisher exact test
   C. McNemar test
   D. Mantel–Haenszel test
   E. Student's t-test

5. An investigator in pediatric cardiology would like to use a statistical method to compare groups that have clinical data with normal distributions. Of the following, which statistical test should be used to analyze such parametric data?

   A. Wilcoxon signed-rank test
   B. Mann–Whitney *U*-test
   C. Wilcoxon rank sum test
   D. Kruskal–Wallis test
   E. Analysis of variance (ANOVA) test

6. A pediatric cardiologist wishes to understand the relationship between prevalence of congenital heart disease in his home city and the positive predictive value (PPV) and negative predictive value (NPV) of newborn pulse oximetry congenital heart disease screening. Which of the following is the relationship between these parameters?

   A. As prevalence increases, both PPV and NPV increase as well
   B. As prevalence increases, no change occurs in PPV and NPV
   C. As prevalence increases, PPV increases and NPV decreases
   D. As prevalence decreases, PPV increases and NPV decreases
   E. Prevalence changes do not affect PPV and NPV of a test

7. The graph in **Figure 17.1** depicts which of the following?

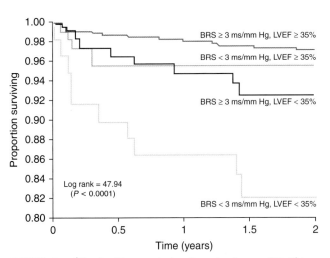

FIGURE 17.1 (Used with permission from La Rovere MT, Bigger Jr JT, Marcus FI, et al., Baroreflex sensitivity and heart-rate variability in prediction of total cardiac mortality after myocardial infarction. ATRAMI Investigators. *Lancet.* 1998;351:478–484.)

   A. Kaplan–Meier survival curve
   B. Linear regression curve
   C. Logistic regression curve
   D. Poisson regression curve
   E. Correlation curve with Spearman coefficient

8. **Figure 17.2** depicts normal and disease populations with frequency on the *y*-axis and the diagnostic test value on the *x*-axis. The cut point is indicated by the vertical black line, above which we consider the test to be abnormal and below which we consider the test to be normal. TN is true negatives and TP is true positives. The area at which the arrow is pointing represents which of the following?

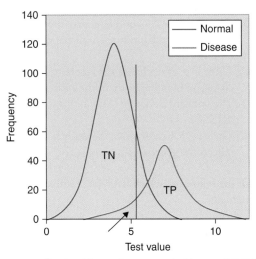

FIGURE 17.2 (Derived from gim.unmc.edu/dxtests/ROC1.htm)

   A. False negatives
   B. False positives
   C. Positive predictive value (PPV)
   D. Negative predictive value (NPV)
   E. Sensitivity/specificity

9. A normal or Gaussian distribution is a well-recognized curve that reflects a continuous probability distribution that is bell shaped (unimodal) and symmetrical about the mean with two parameters, the mean (μ) and the variance (σ^2). Which of the following continuous probability distributions most closely resembles the normal or Gaussian distribution?

   A. *t*-distribution
   B. χ^2 distribution
   C. *F*-distribution
   D. Binomial distribution
   E. Poisson distribution

10. The mean systolic blood pressure before an antihypertensive medication was given for a group of 50 patients was 165 mm Hg. The mean decrease in blood pressure after the medication was administered was 20 mm Hg. The 95% confidence interval (CI) was −5 to 45 mm Hg. Which of the following statements is ***correct***?

   A. The CI can be decreased with a smaller sample of patients

   B. One can be 95% confident that the treatment can lower the blood pressure in all patients by at least 20 mm Hg

   C. There is a >5% chance that there would be no true change in blood pressure in the entire population

   D. The standard deviation (SD) in this study is the same as the CI

   E. There is 95% chance that the study sample accurately reflects the general population

11. Of the following, which is a type of inferential statistical method?

   A. Arithmetic mean
   B. Mode
   C. Student's *t*-test
   D. Median
   E. Histogram

12. Which of the following statements regarding hypothesis testing is ***true***?

   A. A type I error (α error) occurs when a null hypothesis that is correct is accepted

   B. A type II error (β error) occurs when a hypothesis that is incorrect is rejected

   C. A type III error is a study design that produces the wrong answer to the right question

   D. The *P* (probability) value is the probability that defines how likely it is that the null hypothesis is false

   E. The *P*-value is the probability of an observed difference occurring solely by chance

13. Which of the following would ***increase*** the power of a study?

   A. Smaller significance level
   B. Larger effects
   C. Increased variability of the observations
   D. Smaller sample size
   E. Increased variance

14. An economic assessment method is utilized in which the costs and consequences of alternative cardiac interventions are expressed in costs per unit of health outcome. This commonly used methodology is applicable to health programs as well as health services to help determine the preferred action that requires the least cost to produce a given level of effectiveness. Which of the following is this assessment tool?

   A. Cost-effectiveness analysis (CEA)
   B. Cost-utility analysis (CUA)
   C. Cost-benefit analysis (CBA)
   D. Cost-minimization analysis (CMA)
   E. Cost-value analysis (CVA)

15. A meta-analysis is a technique where results from a number of studies that are similar in nature are gathered to give one overall estimate of the effect. Which of the following is a disadvantage of this technique?

   A. Refinement and reduction of large amount of information

   B. Efficiency relative to a new study
   C. Publication bias for statistically significant studies
   D. Power to detect effects of interest
   E. Precision greater than a single study

For Questions 16 to 19, use the following scenario: In a prospective cohort study for a new antiarrhythmic agent in a total of 930 participants, the investigators found that 16 of 465 children (3.4%) in the treatment group had arrhythmias; while in the placebo group, 23 of 465 children (4.9%) had arrhythmias.

16. What is the ***relative risk*** in this study?
   A. 1.44
   B. 0.44
   C. 0.69
   D. 0.31
   E. 1.50

17. What is the ***relative risk reduction (RRR)*** in this study?
   A. 44%
   B. 31%
   C. 69%
   D. 144%
   E. 1.5%

18. What is the ***absolute risk reduction (ARR)*** in this study?
   A. 44%
   B. 31%
   C. 69%
   D. 144%
   E. 1.5%

19. What is the *number of patients need to be treated (NNT)* for one to get benefit of this drug?

    A. 67
    B. 15
    C. 20
    D. 29
    E. 144

20. In a typical receiver operating characteristic (ROC) curve, what is the significance of the upper left corner or coordinate (0,1)?

    A. 100% sensitivity and specificity
    B. 0% sensitivity and 100% specificity
    C. 100% sensitivity or 0% specificity
    D. 0% sensitivity and specificity
    E. 50% sensitivity and 50% specificity

21. The measure of precision of the sample mean or how close the sample mean is likely to be to the population mean is termed as which of the following?

    A. Variance
    B. Coefficient of variation
    C. Standard deviation to the mean
    D. Standard deviation (SD)
    E. Standard error of the mean (SEM)

22. **Figure 17.3** shows the relationship between accuracy and precision to be which of the following?

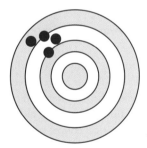

FIGURE 17.3

    A. Accurate and precise
    B. Not accurate but precise
    C. Accurate but not precise
    D. Neither accurate nor precise
    E. Figure does not display this relationship

23. Some children with supraventricular tachycardia were treated with digoxin while others were treated with propranolol. The results in a contingency table are shown in **Table 17.1**.

TABLE 17.1 Digoxin versus Propranolol for SVT

	Digoxin	Propranolol	Total
No SVT	30 (60%)	34 (67%)	64 (64%)
Some SVT	20 (40%)	16 (33%)	36 (36%)
Total	50 (100%)	50 (100%)	100 (100%)

$$\chi^2 = 2.3$$

What additional information is necessary for the calculation of *P*-value?

    A. Degrees of freedom (df)
    B. SEM
    C. Variance
    D. Power
    E. Covariance

24. Which of the following statements regarding the correlation coefficient *r* is *true*?

    A. It is dimensionless
    B. When $r = 0$, there is perfect correlation
    C. A correlation between x and y implies that there is a cause-and-effect relationship
    D. The correlation coefficient *r* can be calculated when there are several outliers
    E. A nonlinear relationship does not imply that a correlation coefficient cannot be calculated

For Questions 25 to 28, use the following scenario: *A cardiologist reviews the database for elevated (>100 pg/mL) serum BNP in his cardiac patients and tabulated the data in* **Table 17.2**. *Of note, complete questions 25 to 28 prior to reviewing answers.*

TABLE 17.2 Cardiac Disease and BNP

	Cardiac Disease		
BNP >100 pg/mL	+	−	Total
+	50	5	55
−	25	100	125
Total	75	105	180

25. What is the *positive predictive value (PPV)* for BNP >100 pg/mL for cardiac disease in this patient population?

    A. 50/55
    B. 50/75
    C. 5/105
    D. 100/125
    E. 100/105

26. What is the *negative predictive value (NPV)* for BNP >100 pg/mL for cardiac disease in this patient population?

    A. 50/55
    B. 50/75
    C. 5/105
    D. 100/125
    E. 100/105

27. What is the *sensitivity* for BNP >100 pg/mL for cardiac disease in this patient population?

    A. 50/55
    B. 50/75
    C. 5/105
    D. 100/125
    E. 100/105

28. What is the *specificity* for BNP >100 pg/mL for cardiac disease in this patient population?

    A. 50/55
    B. 50/75
    C. 5/105
    D. 100/125
    E. 100/105

29. What type of bias occurs when a spurious association is noted due to a failure to adjust fully for factors leading to an erroneous conclusion?

    A. Observer bias
    B. Confounding bias
    C. Selection bias
    D. Information bias
    E. Allocation bias

30. In an observation study, which of the following is *not* a criterion for concluding causation in addition to an association?

    A. Temporality
    B. Dose–response
    C. Repetition in a different population
    D. Consistency with other studies
    E. Expert consensus

31. A pediatric cardiologist is conducting a research project on the use of a new drug for heart failure in children. He is being very truthful to the parent regarding the possible side effect of hypotension with the use of this new drug. He is abiding by which principle of the Belmont report?

    A. Respect for persons
    B. Beneficence
    C. Justice
    D. Lack of conflict of interest
    E. Scientific reasoning

32. An independent group of experts that continuously monitors data from various aspects of a clinical trial to ensure patient safety as well as validity and scientific merit is which of the following?

    A. Institutional Review Board (IRB)
    B. Ethics Committee
    C. Data Safety Monitoring Board (DSMB)
    D. Independent Ethics Board
    E. Clinical Trials Safety Committee

33. Which of the following is a statistical term to describe the consistency of a set of measurements/measurement tool or its repeatability/reproducibility?

    A. Precision
    B. Accuracy
    C. Reliability
    D. Validity
    E. Power

34. A pediatric cardiologist is studying the efficacy of a new antiarrhythmic agent in the treatment of junctional ectopic tachycardia. He is interested in a randomized, double-blind placebo-controlled trial. To calculate the number of patients needed for the study with a power of 0.80 and a statistical significance of 0.05, he needs which additional information?

    A. Standardized difference
    B. Standard error of the mean
    C. Confidence Interval
    D. Bias
    E. Expected mean

35. Which of the following statements is an advantage of a cohort study?

    A. Not suited for the study of rare diseases because a large number of subjects are required
    B. Not suited when the time between exposure and disease manifestation is very long, although this can be overcome in historical cohort studies
    C. Exposure patterns, for example, the composition of oral contraceptives, may change during the course of the study and make the results irrelevant
    D. Maintaining high rates of follow-up can be difficult
    E. Permits calculation of incidence rates (absolute risk) as well as relative risk

36. A cardiology researcher has a research project and needs to find a statistical method that allows paired comparisons of two nonnormally distributed patient populations. Which of the following would be the *correct* choice?

    A. Wilcoxon signed-rank test
    B. Mann–Whitney *U*-test
    C. Wilcoxon rank sum test
    D. Kruskal–Wallis test
    E. ANOVA

37. Which of the following is a statistical test used for two large (>5) groups of unpaired categorical data?

    A. One-way ANOVA
    B. χ^2 test
    C. McNemar test
    D. Fisher exact test
    E. Wilcoxon rank sum test

38. Data can be categorized into categorical or numerical data. Which of the following data is an example of a categorical type of data called ordinal data?

    A. Severity of AV valve regurgitation
    B. Single ventricle and biventricular surgical strategies
    C. Blood pressure measurements before and after angiotensin-converting enzyme (ACE) inhibitors
    D. Number of reinterventions after Norwood procedure
    E. Antiarrhythmic agent for supraventricular tachycardia

39. A pediatric cardiologist is interested in prospectively studying the relationship between neonatal surgical cardiopulmonary bypass time and fine motor development at ages 5 and 10. He will be enrolling neonates in this study. This type of study is which of the following?

    A. Case-control study
    B. Cohort study
    C. Case series
    D. Retrospective study
    E. Historical cohort study

40. A pediatric cardiologist is interested in studying intravenous milrinone in pediatric septic shock and is organizing a randomized controlled multicenter trial involving over 300 children with septic shock. He is primarily interested in assessing the benefit of milrinone compared to traditional inotropic agents. This phase of the clinical trial would be considered as which of the following?

    A. Phase 0
    B. Phase I
    C. Phase II
    D. Phase III
    E. Phase IV

41. A chi-squared (χ^2) test is most closely related to which of the following statistical tests?

    A. ANOVA
    B. Student's t-test
    C. Kolmogorov–Smirnov test
    D. Wilcoxon signed-rank test
    E. Fisher exact test

42. The department of public health is interested in knowing the prevalence of congenital heart disease in the city. Which of the following is the correct definition for **prevalence** of congenital heart disease?

    A. Number of new cases of the disease that occur in a population during a period of time/sum for each individual in the population of the length of time at risk of getting the disease
    B. Number of individuals who get the disease during a certain period/number of individuals in the population at the beginning of the period X
    C. Existing number of individuals having the disease at a specific time/number of individuals in the population at that point in time
    D. Number of new cases of the disease that occur in a population during a period of time/number of individuals in the population at the beginning of the period X
    E. Number of individuals who get the disease during a certain period/sum for each individual in the population of the length of time at risk of getting the disease

43. A review article on the most current heart failure management discussed a myriad of medical therapies. The use of a particular beta blocker is discussed and "**Level C**" is included at the end of the discussion. This designation is interpreted as which of the following?

    A. Fair scientific evidence that risks outweigh the benefit
    B. Scientific evidence is lacking, or of poor quality, or conflicting
    C. Fair scientific evidence (benefit and risk too close)
    D. Good scientific evidence (benefits substantially outweigh risk)
    E. Fair scientific evidence (benefits outweigh the risk)

For Questions 44 to 47, use the following scenario: An athlete in a high-school football game recently collapsed and died from hypertrophic cardiomyopathy. An electrocardiogram (ECG) screening program to identify hypertrophic cardiomyopathy in a local high school for all student athletes yielded: 21 positive ECGs for hypertrophic cardiomyopathy with only one of those 21 truly being positive by echocardiogram and 786 negative ECGs for hypertrophic cardiomyopathy and only one of those 786 truly being positive by echocardiogram.

44. What is the screening ECG **sensitivity** for hypertrophic cardiomyopathy in this study?

    A. 1/805
    B. 1/21
    C. 1/2
    D. 1/786
    E. 1/807

45. What is the screening ECG *specificity* for hypertrophic cardiomyopathy in this study?

    A. 20/805
    B. 785/805
    C. 785/786
    D. 20/807
    E. 785/807

46. What is the screening ECG *positive predictive value (PPV)* for hypertrophic cardiomyopathy in this study?

    A. 1/21
    B. 1/805
    C. 1/2
    D. 20/805
    E. 21/807

47. What is the screening ECG *negative predictive value (NPV)* for hypertrophic cardiomyopathy in this study?

    A. 785/786
    B. 1/786
    C. 785/805
    D. 1/805
    E. 1/2

For Questions 48 to 51, use the following scenario:
The efficacy and safety of an angiotensin receptor blocker in Duchenne muscular dystrophy patients with severe heart failure is being studied in a multi-institutional study. In the treated group, 5 of 200 patients had hospital admission for exacerbations of heart failure while 25 of the 250 in the untreated group were hospitalized.

48. What is the relative risk (risk ratio)?

    A. 2.5/10
    B. 5/200
    C. 5/250
    D. 25/250
    E. 25/450

49. What is the *relative risk reduction (RRR)* for the treated group?

    A. 25%
    B. 75%
    C. 50%
    D. 7.5%
    E. 2.5%

50. What is the *absolute risk reduction (ARR)* in this study?

    A. 25%
    B. 75%
    C. 50%
    D. 7.5%
    E. 2.5%

51. What is the *number needed to treat (NNT)* in this study?

    A. 13.3
    B. 7.5
    C. 4
    D. 2
    E. 25

52. You are investigating whether the use of thiazide diuretics plus angiotensin converting enzyme inhibitors in the treatment of children with hypertension results in higher rates of long-term blood pressure control compared to thiazide diuretics alone. Which study would yield the *most* reliable results?

    A. Interrupted time series study
    B. Double-blind, placebo-controlled trial
    C. Retrospective case-control study
    D. Observational prospective study
    E. Cross-sectional studies

53. You received a grant for research and wish to conduct a study to investigate the role of maternal diabetes as a risk factor for congenital heart disease. You must decide whether to do a case-control or a cohort study. After comparing the advantages of each type of study, you determine that a case-control study would be the better option. Which *best* describes a case-control study?

    A. Allows for the study of one potential risk factor at a time
    B. Allows for calculation of rates of disease in exposed and unexposed
    C. Well suited for conditions with a short latency
    D. Relies on recall or records of past events
    E. Well suited for rare conditions

54. You have a patient who presents to clinic with the chief complaint of chest pain. You review the current literature and find an article about the prevalence of chest pain in children and adolescents in your area. In this study, an anonymous survey was sent out to families with children 5 to 18 years of age registered within the local school district. This survey included various demographic and clinical questions, one of which asked about the presence of chest pain within the last 6 months. Which of the following *best* describes the study design used above?

A. Prospective cohort study
B. Census
C. Retrospective cohort study
D. Cross-sectional study
E. Observational prospective study

55. A child is referred to your practice for the diagnosis of aortic coarctation with a peak instantaneous pressure gradient of 30 mm Hg. The family has consented to participate in a multi-institutional study looking at the efficacy of surgical repair versus balloon angioplasty. The medical student working with you asks why it is important to accrue a large number of participants. The correct response to this medical student's question would be:

A. Increasing the sample size improves the ability to detect adverse events
B. The likelihood of a type II error increases with increased sample size
C. The larger the sample size, the less likely a type I error is made
D. A larger sample size decreases the power of a study
E. The larger the detectable difference in effect, the larger the sample size required

56. The parents of a patient ask if treatment with an angiotensin II receptor blocker in addition to a beta blocker improves protection against progressive aortic root dilation in children with Marfan syndrome. You find a study where researchers investigated whether angiotensin II receptor blockers were a protective factor against progressive aortic root dilation 10 years after diagnosis in patients concurrently on beta blockers. Participants were identified as to whether they were on an angiotensin II receptor blocker plus beta blocker or beta-blocker monotherapy and then followed at 1-year intervals for a total of 10 years. Which of the following statements is *true* regarding this study?

A. The patients were studied retrospectively
B. The cohort was biased by the healthy entrant effect
C. This represents a type of prospective cohort study
D. The natural epidemiology of aortic root dilation in patients with Marfan syndrome could be studied in this cohort
E. This represents a case-control study

57. A 16-year-old female presented to the emergency department (ED) 2 days ago with syncope. Her description of the syncopal episode was consistent with vasovagal syncope. An ECG obtained in the ED showed prolongation of the QTc interval to 460 ms. She was diagnosed with long QT syndrome and the ED provider recommended initiation of beta-blocker therapy. Her mother requested an evaluation by pediatric cardiology prior to starting this treatment. In your office, the patient is appropriate with normal vital signs. Her repeat ECG is normal with QTc of 400 ms. You recommend no treatment for QT prolongation. Of the following, which limitation of the testing performed in the ED *best* supports your action?

A. Generalizability
B. Negative predictive value
C. Sensitivity
D. Specificity
E. Validity

58. In your effort to help older adolescents with hyperlipidemia, you seek studies of effective nutrition strategies in college-age students. You find one where 336 subjects were studied. In this study, 154 were allocated to food intake recording, weekly weigh-ins, and weekly group education; while the remaining 182 were allocated to a wait-list control arm. At 4 months, the intervention group showed improved cholesterol management than the wait-listed group (mean 162 [95% CI 149 to 173] vs. 189 [95% CI 179 to 197]); $P = 0.007$. The authors concluded that, at least compared to the wait-list, a structured consultation program resulted in significantly improved short-term cholesterol management. Which of the following statements *best* describes the 95% CI for cholesterol levels in the intervention group?

A. 95% of sample participants in the intervention group achieved a cholesterol level 149 to 173
B. If this study was repeated, there is a probability of 0.95 that the sample mean cholesterol level for the intervention group was between 149 and 173
C. 95% of the population would achieve a cholesterol level between 149 and 173 if they received the intervention
D. There is a probability of 0.95 that the population mean cholesterol level at 4 months with the intervention would be between 149 and 173
E. There is a 95% chance that the results of the study are accurate

59. You propose to your colleagues a study regarding risk factors for sudden death in patients with hypertrophic cardiomyopathy. Your plans include data collection with a survey of parents regarding the presence of chest pain in their child prior to their sudden death event. This type of data collection is *most* vulnerable to:

    A. Lead-time bias
    B. Selection bias
    C. Recall bias
    D. Length bias
    E. Referral bias

60. You are doing a preoperative evaluation of a patient with atrioventricular septal defect and note that the patient is anemic with a hemoglobin level of 9.7 g/dL. You do a literature search to find the prevalence of anemia in children with AV canal defects and find a study looking at children with either a ventricular septal defect (VSD) or AV canal defect and their rates of anemia. In this study, they found an odds ratio of 0.21 (95% CI 0.07 to 0.68) for the risk of anemia in patients with AV canal defects. Based on this information, which statement is *true*?

    A. The *P*-value is likely to be >0.05
    B. The risk of anemia is lower in children with AV canal defect
    C. Children with anemia are more likely to have an AV canal defect than a VSD
    D. The odds of having anemia are lower in a child with a VSD
    E. 21% of patients in the study have an AV canal defect

61. A medical student rounding with the cardiology team asks about the use of sirolimus for immunosuppression in children after undergoing heart transplant. You present the student with a study showing the incidence of rejection in children both prior to and following sirolimus initiation. Sixty children were included in this study and all were 2 years status post initial heart transplant. The average number of rejection episodes was found to be 3.2 +/− 0.7 prior to initiation of sirolimus. After initiation of sirolimus, the children were followed for another 2 years and the average number of rejections episodes was 2.7 +/− 0.4. Which type of statistical analysis would be *most* appropriate in this study?

    A. Paired Student's *t*-test
    B. Wilcoxon signed-rank test
    C. Chi-squared
    D. Odds ratio
    E. Kaplan–Meier curve

62. A pediatric cardiology fellow performs a case-control study to evaluate the association between children with a history of prosthetic valve replacement surgery and subsequent endocarditis. They obtain the results presented in **Table 17.3**.

TABLE 17.3 A Case-Control Study in Cardiology: Results

	Endocarditis Present	No Endocarditis Present
Prosthetic valve replacement	10	40
No prosthetic valve replacement	2	48

What is the **odds ratio** for the development of endocarditis in patients with a previous valve replacement compared to those without history of valve replacement?

A. $(10 \times 48)/(40 \times 2)$
B. $(40 \times 2)/(10 \times 48)$
C. $(2 \times 48)/(40 \times 10)$
D. $(2 \times 10)/(40 \times 48)$
E. $(10 \times 40)/(2 \times 48)$

63. A new antiarrhythmic medication has been developed and it is going to be compared to standard treatment for neonatal supraventricular tachycardia. The research team anticipates using a χ^2 analysis to evaluate their findings. Based on this information, which statement is *false*?

    A. This study involves the collection of continuous data
    B. Each group must be completely independent of the others for the intervention of interest
    C. Expected values in each cell of a 2 × 2 table must be at least 5
    D. The *P*-value calculated from the χ^2 analysis tells you how likely it is that the outcomes observed could have been found by chance
    E. χ^2 analysis is used to evaluate nominal data

64. When creating a Kaplan–Meier survival curve for patients with Down syndrome who died from a cardiovascular cause after AV canal repair, it is important to remember that noncensored patients will include:

    A. Patients who died from a cardiovascular cause
    B. Patients who withdrew from the study
    C. Patients lost to follow-up
    D. Patients still alive at the end of the study period
    E. Patients who experienced a different event making further follow-up impossible

65. You are evaluating a new medication for the treatment of heart failure and would like to test its ability to improve cardiac function in patients with myocarditis. You have a study in which patients with newly diagnosed myocarditis are randomized to receive either placebo or the new medication. There are 50 patients in the treatment group and 50 in the placebo group. The ejection fraction (EF) is followed for each patient for 6 months. The average EF in patients on treatment at 6 months is 51% (±6%) versus 40% (±5%) in the placebo group. After the therapeutic trial, the number of patients with decreased heart function in the treatment group is 18 and the number of patients with decreased heart function in the placebo group is 35. What is the *number needed to treat (NNT)* with this new medication to maintain cardiac function in patients with myocarditis?

   A. 3
   B. 9
   C. 11
   D. 50
   E. 100

66. A pediatric cardiologist would like to evaluate how fellows self-evaluate their catheterization procedures. She instructs both pediatric cardiology staff and fellows to score their catheterization procedures based on a standardized scoring system and then she compares their evaluations. What would be the *best* test to analyze these data?

   A. Sensitivity
   B. Kappa statistic
   C. Regression analysis
   D. Receiver operating curve
   E. Beta factor

67. A study designed to look at mortality in children with interrupted aortic arch utilizes chi-squared analysis to describe mortality rates in children with interrupted arch as compared to those with coarctation of the aorta. As you review the results section of this study, you notice that there were only 10 patients in the interrupted aortic arch group with 3 deaths and 25 patients in the coarctation group with 4 deaths. What would have been the most appropriate type of test to use for analysis of the data in this study?

   A. Fischer exact test
   B. The most appropriate test was already used
   C. Kruskal–Wallis test
   D. ANOVA
   E. Student's *t*-test

68. A multi-institutional study comparing the use of an angiotensin II receptor blocker, an angiotensin converting enzyme inhibitor, and a beta blocker for the management of heart failure is conducted. The authors decide to analyze the data using ANOVA analysis. What is a potential concern with the use of ANOVA analysis in this study?

   A. If P is <0.05, this study demonstrates a difference among the groups, but not specifically between which groups the difference occurs or how big the difference is
   B. ANOVA analysis requires four or more different groups
   C. ANOVA will underestimate the difference between the groups
   D. ANOVA analysis is very time consuming and does not provide clinically relevant data
   E. There is a very high incidence of false-positive results using ANOVA

69. You are studying the mean blood pressure values in children with body mass index (BMI) >85th percentile randomized to treatment with lisinopril, weight management regimen, or placebo medication. This study includes 30 participants with 10 patients in each group. The distribution of the data for the group of patients given lisinopril is shown in **Figure 17.4**.

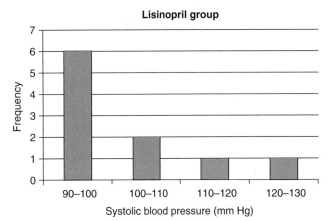

FIGURE 17.4

What would be the best test to compare the mean blood pressures between the groups?

   A. Kruskal–Wallis test
   B. ANOVA
   C. χ^2 test
   D. Student's *t*-test
   E. Wilcoxon signed-rank test

70. The incidence of all forms of congenital heart disease in the United States is about 1% of all live births per year or 100/10,000 live births per year, and it has not changed appreciably over the last six decades. One estimate of the number of people living with congenital heart disease in the United States in 2010 was 2.4 million people. With a US population size of 309.3 million in the 2010 census, what is the prevalence of congenital heart disease and how would you determine the average duration of disease?

A. 129/10,000 people, and incidence = prevalence × duration of disease (avg.)
B. 129/10,000 people, and prevalence/incidence = duration of disease (avg.)
C. 78/10,000 people, and incidence = prevalence × duration of disease (avg.)
D. 78/10,000 people, and prevalence = incidence × duration of disease (avg.)
E. 100/10,000 people, and prevalence = incidence × duration of disease (avg.)

71. You have designed a research study to determine the risk of mortality based on pulmonary artery pressure measured by catheterization prior to the Fontan surgery. Based on preliminary data, you determine that you will enroll 100 patients to reach a statistically significant predictor of mortality, but your statistician says that you are underpowered to answer that question. Which of the following would increase the power of your study?

A. Increased variance of the pressure measurement
B. Decreased standard error of the mean
C. Increased confidence interval
D. Smaller sample size
E. Lower *P*-value

For Questions 72 to 74, use the following scenario as well as Table 17.4: You have designed a therapy that improves Fontan circulation. After 6 months of therapy, 125/500 have normal exercise performance on the new therapy, whereas 50/500 have normal exercise performance on placebo.

TABLE 17.4 Exercise Performance Outcomes for Novel Fontan Therapy

	Decreased Exercise Performance	Normal Exercise Performance
Treatment	375	125
Placebo	450	50

72. What is the **absolute risk** (incidence rate) of poor exercise performance on the new therapy?

A. 90%
B. 25%
C. 75%
D. 10%
E. 15%

73. What is the **absolute risk reduction** on therapy versus placebo?

A. 25%
B. 50%
C. 15%
D. 75%
E. 10%

74. What is the **number needed to treat** to see an effect of the therapy on exercise performance?

A. 85 patients
B. 67 patients
C. 75 patients
D. 6.7 patients
E. 4 patients

75. How would you describe the accuracy and precision of test A versus test B in **Figure 17.5**?

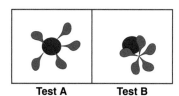

Test A　　**Test B**

FIGURE 17.5 This figure demonstrates the results of a study evaluating two new blood tests. The red area is the range of true values for the gold standard test.

A. Test A is more accurate and more precise than test B
B. Test A is less accurate but more precise than test B
C. Test A is less accurate and less precise than test B
D. Test A is more accurate but less precise than test B
E. Test A has similar accuracy but is less precise than test B

76. There is a nuclear power plant in a region of the state where you have noticed an increased number of prenatally diagnosed congenital heart diseases. You decide to study whether exposure to the nuclear power plant causes congenital heart disease. Which type of study design would longitudinally follow those who live near the power plant?

A. Case-control study
B. Cross-sectional study
C. Experimental study
D. Descriptive study
E. Cohort study

77. As an epidemiologist, you want to determine the odds of developing pulmonary hypertension after exposure to a common weight-loss medication. Which matched study design to design type quality is the correct in order to determine the odds of developing pulmonary hypertension and whether it is significant?

A. Cohort design—longitudinal follow-up after exposure
B. Case-control—it is easier for studying a rare exposure
C. Experimental design—dose-response relationship can be determined
D. Case-control—it is easier for studying a rare disease
E. Cohort design—it is easier for studying a common exposure

78. You perform a cross-sectional study evaluating vascular function in patients with intravascular hemolysis and the results are shown in **Figure 17.6**. Vascular dysfunction (low FMD) is associated with a higher concentration of cell-free hemoglobin in the plasma. Which of the following would demonstrate causal inference?

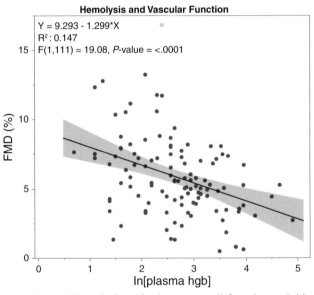

Hemolysis and Vascular Function

$Y = 9.293 - 1.299*X$
$R^2 : 0.147$
$F(1,111) = 19.08$, P-value = <.0001

FIGURE 17.6 The relationship between cell-free hemoglobin and vascular function is demonstrated. The fit line equation, R^2, F value, and P-value are included.

A. Prior vascular function measurements were worse while cell-free hemoglobin was normal, and the addition of intravenous hemoglobin as an oxygen carrier did not alter the vascular function
B. The strength of the association as determined by the significant P-value; < 0.0001
C. Another study with over 10,000 patients did not show an association between cell-free hemoglobin and vascular function
D. The use of intravenous cell-free hemoglobin as an oxygen carrier resulted in worsening vascular function and hypertension
E. Another small molecule present in the bloodstream is highly associated with both measures and is shown to directly cause vascular dysfunction in a dose-dependent manner

79. You aim to determine whether a novel gene marker is expressed in patients with an isolated muscular VSD compared to healthy subjects. You find that a higher proportion of patients with an isolated VSD express this gene marker. However, you also discover that a higher proportion of patients with VSD and the gene marker are from Central America. So, you repeat the study at a center in Canada, a center in Panama, and a center in Africa. If you want to determine whether geographic location is a confounder for the odds of having the gene marker and a VSD, which test would you use?

A. Fisher exact χ^2 test
B. McNemar χ^2 test
C. Cochran–Mantel–Haenszel χ^2 test
D. Pearson χ^2 test
E. Analysis of Variance (ANOVA)

80. Which are the correct matching tests for the **Figure 17.7**?

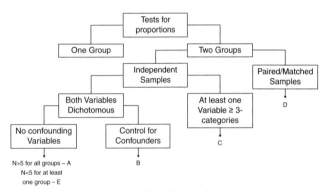

FIGURE 17.7 Categorical statistical tests for proportions.

A. A—Pearson χ^2 test; C—r × c contingency table χ^2 test; E—Fisher exact test
B. A—McNemar χ^2 test; B—Cochran–Mantel–Haenszel χ^2 test; D—Pearson χ^2 test
C. C—r × c contingency table χ^2 test; D—Fisher exact test; B—Cochran–Mantel–Haenszel χ^2 test
D. B—Cochran–Mantel–Haenszel χ^2 test; C—Fisher exact test; D—Pearson χ^2 test
E. A—Fisher exact test; B—r × c contingency table χ^2 test; C—Cochran–Mantel–Haenszel χ^2 test

81. A new blood test has been determined to be a good screening test for a disease when it is positive. A physician is now seeing his patient in clinic and gets a positive test result after sending out the new blood test. Which of the following represents the probability that this patient has the disease?

A. Sensitivity
B. Negative predictive value
C. Positive predictive value
D. Specificity
E. P-value <0.05

82. What is the proper matching of tests for **Figure 17.8**?

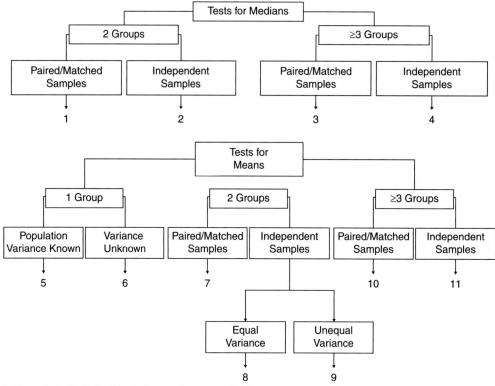

FIGURE 17.8 Statistical tests for continuous variables.

A. 1—Wilcoxon signed-rank test, 2—ANOVA, 3—Kruskal–Wallis test, 8—Welch *t*-test

B. 2—Kruskal–Wallis test, 3—Wilcoxon rank sum test, 7—repeated measures ANOVA, 8—Student's *t*-test

C. 1—Kruskal–Wallis test, 2—Wilcoxon rank sum test, 5—Z-test, 11—one-way ANOVA

D. 2—Wilcoxon rank sum test, 4—Kruskal–Wallis test, 7—paired *t*-test, 10—repeated measures ANOVA

E. 3—Friedman–Kendall–Smith test, 4—Wilcoxon signed-rank test, 6—Z test, 9—Welch test

83. You are evaluating surgical outcomes in a group of patients with tetralogy of Fallot and another group with transposition of the great arteries. One of the variables included in the analysis is preoperative oxyhemoglobin saturation. You determine that the distribution of oxyhemoglobin saturation is not normal. Which test should you use to determine if there is a difference in preoperative saturation between these two groups?

A. Analysis of variance (ANOVA)

B. Kruskal–Wallis test

C. Paired *t*-test

D. Wilcoxon rank sum test

E. Student's *t*-test

Answers

1. (D) Data from variables can be categorical (qualitative) or numerical (quantitative).

Categorical data include (1) nominal data that describe data that can be in categories but have no particular order or magnitude differences (such as blood groups) and (2) ordinal data that are data that can be allocated to an ordered set of categories (such as AHA classes I to IV or severity of AV valve regurgitation from mild to severe).

Numerical data include (1) discrete data that can only be certain whole numbers (such as number of surgeries or catheterizations) and (2) continuous data that can be any numerical value (such as cardiac indices or pulmonary vascular resistances). Pulmonary vascular resistance, therefore, would be numerical data of a continuous nature.

2. (A)
Case-control studies:
Advantages:

1. Permit the study of rare diseases.
2. Permit the study of diseases with long latency between exposure and manifestation.
3. Can be launched and conducted over relatively short time periods.
4. Relatively inexpensive as compared to cohort studies.
5. Can study multiple potential causes of disease.

Disadvantages:

1. Information on exposure and past history is primarily based on interview and may be subject to recall bias.
2. Validation of information on exposure is difficult, incomplete, or even impossible.
3. By definition, concerned with one disease only.
4. Cannot usually provide information on incidence rates of disease.
5. Generally incomplete control of extraneous variables.
6. Choice of appropriate control group may be difficult.
7. Methodology may be hard to comprehend for nonepidemiologists and correct interpretation of results may be difficult.

Cohort studies:[1]
Advantages:

1. Allow complete information on the subject's exposure, including quality control of data, and experience thereafter.
2. Provide a clear temporal sequence of exposure and disease.
3. Give an opportunity to study multiple outcomes related to a specific exposure.
4. Permit calculation of incidence rates (absolute risk) as well as relative risk.
5. Methodology and results are easily understood by nonepidemiologists.
6. Enable the study of relatively rare exposures.

---

[1]Data from Metric O. Cohort and Case–Control Studies, WHO.

Disadvantages:

1. Not suited for the study of rare diseases because a large number of subjects are required.
2. Not suited when the time between exposure and disease manifestation is very long, although this can be overcome in historical cohort studies.
3. Exposure patterns, for example, the composition of oral contraceptives, may change during the course of the study and make the results irrelevant.
4. Maintaining high rates of follow-up can be difficult.
5. Expensive to carry out because a large number of subjects are usually required.
6. Baseline data may be sparse because the large number of subjects does not allow for long interviews.

3. (B) A clinical trial is research involving administration of a test regimen to humans to evaluate both efficacy and safety. The several phases of a clinical trial are (1) phase I—safety and pharmacologic profiles; (2) phase II—pilot efficacy studies; (3) phase III—extensive clinical trial; and (4) phase IV—studies after FDA approval for distribution.

Phase 0—administration of a single subtherapeutic dose of the drug to a small group (10 to 15 subjects) to gather preliminary data on pharmacokinetics and pharmacodynamics; phase I—a small group (20 to 80 subjects) of volunteers to assess the safety and pharmacokinetic profile of the medication; phase II—a large group (20 to 300 of subjects) to assess safety in a larger group of patients as well as effectiveness of the drug; phase III—randomized controlled multicenter trial on a relatively large group (300 to 3,000 or more subjects) depending on the medical condition and to assess the effectiveness of the drug in comparison with an accepted therapy; and phase IV—involves safety surveillance and ongoing technical support of a drug after permission for it to be distributed.

4. (B) The Fisher exact test is used when the numbers in the contingency table of categorical variables are relatively small while the McNemar test is used for two groups with paired data. The Mantel–Haenszel test is an extension of the χ^2 test used when comparing several two-way tables (such as for meta-analysis studies). χ^2 test is a measure of the difference between actual and expected frequencies with categorical variables.

5. (E) Parametric tests are used to compare samples of normally (or Gaussian) distributed data. These tests include (1) the Student's t-test (used to compare two samples to test the probability that the samples come from a population with the same mean value) and (2) the ANOVA (used to compare the means of two or more samples to see whether they are derived from the same population). The analysis of covariance (ANCOVA) is an extension of ANOVA to accommodate continuous variables. *Note:* The Kolmogorov–Smirnov test is used to test the hypothesis that the collected data are from a normal distribution so that the parametric statistics can be used.

Nonparametric tests are used when the data are not normally distributed so that the above tests are not appropriate. These tests include (1) the Wilcoxon signed-rank test (for comparing the difference between paired groups, as in t-test for parametric data); (2) the Mann–Whitney U-test or the Wilcoxon rank sum test (for comparing two sets of data that are derived from two different sets of subjects); and (3) the Kruskal–Wallis test (for comparing two or more independent groups, as in ANOVA for parametric data).

6. (E) Prevalence of a disease describes what proportion of the population has the disease at a specific point in time (disease burden of a specific population). The prevalence of a disease depends on both the incidence and duration of the disease (prevalence = incidence × duration of disease). Of note, incidence describes the occurrence frequency of new cases during a time period. Prevalence can be considered to be similar to pretest probability; the more disease in the population, the higher likelihood of getting a positive test. Thus, as prevalence increases, PPV increases and NPV decreases. The opposite is true for decreasing prevalence; PPV decreases and NPV increases.

7. (A) Correlation is often confused with "regression," which quantifies the association between two variables. Regression analysis is used to delineate how one set of data relates to another through a best fit line, in which the regression coefficient is the slope of the line. While this describes a simple linear regression, other types of regression include (1) logistic regression (variation of linear regression when there are only two possible outcomes); (2) Poisson regression (variation of regression calculations to allow for frequency of rare events); and (3) Cox proportional hazards regression model (used in survival analysis to investigate the relationship between an event and several variables).

The most common survival curve method is the Kaplan–Meier curve, which graphically displays the survival of a cohort with calculation of survival estimates upon each death or event (as seen in **Figure 17.1**). This figure depicts Kaplan–Meier event-free survival curves for arrhythmic events according to the combination of left ventricular ejection fraction (LVEF) with nonsustained ventricular tachycardia and baroreflex sensitivity (BRS). The total population has been divided into four groups after dichotomization of LVEF according to <35% and >35% and BRS and SD of normal intervals according to the ATRAMI cutoff values of <3 ms/mm Hg and >3 ms/mm Hg. The probability value refers to differences in event rate between subgroups. A nonparametric test to compare the survival between two potential Kaplan–Meier curves is the log rank test.

8. (A) The sensitivity and specificity of a diagnostic test depends on more than just the "quality" of the test; they also depend on the definition of what constitutes an abnormal test. Look at the idealized graph in **Figure 17.9** showing the number of patients with and without a disease arranged according to the value of the diagnostic test. These distributions overlap; the test (like most) does not distinguish normal from disease with 100% accuracy. The area of overlap between these two distributions represents where the test cannot distinguish normal from disease.

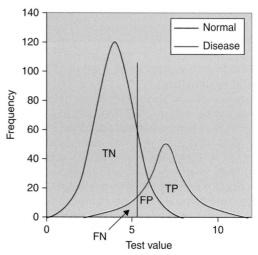

FIGURE 17.9 The normal distribution. (From http://en.wikipedia.org/wiki/File:The_Normal_Distribution.svg)

In practice, we choose a cutoff (indicated by the vertical black line) above which we consider the test to be abnormal and below which we consider the test to be normal. The position of the cut point will determine the number of true positive, true negatives, false positives, and false negatives. We may wish to use different cutoffs for different clinical situations if we wish to minimize one of the erroneous types of test results. The arrow points to the false negatives.

9. (A) A normal or Gaussian distribution is a well-recognized curve (**Figure 17.10**). This reflects a continuous probability distribution that is bell shaped (unimodal) and symmetrical about the mean with two parameters, the mean (μ) and the variance (σ^2). The SD is the measure of dispersion or variability in a sample. The SD is used for data that are normally distributed (±1 SD = 68.2%, ±2 SD = 95.4%, and ±3 SD = 99.7% of data). The mean and the median of a normal distribution are equal.

Note: A quick check to see whether a distribution is normally distributed is to see whether two SD away from the mean are still within the possible range for the variable.

The t-distribution is similar to the normal distribution but more spread out with longer tails.

Examples of continuous probability distributions that are not normal include the χ^2 distribution (a right skewed distribution characterized by degrees of freedom); the F-distribution (also skewed to the right and used for comparing two variances); and the lognormal distribution (highly skewed to the right as it is the probability distribution of a random variable whose log follows the normal distribution). The binomial and Poisson distributions are types of discrete probability distributions.

10. (C) CI is the range that is likely to contain the true population mean value that would be present (if the data for the whole population is obtained). A 95% CI means that there is 95% chance that the population value lies within the stated limits. The SD indicates the variability in a sample. In a normal distribution, 95% of the distribution of the sample means it is within 1.96 SD of the population mean. The SD is

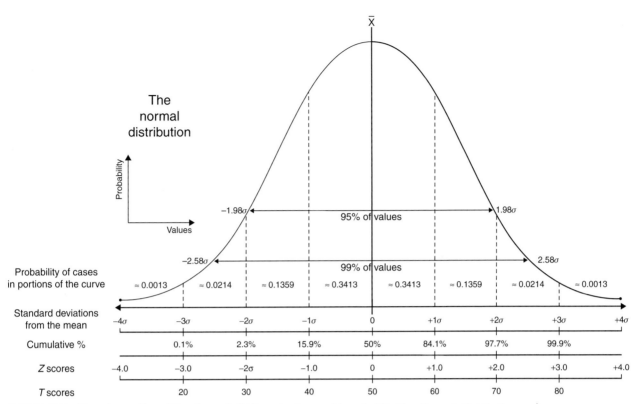

FIGURE 17.10 (From https://en.wikipedia.org/wiki/Standard_score#/media/File:The_Normal_Distribution.svg)

the standard error of the mean (SEM) and the 95% CI for the mean is calculated by: sample mean − 1.96 × SEM to sample mean + 1.96 × SEM.

The size of the CI would be related to the sample size of the study (the larger the study population, the narrower the CI). Importantly, when assessing the averages or means of two groups and the CI includes zero, then no difference between the populations is detected (null hypothesis cannot be rejected). If using relative risk or odds ratio rather than means of two groups and the CI includes one, then no difference between the populations is detected (null hypothesis cannot be rejected). Therefore, in this case, the CI includes zero and no true difference can be stated; thus, the P-value would likely be >0.05 (5%).

11. (C) There are two types of applied statistics. Descriptive statistics (means, medians, modes, SD, quartiles, and histograms) describe the data in a sample. Inferential statistics are statistical methods that estimate whether the results suggest a real difference between populations (such as the Student's t-test, ANOVA, and the χ^2 test).

12. (E) A type I error (α error) occurs when a null hypothesis that is correct is rejected (declaring that there is a difference when there is not). A type II error (β error) occurs when a hypothesis that is incorrect is accepted (declaring that a difference does not exist when in fact it does). The chance of making a type I error is the same as the P-value. *Note:* A type III error is a study design that produces the right answer to the wrong question.

The P (probability) value is the probability that defines how likely it is that a hypothesis (usually the null

hypothesis) is true (that there is no difference between two treatments). The P-value is therefore the probability of an observed difference occurring solely by chance. The usual P-value at the significance level is 0.01 to 0.05. *Note:* A method used to adjust the P-value for multiple testing is the Bonferroni adjustment.

13. (B) The power of a study is the probability that it would detect a statistically significant difference. As the β value is the probability of accepting a hypothesis that is false, the power of the study (1 − β) is therefore the probability of rejecting the null hypothesis when it is false. Or in other words, power is the probability of avoiding a type II error. The power of a study should be at least 80% and is increased by several factors including larger significance level, larger effects, decreased variability or variance of the observations, and larger sample size.

14. (A) A CEA is an economic assessment method in which the costs and consequences of alternative interventions are expressed in costs per unit of health outcome. This commonly used methodology is applicable to health programs as well as health services to help determine the preferred action that requires the least cost to produce a given level of effectiveness.

Another economic tool is the CUA, which uses quality-of-life measurements expressed as utilities (such as QALY) in the value equation. A disability-adjusted life year (DALY) is also a measure used but is for the overall "burden of disease." It quantifies the impact of not only premature death as in QALY but also disability on a population by combining them into a single, comparable metric.

A third economic assessment methodology is the CBA, which seeks to translate all relevant healthcare considerations into monetary terms by analyzing economic and social costs of medical care and benefits of reduced loss of net earnings due to prevention of premature death or disability.

Other less common methods of economic evaluation include cost-consequence analysis (CCA), CMA, and even CVA.

15. (C) A meta-analysis is a technique in which results from a number of studies that are similar in nature are gathered to give one overall estimate of the effect. The formal steps include the following: (1) decide on effect of interest, (2) check for statistical homogeneity, (3) estimate the average effect of interest with CIs, and (4) interpret the results and present the findings (forest plot). The advantages include refinement and reduction, efficiency, generalizability and consistency, reliability, and power and precision. The disadvantages include publication bias, clinical heterogeneity, quality differences, and lack of independence of study subjects.

A systemic review (such as the international network called the Cochrane collaboration with its Cochrane database of systematic reviews) often uses meta-analysis techniques to render well-informed clinical decisions; it is an essential part of evidence-based medicine. Major disease categories will often have a sufficient number of randomized clinical trials for a meta-analysis to be carried out to determine the value of such an intervention.

For **Answers 16 to 19,** Table 17.5 was created from the question stem.

TABLE 17.5 Antiarrhythmic and Placebo Cohort

	Arrhythmia	No Arrhythmia	Total
Antiarrhythmic agent group	16	449	465
	(A)	(B)	
Placebo group	23	442	465
	(C)	(D)	
	39	891	930

16. (C) Relative risk (also risk ratio), used in prospective **cohort** studies, represents the ratio of the probability of an event occurring in an exposed group to the probability of the event occurring in a nonexposed group. It is calculated by dividing the risk in the treated or exposed group by the risk in the control or unexposed group (as in odds ratio, relative risk can be <1, 1, or >1 and given with their 95% CI—if the CI includes 1, it is not statistically significant). Relative risk is calculated by: A/(A+B) ÷ C/(C+D). In this case, the relative risk is 0.034/0.049 or 3.4%/4.9% = 0.69.

17. (B) The RRR is the proportion by which the intervention reduces the event rate (risk) in the experimental group (treatment) compared to the control group (placebo). Relative risk reduction is calculated by: 1 – relative risk. In this case, 1 – 0.69 = 0.31 or 31% relative risk reduction in arrhythmias occurring in the treatment group when compared to the placebo group. Of note, RRR can also be calculated as: ARR ÷ C/(C+D).

18. (E) The ARR is the absolute difference between the event rates in the intervention (treatment) versus control (placebo) groups. Absolute risk reduction is calculated by: C/(C+D) − A/(A+B). In this case, the ARR is 0.049 − 0.034 = 0.015 or 1.5%.

19. (A) The NNT is the number of patients who need to be treated for one to get benefit; in other words, the effectiveness of an intervention. NNT is calculated by: 1/ARR. The inverse of the NNT equals the ARR. In this case, the NNT is 1/0.015 = 67. Thus, 67 patients will need to be treated with the new antiarrhythmic agent in order to prevent one adverse outcome (arrhythmia).

20. (A) The ROC curve is a two-way plot of the sensitivity (true-positive rate) against 1 – the specificity (false-positive rate) for different cutoff values for a continuous variable in a diagnostic test[2]. The upper left corner or coordinate (0,1) is called the perfect classification (100% sensitivity or no false negatives, and 100% specificity or no false positives) (**Figure 17.11**).

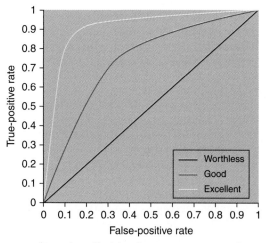

FIGURE 17.11 (From http://celebrating200years.noaa.gov/magazine/tct/tct_side1.html)

21. (E) The variance is the square of the SD while coefficient of variation is the ratio of the SD to the mean. While the SD is a measure of spread away from the mean and is equal to the square root of the variance, the SEM is a measure of precision of the sample mean or how close the sample mean is likely to be to the population mean.

---

[2]See website with moving description of all the above at www.anaesthetist.com/mnm/stats/roc/Findex.htm

22. (B) Accuracy is the degree of closeness of measurements to that quantity's true value while precision is the reproducibility of a study result with the study to be repeated under the same circumstances (measured by standard error of measurement) (**Figure 17.12**).

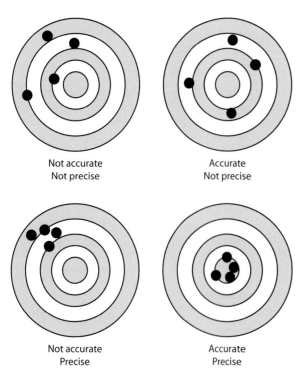

Not accurate
Not precise

Accurate
Not precise

Not accurate
Precise

Accurate
Precise

FIGURE 17.12 Tests for proportions using categorical variables.

23. (A) Chi-squared (χ^2) test is a measure of the difference between actual and expected frequencies with *categorical* variables; a contingency table is set up to calculate the χ^2 value. If there is no difference between actual and expected frequencies, then χ^2 would be 0. The larger the difference, the bigger the χ^2 value (but it is easier to note the P-value that accompanies the χ^2 value). The df is the number of independent comparisons that can be made between members of the sample and is used with χ^2 value to calculate the P-value. In this case, the df (of 1) is needed to calculate the P-value. The χ^2 test is sometimes used with Yates continuity correction to improve the accuracy of the P-value.

The Fisher exact test is used when the numbers in the contingency table of categorical variables are relatively small (<5) while the McNemar test is used for two groups with paired data. The Mantel–Haenszel test is an extension of the χ^2 test used when comparing several two-way tables (such as for meta-analysis studies).

24. (A) Correlation coefficient is the strength of the linear relationship between two variables and it measures the strength of an association between two variables without assuming cause-and-effect. This relationship is denoted by the letter r that ranges from −1 to +1 (R^2 is sometimes given to correct for negatively correlated relationships); 1 = strong positive relationship, −1 = strong negative relationship, and 0 = no relationship. The coefficient r cannot be calculated

when there is neither a nonlinear relationship nor when there are multiple outliers.

When the degree of linear relationship is extended to several variables, it is known as multiple correlation coefficient. The Pearson correlation coefficient "r" is used if the values are sampled from a normally distributed population (if not, the Spearman correlation coefficient "rs" is used).

For **Answers 25 to 28**, see Table 17.6.

TABLE 17.6 Disease and Test Result

Test Result	Disease		Total
	Present	Absent	
Positive	A	B	A + B
Negative	C	D	C + D
Total	A + C	B + D	A + B + C + D

25. (A) PPV is the probability that patients with a positive screening test truly have the disease. It is calculated by: number of diseased who screened positive ÷ total number of those who screened positive. As in **Table 17.6**, PPV = A/(A+B). Of note, there is interdependence between sensitivity and specificity (see **Figure 17.11**).

26. (D) NPV is the probability that patients with a negative screening test truly do not have the disease. It is calculated by: number of healthy (no disease) who screened negative ÷ total number of those who screened negative. As in **Table 17.6**, NPV = D/(C+D). Of note, there is interdependence between sensitivity and specificity (see **Figure 17.11**).

27. (B) Sensitivity is the ability of a test to detect disease when disease is truly present (true positive). It is calculated by: number of diseased who screened positive ÷ total number of diseased. As in **Table 17.6**, Sensitivity = A/(A+C).

28. (E) Specificity is the ability of a test to successfully rule-out disease when no disease is present (true negative). It is calculated by: number of healthy who screened negative ÷ total number of healthy. As in **Table 17.6**, Specificity = D/(B+D).

29. (B) Bias occurs when there is a systematic difference between the result of a study and the true result. It occurs when a systematic error is introduced into the study which results in selecting one outcome over the other. Types of bias include: observer bias (observer inaccurately assesses variable), confounding bias (spurious association), selection bias (selected study subjects not representative of true population), information bias (measurements incorrectly recorded), publication bias (only positive results are published), and others like recall bias (inaccurate remembering of facts or omitting details by subjects), and/or allocation bias (systematic difference in how subjects are assigned to comparison groups).

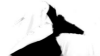

30. (E) An association is any relationship between two measured quantities that relates them to be statistically dependent, whereas correlation defines a linear relationship between the two quantities. Causation in addition to association includes the following criteria: temporality, strength of causality, dose–response, repetition in a different population, consistency with other studies, and biologic plausibility.

31. (A) The Belmont report elucidates three principles of research ethics: (1) respect for persons: protecting the autonomy of all people and treating them with courtesy and respect and allowing for informed consent (researchers must be truthful and conduct no deception); (2) beneficence: the philosophy of "do no harm" while maximizing benefits for the research project and minimizing risks for the research subjects; and (3) justice: ensuring reasonable, nonexploitative, and well-considered procedures are administered fairly and equally.

32. (C) The IRB, also known as the ethical review board, is a committee that is designated to approve and review research involving human subjects to protect the rights and welfare of human research subjects. The DSMB is an independent group of experts that continuously monitors the data from various aspects of a clinical trial to ensure patient safety as well as validity and scientific merit of the trial. The difference between the IRB and the DSMB is that the IRB is primarily responsible for the review of clinical protocols and related documents while the DSMB's main responsibility is to review the trial safety and efficacy data.

33. (C) Reliability is the consistency of a set of measurements/measurement tool, or the repeatability/reproducibility of such a methodology (inversely related to random error). Validity is the extent to which the study measures what it is intended to measure so that validity is a measurement of systematic error or bias (examples are confounding and selection bias). Accuracy is the degree of a measurement closeness to that quantity's true or accepted value; while precision is the closeness of two or more measurements to each other when repeated under the same circumstances (measured by standard error of measurement). Power is the probability of correctly rejecting the null hypothesis when the null hypothesis is false.

34. (A) Calculation of a minimal sample size involves the following parameters: power (usually 0.80); significance level (usually 0.01 or 0.05); variability of the observations (or the standard deviation); and the smallest effect of interest (the standardized difference).

35. (E)
Cohort studies:[3]
Advantages:

1. Allow complete information on the subject's exposure, including quality control of data, and experience thereafter.

2. Provide a clear temporal sequence of exposure and disease.
3. Give an opportunity to study multiple outcomes related to a specific exposure.
4. Permit calculation of incidence rates (absolute risk) as well as relative risk.
5. Methodology and results are easily understood by nonepidemiologists.
6. Enable the study of relatively rare exposures.

Disadvantages:

1. Not suited for the study of rare diseases because a large number of subjects are required.
2. Not suited when the time between exposure and disease manifestation is very long, although this can be overcome in historical cohort studies.
3. Exposure patterns, for example, the composition of oral contraceptives, may change during the course of the study and make the results irrelevant.
4. Maintaining high rates of follow-up can be difficult.
5. Expensive to carry out because a large number of subjects are usually required.
6. Baseline data may be sparse because the large number of subjects does not allow for long interviews.

Case-control studies:
Advantages:

1. Permit the study of rare diseases.
2. Permit the study of diseases with long latency between exposure and manifestation.
3. Can be launched and conducted over relatively short time periods.
4. Relatively inexpensive as compared to cohort studies.
5. Can study multiple potential causes of disease.

Disadvantages:

1. Information on exposure and past history is primarily based on interview and may be subject to recall bias.
2. Validation of information on exposure is difficult, or incomplete, or even impossible.
3. By definition, concerned with one disease only.
4. Cannot usually provide information on incidence rates of disease.
5. Generally incomplete control of extraneous variables.
6. Choice of appropriate control group may be difficult.
7. Methodology may be hard to comprehend for nonepidemiologists, and correct interpretation of results may be difficult.

36. (A) Nonparametric tests are used when the data are not normally distributed. These tests include (1) the Wilcoxon signed-rank test (for comparing the difference between *paired* groups, as in the *t*-test for parametric data or normally distributed); (2) the Mann–Whitney *U*-test or the Wilcoxon ranks sum test (for comparing two sets of data that are derived from two *different* sets of subjects); and (3) the Kruskal–Wallis test (for comparing two or more independent groups, as in ANOVA for parametric data or normally distributed).

---

[3]From Metric O. Cohort and Case–Control Studies, WHO.

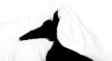

37. (B) See **Table 17.7**.

TABLE 17.7 Summary of Statistical Methods

	Numerical Data	**Categorical Data**
Single group	One-sample *t*-test or sign test[a]	Test of single proportion or sign test[a]
Two groups, paired	Paired *t*-test or Wilcoxon signed-rank test[a]	McNemar test
Two groups, unpaired	Unpaired *t*-test or Wilcoxon rank sum test[a] (Mann–Whitney *U*-test)	χ^2 test or Fisher exact test[a] (<5)
Multiple (>2) groups	ANOVA (one way) or Kruskal–Wallis test[a]	χ^2 test

[a]Nonparametric tests (relevant for populations that do not have a normal distribution).
[b]Used when expected frequencies are small.

38. (A) Categorical data include (1) nominal data that describe data that can be in categories but have no particular order or magnitude differences (such as single ventricle and biventricular surgical strategies or antiarrhythmic agent for supraventricular tachycardia), and (2) ordinal data are data that can be allocated to an ordered set of categories (such as severity of AV valve regurgitation from mild to severe).

Numerical data include (1) discrete data that can only be certain whole numbers (such as number of reinterventions after Norwood procedure) and (2) continuous data that can be any numerical value (such as blood pressure measurements before and after ACE inhibitors).

39. (B) A cohort study (also termed follow-up, longitudinal, or prospective study) is a prospective observational study with study subjects (cohort) assigned to an exposure or condition category and then all followed for a defined observation period to see whether they develop disease. A historical cohort study, as the name implies, is a group of patients from the past and would not involve active enrollment of new study subjects.

A case-control study is a retrospective study that studies the relationship between risk factor and outcome and uses relevant exposure or condition information from a sample of individuals with the disease or condition (cases) rather than examining the entire population. A case series refers to the qualitative study of a single patient or small group of patients with a similar disease.

40. (C) This study fits phase III criteria. Phase 0—administration of a single subtherapeutic doses of the drug to a small group (10 to 15 subjects) to gather preliminary data

on pharmacokinetics and pharmacodynamics; phase I—a small group (20 to 100 subjects) of volunteers to assess the safety and pharmacokinetic profile of the medication; phase II—a large group (100 to 300 of subjects) to assess safety in a larger group of patients as well as effectiveness of the drug; phase III—randomized controlled multicenter trial on a relatively large group (300 to 3,000 or more subjects) depending on the medical condition and to assess the effectiveness of the drug in comparison with an accepted "gold standard" therapy; and phase IV—involves safety surveillance and ongoing technical support of a drug after permission for it to be distributed.

41. (E) The Fisher exact test is used when the numbers in the contingency table of categorical variables are relatively small, while the χ^2 test is a measure of the difference between actual and expected frequencies with categorical variables with larger (>5) populations. Both are tests used for categorical data. The other tests are all used for numerical data.

Parametric tests are used to compare samples of normally (or Gaussian) distributed data. These tests include (1) the Student's *t*-test (used to compare two samples to test the probability that the samples come from a population with the same mean value) and (2) the ANOVA (used to compare the means of two or more samples to see whether they are derived from the same population). The Kolmogorov–Smirnov test is used to test the hypothesis that the collected data are from a normal distribution, so that the parametric statistics can be used. Nonparametric tests are used when the data are not normally distributed, so that the above tests are not appropriate. These tests include the Wilcoxon signed-rank test (for comparing the difference between paired groups, as in *t*-test for parametric data).

42. (C) Incidence describes the frequency of occurrence of new cases during a time period, whereas prevalence describes what proportion of the population has the disease at a specific point in time. The prevalence P depends on both the incidence I and duration D of the disease ($P = I \times D$).

Incidence is useful to explore causal theories or to evaluate effects of preventive measures, whereas prevalence is relevant to planning of health services or assessing need for medical care in a population. Lastly, while chronic diseases can have lower incidence than prevalence, acute illnesses can be the opposite.

Incidence:
Incidence (*I*) (also incidence rate or incidence density) (person-time units):

$$I = \frac{\text{Number of new cases of the disease that occur in a population during a period of time}}{\text{Sum for each individual in the population of the length of time at risk of getting the disease}}$$

whereas

Cumulative incidence (CI) (also cumulative incidence rate or incidence proportion) (0–1 or %):

$$CI = \frac{\text{Number of individuals who get the disease during a certain period}}{\text{Number of individuals in the population at the beginning of the period}}$$

Prevalence:

Prevalence (*P*) (also prevalence rate, point prevalence rate, or prevalence proportion) (0–1 or %):

$$P = \frac{\text{Existing number of individuals having the disease at a specific time}}{\text{Number of individuals in the population at that point in time}}$$

43. (C) A designation from level A to I as described by the US Preventive Services Task Force can be made for each review: (1) level A—good scientific evidence (benefits substantially outweigh risk); (2) level B—fair scientific evidence (benefits outweigh the risk); (3) level C—fair scientific evidence (benefit and risk too close); (4) level D—fair scientific evidence that risks outweigh the benefit; and (5) level I—scientific evidence is lacking, or of poor quality, or conflicting.

*For **Answers 44 to 47**, please see the filled in 2 × 2 Table 17.8 from the question stem.*

TABLE 17.8 Hypertrophic Cardiomyopathy and ECG

ECG	Hypertrophic Cardiomyopathy		
	Present	Absent	Total
Positive	1	20	21
Negative	1	785	786
Total	2	805	807

44. (C) Please see Answer 27 for explanation of sensitivity.

45. (B) Please see Answer 28 for explanation of specificity.

46. (A) Please see Answer 25 for explanation of PPV.

47. (A) Please see Answer 26 for explanation of NPV.

*For **Answers 48 to 51**, Table 17.9 was created from the question stem.*

TABLE 17.9 Angiotensin Receptor Blocker and Hospitalization

	Hospitalized	Not Hospitalized	Total
Treated group	5	195	200
	(A)	(B)	
Untreated group	25	225	250
	(C)	(D)	
	30	420	450

48. (C) Relative risk (also risk ratio), used in prospective **cohort** studies, represents the ratio of the probability of an event occurring in an exposed (treated) group to the probability of the event occurring in a nonexposed (not treated) group. It is calculated by dividing the risk in the treated or exposed group by the risk in the control or unexposed group (as in odds ratio, relative risk can be <1, 1, or >1 and given with their 95% CI—if the CI includes 1, it is not statistically significant). Relative risk is calculated by: A/(A+B) ÷ C/(C+D). In this case, the relative risk is 0.025/0.1 or 2.5%/10% or 0.25.

49. (B) The RRR is the proportion by which the intervention reduces the event rate (risk) in the experimental group (treatment) compared to the control group (placebo or not treated). Relative risk reduction is calculated by: 1 − relative risk. In this case, 1 − 0.25 = 0.75 or 75% relative risk reduction in arrhythmias occurring in the treatment group when compared to the placebo group. Of note, RRR can also be calculated as: ARR ÷ C/(C+D).

50. (D) The ARR is the absolute difference between the event rates in the intervention (treatment) versus control (placebo or not treated) groups. ARR is calculated by: C/(C+D) − A/(A+B). In this case, the ARR is 0.1 − 0.025 = 0.075 or 7.5%.

51. (A) The NNT is the number of patients who need to be treated for one to get benefit; in other words, the effectiveness of an intervention. NNT is calculated by: 1/ARR. The inverse of the NNT equals the ARR. In this case, the NNT is 1/0.075 = 13.3. Thus, approximately 13 to 14 patients will need to be treated with the new angiotensin receptor blocker agent in order to prevent one adverse outcome (hospitalizations for exacerbation of heart failure).

52. (B) Reliability is the degree to which a study produces stable and consistent results. One way to improve reliability is to minimize bias within the study. Randomization refers to the practice of randomly assigning enrolled patients in one of the treatment or control groups. Double blinding involves designing the study in such a way that providers administering the intervention, those measuring the outcomes, and patients receiving the therapy are not aware of which patients are in the treatment group and which are in the control group. Both randomization and double blinding can minimize the susceptibility bias which occurs when differences in the subjects at baseline between the compared groups cause differences in outcomes beyond what the difference in interventions would cause otherwise. Use of a placebo control group is also important to assure changes that would not be seen in the study groups regardless of the intervention.

53. (E) Case-control studies involve reviewing risk factors for those patients who have the disease of interest and comparable control patients who do not. This type of study is used to determine the likelihood that various risk factors are more (or less) associated with the cases versus the controls. Cohort studies entail prospectively following those patients with a given exposure and those without. Some of the advantages of case-control study include the ability to

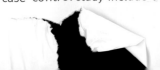

study multiple risk factors and rare conditions making it appropriate for the use of evaluating congenital heart disease in children of diabetic mothers.

54. (D) A cross-sectional study involves the collection and analysis of data collected from a population at one specific point in time. In the study described, a representative cohort of families was surveyed to help determine the prevalence of chest pain in the pediatric population. A census would not be a type of study design and therefore, it is not the correct answer. A retrospective cohort study would involve the review of records from a cohort of patients described, but that was not done in this case. A prospective cohort study would involve following a group of patients forward in time to determine which of them developed disease rather than a point in time analysis as described in this study. A cross-sectional study is very useful for determining prevalence of a disease making it an appropriate study design choice for the clinical question of interest.

55. (A) The more participants that enroll in a study, the higher the sensitivity is for detecting adverse events. Type II error refers to the inability to reject the null hypothesis when a difference between study groups truly exists. In other terms, this can be thought of as a false-negative finding. One way to decrease this risk is to increase the sample size studied, thereby increasing the power and the ability to find a difference if one truly exists. Type I error refers to the rejection of the null hypothesis when a true difference does not exist (i.e., false-positive study results). The probability at which the significance cutoff value occurs can be adjusted up or down but it is typically set at 0.05 (5% chance that the results are related to chance alone rather than a true difference).

56. (C) A prospective cohort study is a type of study design in which patients with exposure to the intervention of interest (angiotensin II receptor blocker therapy) and those without are followed forward in time for the development of the measured outcome (aortic root dilation). This is not a retrospective study because patients were followed forward in time rather than review of previous records. This study would not be useful to determine the natural epidemiology of aortic root dilation in Marfan syndrome because there is an intervention. The healthy entrant effect refers to a lower morbidity/mortality in patients entering a study than the general population due to the design of the study. The healthy entrant effect is not a factor in this study. This is not a case versus control study as both participating cohorts had Marfan syndrome.

57. (D) Specificity refers to the ability of a test to correctly identify those without the disease. In this case, transient QT prolongation can be seen in patients following syncope; so an ECG showing QT prolongation in a patient following syncope is not specific for the diagnosis of long QT syndrome. A negative predictive value refers to the ability of a negative test to truly predict patients without the disease. Reliability refers to the ability of a test (ECG) to demonstrate the same (QTc) value on repeat checks and validity refers to a test's ability to demonstrate an accurate (QTc) value. Neither reliability nor validity is in question for the ECG obtained in the ED.

58. (D) Studies are comprised of a representative sample of the population of interest which in this case is older adolescents with hyperlipidemia. Data are collected on these patients and a mean value is determined based on the measured outcome (cholesterol level). A 95% CI is calculated around the mean value for each group. The 95% CI is the range of values that are 95% certain to contain the true mean for a population based on data from the representative cohort. It does NOT represent the values between which 95% of the sample or population values fall. In this case, the 95% confidence values for cholesterol level in adolescents with the intervention (food intake recording, weekly weigh-ins, and weekly group education) were 149 to 173.

59. (C) Recall bias is a type of systematic error which occurs as a result of inaccurate recollection of events by study participants when asked to describe events from the past. This is particularly challenging and prone to bias for events with a significant emotional component such as the death of a child. Lead-time (aka length) bias refers to the inaccurate perception that a given test improves survival time for an illness; when in reality, survival is not prolonged, but rather a patient is recognized as having the disease at an early point in the disease course. Selection bias is another type of systematic error which results from the nonrandom collection of participants in a study such that certain traits are selected for. Referral bias is the bias created when only a subset of the population is included in the study. This typically happens when the center performing the study is a tertiary referral center and the patients who are referred to the center represent the most complicated subset of patients and not the disease pattern seen in the general community. This creates a study cohort which is not truly representative of the population of interest.

60. (B) The odds ratio statistically describes the association between an exposure and the risk of the outcome of interest. In this case, the odds ratio describes the association between having an AV canal defect and the risk of anemia. Since the odds ratio is <1, this indicates a decreased risk for anemia in patients with AV canal defect. An odds ratio >1 indicates an increased association. This odds ratio is likely to be statistically significant ($P < 0.05$) because the 95% confidence interval does not include 1.

61. (A) This study describes the use of a continuous variable (number of rejection episodes) both pre- and postintervention (initiation of sirolimus) in the same patient. Because this is a continuous variable with sample size >25, you can use a parametric test which in this case would be Student's *t*-test. The correct answer is to use the paired Student's *t*-test because each patient is studied both before and after the intervention thereby providing two matched cohorts. The Wilcoxon signed-rank test is a nonparametric test used to compare cohort means in samples that are nonnormally distributed or with low number of participants. Chi-squared is an analysis used to compare categorical outcomes rather than continuous variables. An odds ratio demonstrates the odds of developing a given outcome in those patients with a particular exposure and those without.

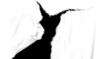

A Kaplan–Meier curve is a method to display survival results graphically and not a form of statistical analysis.

62. (A) This is a case-control study, in which the cases were defined first and the exposure was determined retrospectively, so the estimate of relative risk is the odds ratio. In this case, the odds ratio describes the odds of the outcome of interest (endocarditis) in those patients with the exposure (valve replacement). It is calculated by the equation $(A \times D)/(B \times C)$. See **Table 17.10**. It is important to know the difference between an odds ratio as an estimate of relative risk (case-control study) and directly determining the relative risk of developing a disease/outcome (cohort study).

TABLE 17.10 A Case-Control Study in Cardiology: Determination of the Odds Ratio

	Endocarditis Present	No Endocarditis Present
Prosthetic valve replacement	$A = 10$	$B = 40$
No prosthetic valve replacement	$C = 2$	$D = 48$

63. (A) Chi-squared analysis is used to statistically evaluate nominal data but is not the appropriate test for continuous data. To use chi-squared analysis, several assumptions must be fulfilled including random and completely independent study groups, all cells of the table must have an expected value of >5, and data must be able to be arranged in a table form (i.e., nominal data). We generally define a statistically significant P-value as <0.05, which means that there is less than a 5% chance that the data distribution seen in the study could have occurred by random chance.

64. (A) In a survival curve, patients are defined as being censored or noncensored. Those patients who dropped out of the study for reasons other than the outcome of interest, which in this case is cardiovascular death, are censored. This can be due to withdrawal from the study, being lost to follow up, unable to continue in the study due to a different event, or being alive at the end of the study period. Those patients who had the event of interest (cardiovascular death in this case) are defined as being noncensored.

65. (A) In order to reliably calculate the number needed to treat (NNT), the data should be a distinct event/integer; thus, continuous data is less than ideal but an estimate can sometimes be made from continuous data. The NNT is the number of patients who need to be treated for one to get benefit; in other words, the effectiveness of an intervention. NNT is calculated by: 1/ARR. The inverse of the NNT equals the ARR. Additionally, the ARR is the absolute difference between the event rates in the intervention (treatment) versus control (placebo or not treated) groups. Absolute risk reduction is calculated by: C/(C+D) − A/(A+B). In this case, the ARR is 35/50 − 18/50 = 17/50 or 0.34 (34%). Therefore, 1/0.34 or ~3 is the NNT. Thus, approximately 3 patients will need to be treated with the new medication in order to improve function.

66. (B) The kappa statistic demonstrates agreement between two groups when there is no clear gold standard. The kappa statistic can range from −1 (negative association) to 1 (positive association) with 0 demonstrating no association between the two groups. Sensitivity calculations and a receiver operating curve can be used to evaluate a test when there is a clear gold standard, but this type of analysis would not be appropriate in this study. Regression analysis can demonstrate the relationship between a dependent variable and one or more independent variables; however, in this study, the two scores cannot be defined as dependent and independent, so this would not be the appropriate statistical analysis.

67. (A) The Fischer exact test is a nonparametric test used to analyze categorical data with sample sizes that are too small to allow for the use of the χ^2 analysis. For χ^2 analysis to be used, there must be more than five patients in each cell and this would not be the case for the study described, hence it would not be appropriate to utilize this test for the data presented. The Student's t-test is for continuous data which were not reported in this study. ANOVA analysis is used to compare the mean values from three or more groups, and the Kruskal–Wallis test is the nonparametric equivalent of the ANOVA analysis.

68. (A) ANOVA analysis is a parametric test used to compare group means when there are three or more independent groups in a study. If the P-value calculated using ANOVA analysis is statistically significant (typically defined as $P < 0.05$), this indicates that there is a difference in the group means among the multiple study groups, but not specifically where the difference lies or how great a difference there is. Additional analysis comparing each group to the other is required to tease out the exact difference.

69. (A) The graph shown demonstrates a skewed distribution of the data; not normally distributed. Although the distribution for the other two groups is not shown, you can assume that these are likely not normally distributed as well due to the small number of patients in each group. The Kruskal–Wallis test is used to compare the mean values among multiple groups when ANOVA testing is not appropriate, such as this case in which the data are not normally distributed. χ^2 analysis is used to evaluate categorical data rather than group means and therefore, it would not be appropriate to use. Student's t-test is for analyzing two mean values, but in this case there are three groups again making this an incorrect test to choose.

70. (D) Incidence describes the frequency of occurrence of new cases during a time period, whereas prevalence describes what proportion of the population has the disease at a specific point in time. The prevalence P depends on both the incidence I and duration D of the disease ($P = I \times D$). Incidence is useful to explore causal theories or to evaluate effects of preventive measures, whereas prevalence is relevant to planning of health services or assessing need for medical care in a population. Lastly, while chronic diseases can have a lower incidence than prevalence, acute illnesses can be the opposite. In this case, the prevalence is 2.4 million people with congenital heart disease per 309.3 million people in the United States, which is 78/10,000.

71. (B) Power is increased if there is smaller variance in the data, larger separation between the group means, or increased sample size; because the standard error of the mean is decreased when there is smaller variance and increased sample size. Remember that the standard error is calculated by the standard deviation divided by the square root of the sample size. (**A**), (**C**), and (**D**) would increase the standard error, which would decrease the power. The *P*-value does not determine the power of your findings. The variance and sample size, and thus the standard error of the mean will affect both the *P*-value and the power but the *P*-value does not determine power.

*For **Answers 72 to 74**, please refer to **Table 17.4**.*

72. (C) The absolute risk focuses on one group only, either the treatment or the placebo. Therefore, the absolute risk of decreased exercise performance in the treatment arm is A/(A + B) or 375/(375 + 125), which is 75%. The absolute risk of the placebo group is 450/(450 + 50) or 90%. This may be confused with either absolute risk reduction or the relative risk (incidence rate ratio).

73. (C) The absolute risk reduction is the difference between the absolute risk in the untreated group and the treated group. This is also called the preventable risk difference. In this case, the absolute risk reduction is 90% − 75%, which is 15%. This may be confused with relative risk, which is calculated by the ratio of absolute risk in the treatment group ÷ Placebo group or A/(A + B) ÷ C/ (C + D). The relative risk gives the reader an idea of the absolute risk in both groups; however, it can also hide extreme values such as a low or high absolute risk.

74. (D) The number needed to treat is an estimate of the number of patients who would need to be on a treatment in order to prevent one patient from having a bad outcome or in this case, decreased exercise performance. From our data above, the absolute risk reduction was 0.15 (15%), so the number needed to treat is 1 ÷ 0.15, which is 6.7.

75. (D) Precision is how similar the values are for each measurement. Accuracy is how close each measurement is to the true value. Precision can also be described mathematically by how many places past the decimal point a test can measure a value. For example, the ability to measure the pulmonary artery to the millimeter is more precise than a measurement that can only be measured to the centimeter.

76. (E) In a cohort study design, the exposure is defined first and then the participant is followed over time to determine whether they develop a disease or other outcome. A cohort study is a prospective study and is good for assessing rare exposures. In a cohort study, the incidence rate and relative risk of getting a disease can be determined. A case-control study is a retrospective study that starts by defining a group of people with a disease and a group without a disease, and then evaluating their history for certain exposures. The odds of having an exposure is determined NOT by a relative risk of developing a disease. The incidence rate and relative risk CANNOT be determined in a case-control study. An experimental study is determined by the intervention first and then patients with a certain condition are assigned to either receive the intervention or not. A placebo-controlled drug study is an example of an experimental study design. A descriptive study does not test hypotheses, it is more often hypothesis generating.

77. (D) Pulmonary hypertension is a rare disease and the most commonly used study design for a rare disease is a case-control study. A case-control study defines cases with a disease and a control group without the disease then looks back in time for an exposure. In a case-control study, the odds of having an exposure can be determined as an estimate of relative risk; however, the incidence rate of the disease and the relative risk of developing the disease are NOT determined with this study design. If the incidence of developing pulmonary hypertension is high enough, then answer (**A**), cohort design, would be the best study design.

78. (D) Association is NOT causation. The best way to determine causation is through an experimental study design. Sometimes an experimental design is not possible; therefore, other relationships can be determined. Temporal and dose response relationships can support causation. Answer (**A**) would work against establishing a temporal or dose response relationship as support for causation. Answer (**B**), the strength of a linear association is determined by the correlation coefficient (r) not the *P*-value. The *P*-value is the probability that the results are due to chance, not the strength of the association. Answer (**C**), increasing the number of participants in a study can increase the power of the study; therefore, a larger well powered study that does not support the initial association would not support causation.

79. (C) The Cochran–Mantel–Haenszel χ^2 test assesses the association between an exposure and a dichotomous outcome, while accounting for confounder variables. The exposure and the outcome should be dichotomous. The McNemar χ^2 test is a paired analysis for dichotomous exposure/outcome sets; it tests for a difference between proportions of exposure/outcomes before and after some intervention or event. It is the nonparametric equivalent to a paired *t*-test. The Pearson χ^2 test is the most commonly used test to determine if an exposure and disease are related; it specifically tests whether there is a significant relationship between an exposure and outcome by looking at the observed relationship versus what is expected if there is no relationship. The data in this example are nominal/categorical data, an ANOVA is a test for differences between groups when there is more than two groups with normally distributed, continuous data. Fisher exact χ^2 test is a specific χ^2 test that is used when there is a group with less than five data points.

80. (A) See **Figure 17.13**. Testing whether an observed proportion is significantly different from what is expected can

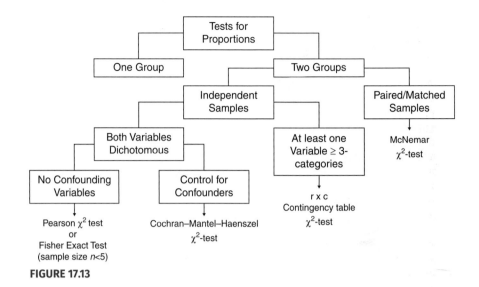

FIGURE 17.13

be accomplished by using a Chi-squared test. The type of Chi-squared test used for analysis of proportions is determined by (1) the number of groups, (2) whether groups are matched or independent, (3) whether the results are dichotomous or have ≥3 categories, and (4) whether confounding variables are included in the analysis. Pearson Chi-square assumes that each outcome has ≥5 participants. If there are <5 participants with a certain outcome, then Fisher exact test would be the appropriate test to determine whether the observed proportion of participants with that outcome is different than expected. When the study design tests for potentially confounding variables, a Cochran–Mantel–Haenszel test is used. When an outcome has ≥3 categories, an r × c contingency table should be used to account for each outcome category. McNemar test is used when testing

for a difference between outcomes that are paired (not independent).

81. (C) The question states that the blood test has been determined to be a good screening test, which means the test is sensitive. Once the test is placed into clinical practice, a practitioner will want to know whether the positive test actually predicts the disease/outcome of interest, which is the positive predictive value. The positive predictive value is the probability that the positive test predicts whether a disease/outcome is truly present; minimizing false-positive tests improves the positive predictive value. The sensitivity of a test is the probability that someone with a disease will have a positive test; minimizing false-negative tests improves the sensitivity. The negative predictive value is the

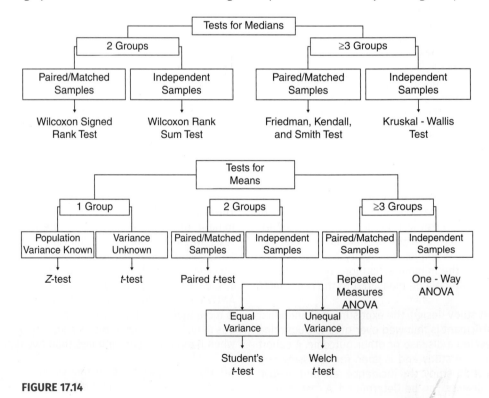

FIGURE 17.14

probability that a participant with a negative test does not have a disease/outcome; minimizing false-negative tests improves the negative predictive value. The specificity of a test is the probability that someone who does not have the disease has a negative test; minimizing false-positive tests improves the specificity. The *P*-value is the probability that the findings of the study, in this case a test of proportions, is due to chance alone.

82. (D) See **Figure 17.14**. Picking the right test for determining a group-wise difference for continuous data first depends on the distribution of the data, whether it is normally distributed or not, and then the number of groups, whether the samples are independent measures or paired and whether the variance in the outcome will determine which type of test should be used. Testing for a difference between two groups with dependent/paired outcomes would utilize Wilcoxon signed-rank test and paired *t*-test for nonparametric and normally distributed data, respectively. For a difference between two groups with independent data, Wilcoxon rank sum, Student's t-test, and Welch *t*-test would be used for nonparametric, normally distributed data with equal variance and normally distributed

data with unequal variance, respectively. For group-wise comparisons between three groups, (1) ANOVA, (2) repeated measures ANOVA, (3) Kruskal–Wallis, and (4) Friedman–Kendall–Smith test would be used for normally distributed data with independent samples, normally distributed data with paired samples, nonparametric data with independent samples, and nonparametric data with paired samples, respectively.

83. (D) See **Figure 17.14.** The test for a difference between two groups with data that are not normally distributed is the Wilcoxon rank sum test. The equivalent test for the difference between two groups with data that are normally distributed is Student's *t*-test. The Kruskal–Wallis test is the test for a difference between groups with data that is not normally distributed and when there are three or more groups. The equivalent test for normally distributed data and testing the difference between three or more group means is an ANOVA. A paired *t*-test is used for testing the difference between two groups of data that are not independent groups. An example of a study design that uses a paired *t*-test is a study that evaluates normally distributed data prior to and following an intervention.

SUGGESTED READINGS

Ahlbom A, Norell S. *Introduction to Modern Epidemiology.* Epidemiology Resources Inc; 1990.

Harris M, Taylor G. *Medical Statistics Made Easy.* Taylor and Francis; 2004.

Last JM. *A Dictionary of Epidemiology.* Oxford University Press; 2001.

Petrie A, Sabin C. *Medical Statistics at a Glance.* Blackwell Publishing; 2005.

Van Dorn CS, Johnson JN, Taggart NW, et al. QTc values among children and adolescents presenting to the emergency department. *Pediatrics.* 2011;128(6):e1395–e1401.

CHAPTER 18

Classic Images in Congenital Heart Disease

Benjamin W. Eidem, Robert E. Shaddy, Paul F. Kantor, Bryan C. Cannon, and Frank Cetta

Questions

1. The arrow in **Figure 18.1** demonstrates a "ring sign." What causes this?

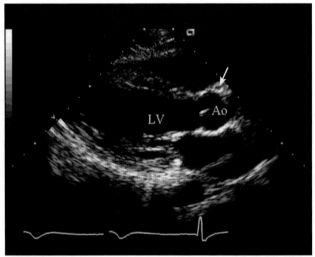

FIGURE 18.1

A. Anomalous origin of left coronary artery from pulmonary artery (ALCAPA)
B. Anomalous origin of right coronary artery from pulmonary artery (ARCAPA)
C. High, anterior, and leftward origin of the right coronary artery
D. Origin of the right coronary artery from the right sinus of Valsalva
E. Origin of the left coronary artery from the left sinus of Valsalva

2. **Figure 18.2A,B** demonstrate a newborn with which cardiac lesion?

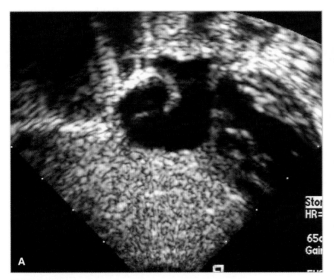

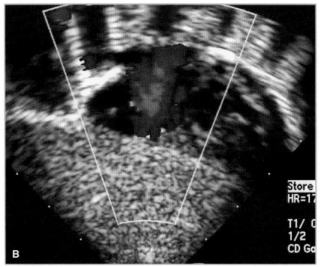

FIGURE 18.2

    A. Tetralogy of Fallot
    B. Membranous VSD
    C. Infracardiac TAPVC
    D. TAPVC to the coronary sinus
    E. Large secundum ASD

3. The patient with the echo image shown in **Figure 18.3** was diagnosed with LV noncompaction (LVNC). What would be the next best decision in this patient's management?

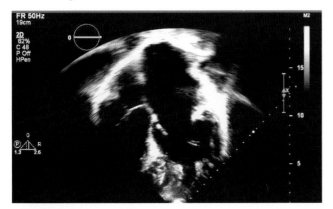

FIGURE 18.3

    A. Take a careful family history to assess risk for sudden death
    B. Place a Holter monitor
    C. Perform MRI to confirm diagnosis of LVNC
    D. Perform genetic testing for LVNC
    E. Obtain a second opinion on the echo reading

4. **Figure 18.4** shows two vessels on either side of a dilated aortic root.

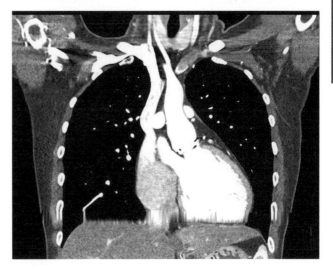

FIGURE 18.4

What congenital cardiac lesion does this patient most likely have?

    A. Tetralogy of Fallot
    B. d-TGA
    C. Bicuspid aortic valve
    D. Marfan syndrome
    E. Turner syndrome

CHAPTER 18

5. **Figure 18.5** depicts a patient who most likely had which surgery?

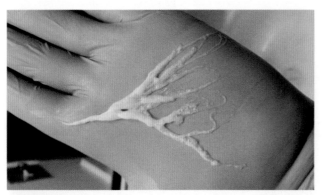

FIGURE 18.5

    A. Classic Blalock–Taussig–Thomas shunt
    B. Mustard
    C. Baffes
    D. Arterial switch
    E. Fontan

6. The patient who has the chest radiograph shown in **Figure 18.6** has what chance of having congenital heart disease?

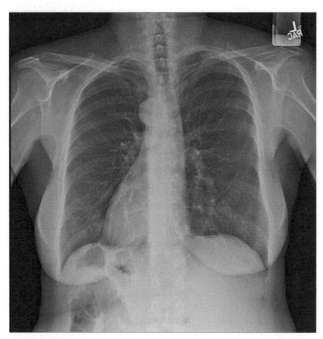

FIGURE 18.6

    A. >95%
    B. 75%
    C. 50%
    D. 25%
    E. <1%

7. A 12-year-old male presented with acute stroke-like symptoms. He experienced recurrent fever, unintentional weight loss, and dizziness over the past 3 months. Physical examination discloses the skin findings shown in **Figure 18.7**.

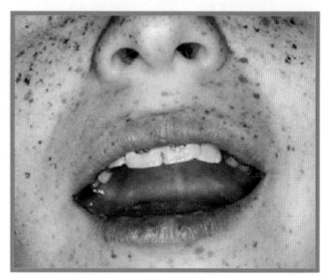

FIGURE 18.7

What is his most likely genetic disorder?

    A. Gorlin syndrome
    B. Tuberous sclerosis
    C. Neurofibromatosis
    D. Carney complex
    E. None of the above

8. **Figure 18.8** depicts an issue with which embryonic arch?

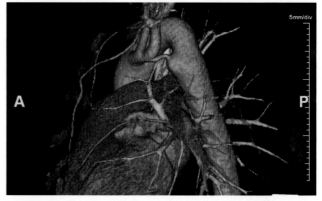

FIGURE 18.8

    A. I
    B. III
    C. IV
    D. VI
    E. X

9. The patient depicted in **Figure 18.9** had which valve replaced?

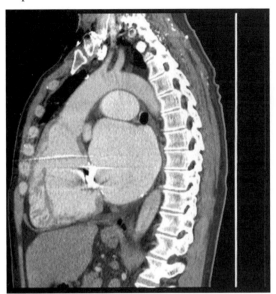

FIGURE 18.9

A. Aortic
B. Pulmonary
C. Mitral
D. Tricuspid
E. No valve was replaced

10. Which of the following congenital cardiac lesions is the *least* likely to cause the chest radiograph finding shown in **Figure 18.10**?

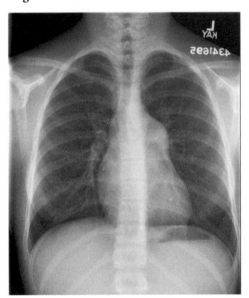

FIGURE 18.10

A. ASD
B. VSD
C. PDA
D. AP window
E. Bicuspid aortic valve

11. You are asked to evaluate a postoperative patient who had chest tubes removed approximately 1 hour ago. He is doing well except for complaining of some mild incisional pain. Oxygen saturation in room air is 100%. Based on this chest radiograph (**Figure 18.11**), what is the next best course of action?

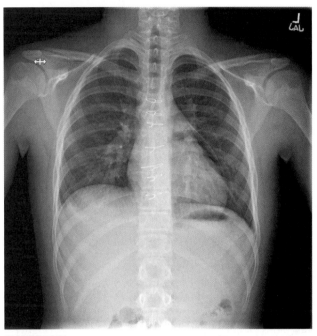

FIGURE 18.11

A. Obtain stat echocardiogram
B. Reinsert chest tube
C. Prescribe ibuprofen
D. Do nothing, observe

12. You are asked to evaluate a postoperative patient who had chest tubes removed approximately 1 hour ago. He is tachypneic and tachycardiac. Oxygen saturation in room air is 88%. Based on this chest radiograph (**Figure 18.12**), what is the next best course of action?

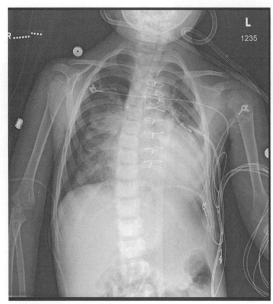

FIGURE 18.12

A. Obtain stat echocardiogram
B. Reinsert chest tube

C. Prescribe ibuprofen
D. Do nothing, observe

13. This Doppler signal from the abdominal aorta (**Figure 18.13**) is *most* consistent with which of the following:

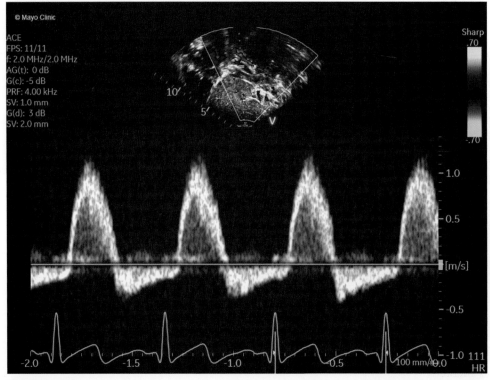

FIGURE 18.13

A. Mild aortic valve insufficiency
B. Coarctation of the aorta
C. Large patent ductus arteriosus

D. Severe aortic valve stenosis
E. Hypertension

14. This classic chest x-ray (CXR) (**Figure 18.14A,B**) is *most* likely to be found in which of the following cardiac lesions?

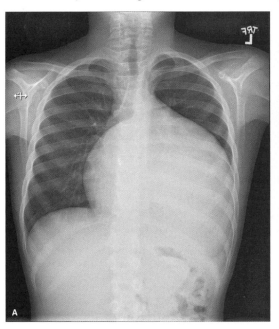
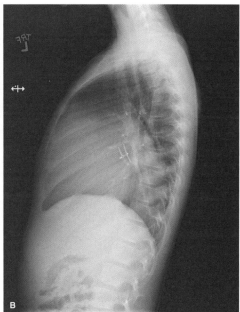

FIGURE 18.14

    A. Ebstein anomaly
    B. Coarctation of the aorta
    C. D-transposition of the great arteries
    D. Tetralogy of Fallot
    E. Total anomalous pulmonary venous connection

15. In which congenital cardiac lesion would you *most* likely have the imaging finding shown in **Figure 18.15**?

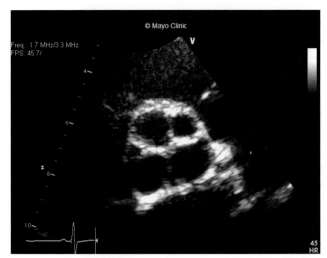

FIGURE 18.15

    A. Tetralogy of Fallot
    B. Truncus arteriosus
    C. Coarctation of aorta
    D. Ebstein anomaly
    E. Shone syndrome

16. These echocardiographic images (**Video 18.1A,B**) are *most* likely to be found in which congenital heart anomaly?

    A. Asplenia syndrome
    B. Scimitar syndrome
    C. Sinus venosus atrial septal defect with anomalous right-sided pulmonary veins
    D. Polysplenia syndrome
    E. Infracardiac total anomalous pulmonary venous connection

CHAPTER **18**

17. This classic chest x-ray (CXR) (**Figure 18.16**) would *most* commonly be found in which of the following cardiac anomalies?

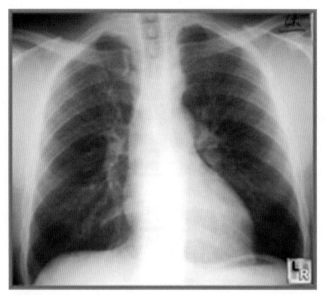

FIGURE 18.16

A. Interruption of the aortic arch
B. Systemic hypertension
C. Left ventricle to aorta tunnel

D. Coarctation of the aorta
E. Aortopulmonary window

18. This pulsed-wave Doppler (**Figure 18.17**) is *most* consistent with:

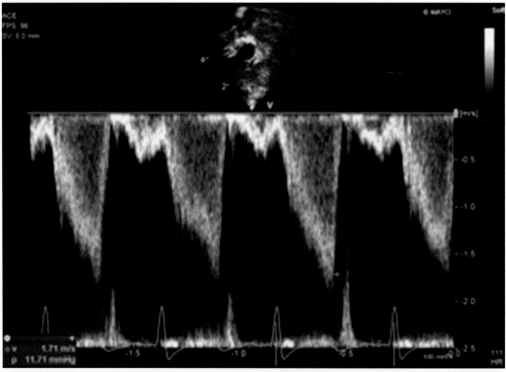

FIGURE 18.17

A. Dynamic RV outflow tract (RVOT) obstruction
B. Pulmonary hypertension
C. Pulmonary valve stenosis

D. Pulmonary venous obstruction
E. Normal pulmonary flow

19. The following echocardiographic clip (**VIDEO 18.2**) is most characteristic of which of the following syndromes?

    A. Holt–Oram syndrome
    B. DiGeorge syndrome
    C. Shone syndrome
    D. Turner syndrome
    E. Marfan syndrome

20. This mobile structure in **VIDEO 18.3A,B** is most likely which of the following?

    A. Chiari network
    B. Eustachian valve
    C. Thebesian valve
    D. Ruptured sinus of Valsalva
    E. Gerbode defect

21. The following histologic images (**Figure 18.18A,B**) best represent:

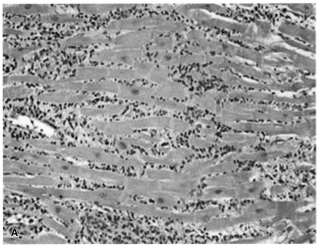

FIGURE 18.18

    A. Acute cellular cardiac rejection
    B. Vaso-occlusive crisis of sickle cell anemia
    C. Libman–Sacks endocarditis
    D. Hypertrophic cardiomyopathy
    E. Acute rheumatic fever

22. These histologic photographs (**Figure 18.19**) depict:

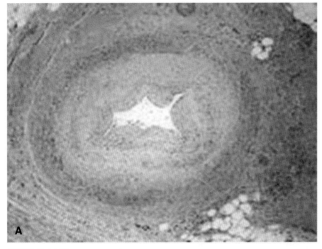
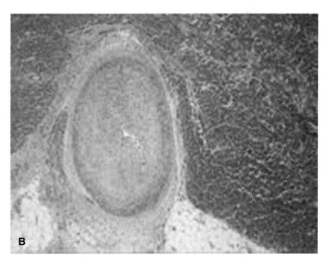

FIGURE 18.19

    A. Acute cardiac allograft rejection
    B. Bridging hepatic fibrosis
    C. Hypotensive arterial vasoconstriction
    D. Coronary allograft vasculopathy
    E. Thrombotic vascular occlusion

CHAPTER **18**

23. The following heart rhythm image (**Figure 18.20**) best represents:

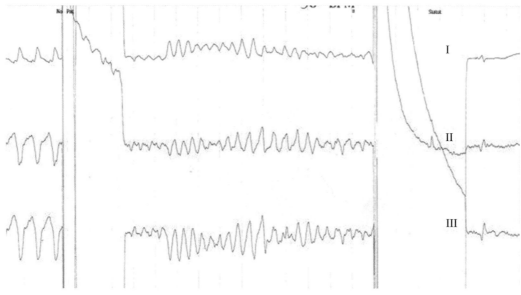

FIGURE 18.20

A. ICD shock of ventricular tachycardia and ventricular fibrillation

B. Spontaneous resolution of supraventricular tachycardia

C. Abrupt onset of atrial fibrillation

D. Pacing of second-degree heart block, type 2

E. Vasovagal syncope due to bradycardia

24. The following echocardiographic images (**Figure 18.21**) are representative of:

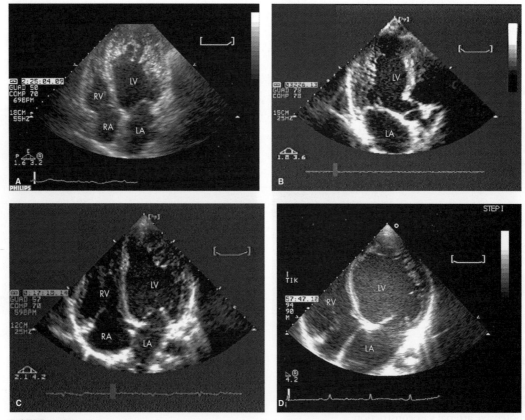

FIGURE 18.21

A. Hypertrophic cardiomyopathy

B. Left ventricular noncompaction

C. Mural left ventricular thrombus

D. Bacterial endocarditis

E. Mitral stenosis

25. The following echocardiographic image (**Figure 18.22**) best represents:

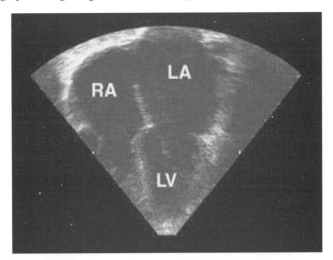

FIGURE 18.22

A. Dilated cardiomyopathy
B. Congenital mitral stenosis
C. Normal variant

D. Hypoplastic right ventricle
E. Restrictive cardiomyopathy

26. A 17-year-old patient complains of recurrent chest pain while playing baseball. Following an evaluation by his pediatric cardiologist, he is referred for a CT angiogram which reveals the **Figure 18.23A,B**.

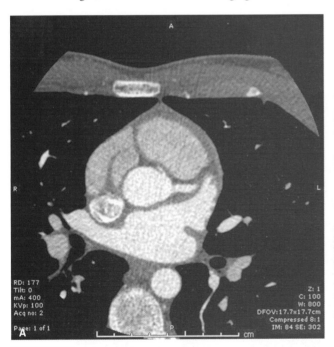 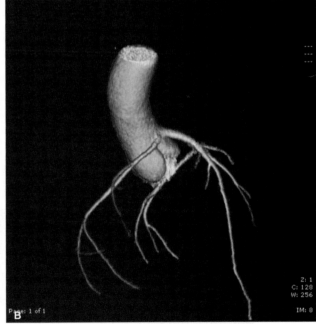

FIGURE 18.23

Select the best first step in management for this patient.

A. Obtain an interventional catheterization consultation
B. Commence treatment with a cardioselective beta blocker
C. Refer for surgical correction

D. Obtain an exercise stress test looking for evidence of inducible ischemia on ECG
E. Restrict from baseball and counsel frequent follow-up

27. A 3-year-old child presents with a persistent slow heart rate and a junctional escape rhythm of 60 bpm is recorded. The chest x-ray shown in **Figure 18.24** is most consistent with which of the following in this child?

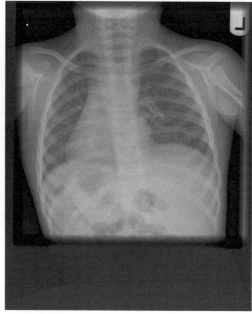

FIGURE 18.24

A. Situs inversus totalis
B. Edwards syndrome (trisomy 18)
C. Scimitar syndrome

D. Heterotaxy syndrome with left atrial isomerism
E. Down syndrome

28. What congenital heart anomaly is most consistent with the chest x-ray (CXR) and levophase CT angiogram demonstrated in **Figure 18.25A,B**?

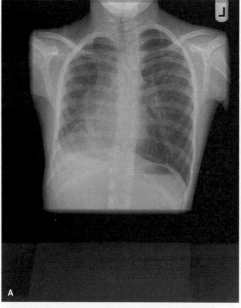
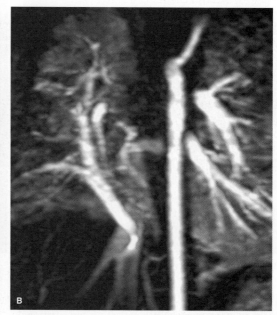

FIGURE 18.25

A. Scimitar syndrome
B. Tetralogy of Fallot with pulmonary atresia
C. Interrupted aortic arch type B

D. Diffuse aortic hypoplasia
E. Total anomalous pulmonary venous return

29. A 7-year-old patient presents with fatigue on mild exertion and describes two pillow orthopnea. On auscultation, a prominent S_4 is auscultated. The ECG shown in **Figure 18.26** is recorded.

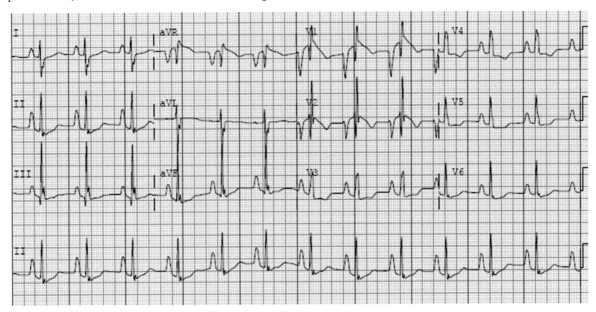

FIGURE 18.26

Of the following diagnoses, which is most consistent with this presentation?

A. Coarctation of the aorta

B. Mitral stenosis

C. Aortic stenosis

D. Restrictive cardiomyopathy

E. Total anomalous pulmonary venous return

30. The chest radiograph and subsequent angiogram (**Figure 18.27A,B**) were obtained from an 8-hour-old newborn infant who presented with cyanosis and respiratory distress.

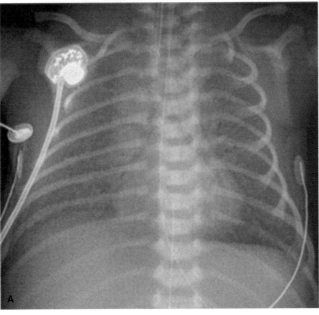

FIGURE 18.27

What does this levophase angiogram image demonstrate?

A. Thrombosis of the ductus venosus

B. Dilated aortopulmonary collateral vessel

C. Vertical venous confluence with infrahepatic obstructed pulmonary venous return

D. Scimitar vein

E. Coronary sinus obstruction with collateral veins

CHAPTER **18**

31. A 23 year old with complex congenital heart disease presents with a 1-week history of fatigue. The ECG shown in **Figure 18.28** is obtained.

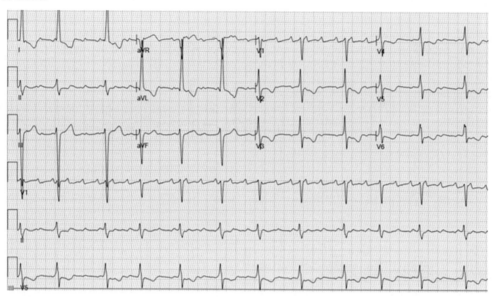

FIGURE 18.28

The therapy most likely to benefit this patient is:

A. IV adenosine

B. DC cardioversion

C. Oral beta blocker

D. Structured exercise program

E. Chronic resynchronization pacing therapy

32. A 26 year old with complex congenital heart disease presents with the ECG shown in **Figure 18.29**.

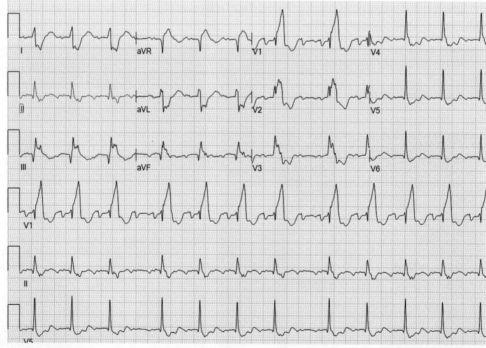

FIGURE 18.29

The patient is at most risk for:

A. Pulmonary fibrosis

B. Renal failure

C. AV block

D. Stroke

E. Pulmonary hypertension

Answers

1. (C) See **Figure 18.30**. Anomalous origin of the RCA (AORCA) from the left sinus or anomalous origin of the LCA (AOLCA) from the right sinus can cause this ring sign. Also, a high, anterior, and leftward origin of the RCA (a benign anomaly) can give the same appearance as the RCA that crosses anteriorly over the aortic root. Answer (**D**) and (**E**) are normal.

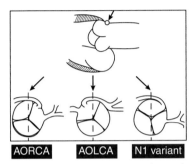

FIGURE 18.30 Interarterial course of CA (*arrow*). Please note: this is a parasternal long axis image with the ring anterior to the right cusp. (Derived from Jureidini, et al. JASE 2003.)

2. (C) These are subcostal echo images in the frontal plane which show a classic "whale-tail" sign consistent with TAPVC to the coronary sinus.

3. (E) This is not LVNC. Look at the crux of the heart. This is congenitally corrected TGA and the image demonstrates AV discordance. Hypertrabeculation is normal for a morphologic RV.

4. (B) This patient had d-TGA and a subsequent arterial switch with a LeCompte maneuver. The two vessels that straddle the ascending aorta are the RPA and LPA. See the horizontal cut from same patient in **Figure 18.31**.

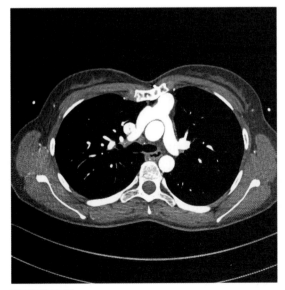

FIGURE 18.31

5. (E) This is a pulmonary cast that a patient with plastic bronchitis (PB) coughed up during rounds one day. A small percentage (<5%) of patients after Fontan are afflicted with PB.

6. (E) The chest radiograph demonstrates situs inversus totalis. The risk of CHD is the same as the general population, 0.8%.

7. (D) He likely had a stroke due to embolization of an atrial myxoma and has Carney complex. Carney complex is an association of myxomas, spotty pigmentation, and endocrine over-reactivity. Inheritance is autosomal dominant (PRKAR1A [PRKACA, PRKACB]) and 70% of cases are familial. Gorlin syndrome is associated with fibromas. Tuberous sclerosis is associated with rhabdomyomas. Various congenital defects have been reported with neurofibromatosis.

8. (C) This MRI demonstrates a double aortic arch, an issue with persistence of a right fourth arch.

9. (D) The patient has congenitally corrected TGA. This lateral CT view demonstrates the inflow/outflow of the systemic morphologic RV. The anterior aortic valve and the replaced tricuspid valve are separated by an infundibulum.

10. (E) The main pulmonary artery shadow is dilated. All of the lesions listed can cause this except an isolated bicuspid aortic valve.

11. (D) The patient has a small pneumopericardium shortly after removal of a chest tube. Since he is hemodynamically stable, observation is all that is needed. A repeat chest x-ray in 24 hours would be prudent. Echocardiogram images with a large pneumopericardium will frequently be of poor quality due to air artifact.

12. (B) There is a large right pneumothorax. The patient is asymptomatic and oxygen saturations are reduced. A chest tube should be reinserted.

13. (C) This Doppler pattern in the abdominal aorta depicts holodiastolic reversal of flow. This pattern is consistent with abnormalities that have a large runoff including a large PDA, severe aortic valve insufficiency, an aortopulmonary window, and a large cerebral arteriovenous malformation.

14. (A) This CXR is from a patient with Ebstein anomaly with severe dilatation of the right atrium and atrialized right ventricle resulting in severe cardiomegaly. Some have compared this classic CXR to a basketball within the chest. Other "classic" CXRs include coarctation of the aorta (figure of 3 sign), D-TGA (an egg on a string), tetralogy of Fallot (a boot shaped heart), and TAPVC (snowman sign).

15. (B) This is a quadricuspid semilunar valve that most commonly is found in truncus arteriosus. The truncal valve has been reported to have from one to six cusps, with the quadricuspid valve morphology being the second most common.

16. (D) The first Video clip (Video E4A) demonstrates a prominent azygos vein (blue color Doppler flow) located posterior to the abdominal aorta with its flow in the opposite direction to the abdominal aorta (red color Doppler flow). The second Video clip (Video E4B) demonstrates absence of the intrahepatic portion of the inferior vena cava. Interruption of the IVC with azygos vein continuation to the SVC is most commonly found in polysplenia.

17. (D) This classic CXR is the "figure of 3 sign" and is most commonly found in patients with coarctation of the aorta.

18. (A) This Doppler signal demonstrates late peaking obstruction which is most characteristically found in patients with tetralogy of Fallot with dynamic RVOT obstruction.

19. (E) This echocardiographic clip demonstrates both mitral valve prolapse and dilatation of the aortic root which are both hallmarks of Marfan syndrome.

20. (A) This membrane is present near the tricuspid valve orifice on the floor of the right atrium. This membrane is a Chiari network and is believed to represent the incomplete embryonic absorption of the thebesian valve (valve of the coronary sinus).

21. (A) This photomicrograph is from an endomyocardial biopsy sample from a patient undergoing acute cellular rejection. There is infiltration of the myocardium with white blood cells, and architectural disruption of the myocytes.

22. (D) These photomicrographs show the marked concentric intimal thickening and luminal narrowing of the coronary arteries that is seen in severe coronary allograft vasculopathy.

23. (A) This ECG tracing shows a wide complex tachycardia (far left frame) followed by ICD shock (vertical line), ventricular fibrillation (middle frame), and ICD shock (vertical line), with resumption of sinus rhythm (far right frame).

24. (B) These four echocardiographic images show four different phenotypes of left ventricular noncompaction: apical (A), septal (B), Free wall (C), and free wall with LV dilation (D).

25. (E) This echocardiographic four-chamber view demonstrates the classic features of restrictive cardiomyopathy, including enlargement of both right and left atria, with normal size of the ventricular chambers.

26. (D) The CT angiography demonstrates anomalous origin of the right coronary artery (RCA) from the left sinus of Valsalva. The RCA appears to have a narrow orifice and a probable intramural course. In the presence of reversible ischemia on exercise, it is an indication of surgical reimplantation. However it is important to demonstrate that there is evidence of ischemia before committing to surgery for correction of anomalous origin of the RCA.

27. (D) There is dextrocardia, abdominal situs inversus, and thoracic situs ambiguus, with bilateral symmetric bronchi, consistent with left atrial isomerism. This could be mistaken for situs inversus, except that the air bronchogram is symmetric, and the escape rhythm is consistent with sinus node dysfunction, which is most common in left atrial isomerism. None of the other stated anomalies are commonly associated with this appearance and presentation.

28. (A) The CXR shows hypoplasia of the right lung with cardiac dextroposition. There is a suggestive shadow of a Scimitar vein. The levophase CT angiogram demonstrates normal pulmonary venous return on the left, with anomalous pulmonary venous return of the right lung, to a Scimitar vein reaching the infradiaphragmatic IVC.

29. (D) The ECG shows massive left atrial and substantial right atrial enlargement. An S_4 suggests elevated late diastolic filling pressures in the LV. There is also evidence of LV strain. In the absence of a diastolic inflow murmur, mitral stenosis is unlikely. The other diagnoses are not consistent with the clinical information given.

30. (C) The catheter course runs up the IVC, and crosses the tricuspid valve, reaching the main pulmonary artery, with the levophase of a pulmonary angiogram shown. Pulmonary venous return reaches a vertical vein, which descends below the diaphragm and empties into a dilated hepatic vein. This patient therefore has infradiaphragmatic obstructed total anomalous pulmonary venous return. None of the other options offered are consistent with this clinical picture or appearance.

31. (B) The ECG shows intra-atrial reentry tachycardia (IART or scar flutter). This arrhythmia is best terminated by DC cardioversion. IV adenosine will block the AV node and make the IART waves more visible, but typically does not terminate the arrhythmia. Oral beta blockers may slow the ventricular response rate, but are unlikely to terminate the tachycardia. There is no indication for chronic resynchronization (biventricular) pacing and an exercise program will not help with symptoms caused by this arrhythmia.

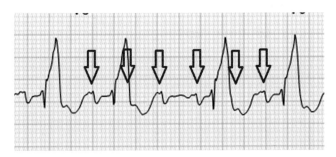

FIGURE 18.32

32. (D) This patient has atrial flutter (intra-atrial reentrant tachycardia—see *arrows* in **Figure 18.32**). Just like patients with atrial fibrillation, patients with IART are at risk for a stroke, especially with a dilated atrium or poor ventricular function. Patients should ideally be anticoagulated for 3 weeks prior to cardioversion or at minimum have a TEE to look for thrombus prior to the cardioversion. Patients may have underlying sinus node dysfunction, but the ECG shows no evidence of AV block.

Index

Note: Page number followed by f and t indicates figure and table respectively.